BSAVA Manual of Canine and Feline Fracture Repair and Management
second edition

Editors:

Toby J. Gemmill
BVSc MVM DSAS(Orth) DipECVS MRCVS
Willows Referral Service, Highlands Road,
Shirley, Solihull, West Midlands B90 4NH, UK

Dylan N. Clements
BSc BVSc PhD DSAS(Orth) DipECVS MRCVS
Royal (Dick) School of Veterinary Studies
and The Roslin Institute,
The University of Edinburgh, Hospital for Small Animals,
Easter Bush Veterinary Centre, Roslin,
Midlothian EH25 9RG, UK

Published by:

British Small Animal Veterinary Association
Woodrow House, 1 Telford Way,
Waterwells Business Park, Quedgeley,
Gloucester GL2 2AB

A Company Limited by Guarantee in England
Registered Company No. 2837793
Registered as a Charity

Figures 2.3 (part), 4.2, 4.3, 4.4, 4.6, 4.8, 4.10, 4.11, 5.3, 7.2, 11.2, 11.3, 11.4, 11.5, 11.6, 11.7, 11.8, 11.9, 11.11, 11.12, 11.13, 11.14, 11.15, 11.17, 11.18, 11.21, 13.6, 15.15, 15.17, 15.19, 15.21, 17.7, 17.8, 18.13, 19.1, 19.14, 19.15, 19.17c, 19.19, 20.6, 20.28a, 20.31, 20.32, 20.33, 20.36, 20.38, 20.39, 21.4, 21.14, 21.15, 21.17, 21.19, 21.20, 21.23, 21.24, 21.25, 21.26, 21.27, 21.29, 21.30, 21.34, 21.35, 21.36, 21.41, 21.42, 21.47, 22.7, 22.13, 22.16, 22.17, 22.20, 22.21, 23.1, 23.7, 23.11, 23.15, 23.18, 23.19, 23.21, 23.22, 23.23, 23.24, 23.25, 23.28, 24.8c, 25.2d, 25.6, 26.7, 26.15, 26.16, 26.17, 26.18, 26.19, 27.6d, 27.7, 27.9, 27.10, 27.11, 27.12, 29.5 and 31.3 were drawn by S.J. Elmhurst BA Hons (www.livingart.org.uk) and are printed with her permission.

Figures 2.3 (part), 2.5, 2.6, 4.5, 10.10, 10.15, 10.16, 10.30, 11.10, 11.16, 11.19, 11.20, 17.1, 17.2, 17.4, 17.15, 18.6, 18.12, 18.14, 18.16, 18.17, 18.18, 18.19, 18.20, 18.21, 18.22, 18.24, 19.7, 19.11, 19.13, 19.16, 19.17a, 19.17b, 19.18, 19.20, 19.21, 20.1, 20.7, 20.29, 20.30, 20.35, 20.37, 21.1, 21.2, 21.3, 21.5, 21.8, 21.12, 21.13, 21.16, 21.18, 21.28, 21.31, 21.32, 21.33, 21.37, 21.38, 21.43, 21.45, 21.46, 23.10, 23.12, 23.13, 23.14, 23.16, 23.17, 23.26, 23.27, 23.29, 24.6, 24.8a, 24.8b, 24.11, 24.13, 24.19, 24.21, 24.22, 24.25, 24.27, 25.1, 25.2a. 25.2b, 25.2c, 25.3, 25.7, 25.10, 25.11, 25.15, 25.17, 25.18, 25.20, 25.22, 25.23, 25.24, 25.25, 25.26, 25.27, 25.28, 25.29, 25.30, 25.31, 25.32, 25.33, 27.6a, 27.6b, 27.6c, 27.8, 29.3, 29.4, 29.6, 30.1, 30.11, 30.13 and 30.17 were drawn by Vicki Martin Design, Cambridge, UK and are printed with her permission.

A catalogue record for this book is available from the British Library.

ISBN 978 1 905319 68 8

The publishers, editors and contributors cannot take responsibility for information provided on dosages and methods of application of drugs mentioned or referred to in this publication. Details of this kind must be verified in each case by individual users from up to date literature published by the manufacturers or suppliers of those drugs. Veterinary surgeons are reminded that in each case they must follow all appropriate national legislation and regulations (for example, in the United Kingdom, the prescribing cascade) from time to time in force.

Printed in the UK by Severn, Gloucester GL2 5EU
Printed on ECF paper made from sustainable forests

17391PUBS22

Titles in the BSAVA Manuals series

Manual of Avian Practice: A Foundation Manual
Manual of Backyard Poultry Medicine and Surgery
Manual of Canine & Feline Abdominal Imaging
Manual of Canine & Feline Abdominal Surgery
Manual of Canine & Feline Advanced Veterinary Nursing
Manual of Canine & Feline Anaesthesia and Analgesia
Manual of Canine & Feline Behavioural Medicine
Manual of Canine & Feline Cardiorespiratory Medicine
Manual of Canine & Feline Clinical Pathology
Manual of Canine & Feline Dentistry and Oral Surgery
Manual of Canine & Feline Dermatology
Manual of Canine & Feline Emergency and Critical Care
Manual of Canine & Feline Endocrinology
Manual of Canine & Feline Endoscopy and Endosurgery
Manual of Canine & Feline Fracture Repair and Management
Manual of Canine & Feline Gastroenterology
Manual of Canine & Feline Haematology and Transfusion Medicine
Manual of Canine & Feline Head, Neck and Thoracic Surgery
Manual of Canine & Feline Musculoskeletal Disorders
Manual of Canine & Feline Musculoskeletal Imaging
Manual of Canine & Feline Nephrology and Urology
Manual of Canine & Feline Neurology
Manual of Canine & Feline Oncology
Manual of Canine & Feline Ophthalmology
Manual of Canine & Feline Radiography and Radiology: A Foundation Manual
*Manual of Canine & Feline Rehabilitation, Supportive and Palliative Care: Case Studies in
    Patient Management*
Manual of Canine & Feline Reproduction and Neonatology
Manual of Canine & Feline Shelter Medicine: Principles of Health and Welfare in a Multi-animal Environment
Manual of Canine & Feline Surgical Principles: A Foundation Manual
Manual of Canine & Feline Thoracic Imaging
Manual of Canine & Feline Ultrasonography
Manual of Canine & Feline Wound Management and Reconstruction
Manual of Canine Practice: A Foundation Manual
Manual of Exotic Pet and Wildlife Nursing
Manual of Exotic Pets: A Foundation Manual
Manual of Feline Practice: A Foundation Manual
Manual of Ornamental Fish
Manual of Practical Animal Care
Manual of Practical Veterinary Nursing
Manual of Psittacine Birds
Manual of Rabbit Medicine
Manual of Rabbit Surgery, Dentistry and Imaging
Manual of Raptors, Pigeons and Passerine Birds
Manual of Reptiles
Manual of Rodents and Ferrets
Manual of Small Animal Practice Management and Development
Manual of Wildlife Casualties

For further information on these and all BSAVA publications, please visit our website: **www.bsava.com**

Contents

Contributors

Ralph H. Abercromby
BVMS CertSAO MRCVS
Anderson Abercromby Veterinary Referrals,
1870 Building, Jayes Park Courtyard,
Forest Green Road, Ockley,
Surrey RH5 5RR, UK

Angus A. Anderson
BVetMed PhD DSAS(Orth) MRCVS
Anderson Abercromby Veterinary Referrals,
1870 Building, Jayes Park Courtyard,
Forest Green Road, Ockley,
Surrey RH5 5RR, UK

Gareth I. Arthurs
PGCertMedEd MA VetMB CertVR CertSAS DSAS(Orth) FHEA MRCVS
Queens Veterinary School Hospital,
University of Cambridge,
Madingley Road,
Cambridge CB3 0ES, UK

Steve R. Bright
BVMS CertSAS DipECVS MRCVS
Manchester Veterinary Specialists,
Priestley Road, Worsley,
Manchester M28 2LY, UK

Gordon Brown
BVM&S CertSAO MRCVS
Grove Referrals,
Grove House, Holt Road,
Fakenham, Norfolk NR21 8JG, UK

Neil J. Burton
BVSc DSAS(Orth) CertSAS PGCert(TLHE) FHEA MRCVS
Langford Veterinary Services,
University of Bristol,
Langford House,
Langford, Bristol BS40 5DU, UK

Mark A. Bush
MA VetMB CertSAS DSAS(Orth) MRCVS
Dick White Referrals,
Station Farm, London Road,
Six Mile Bottom, Suffolk CB8 0UH, UK

Steven J. Butterworth
MA VetMB CertVR DSAO MRCVS
Weighbridge Referrals,
Kemys Way,
Swansea Enterprise Park,
Swansea SA6 8QF, UK

Ignacio Calvo
LdoVet CertSAS DipECVS FHEA MRCVS
The Royal Veterinary College,
Department of Clinical Sciences and Services,
Hawkshead Lane, North Mymms,
Hatfield, Hertfordshire AL9 7TA, UK

Stephen Clarke
BVM&S DSAS(Orth) DipECVS MRCVS
Willows Referral Service,
Highlands Road, Shirley,
Solihull, West Midlands B90 4NH, UK

D. Gareth Clayton Jones
BVetMed DVR DSAO HonFRCVS DHSMA
Bayswater Referrals,
35 Alexander Street, Bayswater,
London W2 5NU, UK

Dylan N. Clements
BSc BVSc PhD DipECVS DSAS(Orth) MRCVS
Royal (Dick) School of Veterinary Studies and
The Roslin Institute,
The University of Edinburgh, Hospital for Small Animals,
Easter Bush Veterinary Centre, Roslin,
Midlothian EH25 9RG, UK

Jonathan Dyce
MA VetMB DSAO DipACVS MRCVS
Ohio State University Veterinary Medical Center,
Hospital for Companion Animals,
601 Vernon L Tharp Street,
Columbus, OH 43210-1089, USA

Mike Farrell
BVetMed CertVA CertSAS DipECVS MRCVS
Fitzpatrick Referrals,
Halfway Lane,
Eashing, Godalming,
Surrey GU7 2QQ, UK

Toby J. Gemmill
BVSc MVM DSAS(Orth) DipECVS MRCVS
Willows Referral Service,
Highlands Road, Shirley, Solihull,
West Midlands B90 4NH, UK

Sarah L. Girling
BSc BVSc CertSAS DipECVS MRCVS
Fitzpatrick Referrals,
Halfway Lane,
Eashing, Godalming,
Surrey GU7 2QQ, UK

James M. Grierson
BVetMed CertVR CertSAS DipECVS FHEA MRCVS
Anderson Moores Veterinary Specialists,
The Granary, Bunstead Barns,
Poles Lane, Hursley, Winchester,
Hampshire SO21 2LL, UK

Tomás G. Guerrero
PD Dr. med. vet. DipECVS
St. George's University,
School of Veterinary Medicine,
True Blue, Grenada, West Indies

Michael Guilliard
MA VetMB CertSAO FRCVS
Anvil Cottage, Wrinehill Road,
Wybunbury, Nantwich,
Cheshire CW5 7NU, UK

Gawain Hammond
MA VetMB MVM CertVDI DipECVDI FHEA MRCVS
School of Veterinary Medicine,
University of Glasgow,
Bearsden Road,
Glasgow G61 1QH, UK

John E.F. Houlton
MA VetMB DVR DSAO DipECVS MRCVS
Empshill,
Robins Lane, Lolworth,
Cambridge CB23 8HH, UK

Stanley E. Kim
BVSc MS DipACVS
Department of Small Animal Clinical Science,
College of Veterinary Medicine,
University of Florida,
Gainesville, FL 32611 USA

Sorrel J. Langley-Hobbs
MA BVetMed DSAS(Orth) DipECVS FHEA MRCVS
Langford Veterinary Services,
University of Bristol,
Langford House, Langford,
Bristol BS40 5DU, UK

Carlos Macias
Ldo Vet DSAS(Orth) MRCVS
Centro Veterinario de Referencia Bahia de Malaga,
Parque Empresarial Laurotorre, 25,
29130 Alhaurín de la Torre,
Málaga, Spain

W. Malcolm McKee
BVMS MVS DSAO MACVSc MRCVS
Willows Referral Service,
Highlands Road, Shirley,
Solihull, West Midlands B90 4NH, UK

Andy P. Moores
BVSc DSAS(Orth) DipECVS MRCVS
Anderson Moores Veterinary Specialists,
The Granary, Bunstead Barns,
Poles Lane, Hursley, Winchester,
Hampshire SO21 2LL, UK

Bill Oxley
MA VetMB DSAS(Orth) MRCVS
Willows Referral Service,
Highlands Road, Shirley,
Solihull, West Midlands B90 4NH, UK

Rob Pettitt
BVSc PGCertLTHE DSAS(Orth) FHEA MRCVS
Small Animal Teaching Hospital,
School of Veterinary Science,
University of Liverpool,
Leahurst Campus, Chester High Road,
Neston, Wirral CH64 7TE, UK

Jonathan J. Pink
BSc BVetMed CertSAS DipECVS MRCVS
Willows Referral Service,
Highlands Road, Shirley,
Solihull, West Midlands B90 4NH, UK

Alessandro Piras
DVM SVS
Referral Centre and Canine Sport Medicine,
Russi, Via Faentina Nord,
125/6, 48026 Russi, RA, Italy

Antonio Pozzi
Prof. Dr.med.vet. DipECVS DipACVS DipACVSMR
Department for Small Animals,
Vetsuisse Faculty Zurich,
Winterthurerstrasse 258c,
8057 Zurich, Switzerland

Rob Rayward
MA VetMB DSAS(Orth) MRCVS
Coast Veterinary Referrals,
Unit 2 Glennys Estate,
158 Latimer Road, Eastbourne,
East Sussex BN22 7ET, UK

Harry W. Scott
BVSc CertSAD CBiol FRSB DSAS(Orth) CCRP FRCVS
Southern Counties Veterinary Specialists,
Unit 6, Forest Corner Farm,
Hangersley, Ringwood,
Hampshire BH24 3JW, UK

Russell Yeadon
VetMB MA CertSAS DipECVS MRCVS
Fitzpatrick Referrals,
Halfway Lane,
Eashing, Godalming,
Surrey GU7 2QQ, UK

Foreword

Fracture fixation has been on the fast-track in the recent past and many new advances have taken place since the last edition of this manual. The downside of the expansion of the field is the greater amount of information, knowledge and training that a veterinary surgeon requires to accomplish acceptably good results from fracture repair, as the bar has been raised considerably.

With this manual the editors have collected a wealth of information which addresses the needs of the busy veterinary surgeon who wishes to understand modern fracture fixation. They have also made available a massive body of practical experience, shared from an impressive array of contributors. The format is the same as with the earlier manual which proved so user friendly in the past.

Successful fracture management is achieved through an understanding of fundamental principles and their correct application. This manual seeks to provide these principles and demonstrates how they can be best used in various situations. It is worth remembering that, even with increasing complexity, the surgeon should be seeking the simplest solution that addresses the problems provided by the fracture. This approach gives the best chance of a successful outcome.

The editors should be congratulated as once more this excellent source of practical information can be returned to pride of place on practice bookshelves.

Stuart Carmichael BVMS MVM DSAO MRCVS
Professor of Veterinary Science,
University of Surrey

Preface

The original *BSAVA Manual of Small Animal Fracture Repair and Management*, edited by Andrew Coughlan and Andrew Miller, has for many years been an essential text for veterinarians undertaking orthopaedic surgery in small animal practice. The style of the original manual, published in 1998, was unique at the time, providing the perfect balance of a detailed yet readable text with clear colour illustrations to explain the nuances of operative techniques. There can be few veterinary surgeons performing orthopaedic surgery in recent years who have not referred to the manual at some point for guidance. Indeed, such was the impact of the original manual that that its format was used as a template for subsequent BSAVA Manuals covering other areas of veterinary medicine in the years to come.

As in other fields, fracture surgery has developed rapidly since the first edition of the manual was published. Advances in imaging modalities and implant systems have led to significant improvements in our ability to treat patients with fractures. The continual re-appraisal of the basic principles underpinning treatment of fractures has also changed the way in which many cases are managed. As a result many fractures which were once deemed irretrievable can now be treated successfully. For the busy practitioner, keeping abreast of these changes can be daunting, and the time had come to collate these developments and advances in the form of a new manual.

With this new manual we aimed to keep the vernacular of the first edition, using the same clear format with chapters organized into sections covering basic principles, different anatomical regions and complications. Chapters from the original manual have been extensively re-written to convey the advances which have occurred over the past two decades, and several new chapters have been introduced covering emerging areas such as minimally invasive fracture surgery. The original line drawings that were such a benefit in the previous edition of the manual have been retained and expanded, giving practitioners rapid access to essential information when faced with specific fractures. In addition, the clinical images and case examples have been expanded to give context to the concepts being presented.

A panel of renowned authors from the UK and overseas have contributed to this manual, bringing with them a huge wealth of practical experience and making its content internationally applicable. We hope that the new manual will be of value and interest to anyone involved in the management of small animals with fractures, including veterinary nurses, undergraduates, general practitioners, residents, diagnostic imagers and specialist orthopaedic surgeons.

As editors we would like to extend our sincere thanks to everyone who has contributed to this edition of the manual, including all the authors and the editorial team at BSAVA. Lastly we would also like to thank our families for their support whilst the manual was in production. We hope you will find the new manual as inspiring to use as we ourselves found the original nearly 20 years ago.

Toby Gemmill and Dylan Clements
January 2016

Chapter 1

History of fracture treatment

Toby Gemmill

There is evidence that attempts have been made to treat fractures since 4000 years BC. Early medical practitioners appreciated that, if left unsupported, fractures either would not heal or would develop significant malunions, compromising future use of the limb. Therefore, attempts were made to realign broken bones and maintain their reduction during the healing period, using various forms of splints and bandages. Wooden splints were used by the Egyptians around 5000 years ago (Elliot Smith, 1908) but, whilst it appears these splints were often effective at facilitating bone healing, limb shortening due to overriding of fragments was common. Splinting of fractures was also used by other civilizations with some success, notably in India where bamboo splints were used and in ancient Greece where support was provided using bandages impregnated with resin or wax that subsequently set hard.

The ancient civilizations declined and, for over 1000 years during the Dark Ages, there was very little advancement in the management of fractures. However, scientific thinking was revived in the 15th and 16th centuries during the Renaissance in Europe. Despite advances in anatomical understanding, fracture treatment was still limited to the use of external coaptation. Attempts were made to overcome the problem of limb shortening by using traction devices (Figure 1.1); however, the results were still somewhat unpredictable. Patients were often confined to their beds for several months during the healing period, and poor limb use and deformities were common sequelae to fractures managed in this way. Operative treatment of

1.1 Application of an extension device to a fractured arm by Gersdoff in 1517.
(Reproduced from Guthrie (1958) with permission from the publisher)

fractures, usually performed on soldiers following battle-field injuries, was generally limited to amputations. However, mortality associated with these procedures was high and, due to the excruciating pain of surgery, patients often preferred to choose near certain death from their injuries rather than elect for any form of operative treatment.

A number of important innovations occurred during the 19th century. Firstly, in 1846 Morton demonstrated that general anaesthesia could be performed relatively safely with the careful administration of ether. In the same year, Liston performed the first operation on a patient under anaesthesia; a mid-femoral limb amputation. Secondly, improved understanding of microbial infections led to the development of a system of antisepsis by Lister (1867), who used carbolic acid on instruments and wounds and demonstrated that this could reduce the risk of postoperative infections. Finally, X-rays were discovered by Röntgen in 1895, which enabled the detailed *in vivo* assessment of bone injury and healing for the first time. Cases with poor results could be better investigated and explanations given for failures. These vital discoveries led to a more widespread consideration of operative techniques for fracture management, which began to be developed in the late 19th and early 20th centuries.

Treatment of fractures in animals

The concept of animal welfare is relatively modern; for many centuries animals with fractures would be abandoned or euthanased, often using somewhat barbaric techniques. A notable exception was the horse, which clearly had value for use in work or war. Forms of farriery existed in ancient Greece, and the Romans used a metal device known as a 'hipposandal' to protect horses' hooves. Fractures of the distal phalanx could be managed by simple rest, and attempts were made to manage more proximal limb fractures using external splints with the horses suspended in slings, often for many months (Gibson, 1729).

The treatment of femoral fractures in dogs using an external wooden splint was described by Blaine in 1824. Subsequently, alternative materials such as plaster of Paris or sodium silicate were used. For the proximal limb, where poor reduction and overriding of the fracture were concerns, attempts were made to apply traction, either by suspending dogs by their hindlimbs during the healing period (Steiner, 1928), or by using traction devices such as the Schroeder–Thomas splint. However, the results were often very poor. Ultimately, as with human orthopaedics, it was the development of anaesthesia, antisepsis and radiography that led to the consideration of operative management for fractures.

External skeletal fixation

The first use of external skeletal fixation (ESF) is attributed to Jean-François Malgaigne in the 1840s, who described the use of a simple spike held by a strap to prevent displacement of tibial fractures. He subsequently devised an external clamp with four prongs, which was used to stabilize fractures of the patella and olecranon (Figure 1.2).

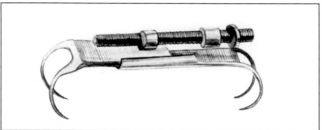

1.2 Malgaigne's clamp (1849) used for fractures of the patella and olecranon. The prongs projected through the skin.
(Reproduced from Venable and Stuck (1947) with permission from the publisher)

The first widely available fixators were devised by Clayton Parkhill at the University of Colorado and Albin Lambotte at the Stuyvenberg Hospital in Antwerp. The Parkhill device consisted of steel bone screws attached to a plate spanning the fracture. Two screws were placed either side of the fracture, which was then stabilized by clamping the plates together (Figure 1.3). Parkhill reported 100% success with the use of the device in 14 patients in 1897. Entirely independently, Lambotte had also devised a system using two plates clamped on to four bone screws, two either side of the fracture. He reported success in a variety of patients, recognizing some of the inherent advantages of ESF, including that 'the apparatus can be easily installed, has great rigidity, open wounds can be addressed, it can be completely removed without difficulty and the limb can be mobilized during the healing process'.

Several surgeons subsequently developed variations on these early systems during the early part of the 20th century. However, a common problem was that the constructs created were not particularly stable; thus patients were confined to their beds for the entire healing period. In 1938, Raoul Hoffman described a more rigid system using three pins in each bone fragment. The Hoffman frame was more adjustable, allowing easier fracture reduction as well as fracture compression or bone lengthening. The system was widely used throughout Europe, but less well known

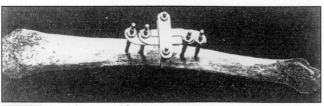

1.3 An early external fixation apparatus.
(Reproduced from Parkhill (1897) with permission from the *American Surgical Association*)

in the USA. Again in the 1930s, but entirely independently from Hoffman, Roger Anderson from Seattle described the use of a very similar system in North America.

The first significant use of ESF in animals was described by Otto Stader. After an initial period during which he became recognized as an expert in cattle infertility, he developed an interest in small animal fracture treatment and introduced the 'Stader splint' in 1937. This was a more robust frame that was widely used in dogs and subsequently introduced in humans. The Stader splint was refined and commonly used by human trauma surgeons during World War II. After the war, a similar system was developed and used successfully on dogs by Schroeder and Leighton at the Angel Memorial Animal Hospital in Boston.

Another significant advance was made with the introduction of the Kirschner–Ehmer (KE) system in the 1940s. The KE system was more versatile than its predecessors, allowing greater variation in the angulation with which pins could be inserted. Concerns regarding inadequate stability led to refinement of the initial frame types, with the more modern frame configurations gradually evolving. Due to its versatility, the KE system has been the most widely used ESF system in veterinary practice for the past 60 years, and has formed the basis for many subsequent systems.

Following World War II, a number of authorities questioned the continued use of ESF in humans and animals with reference to common complications such as infection, soft tissue morbidity and non-union. This coincided with the development of highly successful internal fixation techniques in the 1950s and 1960s, and subsequently the use of ESF declined. However, it became clear during the late 1960s and 1970s that internal fixation was not the panacea that had initially been suggested. In particular, the complication rate following treatment of comminuted or open fractures with plates and screws was often very high, mainly due to a failure to appreciate the importance of the soft tissues and fracture site biology during their application. The huge number of casualties during wars in the 1970s and 1980s provided large caseloads for trauma surgeons, and the use of ESF began to regain favour as its advantages for the stabilization of open and comminuted fractures began to be understood. In field conditions, it was found that fractures could be rapidly stabilized with minimal compromise to biology. Technical advances in the design and application of ESF apparatus led to further improvements in outcome, and the use of ESF steadily increased. The increased popularity in human orthopaedics was mirrored in veterinary practice, and a number of publications in the 1980s and early 1990s reported and supported the use of ESF for more complex fractures, predominantly using the KE system.

Throughout the 1990s and 2000s several companies sought to develop their own ESF systems in an attempt to circumvent some of the inherent disadvantages of the original KE system. Modern systems have significant advantages, including allowing the use of transfixation pins of different sizes in different areas of the bone and the placement of additional clamps in between existing clamps on a frame. In some systems, the connecting bars are made from lightweight radiolucent materials, such carbon fibre or acrylic composites (Figure 1.4), decreasing the overall weight of the apparatus and permitting better postoperative radiographic assessment of bone alignment and healing. Improvements in the mechanical strength of the fixation components have allowed more simple frames (type 1a or 1b) to be used in preference to complex frames (type 2 or 3) (see Chapter 4 for further information).

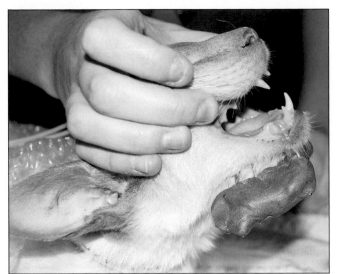

1.4 An acrylic pin external fixator used to treat a mandibular fracture in a cat. Following reduction of the fracture, transfixation pins are driven into the mandible. Acrylic is then moulded around the pin ends; the acrylic sets to create a hard bond between the pins.

This simplifies surgery and allows better use of 'safe corridors' for transfixation pin placement, which helps to reduce morbidity and complication rates. The smooth transfixation pins initially used with ESF systems have now been largely replaced by pins with a positive, negative or tapered thread; this improves the integrity of the pin–bone interface and maximizes the resistance of pins to pull-out.

The use of circular or ring fixators, where bone fragments are stabilized using small tensioned wires, was pioneered by Gavril Ilizarov, a Russian surgeon working in relative isolation from the West in Siberia. During the 1940s he devised the circular fixator system and developed techniques for distraction osteogenesis to improve treatment of fractures, orthopaedic complications and limb deformities. It is rumoured that distraction osteogenesis was discovered purely by chance when a patient mistakenly distracted their circular fixator rather than compressing it, and new bone developed in the enlarging fracture gap. Ilizarov rose to prominence in Russia after successfully treating a celebrated national athlete who had sustained an open tibial fracture in a motorcycle accident; the fracture had previously failed to heal despite some 20 operations. Ilizarov subsequently went on to establish a huge hospital and research centre in Kurgan, Siberia.

Despite great success within Russia, Ilizorav's work was largely unknown in the West until a famous Italian explorer and mountaineer, Carlo Mauri, sought treatment for an infected non-union fracture of his tibia. The fracture was successfully treated, and Mauri facilitated the attendance of Ilizarov at an Arbeitsgemeinschaft für Osteosynthesefragen (AO) meeting in Italy in 1961. This led to the emergence and acceptance of circular fixation, first in Italy, and then worldwide, throughout the 1970s and 1980s. The first report of circular ESF in animals was from Antonio Ferretti in 1984. The unique advantages and versatility of circular ESF led to an explosion of interest and the development of several veterinary systems by different companies. More recently, systems have been introduced which allow the use of both circular and linear components within the same frame (Figure 1.5). These 'hybrid' frames confer advantages of both the circular and linear systems and, if used appropriately, can simplify application and lead to decreased complication rates.

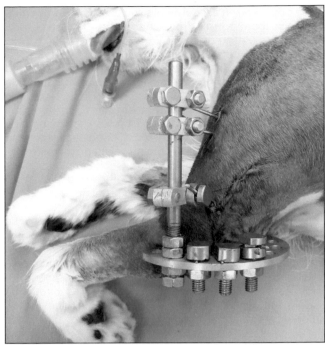

1.5 A hybrid external skeletal fixator used to stabilize a comminuted distal humeral fracture in a cat. The ring is secured to the bone distally using tensioned wires; the hybrid post extends proximally allowing the use of linear components on the proximal humerus.
(Courtesy of D Clements)

Internal fixation

Despite some success with early ESF systems, it soon became clear that they were commonly associated with a plethora of complications, especially soft tissue problems such as pin tract discharge. As a result of these problems, and the high complication rates associated with the use of external coaptation, many surgeons began to explore the use of internal fixation techniques.

Orthopaedic wire

Wire sutures, or interfragmentary wires, were used in humans in the late 19th and early 20th centuries. Forms of cerclage wiring were also used. Some success was recorded, but concerns existed regarding erosion of the bone adjacent to the wires. This was initially attributed to pressure necrosis, but it subsequently became apparent that electrolysis of the wire and metal corrosion were to blame; this problem was resolved following the identification and introduction of biologically inert materials, forerunners to materials such as 316L stainless steel that are used today. The use of cerclage wire to treat long oblique fractures in dogs was described by Turnbull in 1949, although complications were common; Hinko and Rhinelander (1975) refined the application techniques and achieved better results.

Intramedullary devices

Intramedullary devices were used in the late 19th and early 20th centuries to treat long bone fractures. Short pegs of ivory, bone and nickel-plated steel were tried both in humans and dogs, but with only limited success. The pegs were difficult to insert and failed to provide rigid stabilization of the fracture. However, a variation on the use of these pegs, known as 'dowel pinning', is still used by some surgeons today to treat metacarpal and metatarsal fractures in cats (Zahn *et al.*, 2007).

The use of pins spanning the full length of the bone was popularized in the early 1940s by Kuntscher, who stabilized experimentally created femoral fractures in dogs using V- or trefoil-shaped nails. This technique became relatively widespread in human medicine in the 1940s and 1950s. In dogs, round profile Steinmann pins proved more popular as they were easier to insert and were cheaper. However, problems relating to poor rotational stability became apparent. Techniques such as stack pinning were developed and threaded pins were used in an attempt to overcome this problem, but complications due to rotational instability persisted. In addition, intramedullary pins did little to prevent the axial collapse of comminuted fractures.

In the human field, interlocking nails were developed in the 1980s to overcome the problems of poor rotational stability and axial collapse. These devices consisted of a large diameter pin or nail with holes drilled through it (Figure 1.6). Having placed the nail in the medullary canal, screws could be drilled perpendicular to the nail into the bone and through the holes, thus interlocking with the nail. This construct effectively resisted all disruptive forces at the fracture site and their use became widespread for the treatment of femoral, humeral and tibial fractures. The screws were placed using special aiming jigs or under fluoroscopic guidance. An additional advantage of interlocking nails was that they could be placed in a minimally invasive fashion through small incisions away from the fracture site.

In small animals, interlocking nails were first used in the 1990s (Dueland *et al.*, 1996; 1999), with some success, although problems such as screw or nail breakage were not uncommon. These problems have largely been addressed as the design of the implants has evolved. Recent innovations include the development of solid bolts rather than screws to reduce implant breakage, and the

manufacture of an 'angle-stable' system, which improves stability at the fracture site by preventing movement at the nail–bolt interface (Déjardin *et al.*, 2014). Interestingly, smooth intramedullary pins are still routinely used in small animal fracture surgery, without modifications to their profile, although they are now most commonly used in combination with other forms of fixation such as ESF or bone plates to create constructs which can neutralize all disruptive forces at the fracture site.

Plates and screws

The use of metal plates and screws was first described in humans by Hansmann in 1886. The ends of the screws were left long, protruding from the skin, to allow simple removal. Lane (1907) developed a system that was entirely contained under the skin, simplifying patient care; use of these plates was described in dogs by Larsen in 1927. The plates often broke due to cyclic fatigue (Figure 1.7), and the original Lane plates were subsequently replaced by much larger and stronger implants such as the Sherman and Venable plates. Complications in early cases were very common and included osteolysis, plate loosening, wound breakdown and non-union. It became apparent that many of these problems were due to electrolysis and corrosion of the metals used to manufacture the implants as had been noted with orthopaedic wire. Subsequently, more biologically inert materials were introduced and complications relating to metal corrosion decreased. However, other complications persisted, and limb function following fracture treatment was often poor, even if the bone healed.

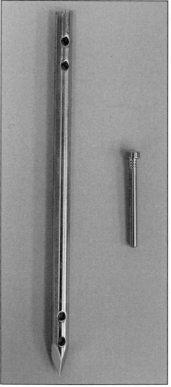

1.6 An interlocking nail (left) and a transfixation bolt (right). The nail is placed in the medullary canal; holes are then drilled through the bone, aligning with the holes in the nail, and bolts are placed to interlock with the nail.

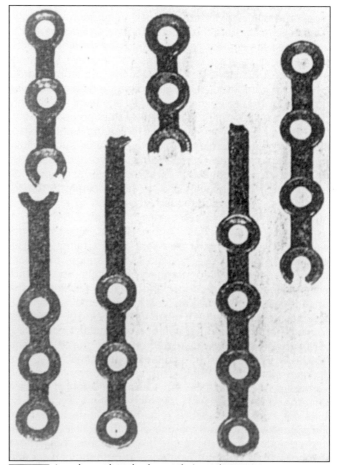

1.7 Lane bone plates broken at their weakest point. (Reproduced from Sherman (1912) with permission from *Surgery, Gynecology and Obstetrics*)

In response to the suboptimal outcomes following fracture treatment, a group of Swiss doctors formed the Arbeitsgemeinschaft für Osteosynthesefragen (AO) group in 1958. This translates as 'Association for the Study of Internal Fixation'. This group realized the vital importance of the interaction of the bone and surrounding soft tissues in promoting fracture healing. They also noted that the most important outcome measure following fracture treatment should be limb function, rather than simply healing of the fracture; therefore, they emphasized the importance of early mobilization of fractured limbs. Extensive research was carried out in their laboratories in Davos, and the defining principles of fracture management developed. These principles have remained valid ever since:

- Accurate reduction of fracture fragments
- Preservation of fracture site biology and blood supply
- Rigid internal fixation
- Early return to function to minimize fracture disease.

Application of these principles led to a marked improvement in patient outcomes, and the AO techniques were soon introduced into small animal orthopaedics; the AOVET group was formed in 1969. The use of bone plates and screws was facilitated by the widespread introduction of antibiotics in the 1950s and 1960s, which decreased the risk of infection that had been previously been associated with internal fixation techniques.

The AO group also developed new implants and instruments to allow effective stabilization of fractured bones. The most important of these was the dynamic compression plate (DCP), which circumvented the need for cumbersome devices to achieve interfragmentary compression. The DCP and its subsequent variations (such as the low contact DCP or 'LC-DCP') were widely used in both humans and small animals in the latter part of the 20th century, and are still commonly used today.

A recent development in bone plate technology was the introduction of angle-stable or locking plates (Perren, 2002). The key feature of these systems is that, rather than compressing the plate against the bone and achieving stability by friction, the head of the screw directly engages or 'locks into' the plate. The device functions mechanically in a similar manner to an external skeletal fixator but is applied under the skin, avoiding the morbidity that can be associated with percutaneous pin placement. Locking plates can confer several advantages when compared with traditional plates and screws, including better preservation of periosteal vascularity and improved mechanical strength, especially in soft, osteoporotic bone such as that which is commonly encountered in elderly humans. However, locking plates can also have several disadvantages, including an inability to angle screws away from adjacent joints or other vital structures and unique mechanisms of failure, such as multiple screw shearing and 'bone slicing' where rigid screws cut through bone. Therefore, it is imperative that locking systems are used correctly, and in many cases it may still be more appropriate to use traditional DCPs. More recent developments in locking plate technology have included the introduction of 'combi' plates, such as the locking compression plate, which can accept either locking or conventional cortex screws, and the development of variable angle locking plates (see Chapter 10). Currently, precise guidelines regarding the use of different systems have not been developed for small animals. Therefore, the surgeon must consider the advantages and disadvantages of each system to allow the most appropriate implants to be selected for each case.

Changes in philosophy

The introduction of AO principles and implants in the 1960s and 1970s led to vastly improved outcomes in both human and small animal fracture patients. However, it became clear that whilst simple fractures often healed uneventfully, complications were not uncommon in patients with comminuted fractures. Despite meticulous anatomical reconstruction and rigid fixation, comminuted fractures were often slow to heal and delayed construct failure was seen frequently (Figure 1.8). In addition, infections were common, especially following treatment of open fractures. Researchers realized that these complications could be attributed to biological damage at the time of surgery, caused by excessive manipulation of fragments in an attempt to achieve perfect anatomical reduction. This damage increased the risk of infection and led to delayed healing, cyclic implant fatigue and eventual implant failure.

These concerns led to a reappraisal of the AO principles in the 1980s and 1990s. For comminuted fractures, it was recognized that preservation of biology should be emphasized above anatomical reconstruction of the fracture fragments. This led to the development of so-called 'biological treatment' of comminuted fractures. Using this strategy, the length and alignment of the bone was restored without individual fragment reconstruction, and robust bridging fixation was applied. The fracture then healed by callus formation (Johnson et al., 1996; Dudley et al., 1997). Simple fractures were usually still treated by reconstruction and compression, with the aim of achieving primary bone healing.

Paradoxically, the development of 'biological treatment' actually led to an initial increase in use of ESF constructs for the treatment of comminuted long bone fractures. The ESF constructs could be applied with closed fracture reduction and the implants could be positioned away from the fracture site to improve preservation of the biology. However, despite improvements in ESF technology, complications inherent to ESF (such as pin tract discharge) remained common.

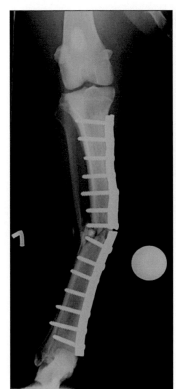

1.8 Cyclic fatigue of a plate. A mildly comminuted fracture in a 5-year-old Labrador Retriever was treated by open reduction, anatomical reconstruction and application of a compression plate. Individual fragments were repositioned prior to application of the plate, compromising their vascularity. Despite good limb function following the initial surgery, the bone did not heal and the construct failed 3 months postoperatively.

Consequently, robust internal fixation techniques were revisited and new solutions developed, such as the pin–plate combination (Figure 1.9). This construct was shown to be far more durable than bridging plate fixation alone (Hulse *et al.*, 1997). The refinement of surgical techniques to preserve the healing capacity of the soft tissues at the injured site has continued over the last 20 years, with particular reference to the placement of the fixation apparatus. For example, the widely adopted 'open but do not touch' (OBDNT) technique uses an open approach to place the fixation apparatus, but fracture reduction and implant placement is performed without direct manipulation of the fragments or disturbance of the haematoma at the fracture site. More recently, further development of the biological approach to fracture stabilization has occurred, where no approach to the fracture site is performed at all: following closed reduction the implants are placed through small incisions made remote from the fracture site. This strategy is known as *minimally invasive osteosynthesis* (see Chapter 15).

As our understanding has improved it has become apparent that it is not possible to divide cases into those that should be treated 'biologically' and those that should be treated by reconstruction and interfragmentary compression. In reality all of the basic AO principles should be applied to every case; the principles are as valid today as they were 50 years ago. However, it is now clear that greater emphasis should be placed on certain principles in different fracture situations. In the future it is likely that, as our understanding continues to improve and new implants are developed, the application of basic principles will continue to evolve. As the writer Khalil Gibran speculated, *'Progress lies not in enhancing what is, but in advancing toward what will be'*.

References and further reading

Blaine D (1824) *Canine Pathology, 2nd edn.* Boosey and Sons, London

Déjardin LM, Cabassu JB, Guillou RP *et al.* (2014) *In vivo* biomechanical evaluation of a novel angle-stable interlocking nail design in a canine tibial fracture model. *Veterinary Surgery* **43**, 271–281

Dudley M, Johnson AL, Olmstead M *et al.* (1997) Open reduction and bone plate stabilization, compared with closed reduction and external fixation, for treatment of comminuted tibial fractures: 47 cases (1980–1995) in dogs. *Journal of the American Veterinary Medical Association* **211**, 1008–1012

Dueland RT, Berglund L, Vanderby R Jr and Chao EY (1996) Structural properties of interlocking nails, canine femora, and femur-interlocking nail constructs. *Veterinary Surgery* **25**, 386–396

Dueland RT, Johnson KA, Roe SC, Engen MH and Lesser AS (1999) Interlocking nail treatment of diaphyseal long-bone fractures in dogs. *Journal of the American Veterinary Medical Association* **214**, 59–66

Elliot Smith G (1908) The most ancient splints. *British Medical Journal* **1**, 732–736

Gibson W (1729) *The Farrier's New Guide, 6th edn.* Osborn and Longman, London

Guthrie D (1958) *A History of Medicine (with supplements).* Thomas Nelson and Sons, London

Hinko PJ and Rhinelander FW (1975) Effective use of cerclage in the treatment of long bone fractures in dogs. *Journal of the American Veterinary Medical Association* **166**, 520–524

Hulse D, Hyman W, Nori M and Slater M (1997) Reduction in plate strain by addition of an intramedullary pin. *Veterinary Surgery* **26**, 451–459

Johnson AL, Seitz SE, Smith CW, Johnson JM and Schaeffer DJ (1996) Closed reduction and type-II external fixation of comminuted fractures of the radius and tibia in dogs: 23 cases (1990–1994) *Journal of the American Veterinary Medical Association* **209**, 1445–1448

Lane WA (1907) Clinical remarks on the operative treatment of fractures. *British Medical Journal* **1**, 1037–1038

Lister J (1867) On the antiseptic principle in the practice of surgery. *The Lancet* **90**, 353–356

Parkhill C (1897) A new apparatus for the fixation of bones after resection and in fractures with a tendency to displacement. *Transactions of the American Surgical Association* **15**, 251–256

Perren SM (2002) Evolution of the internal fixation of long bone fractures. The scientific basis of biological internal fixation: choosing a new balance between stability and biology. *Journal of Bone and Joint Surgery (British Volume)* **84**, 1093–1110

Pettit GD (1992) History of external skeletal fixation. *Veterinary Clinics of North America* **22**, 1–10

Sherman WO (1912) Vanadium steel bone plates and screws. *Surgery, Gynecology and Obstetrics* **14**, 629–634

Stader O (1937) A preliminary announcement of a new method of treating fractures. *North American Veterinarian* **18**, 37–38

Steiner AJ (1928) Treating femur and pelvic fractures. *Journal of the American Veterinary Medical Association* **73**, 314

Turnbull NR (1949) Fractures of the humerus and femur repaired by intramedullary pins. *Veterinary Record* **63**, 678

Venable CS and Stuck WG (1947) *The Internal Fixation of Fractures.* Blackwell Science, Oxford

Zahn K, Kornmayer M and Matis U (2007) Dowel pinning for feline metacarpal and metatarsal fractures. *Veterinary and Comparative Orthopaedics and Traumatology* **20**, 256–263

1.9 Pin–plate fixation. (a) A severely comminuted tibial fracture in a 6-year-old terrier was reduced in a minimally invasive fashion and (b) stabilized using an intramedullary pin and a medial plate. The fracture healed uneventfully.

Chapter 2

Fracture classification and description

Gareth Clayton Jones

Classification of fractures is useful for a variety of reasons. Accurate description of a fracture enables surgeons to plan and discuss methods of treatment and prognosis, and allows more effective comparison of outcomes. In larger hospitals, planning for patient requirements or ordering of implants in quantity can also be facilitated. The use of a similar fracture classification system for small animals and humans could provide a basis for comparative studies.

Many of the terms still in use today are historical. Initially, verbal description was essential for recording and communication as the only alternative was to draw diagrams. The difficulty with verbal description is that there is no universally agreed definition of the terms commonly employed. For example, it can be unclear how angulated a fracture line may be for the fracture still to be described as 'transverse'. Lack of a common language adds to the problem. However, the value of exchange of information is obvious, especially with regard to uncommon fracture types where individual surgeon experience may be very limited.

Since the discovery of X-rays and the development of other imaging modalities, electronic transmission and storage of data has become much easier. Rapid transfer of information about individual cases is possible, and advice can be sought from specialists across the world. In addition, three-dimensional printers are now readily available, which can allow examination of an actual model of the affected bone. However, for analysis of large numbers of cases a classification system is required, and placing fractures into alphanumerical groups according to agreed definitions has become the international method of choice. The problem with such systems is that a decision is needed at the outset as to how much information is required and therefore how complex the coding system should be. Although more complex systems allow for storage of more information, their use makes it more difficult for the user to code the data and therefore the opportunity for variation is greater.

As yet, no single system of classification has been adopted for small animals. A system has been developed for human patients by the Arbeitsgemeinschaft für Osteosynthesefragen/Association for the Study of Internal Fixation (AO/ASIF) (Müller *et al.*, 1990; AO/ASIF, 1996), which classifies fractures according to the affected bone, location and pattern of the fracture, and the degree of fragment contact. This system uses alphanumeric classification combined with electronically stored images. A similar system is available for equine fractures (Fackelman *et al.*, 1993).

Methods of fracture description

Early methods relied on anatomical descriptions of fractures identified by palpation, such as humeral, femoral or wrist; or used eponymous descriptions named after the first observer (or patient). Common names still used for human fractures are Colles' (distal radius and ulna), Pott's (lower tibia and fibula) and Monteggia (ulnar fracture with radial head luxation). These are occasionally used in veterinary practice but are of limited value unless all involved are familiar with the descriptions.

Early classification divided fractures into 'simple' (closed) or 'compound' (open). Prior to the development of antiseptic treatment and, later, aseptic techniques and antibiotics, this classification could predict whether the patient lost the limb, or even lived or died. 'Simple' did **not** imply ease of treatment.

A few general descriptions remain in contemporary use:

- **Open** (compound) fractures are now generally classified into types based on the degree of tissue damage; this has clinical relevance from the point of view of treatment and prognosis (see Chapter 12). 'Compound' does not indicate the number or type of fragments present, although the term is commonly misused to imply a difficult or very fragmented fracture. The number of fragments does not directly affect the classification, but in general the number of fragments relates to the amount of trauma and thus the amount of tissue damage, hence the classification awarded
- **Pathological** (secondary) fractures are those in which there is an underlying disease process affecting the bone strength such as a generalized bone dystrophy or a localized lesion such as a bone tumour (see Chapter 13). In these cases the bone breaks with a lower force than would be required to fracture a healthy bone (Figure 2.1)
- **Complicated** fractures are those in which there is major blood vessel, nerve or joint involvement. Such fractures may result in permanent defective limb function or even loss of all or part of the limb
- **Comminuted** fractures have several fragments (more than two)
- **Multiple** fractures are those in which there are fractures at more than one level in the bone, or fractures of more than one bone in the patient.

Various criteria are used to specify fractures more accurately.

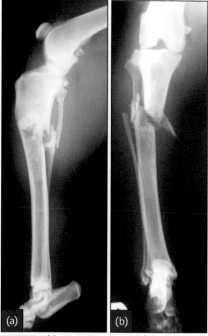

2.1 (a) Mediolateral and (b) caudocranial radiographs of the tibia of a 6-year-old crossbred dog which sustained a spontaneous tibial fracture whilst walking. A highly comminuted transverse fracture of the proximal tibial diaphysis and a marginally oblique fracture of the fibula are observed. The high-energy appearance of the fracture, its unusual location and lysis of the distal tibial fracture fragment adjacent to the fracture site with coarsened trabecular pattern are consistent with a pre-existing neoplastic process producing a pathological fracture.
(Courtesy of D Clements)

Anatomical location

The shaft of long bones (diaphysis) is conventionally divided into thirds: proximal, middle and distal.

General location

Location can also be described as:

- Articular
- Capital
- Subcapital
- Physeal
- Metaphyseal
- Diaphyseal.

Specific location

More detailed anatomical locations include:

- Condylar – lateral or medial
- Trochanteric
- Subtrochanteric
- Basal.

Displacement of fragments

- Greenstick – incomplete fractures in juvenile animals in which the periosteum is largely or completely intact.
- Folded – a form of greenstick fracture resembling an acutely folded cardboard tube.
- Fissure – undisplaced fragments which may displace at surgery or under stress.
- Depressed – fragments invade an underlying cavity, especially parts of the skull.

- Compression – of cancellous bone, often of the vertebral body or involving subchondral bone.
- Impacted – in which one fragment is driven into the cancellous bone of the opposing fragment.

The manner of the displacement of the fragments is often of clinical importance.

Nature of the fracture

- Complete – the cortex is completely broken with separation of the fragments.
- Incomplete – part of the bone remains intact.

The direction of the fracture line

- Transverse – the fracture line is at right angles or up to 30 degrees to the long axis of the bone.
- Oblique – the fracture line is equal to or greater than 30 degrees to the long axis of the bone.
- Spiral – the fracture line runs helically along the bone.
- Longitudinal – the fracture line follows the long axis of the bone.
- Y- or T-fracture – the pattern of fracture lines involving bony condyles, commonly of the distal humerus.

Number or nature of the fragments

- Two-fragment, three-fragment, comminuted (more than two).
- Wedge or butterfly fragment – an intermediate fragment.
- Segmental – two separate fracture lines in the same long bone, resulting in one or more additional fragments of complete bone between them (Figure 2.2).
- Avulsion/apophyseal – pulled by tendon or ligament.
- Chip – fragment at articular margin, often seen following hyperextension injuries.
- Slab – larger fragment with vertical or oblique fracture line in cancellous bone which extends into two articular surfaces.

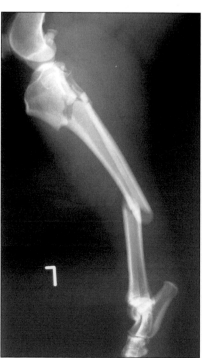

2.2 A mediolateral radiograph of the tibia of a 2-year-old Border Collie with a segmental tibial fracture, comprising a comminuted transverse proximal tibial diaphyseal fracture just below the metaphysis and a marginally oblique, overriding fracture of the distal third of the diaphysis.
(Courtesy of D Clements)

Articular fractures

- Extra-articular – close to a joint but not involving the articular surface: may be intracapsular, such as in femoral neck fractures.
- Partial articular – involving a part of the articular surface with remaining articular cartilage surface still attached to the diaphysis.
- Complete articular – disrupting the articular surface and separating it completely from the diaphysis, for example dicondylar humeral fractures.

Stability after reduction

- Stable after reduction – tend to remain in place without force, so may be treatable by coaptation.
- Unstable after reduction – the fracture collapses as soon as the reducing forces are removed; these may require operative stabilization.

Special classifications

Growth plate or epiphyseal fractures (separations)

The most commonly used is the Salter–Harris system (Salter and Harris, 1963) in which six types of injury are recognized (Figure 2.3):

- Type I – complete, through the zone of hypertrophied cartilage
- Type II – partially includes the metaphysis
- Type III – intra-articular fracture to the zone of hypertrophied cartilage, propagating along the epiphyseal plate to the edge of the bone

- Type IV – intra-articular fracture that traverses the epiphysis, epiphyseal plate and metaphysis
- Type V – crushing injury that causes destruction of growing cells
- Type VI – fracture results in new bone bridges at the periphery of the growth plate.

Special joint fractures

Certain joint fractures, mainly of importance in the racing Greyhound, have been classified to aid prognosis and treatment (see Chapter 25).

Accessory carpal bone (Johnson, 1987):

- Type I – intra-articular avulsion of the distal margin.
- Type II – intra-articular fracture of the proximal margin.
- Type III – extra-articular avulsion of the distal margin.
- Type IV – extra-articular avulsion of the insertion of flexor carpi ulnaris at the proximal palmar surface.
- Type V – comminuted fracture of the body which may involve the articular surface.

Central tarsal bone (Dee et al., 1976):

- Type I – small dorsal slab fracture with minimal displacement.
- Type II – dorsal slab fracture with displacement.
- Type III – one-third to half of the bone fractured in the sagittal plane and displaced medially or dorsally.
- Type IV – combination of Types II and III.
- Type V – severe comminution.

Various combinations of fractures of the tarsus, often involving the calcaneus, central tarsal bone and fifth

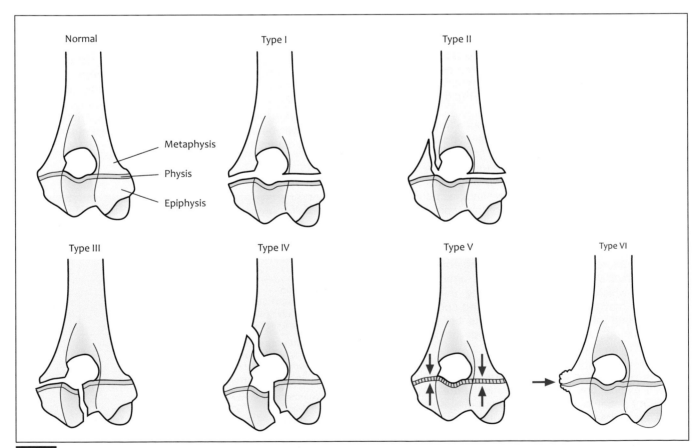

Normal — Metaphysis / Physis / Epiphysis — Type I — Type II — Type III — Type IV — Type V — Type VI

2.3 The Salter–Harris classification of growth plate fractures.

metatarsal bone, are regularly seen concurrently in the Greyhound, but are not classified, although they have been described as **triads** (Newton and Nunamaker, 1985). These fractures may be difficult to assess fully by conventional radiography but, if available, computed tomography (CT) scans can reveal the exact nature of the fracture more accurately (Hercock *et al.*, 2011).

Metacarpal/metatarsal stress fractures (Newton and Nunamaker, 1985): These fractures are primarily seen in Greyhounds and occasionally other hard-working dogs, and are regarded as fatigue fractures, similar to those seen in human athletes or soldiers:

- Type I – painful on palpation at the junction of the proximal third and distal two-thirds of the bone; endosteal and cortical thickening of the bone visible on radiography
- Type II – hairline undisplaced fissure-type fracture
- Type III – complete fracture with palmar/plantar displacement of distal fragment.

Open fractures

Open fractures possess a wound that communicates between the fracture and the outside environment. Usually this is via a visible surface wound, but it could also include a fracture of a skull bone that has penetrated the nose or a sinus cavity. Classification of open fractures is often helpful in determining optimal methods of treatment.

- Type I – a wound produced from inside to outside by the penetration of a sharp fracture fragment end through the overlaying soft tissues. Such a fracture may become open some time following the initiating incident as a result of uncontrolled or unsupported movement. There is usually limited soft tissue injury and the bone fragments are all present, often without comminution.
- Type II – a fracture caused from outside to inside by penetration of a foreign object. There is usually more soft tissue damage with contusion around the skin wound and some mainly reversible muscle damage. Fractures may be more fragmented but there is little if any loss of bone or soft tissue.
- Type III – the most severe form of open fracture in which loss of tissue following penetration by an outside object has resulted. Loss of skin, soft tissue and bone material may have occurred and may be very severe. Some surgeons recognize a subdivision in which loss of the main arterial supply to the limb has occurred, as this often indicates mandatory amputation.

Although not officially recognized, an estimate of the time elapsed since the injury may be helpful in classifying an open fracture. This acknowledges the consequences of bacterial invasion of a wound where, after an initial lag phase in which the bacteria become established, the organisms may begin to multiply, turning contamination of a wound into infection. This relates to the concept of a 'golden period', which should be taken into account, but not relied upon implicitly.

A system for classification of the soft tissue injury has been developed for use in humans (Müller *et al.*, 1992). Certain evaluations in human patients are not made in veterinary patients and so the system may be too complicated for animals, although it could probably be used with a little variation.

Further details of the classification of open fractures are given in Chapter 12.

Fracture classification suitable for computer analysis

The ability to classify fractures for computer analysis can have clear advantages, allowing evaluation and comparison of data as well as easy worldwide cooperation. A number of methods have been suggested but currently no single method has gained acceptance.

A classification of femoral fractures was developed at the University of Michigan (Braden *et al.*, 1995) following a general analysis of fractures by Brinker *et al.* (1990). This system is only applicable to fractures of the femur and has only a limited fracture description. It is based on a paper form which can be scanned and recorded by a computer; thus no computer equipment is required at the originating hospital.

General classification of fractures was developed by Müller *et al.* of the AO group for human fractures (Müller *et al.*, 1990; AO/ASIF, 1996). This has been modified by various workers to create similar methods for small animals and the horse. Two systems for small animals, the Prieur system (Prieur *et al.*, 1990) and the Unger system (Unger *et al.*, 1990), have been described in the literature, although neither has yet been accepted universally. These classifications describe the bone, the location and the type of fracture. Each of the proposed systems creates a four-digit record in a similar way to the human AO system. The Prieur and Unger fracture classification systems can only be used for fractures of the long bones and are not used for fractures involving the skull, vertebral column, pelvis or small limb bones. Neither system discusses associated soft tissue problems, which may be of great importance in determining treatment and outcome.

The Prieur system

This is the simpler system, recording slightly less information. Digits are allocated under each of four fields (bone; location; fracture area; fragment number) (Figure 2.4). The location zones of each bone are determined by drawing a square around the ends, of length and width equal to the widest dimension of the bone end (Figure 2.5). Each fracture is then described by four numbers (Figure 2.6). In spite of its simplicity, the Prieur system has never been widely adopted by the veterinary orthopaedic community.

Field	Number
• **Bone**	
• Humerus	1
• Radius/ulna	2
• Femur	3
• Tibia	4
• **Location**	
• Proximal segment	1
• Middle segment	2
• Distal segment	3
• **Fracture area (percentage of bone length)**	
• <5% (and/or not involving articular cartilage)	1
• 5–25% (specific fractures of femur neck)	2
• >25% (and/or involving articular surface)	3
• **Number of fragments**	
• Two	2
• Three	3
• Four or more	4

2.4 The Prieur system.

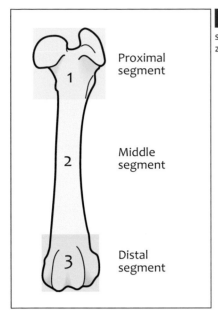

2.5 The Prieur classification system: location of bone zones.

Proximal segment

1

Middle segment

2

Distal segment

3

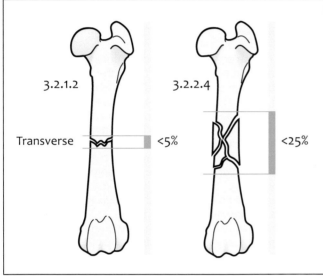

3.2.1.2   3.2.2.4

Transverse   <5%   <25%

2.6 Examples of femoral fractures and their numerical identification using the Prieur classification system.

The Unger system

This identifies fractures in a similar manner to the Prieur system, but records somewhat more data by attempting to identify reducible or non-reducible wedges or the direction of the fracture line. Charts of both letters and numbers for each bone and the codes allocated for various fractures are required with this system, which attempts to record the fractures in a clinically related manner.

Apart from facilitating communication between surgeons regardless of their geographical location, an individual surgeon can obtain significant value from the classification of fractures, because it enables decisions to be made on the method of treatment which would be best employed within practice constraints. In particular, classification helps the surgeon to assess indications for the use of external as opposed to internal fixation, decide when a simple method of external coaptation may be adequate, and may allow better and more accurate prognoses to be given to owners, for example when certain apparently innocuous growth plate injuries are identified.

For any reader wishing to evaluate the human AO system for themselves, or even to develop their own system, Chapters 1.4 and 1.5 of *AO Principles of Fracture Management* (2000) contain further detail and illustrations.

References and further reading

AO/ASIF (1996) *Comprehensive Classification of Fractures*, Pamphlets I and II. Maurice E Müller Foundation, AO/ASIF Documentation Centre, Davos, CH-7270 Switzerland

AO/ASIF (2000) *AO Principles of Fracture Management*, ed. T Ruedi and WM Murphy, pp. 45–76. Thieme, Stuttgart and New York

Braden TD, Eicker SW, Abdinoor D and Prieur WD (1995) Characteristics of 1000 femur fractures in the dog and cat. *Veterinary and Comparative Orthopaedics and Traumatology* **8**, 203–209

Brinker WO, Hohn RB and Prieur WD (1984) *Manual of Internal Fixation in Small Animals*, pp. 85–86. Springer Verlag, Berlin, Heidelberg and New York

Brinker W, Piermattei D and Flo G (1990) *Handbook of Small Animal Orthopaedics and Fracture Treatment*, 2nd edn. WB Saunders, Philadelphia

Dee JF, Dee J and Piermattei DL (1976) Classification, management and repair of central tarsal fractures in the racing Greyhound. *Journal of the American Animal Hospital Association* **12**, 398–405

Fackelman GE, Peutz IP, Norris JC *et al.* (1993) The development of an equine fracture documentation system. *Veterinary and Comparative Orthopaedics and Traumatology* **6**, 47–52

Hercock CA, Innes JF, McConnell F *et al.* (2011) Observer variation in the evaluation and classification of severe tarsal bone fractures in racing Greyhounds. *Veterinary and Comparative Orthopaedics and Traumatology* **24**, 167–256

Johnson KA (1987) Accessory carpal bone fractures in the racing Greyhound. Classification and pathology. *Veterinary Surgery* **16**, 60–64

Müller ME, Allgöwer M, Schneider R and Willenegger H (1992) *Manual of Internal Fixation, abridged 3rd edn*, pp. 118–158. Springer Verlag, Berlin

Müller ME, Nazarian S, Koch P and Schatzker J (1990) *The AO Classification of Fractures of Long Bones*. Springer Verlag, Berlin, Heidelberg and New York

Newton CD and Nunamaker DM (1985) Fractures associated with the racing Greyhound. In: *Textbook of Small Animal Orthopaedics*, pp. 467–477. Lippincott, Philadelphia

Prieur WD, Braden TD and von Rechenberg B (1990) A suggested fracture classification of adult small animal fractures. *Veterinary and Comparative Orthopaedics and Traumatology* **3**, 111–116

Salter RB and Harris WR (1963) Injuries involving the epiphyseal plate. *Journal of Bone and Joint Surgery (American Volume)* **45**, 587–622

Stedman TL (1990) *Stedman's Medical Dictionary, 25th edn*. Williams and Wilkins, Baltimore

Unger M, Montavon PM and Heim UFA (1990) Classification of fractures of long bones in the dog and cat, introduction and clinical application. *Veterinary and Comparative Orthopaedics* **3**, 41–50

Chapter 3

Bone development and physiology

Russell Yeadon

From a surgeon's perspective, it is easy to think of bone as an inert, lifeless, rigid structure. This is not the case; bone must be considered both as a living, elastic tissue and as a complex organ with a range of biological functions and diverse interactions with other organ systems.

Functions of bone are not solely mechanical; they are also engaged in a range of biological roles such as assistance in the control of calcium homeostasis and acid–base balance (Figure 3.1). Although most of these non-mechanical functions are rarely of clinical significance for management of isolated traumatic fractures in small animals, they may become more relevant in cases with pathological fractures, metabolic bone disorders, endocrine dysfunction and various other systemic conditions.

Many of the processes involved in fracture healing are the same as those involved in embryonic bone growth or in bone remodelling in the mature skeleton. Controlling these processes is central to achieving appropriate bone healing and is part of the management of any fracture; this requires a detailed knowledge of the biological requirements of each process. The objective of this chapter is to provide an overview of the mechanisms involved in normal bone development and growth.

Mechanical functions
• Provide body shape and structure • Enable ambulation (e.g. as an attachment site for muscles) • Protection of organs (e.g. in the cranial cavity or thoracic cavity)
Biological functions
• Mineral reservoir (particularly calcium and phosphate) • Role in systemic acid–base balance • Reservoir for haemopoietic cells within bone marrow • Endocrine and biochemical signalling roles • Fatty acid store • Toxin sequestration (e.g. heavy metals, which are absorbed directly into hydroxyapatite)

3.1 The major functions of bone.

Skeletal anatomy

Bones in the body can be loosely divided into groups based on anatomical location and function:

• **Axial skeleton:** skull and hyoid apparatus; vertebral column; ribs and sternum

• **Appendicular skeleton:** thoracic limb; pelvic limb
• **Heterotopic skeleton:** os penis.

For descriptive purposes, bones can be further sub-divided according to their shape, although in many cases this is a largely arbitrary classification, with some variation between sources.

• **Long bones** are the main contributors to limb conformation with examples being the femur, humerus and tibia. These bones typically feature a diaphysis (shaft) with an epiphysis at each end. In juvenile animals, the diaphysis and epiphyses are separated by physeal cartilage from which longitudinal growth primarily originates. At the diaphyseal side of the physis is an area known as the metaphysis that forms a poorly delineated 'interzone' between the epiphysis and diaphysis (Figure 3.2). At skeletal maturity, the cartilaginous component of the physis mineralizes to form a continuous column of bone.
• **Short bones** are found in the carpal and tarsal regions and are typically cuboidal, although some variation in shape is noted.
• **Sesamoid bones** (sometimes grouped with short bones) are generally present within or immediately subjacent to a

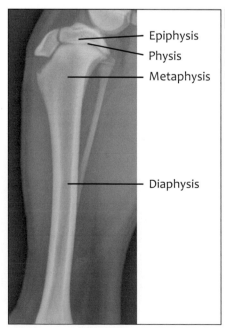

Epiphysis
Physis
Metaphysis
Diaphysis

3.2 Mediolateral radiograph of a juvenile canine tibia demonstrating the main anatomical components of long bones.

BSAVA Manual of Canine and Feline Fracture Repair and Management, 2nd edition. Edited by Toby Gemmill and Dylan Clements. ©BSAVA 2016

tendon. Their main function is to glide over another bone at, or adjacent to, a mobile joint, providing protection to the tendon from frictional or abrasive forces. In some instances, the presence of the sesamoid can improve the biomechanical efficiency of the muscle–tendon unit.

- **Flat bones** comprise most of the major bones of the skull (such as the occipital and frontal bones) where they provide a protective function for the skull contents whilst minimizing weight. Other examples include bones of the limb girdles (such as the scapula) where they mainly serve to provide a large surface area for muscle attachments.

- **Irregular bones** comprise the vertebrae, non-flat bones of the skull (e.g. the zygomatic bone and mandible) and some bones of the pelvis.

Bone embryology

Like other connective tissues such as muscle and fibrous tissue, bone originates from mesodermal layers in the developing embryo. Vertebrate bone develops from three main cell lineages. The lateral plate mesoderm is the main contributor to the appendicular skeleton. The paraxial mesoderm (sclerotome) is the main contributor to the axial skeleton and gives rise to some of the craniofacial skeleton, whilst neural crest cells also make some contribution to the branchial arch derivatives of the craniofacial skeleton.

In each area of future skeletal development, mesenchymal cells condense into nodules of high cellular density. This process of cellular condensation involves complex changes in the extracellular matrix, allowing cell-to-cell communication (particularly at the interface between mesenchymal and epithelial cells), and activating molecular signalling pathways. These changes allow the cells to establish their relative location and orientation, and are the basis of subsequent cellular differentiation. These pathways are not completely understood, but **bone morphogenic proteins (BMPs)** are thought to be one of the critical signalling molecule groups involved in this process. These proteins are diverse in their molecular origins and functions, but those with well recognized functions in bone development (BMP-2 to BMP-7) are part of the transforming growth factor beta (TGF-β) superfamily of proteins. The BMPs are also essential in the promotion of bone healing following fracture.

Bone growth

As bone growth progresses, two distinct mechanisms of bone formation become apparent:

- Intramembranous ossification
- Endochondral ossification.

Intramembranous ossification

Intramembranous ossification involves formation of bone directly from osteogenic mesenchymal cells, mainly on the inner side of the periosteum. Importantly, bone is synthesized directly *without* a cartilage precursor. It accounts for the development of most flat bones, particularly the bones of the skull, and also plays an important role in increasing the width of the diaphysis and metaphyses of long bones.

In intramembranous ossification, the condensations of mesenchymal cells differentiate largely into osteoblasts, with others forming capillaries. This process occurs primarily under the control of two transcription factors, Cbfa 1 (or RUNX2) and oxterix. The osteoblasts secrete a collagen–proteoglycan matrix called **osteoid**, which forms the basic extracellular matrix of bone. This matrix is initially secreted in a completely random orientation with collagen fibrils being secreted 360 degrees around each cell. The fibrous component of this matrix mainly comprises type I collagen with some associated 'ground substance', which includes molecules such as chondroitin sulphate and osteocalcin. This is the basis of **woven bone**. Osteoblasts at this stage are referred to as mesenchymal osteoblasts.

The collagen matrix binds calcium salts from blood delivered by the newly formed capillaries. The process of mineralization is initiated mainly by membrane-bound matrix vesicles, which originate through budding of the cytoplasmic processes of the chondrocytes or osteoblasts, and which subsequently become embedded in the secreted matrix. The membranes of these vesicles are rich in alkaline and acidic phosphatases, which hydrolyze inhibitors of mineralization. The end result is generation of focally high concentrations of calcium (Ca^{2+}) and phosphate (PO_4^{3-}) ions, which precipitate into clusters of crystals. This calcium deposition is further regulated and stabilized by proteins within the ground substance, particularly osteocalcin. The bulk of the calcium bound is stored as **hydroxyapatite** ($Ca_{10}(PO_4)_6OH_2$) mineral crystals. There is typically a time lag of approximately 10 days between formation of osteoid and the process of mineralization. The dry weight of mature bone comprises approximately 65–70% inorganic mineral and 30–35% fibrous proteins (predominantly type I collagen).

Initially there is a small gap of non-mineralized osteoid between the osteoblasts and the mineralizing front. However, as calcification progresses, the osteoblasts become aligned on the surface of the matrix and are then referred to as surface osteoblasts. At this stage, collagen matrix is secreted in parallel fibrils, longitudinally along the woven bone, which serves as a structural scaffold. This creation of layers of osteoid is known as **lamellar bone formation**. When the osteoblasts become completely encapsulated within mineralized bone, they are referred to as **osteocytes** (Figure 3.3). The basic histological structure of osteocytes is similar to that of surface osteoblasts, although as they become deeply embedded in bone their cytoplasmic volume and associated organelles reduce. Osteocytes develop long cytoplasmic processes which extend into canaliculi (small canals) within the mineralized bone; these are involved in intercellular signalling via tight junctions with adjacent osteocytes and osteoblasts. Osteocytes play an important role in bone maintenance and remodelling.

Endochondral ossification

Endochondral ossification involves formation of a cartilage precursor, which subsequently mineralizes to form bone. It is the primary means of longitudinal growth of long bones and formation of the vertebral bodies, ribs, sternebrae and the flat bones of the pelvis.

The initial cellular processes involved in endochondral ossification are architecturally similar to those of intramembranous ossification, specifically the condensation of mesenchymal cells and subsequent secretion of an extracellular matrix (see Figure 3.3). However, molecular signalling pathways, particularly involving a transcription

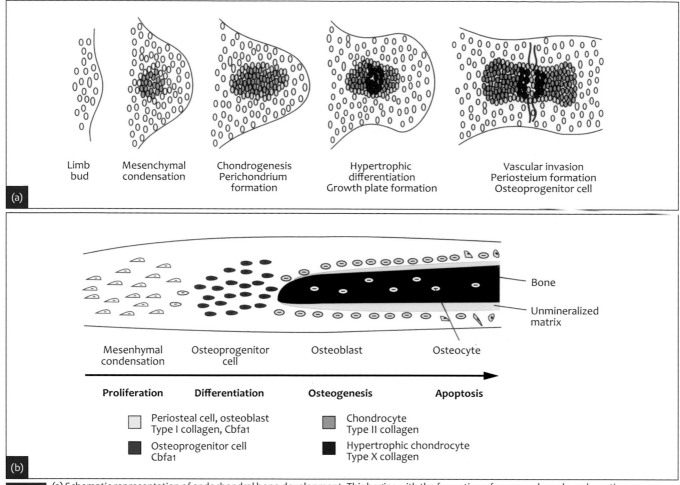

Mesenhymal condensation   Osteoprogenitor cell   Osteoblast   Osteocyte

Proliferation   **Differentiation**   **Osteogenesis**   **Apoptosis**

☐ Periosteal cell, osteoblast
Type I collagen, Cbfa1

☐ Chondrocyte
Type II collagen

■ Osteoprogenitor cell
Cbfa1

■ Hypertrophic chondrocyte
Type X collagen

3.3 (a) Schematic representation of endochondral bone development. This begins with the formation of a mesenchymal condensation, expressing type II collagen (blue). Centrally, cells differentiate into chondrocytes, which hypertrophy and express type X collagen (purple). Progression to the mature growth plate accompanies development of the perichondrium (yellow), vascular invasion and the formation of a centre of ossification containing type I collagen-expressing osteoblasts (yellow). (b) Schematic representation of intramembranous bone development. Undifferentiated mesenchymal cells differentiate into osteoprogenitor cells expressing a transcription factor associated with osteoblast differentiation, Cbfa1 (also known as RUNX2; pink). Osteoprogenitor cells progress to mature osteoblasts that express Cbfa1 and type I collagen (yellow). These cells deposit and mineralize bone matrix. Osteoblasts either die by apoptosis or are embedded in the matrix, becoming osteocytes.
(Reproduced from Ornitz and Marie (2002) with permission from Cold Spring Harbor Laboratory Press and the authors)

factor known as scleraxis, stimulate mesenchymal cells to differentiate into chondrocytes rather than osteoblasts. These chondrocytes secrete a range of cartilage-specific collagens (particularly type X collagen) and proteoglycans, which form a cartilaginous extracellular scaffold.

Long bone development

Long bone growth starts within limb buds, which begin as small tissue proliferations from the lateral plate and paraxial mesoderm in the embryo. Pattern formation and three-dimensional orientation of the limb bud involve a series of processes:

- A cap of epithelium develops at the tip of the limb bud called the apical ectodermal ridge, which is involved in controlling proximal-to-distal orientation of the growing skeletal structures. This effect is believed to be mediated by production of proteins including members of the fibroblast growth factor (FGF) family including FGF-2, 4 and 8
- A similar region of specific mesenchymal cells at the posterior margin of the limb bud known as the zone of polarizing activity is responsible for establishing the anteroposterior orientation of the growing skeletal structures, primarily by transcription of the Sonic hedgehog (Shh) gene
- Synthesis of other proteins including Wnt7a and the transcription factor Lmx-1 are thought to allow for pattern formation in the dorsoventral axis within the limb bud.

As long bone development and maturation progress, a series of structural changes occur in response to the signalling cascades involved in pattern formation. These include formation of both primary and secondary centres of ossification that establish the diaphysis and epiphyses of the bone, respectively. Vascularization of the cartilage matrix appears to be one of the critical steps within this process. The processes of endochondral and intramembranous os-sification occur in conjunction, under the control of a complex set of molecular signalling cascades. These eventually allow the entire cartilage template to be replaced by bone, with cartilage being retained only at the articular surfaces. This series of changes is summarized in Figure 3.4, although it should be noted that there is no consensus about the precise nature and sequence of some parts of the process.

Stage 1	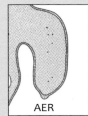	Limb bud formation. Mesenchymal cells are uniformly distributed. Apical ectodermal ridge (AER) forms at the tip of the limb bud, establishing proximodistal pattern formation
Stage 2	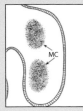	Mesenchymal cells (MC) condense in future areas of bone development
Stage 3	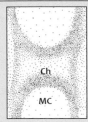	Mesenchymal cells (MC) differentiate into chondrocytes (Ch). Chondrocytes hypertrophy in mid-section of limb, representing future 'interzone' area of joint formation and epiphyses
Stage 4	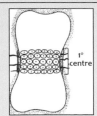	Basic long bone shape becomes established, including epiphyseal shaping. Intramembranous bone formation begins at mid-diaphysis (primary centre of ossification)
Stage 5	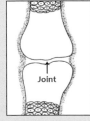	Resorption of cartilage matrix at joint 'interzone'. Smooth articular cartilage surface forms on either side of joint. Vascular invasion of hypertrophic chondrocyte area instigates endochondral bone formation in mid-diaphyseal region, completing the primary centre of ossification
Stage 6	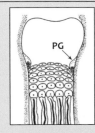	Formation of the physis and of peripheral perichondrial groove (PG) tissue. This tissue varies in precise composition by anatomical location, species and age, but may include a reservoir of chondrocytes (groove of Ranvier), which allows for unrestricted abaxial expansion of the physis during growth, and a fibrous rim (perichondrial ring of LaCroix), which primarily functions to provide mechanical support to the physis
Stage 7	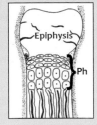	Cartilage of the epiphysis becomes vascularized. Distinct physeal layers become apparent, known respectively as the resting zone, proliferative zone, hypertrophic cartilage zone, calcified cartilage zone and ossification zone, with the resting zone being immediately subjacent to the epiphysis, and the ossification zone comprising the extent of the physis (Ph) adjacent to the diaphysis ▶

Stage 8		Chondrocytes at the centre of the epiphysis undergo hypertrophy to form a spherical mass, known as the secondary centre of ossification
Stage 9	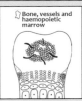	Vascular invasion of developing secondary ossification centre facilitates endochondral ossification with formation of mineralized matrix
Stage 10		Bone formation and marrow cavitation occur within the secondary ossification centre, creating a reservoir for haemopoietic marrow
Stage 11		Increase in size and change in shape of secondary ossification centre progress as the epiphysis develops
Stage 12	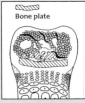	Fat starts to accumulate in the marrow spaces adjacent to secondary ossification centre growth plate
Stage 13	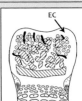	Epiphyseal bone plate forms adjacent to the physis
Stage 14	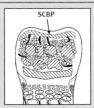	Secondary ossification centre expands to occupy most of the epiphysis, leaving only a thin rim of epiphyseal cartilage (EC) at the periphery
Stage 15	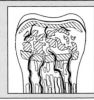	Thinning and ultimate involution of the physis occurs as skeletal maturity approaches. The subchondral bone plate (SCBP) is formed immediately below the articular cartilage layer
Stage 16		Resorption of growth plate occurs at skeletal maturity, with linkage of epiphyseal and metaphyseal circulations. Calcification of the deepest zone of articular cartilage occurs, establishing the final articular contour

3.4 Histological stages in limb, long bone and epiphyseal development.
(Modified from Shapiro (2008) with permission from *European Cells and Materials*)

The precise age at which each stage of bone development occurs varies widely by anatomical location, by species and, of particular note in dogs, by breed. Growth is typically complete at around 7–9 months in smaller breed dogs and at 12–18 months in larger breeds. This has clear clinical implications for the management of fractures in immature animals, and when considering potential genetic, systemic or environmental abnormalities that might interfere with the normal processes involved in bone development.

Bone remodelling

Mechanical bone remodelling is conventionally divided into two subtypes:

- **Endosteal remodelling** – this specifically occurs along the trabeculae (the fine strands of bone matrix) within the cancellous bone and at the axial surface of cortical bone
- **Haversian remodelling** – this occurs within the Haversian canals (and is the process by which these canals are formed) within cortical bone.

This subdivision is largely arbitrary because, in reality, the Haversian system functions as an anatomical extension of the endosteal system and the cellular processes are essentially the same.

Remodelling is a continuous process, with bone resorption and formation occurring in tandem and in balance with each other to replace old bone with new bone as a normal homeostatic process. In adult humans, it is generally accepted that approximately 10% of the total skeletal mass is renewed per year, although figures of up to 30% have been suggested (Sims and Baron, 2002). As previously discussed, bone production is mediated by osteoblast cells and involves secretion of a collagenous matrix known as osteoid, which subsequently becomes mineralized. By contrast, bone resorption is mediated by cells known as **osteoclasts**. These are giant multinucleate cells usually found in contact with a mineralized bone surface, typically within a lacuna (Howship's lacuna) created by the cell's own resorptive processes. Osteoclasts originate from a mononuclear haemopoietic precursor cell with an overlapping ancestry to monocytes and macrophages. There is some evidence that partially differentiated macrophages may actually be able to convert to osteoclasts under specific circumstances.

Much of the intercellular molecular signalling that leads to osteoclast differentiation originates from osteoblasts. Among the most important signalling molecules are the RANK ligand (RANKL; receptor activator of nuclear factor kappa-B (NF-κB) ligand), which is expressed on the osteoblast surface, and M-CSF (macrophage-colony stimulating factor). Osteoblasts also secrete a glycoprotein known as osteoprotegerin (OPG), which functions alongside RANKL. Functions of both the RANKL–OPG and M-CSF pathways are diverse but include stimulation of differentiation of precursor cells into osteoclasts, and the promotion of resorptive activity in differentiated osteoclasts. Control over RANKL, OPG and M-CSF expression by osteoblasts is exerted by various endogenous factors including insulin, prostaglandins and vitamin D, and by exogenous compounds such as bisphosphonate medications.

Osteoclasts are highly developed cells with regard to their cellular structure and function. Attachment to bone is mediated largely by transmembrane integrin adhesion receptors, which bind to specific amino acid sequences within the protein matrix of bone. Cellular adhesion occurs in specific areas of the cell membrane known as podosomes, which allow for high cell motility, permitting the osteoclast to 'walk' along the bone surface as bone resorption progresses.

Bone resorption occurs through a combination of acidification and proteolysis. Acidification is achieved by production of hydrogen (H^+) ions via intracellular carbonic anhydrase II enzyme (which catalyzes the chemical reaction $H_2O + CO_2 \leftrightarrow H^+ + HCO_3^-$). These H^+ ions are then secreted across the cell membrane via proton pumps in the basolateral membrane to create a locally acidic environment immediately between the cell membrane and bone surface. This mainly serves to dissolve hydroxyapatite crystals, exposing the bone matrix. Various secreted enzymes, particularly metalloproteinases (e.g. MMP-9 and MMP-13), can then digest the protein components of the bone matrix.

In endosteal bone remodelling, osteoclasts are located diffusely across the trabecular surfaces, either individually or in clusters of a few cells. By contrast, in the process of Haversian remodelling, groups of osteoclasts act to excavate a tunnel within the cortical bone known as a **cutting cone**. Osteoblasts then produce new bone behind this cone to partially refill the tunnel. The end result is a longitudinal central canal known as an osteon or Haversian canal (oriented along the long axis of the bone), which comprises one or two capillaries and sometimes a nerve fibre, surrounded by concentric lamellae of bone (see Figure 5.3).

Mechanobiology

It has been known since the 18th century that dynamic bone remodelling occurs in response to mechanical stress. This concept was further developed by Julius Wolff in the 1860s into **Wolff's law**. This concept documents adaptations in bone morphology in response to increased mechanical load over time, and was initially used solely to describe these changes within the trabecular bone established by endosteal remodelling. The responses of cortical bone are similar to those of trabecular bone and occur by Haversian remodelling, but endosteal remodelling tends to be more dramatic and more rapid due to the increased bone surface area available for bone resorption and subsequent reformation. The essential premise of Wolff's law is that, with increased repetitive mechanical load, the bone becomes stronger or thicker, specifically related to the orientation of the mechanical force applied. In many anatomical locations, focal areas of well aligned trabecular bone pattern can be seen radiographically as evidence of this process (Figure 3.5). Conversely, with decreased mechanical load the bone becomes weaker or finer, with reduction in both the bone mineral density and the quantity of bone matrix present.

The effects of mechanical stress are mediated at a cellular level by an array of processes, most of which are poorly understood.

- Some effects are known to be generated by direct cyclical mechanical deformation of cells. For example, direct stretching of the osteoblast cell membrane triggers stretch-sensitive ion channels, which influences the secretion of osteoid to occur in alignment to the stress applied.

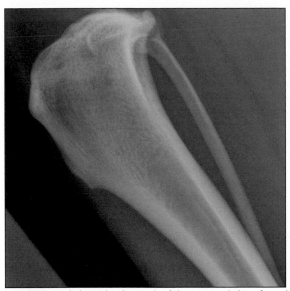

3.5 Mediolateral radiograph of the proximal tibia of an adult dog. The fine 'lace-like' trabecular pattern is visible with clear lines of orientation parallel with lines of mechanical tension within the bone.

- Other effects of mechanical deformation are transferred to the cell less directly. For example, fluid flow within the endosteal spaces and Haversian canals of the bone during elastic deformation is also believed to play a significant role in mechanical transduction to the cellular components of bone. This is probably partially manifested directly by hydrostatic pressure variations, or by the viscoelastic shear forces applied to cell membranes by fluid flow over the cell surface. However, this form of fluid flow is also known to create piezoelectrical currents which are believed to play an important role in cellular signalling pathways with similar effects being reproducible *in vitro* by application of electrical currents to individual cells.
- Further mechanical transduction probably occurs via indirect mechanisms such as the changes in vascular structures within the bone in response to mechanical load, thereby altering local blood flow through the tissue.

The effects of mechanical transduction apply not only at an individual cell level (essentially causing increased osteoblast activity and decreased osteoclast activity); these actions also establish feedback loops between the different cell types which regulate this activity.

Non-mechanical influences on bone structure

Bone development and subsequent remodelling is also affected by a vast array of non-mechanical stimuli, representing various environmental, hormonal and systemic factors.

The endocrine influences on bone are diverse, but the most potent effects are typically caused by general growth regulatory hormones which have effects on multiple organ systems. The most relevant of these are:

- Growth hormone
- Insulin-like growth factor-1
- Sex hormones
- Leptin.

Growth hormone and insulin-like growth factor-1

Growth hormone (GH) is a peptide hormone secreted by somatotropic cells in the anterior pituitary gland, under the influence of growth hormone-releasing hormone from the hypothalamus. Many of the influences of GH on bone are modulated by stimulation of insulin-like growth factor-1 (IGF-1) production by the liver and various other tissues including chondrocytes. IGF-1 is known to be critical in the modulation of bone remodelling, with major effects including promotion of osteoblast proliferation and adhesion at the remodelling bone surface, and co-ordinating the homeostatic mechanisms balancing bone resorption and production. The specific effect of IGF-1 on osteoclasts remains unknown, although osteoclasts are known to have IGF-1 receptors in the cell membrane. The overall effect of increasing levels of GH and IGF-1 is an increasing rate of longitudinal bone growth in juveniles and increasing bone density in adults. In dogs, a single IGF-1 single-nucleotide polymorphism haplotype has been identified on chromosome 15 that is present in almost all small breeds, but is absent from most giant breeds. This sequence variation is believed to be a major contributor to body size in small dogs (Sutter *et al.*, 2007) and illustrates the potency of this mechanism on modulating bone development.

Many systemic hormones have some influence on bone, although in most cases these are likely to be mediated by their effects on the GH–IGF pathway. For example, increased levels of oestrogen and testosterone are known to increase GH secretion, whilst increased levels of glucocorticoids reduce GH secretion. Thyroid hormone also affects this pathway indirectly, and has synergistic effects directly on bone with GH. The GH–IGF pathway is also likely to mediate the bone-related effects of various environmental factors. For example, hypoglycaemia, dietary niacin, fasting and vigorous exercise are known to increase GH secretion. Some of these effects are manifested directly at the level of the hypothalamus or pituitary gland whilst others are probably exerted via other endocrine pathways such as glucocorticoid or leptin stimulation. This clearly creates a highly complex range of feedback pathways.

Sex hormones

Sex hormones, particularly oestrogen and testosterone, inhibit bone resorption and have an influence on macrostructural changes such as timing of physeal closure. In both male and female dogs, early neutering has been shown to delay physeal closure and results in increased adult bone length, although no direct effect on the rate of bone growth has been documented (Salmeri *et al.*, 1991). A similar effect on physeal closure has been noted with neutering in male cats, but not in female cats (Perry *et al.*, 2014). In humans and many other species, gonadectomy is recognized to result in reduced bone density, although this is poorly documented in dogs and cats, and there is some evidence to the contrary in dogs (Ekici *et al.*, 2005). Some of the described effects are understood to be modulated directly at a cellular level via androgen receptors, which exert control over the rate of cell apoptosis or the rate of gene expression. Other effects of these hormones are mediated via indirect feedback mechanisms such as influences on IGF-1 expression.

Leptin

Leptin is an adipose-derived hormone (although it can be produced by a wide range of tissues including the stomach, liver, bone marrow, mammary tissue and skeletal muscle) with its main action being to regulate weight and food intake by suppressing appetite. The mode of action of leptin on bone is somewhat unclear but probably involves both the sympathetic nervous system and expression of a gene known as cocaine- and amphetamine-regulated transcript (*CART*) which appears to decrease RANKL expression by osteoblasts. The net effects of increased leptin levels include loss of cancellous bone but increased mass of cortical bone.

These apparently conflicting actions of leptin are at odds with the conventional understanding of mechanisms of bone regulation, which has stimulated research into alternative signalling mechanisms. In recent years, the roles in bone signalling of a number of neurotransmitters unrelated to leptin have been investigated. A wide range of factors including adrenaline, serotonin, vasoactive intestinal peptide and neuropeptide Y have been implicated although the precise mechanism of action for many of these remains unknown.

Clinical relevance

From a clinical perspective, some of these endocrine pathways have a clear relevance. For example, congenital defects in one or more of these systems can have severe effects on bone growth, such as pituitary dwarfism or congenital hypothyroidism. Similarly, administration of exogenous glucocorticoids or excessive levels of endogenous glucocorticoids (e.g. animals with hyperadrenocorticism) might be expected to lead to abnormalities of bone density or biological activity.

In other circumstances, the clinical relevance of these pathways is less clear, with neutering status and obesity apparently having a less significant effect on bone remodelling in dogs and cats than in some other species, although the potential effects of these mechanisms should still be considered. However, it is generally thought that most of the environmental influences on bone growth such as dietary factors, individual genetic variation and concomitant disease processes are mediated via these endocrine signalling pathways.

Calcium regulatory pathways

The calcium regulatory pathways (Figure 3.6) are relatively well recognized and abnormalities frequently result in significant effects on bone. In the normal animal, decreased levels of serum ionized calcium trigger **parathyroid hormone** (PTH) production from the parathyroid glands. This has three major effects:

- Osteoclast activity is indirectly stimulated. PTH binds osteoblasts, activating the RANKL–OPG signalling system, which then promotes osteoclast activity in bone
- Calcium resorption from the renal distal tubules is stimulated, limiting urinary calcium losses

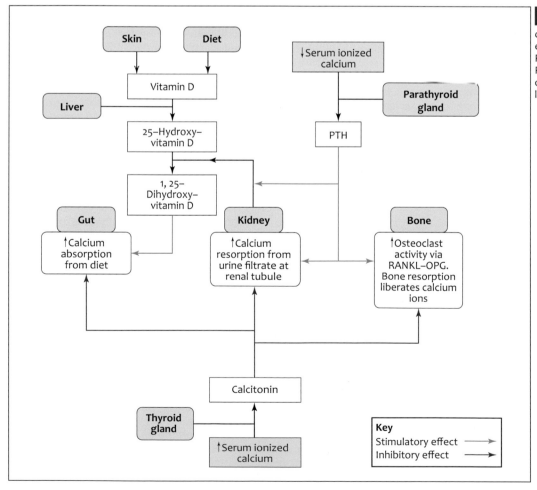

3.6 Flowchart illustrating the major mechanisms of calcium homeostasis and endocrine control pathways. PTH = parathyroid hormone; RANKL–OPC = receptor activator of nuclear factor kappa-B ligand–osteoprotegerin.

- PTH stimulates activation of vitamin D in the kidney. Activated vitamin D (1,25-dihydroxyvitamin D) then acts in the intestine to stimulate absorption of dietary calcium via calbindin. Vitamin D is also believed to have direct effects on stimulation of osteoclast activity, although the majority of its effects are mediated by elevating serum calcium levels.

Calcitonin is a hormone produced by thyroid C-cells in response to stimulation by increasing serum concentrations of ionized calcium and/or serum levels of gastrin. Calcitonin is involved in calcium homeostasis with its main effects being direct osteoclast suppression, including reduction in osteoclast numbers, interference with osteoclast adhesion to the extracellular matrix and decreased secretory cellular activity. The net effect is suppression of bone resorption. There is some evidence that the role of calcitonin is more complex, with wide ranging functions in bone density regulation, and it may also play an important role in the central endocrine cascades, possibly mediating some effects via leptin although this remains unproven. Calcitonin also suppresses intestinal absorption of calcium and inhibits resorption of calcium in the renal tubules allowing a wider role in calcium homeostasis.

Disruption of these calcium regulatory pathways is relatively common in small animal practice, with a range of pathologies such as primary hyperparathyroidism, renal disease or dietary abnormality potentially having substantial effects on bone biology (see Chapter 13). These pathways also represent some potential therapeutic pathways for addressing metabolic bone disease of various causes; this is an area of ongoing development in the human medical field.

References and further reading

Ekici H, Sontas BH, Toydemir SF *et al.* (2005) Effect of prepubertal ovariohysterectomy on bone mineral density and bone mineral content in puppies. *Acta Veterinaria Hungarica* **53**, 469–478

Evans HE (1993) The skeleton. In: *Miller's Anatomy of the Dog, 3rd edn*, pp. 122–218. WB Saunders, Pennsylvania

Gilbert SF (2013) Development of the tetrapod limb. In: *Developmental Biology, 10th edn*, pp. 489–516. Sinauer Associates Inc., Massachusetts

Liedert A, Kaspar D, Augat P *et al.* (2005) Mechanobiology of bone tissue and bone cells. In: *Mechanosensitivity in Cells and Tissues*, ed. A Kamkin and I Kiseleva, pp. 418–433. Academia, Moscow

Ornitz DM and Marie PJ (2002) FGF signaling pathways in endochondral and intramembranous bone development and human genetic disease. *Genes and Development* **16**, 1446–1465

Perry KL, Fordham A and Arthurs GI (2014) Effect of neutering and breed on femoral and tibial physeal closure times in male and female domestic cats. *Journal of Feline Medicine and Surgery* **16**, 149–156

Roberts WE, Roberts JA, Epker BN *et al.* (2006) Remodeling of mineralized tissues, Part I: The Frost legacy. *Seminars in Orthodontics* **12**, 216–237

Salmeri KR, Bloomberg MS, Scruggs SL *et al.* (1991) Gonadectomy in immature dogs: effects on skeletal, physical and behavioural developments. *Journal of the American Veterinary Medical Association* **198**, 1193–1203

Schneider RA, Miclau T and Helms JA (2002) Embryology of bone. In: *Orthopaedics*, ed. RH Fitzgerald, H Kaufer and AL Malkani, pp. 143–146. Mosby, Missouri

Shapiro F (2008) Bone development and its relation to fracture repair. The role of mesenchymal osteoblasts and surface osteoblasts. *European Cells and Materials* **15**, 53–76

Sims N and Baron R (2002) Bone: Structure, function, growth and remodeling. In: *Orthopaedics*, ed. RH Fitzgerald, H Kaufer and AL Malkani, pp. 147–159. Mosby, St. Louis, Missouri

Summerlee AJS (2002) Bone formation and development. In: *Bone in Clinical Orthopaedics, 2nd edn*, ed. G Sumner-Smith, pp. 1–22. AO Publishing, Thieme, Stuttgart

Sutter NB, Bustamante CB, Chase K *et al.* (2007) A single *IGF1* allele is a major determinant of small size in dogs. *Science* **316**, 112–115

Chapter 4

Biomechanical basis of bone fracture and fracture repair

Andy P. Moores

Fracture patterns vary hugely between patients: one dog's tibial fracture may be very different to another's. Even if the fracture pattern is similar, the options for fracture stabilization and how a fixation system is implemented are likely to differ between patients depending on factors such as the age, size and temperament of the dog or cat. With an almost endless variation of fracture configurations and other patient-related factors to consider, it can seem a daunting task to choose an appropriate fixation strategy for an individual patient. A good starting point is to consider the basic mechanical principles that can be applied to any fracture scenario. With a mechanically sound stabilization strategy the chances of a positive outcome for a fracture patient are greatly improved.

Mechanical concepts

In order to appreciate the mechanics of bone and fixation systems it is useful to understand some mechanical terminology. If a large enough force is applied to an object it will deform. The mechanical properties of an object can therefore be defined by a **load–deformation curve**. The response to loading will be dependent on an object's size and shape, as well as its material composition, and as such the curve represents that object's *structural* properties. Simple structures will tend to have a characteristic load–deformation curve with an initial linear response of deformation to load (Figure 4.1). The gradient of the line represents **stiffness**, which is defined as the force required per unit length of deformation and has SI units of newtons/metre (N/m).

$$\text{Stiffness} = \frac{\text{force}}{\text{unit length of deformation}}$$

Most structures will deform elastically when loaded, up to a point. Elastic deformation is reversible once the applied force is removed. For example, a small force can be applied to a Kirschner (K) wire and it will bend, but it will spring back into shape when the force is removed. However, a larger force will result in permanent, or plastic, deformation of the K-wire. On the load–deformation curve the linear section relates to elastic deformation. The point at which the line is no longer straight and the stiffness reduces is known as the **yield point**; this is the point at which plastic deformation occurs.

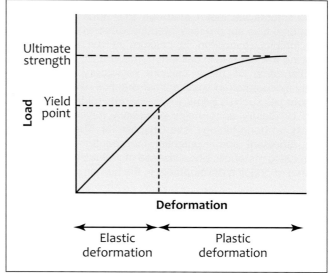

4.1 Load–deformation curve. The gradient of the line represents the stiffness of the structure.

When a force is applied to a material or object, that material or object is described as **stressed**. A long bone is therefore stressed by the forces of gravity (when the animal bears weight) and by the actions of muscles acting on the bone. The effect of the force will depend on the surface area over which the force is distributed: a large force applied over a small area will result in greater stress than a small force applied over a larger area. When an immature dog jumps from a height and lands with a fixed stifle, a large force is distributed across the quadriceps mechanism. The force is equal proximally and distally but the stress is much greater at the relatively small tibial tuberosity, which may fracture, than at the much larger origins of the quadriceps muscles, which are unlikely to be injured. Stress is defined as force per unit area; its SI unit is N/m^2 or pascals (Pa).

$$\text{Stress} = \frac{\text{force}}{\text{area}}$$

When we discuss stress we are usually referring to a force applied perpendicular to the area being measured. In some situations the force may have a component parallel to the plane of contact, which results in **shear stress**.

Metals are examples of **isotropic** materials; they have a very small and randomly oriented internal molecular structure such that their material properties do not vary with the direction of loading. Bone is an **anisotropic** material. Bone has an ordered internal structure with a hydroxyapatite mineral component that provides resistance to compressive forces, and collagen fibres that provide resistance to tension. As well as organization on a molecular level, on a cellular level bone is arranged into osteons, which run longitudinally in the diaphysis. These features mean that the material properties of cortical bone are dependent on the direction of loading; bone as a material is stronger in compression than in tension, and a bone as a structure is stronger when loaded along the long axis than when loaded transversely, especially when loaded in tension.

To describe the intrinsic material properties of an object irrespective of its size or shape it is necessary to eliminate geometric properties from the equation. Rather than using a load–deformation curve we use a **stress–strain curve**. Strain refers to change in length divided by original length (δL/L).

$$\text{Strain} = \frac{\text{change in length}}{\text{original length}}$$

Strain has no units and is reported as a proportion, so a 10 mm fracture gap that deforms by 1 mm represents 10% strain. The linear slope of the stress–strain curve represents Young's modulus of elasticity, which is thus a measure of a *material's* stiffness, rather than a *structure's* stiffness.

$$\text{Young's modulus of elasticity} = \frac{\text{stress}}{\text{strain}}$$

The SI units are pascals, but for many of the materials we might consider, such as bone and implant materials, Young's modulus is reported in gigapascals (GPa), where 1 GPa represents 1 billion or 1×10^9 Pa. Depending on how Young's modulus is calculated, and the type of bone being evaluated, the Young's modulus of bone is typically in the region of 15–20 GPa. Bone is therefore an order of magnitude less stiff than the materials orthopaedic implants are manufactured from; 316L stainless steel has a Young's modulus of around 200 GPa, pure titanium around 110 GPa.

When we are considering the mechanics of implants and bone–implant constructs we must account for geometric factors, i.e. the structural properties as well as the material properties. **Area moment of inertia (AMI)** is a measure of a beam's resistance to bending forces, based on its geometry rather than its material composition (Muir *et al.*, 1995). For our purposes as orthopaedic surgeons, the beam could be rectangular in cross-section and therefore represent the mid-section of a bone plate, or it could be cylindrical and represent a pin, a wire or the shaft of a screw. Since AMI ignores an object's material properties it can only be used to compare structures of the same material. AMI represents how material is distributed with respect to a neutral axis. Material further away from the neutral axis is more efficient at resisting bending forces.

For a rectangular structure:

$$\text{Area moment of inertia} = \frac{bh^3}{12}$$

where b = cross-sectional width and h = cross-sectional height (height is the dimension parallel with the direction of force).

For a cylindrical structure:

$$\text{Area moment of inertia} = \frac{\pi r^4}{4}$$

where r = radius.

We can infer from these equations that small changes in the height or radius will result in large changes in AMI; this can be relevant when choosing implants. Consider a femoral neck fracture for example: a lag screw or screws may be placed to stabilize the fracture. In a medium-sized dog options might include a 3.5 mm cortical screw or a 4 mm cancellous screw. The outer diameter of the 4 mm screw is larger but this would be the weaker option since it is the core diameter, rather than thread diameter, that influences bending strength. For the 4 mm screw the core diameter is 1.9 mm and the AMI is calculated to be 10.2 mm^4. The 3.5 mm screw has a core of 2.4 mm and the AMI is therefore 26.1 mm^4. Thus, the 3.5 mm screw will be more than 2.5 times stronger in bending than the 4 mm screw.

Polar moment of inertia (PMI) is another geometric calculation, which provides a cylindrical object's resistance to torsion if an angular force (or torque) is applied. This is relevant to bones and intramedullary nails exposed to twisting forces.

$$\text{Polar moment of inertia} = \frac{\pi r^4}{2}$$

Therefore, doubling the thickness of a pin or rod results in a 16-fold increase in torsional rigidity.

A force acting on an object will have internal effects; it will result in stress and deformation of the object. There may also be external effects, governed by Newton's laws of motion. For a force applied to the tibial tuberosity by the quadriceps muscle group, the internal effect is stress at the tibial tuberosity resulting in bone strain (but hopefully not fracture). The external effect is movement of the tibia (stifle extension). It is useful for the orthopaedic surgeon to have an understanding of bending moments in relation to the external effect of forces on limbs and fracture constructs. A **moment** is the action of a force that tends to rotate an object about an axis. The magnitude of the moment is the force multiplied by the perpendicular distance between the line of the force and the axis.

$$\text{Moment} = \text{force} \times \text{distance between line of force and axis of rotation}$$

The classic example is the balanced playground see-saw; a 20 kg child 1 m from the centre (fulcrum) of the see-saw will balance a 10 kg child 2 m from the fulcrum, since the moments are equal and opposite. Moments explain the benefit of lever arms, such as the calcaneus. Since the calcaneus places the Achilles tendon away from the central axis of the tibiotarsal joint, the hock extensors do not have to be as strong as they would have to be if they inserted closer to the joint.

Moments also explain several principles of fracture fixation. Consider a plate bridging a fracture gap with a bending force applied (Figure 4.2). The bending force will act to create a moment about the bone–plate junction of the proximal segment, where there is a pivot point. The bending moment is resisted by the opposite bending moment created by the pull-out resistance of the screws and the length of the bone plate. The longer the plate, the greater the bending force that can be resisted: hence the advice to use long plates that span the diaphysis.

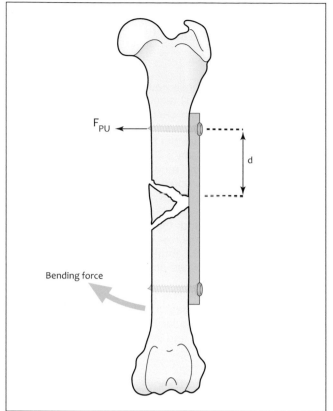

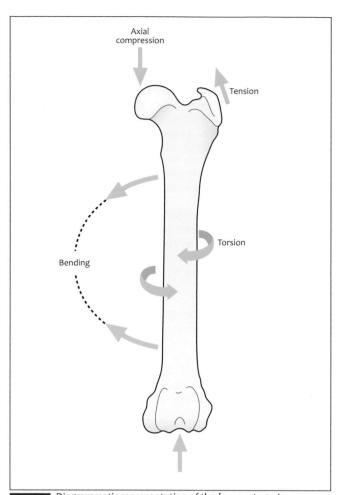

4.2 The effect of a longer plate in resisting a bending force. The medial force on the distal fracture fragment will create a bending moment acting about the distal edge of the proximal fracture fragment. This moment must be resisted by the opposite moment ($F_{PU}d$). The longer the distance between the fracture and first screw (d) is, the greater $F_{PU}d$ will be. F_{PU} = screw pull-out force.

4.3 Diagrammatic representation of the force categories considered when evaluating a fracture, a fixation method or a repaired fracture. Weight bearing and muscle contractions contribute to compressive forces down the long axis. When the bone is at an angle to the ground or when the muscles pull more on one side than on the other, bending will be induced. This may be in any direction. Torsion will occur when the mass of the body changes direction while the limb is bearing weight. Tensile forces exist where soft tissues such as tendons or ligaments attach to the bone.

Forces acting on bones

Bones of the appendicular skeleton are loaded in compression at the joint surfaces and by the tensile forces generated by muscles. The compressive forces are larger than the tensile forces and so the net loading pattern is compression. Bones are not, however, loaded purely in axial compression. The bones of the appendicular skeleton are typically slightly curved and the joint surfaces are often offset from the diaphysis (e.g. the femoral head being offset from the femoral diaphysis). They are also rarely positioned perpendicular to the ground. The diaphyses of long bones are therefore subject to a complex combination of forces, but this can be simplified somewhat for the purposes of fracture planning by considering the dominant bending force that is present. This typically results in the convex aspect of the bone being loaded in tension and the concave aspect in compression. Surgeons should be familiar with the tension and compression surfaces of each bone since the mechanics of bone–implant constructs will vary depending on the surface on which implants are placed. Movement adds additional forces to bones. When a paw is planted on the ground and an animal twists on its leg rotational force (torque) is generated. Long bones are therefore subjected to a combination of compressive, bending, rotational and tensile forces (Figure 4.3). Bones are well adapted to resist these forces. The hollow cylindrical structure of the diaphysis places the majority of the bone's structure away from its neutral axis, thus maximizing the area and polar moments of inertia, without incurring the cost of excessive weight that a solid structure would have.

Fracture of bone

If the energy delivered to bone is greater than the energy that it can absorb, fracture will occur. Bone is a relatively **tough** material, toughness being the ability to absorb substantial energy prior to failure, but toughness of bone varies with the direction of loading. With longitudinal loading, bone is not only tough but it is also considered **ductile**, since the failure (fracture) point of bone is significantly higher than the yield point. This means that there is plastic deformation of bone prior to fracture. Cortical bone is weaker in transverse loading and in this direction of loading it is weaker in tension than in compression. Bone is therefore weakest with tensile loading in the transverse plane, an important consideration when cementless hip prostheses are press-fit into the femoral diaphysis. With this loading pattern, the failure point is close to the yield point and thus bone is considered relatively **brittle** in transverse loading.

Cortical bone also demonstrates **viscoelastic** behaviour: its mechanical properties are dependent on the rate of loading, or **strain rate**. With longitudinal loading, as the strain rate increases, the modulus, yield strength and ultimate strength all increase. As the strain rate increases with normal activity (e.g. with the transition from walking to running) bone also becomes more ductile; although, since the yield point of bone is increased, bone continues to behave in an elastic manner at normal loads despite the increased strain rate. Very high strain rates, however, as may be expected with major trauma, have the opposite effect; cortical bone exhibits a ductile–brittle transition as the strain rate increases.

Cortical bone behaves predictably under certain loading situations (Figure 4.4). The structure of the mineral content of bone is such that pure compressive loads will cause bone to fail by shear, typically at around 45 degrees to the direction of loading. Overloading a long bone in axial compression will therefore result in an oblique fracture. Transverse fractures are created through either pure tension or bending. Bending results in compressive and tensile forces, and since bone is weaker in tension, the bone will fail on the tension side first. The line of tensile failure may propagate across the bone creating a simple transverse fracture or the compression side may fail by shear prior to the tension failure line propagating all the way across the bone, creating comminution on the compression side, often in the form of a single butterfly fragment. If a bending force is coupled with a compressive force the compression side is likely to fail earlier and with a larger butterfly fragment. An uneven bending force may result in an oblique rather than a transverse fracture. Spiral fractures result from torsional forces and have two fracture lines: an angled line which runs around the circumference of the bone and a longitudinal line that joins the two ends of the spiral.

As well as the direction of loading, the rate of loading will influence fracture patterns. Kinetic energy equals ½ x **mass x velocity**^{2}, thus high velocity injuries have much greater energy to dissipate to the bone. This energy is absorbed by the bone and then released when it fractures. The greater the amount of energy released the greater the structural damage caused, not only to the bone but also to the surrounding soft tissues. Thus 'high-energy' fractures result in greater comminution and the predictable fracture patterns described above are less likely to be seen. These fractures will also be associated with greater muscle damage and vascular compromise and are more likely to be open, all of which predispose to bone healing complications. It is essential to recognize the likelihood of severe soft tissue trauma when faced with a highly comminuted fracture and steps should be taken to avoid further soft tissue (and therefore vascular) compromise at surgery.

Mechanics of bone healing

Stability conferred by application of implants or external splints determines the amount of strain at a fracture site, and this in turn governs the nature of cortical bone healing. According to the strain theory of interfragmentary bone healing, a tissue cannot form within an environment that exceeds that tissue's tolerance to strain (Perren, 1979). For example, bone tissue is disrupted (fractured) at strains of more than 2%; therefore, bone cannot form directly in a fracture gap where there is 10% strain. The theory dictates that primary bone healing, as is expected in association with absolute stability provided by compression, can only occur in strain environments less than 2%. Since the compression of bone fragments results in negligible fracture gaps, if there were less than absolute rigidity very high local strains would develop that would impair healing. Secondary bone healing relies on the formation of granulation tissue at the fracture site with a high tolerance to strain (up to 100%). This is then replaced over time with

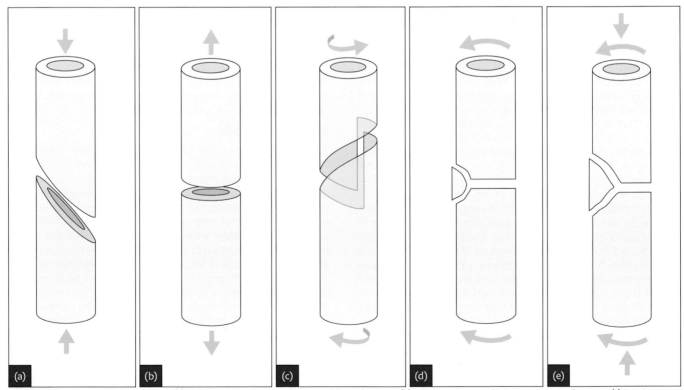

4.4	Fracture patterns of bone. (a) Axial compression results in an oblique fracture. (b) Pure tension results in a transverse fracture. (c) Torsion results in a spiral fracture. (d) Bending results in a transverse fracture with or without a butterfly fragment. (e) Bending in combination with compression will result in a transverse fracture with a larger butterfly fragment.

'soft callus' consisting of fibrous tissue and cartilage. This starts to calcify at the periphery of the callus, extending towards the middle. As bone healing progresses, the tissue in the fracture gap becomes progressively stiffer and the strain environment reduces, enhanced by the periosteal widening of the callus tissue, which increases its AMI. 'Hard callus' forms as the fracture tissues differentiate into woven bone but union can only occur once the strain environment is below 2%. Secondary bone healing occurs when *relative* stability is provided: this is rigid enough to allow for postoperative limb function, but functional loads will result in a small degree of deformation at the fracture site (typically strain of 2–10%). Numerous *in vivo* and *in vitro* studies have shown that the axial micromotion provided by relative stability enhances fracture healing in the early stages. However, in the later stages (from six weeks in ovine studies), continued deformation is detrimental to bone healing. If fracture healing is progressing, the natural increase in stiffness as the fracture heals by callus formation is expected to eliminate deformation, unless excessive external forces are present.

Mechanics of fixation systems

Since one of the primary goals of fracture management is to facilitate limb use during fracture healing, a stabilized fracture will be subjected to the same loads as an intact bone: namely axial compression, bending, rotation and (for avulsion fractures) tension. It is intuitive that any stabilization strategy has to be able to adequately resist these forces in order to provide the stability required to promote uncomplicated bone healing. Some fracture patterns will have a degree of inherent stability against one or more of these forces. A transverse fracture, once reduced, will be resistant to axial compression but will still be vulnerable to bending and rotational forces. An ulnar fracture with an intact radius will have a degree of resistance to axial compression, bending and rotation but, if proximal, will be subject to tensile forces from the triceps muscle. Many diaphyseal fractures, however, are vulnerable to axial compressive, bending and rotational forces, and only three types of fracture fixation are able to resist all of these forces reliably: plating systems, external skeletal fixation (ESF) and interlocking nails.

Whichever fixation system is employed, the surgeon must consider if the system alone will be required to withstand all the forces of weight bearing or if there will be a degree of load sharing between the fixation system and the bone; the resistance of the entire bone–implant construct to the disruptive forces must be considered. Due to load sharing, a reduced transverse fracture will not require as strong fixation as a comminuted fracture that is not reduced. A simple two-piece fracture should always be reduced (to restore alignment of the bone) but for a comminuted fracture the surgeon's priority is to ensure that the main fracture fragments (and thus the joints either end of the bone) are correctly aligned with respect to each other; whether the intermediate fragments are anatomically reduced or not is immaterial as long as the fracture heals. From a mechanical perspective it would be advantageous to reconstruct the entire bone, since this would allow load sharing and would reduce the stresses on the fixation system. However, anatomical reconstruction comes with a biological cost. The additional manipulation of bone fragments and tissues required to reconstruct the fracture anatomically will impair the fracture's vascular supply, since in the early period after trauma the dominant vascular supply to the fracture fragments is the induced extraosseous vascular supply derived from their soft tissue attachments. Additional surgical time and implants will also be required. All these factors increase the risk of infection and bone healing problems. Furthermore, considerable expertise is required to accurately and rigidly stabilize a comminuted fracture. For most comminuted fractures, preservation of the fracture's soft tissue environment will take priority over anatomical reconstruction, since any mechanical advantage gained by reconstruction is outweighed by the biological cost. As there is no load sharing, the fixation system will be exposed to much greater stresses and this will potentially reduce the system's resistance to fatigue failure. The surgeon must therefore employ strategies that allow maximal preservation of the soft tissue environment to encourage early bone healing, and yet at the same time provide fixation that is strong and durable enough to withstand all the forces of weight bearing. In these situations the fixation system will generally provide relative stability rather than absolute stability. Relative stability may be provided by ESF or bridge plating. Absolute stability is usually provided by compressing bone surfaces together; for example, by compression plating or lag screwing.

Intramedullary devices

Intramedullary pins

Since intramedullary pins lie along the central axis of the bone they are well placed to resist bending forces regardless of the plane of bending. Their resistance to bending is a feature of their AMI and their material (typically 316L stainless steel); small increases in diameter will result in large increases in AMI, and a pin that fills most of the medullary cavity at the bone's isthmus will have a very large AMI. The use of an intramedullary pin alone, however, provides no resistance to axial compression or rotation and is therefore not recommended for clinical use. It is often stated that an intramedullary pin can be applied to a transverse fracture with uneven fracture surfaces that interdigitate. Although the transverse nature of this fracture pattern would provide resistance to axial compression, interdigitation should not be relied upon to resist rotational forces.

Interlocking nails

The deficiencies of the intramedullary pin are addressed with the interlocking nail, which is an intramedullary device that is locked to the proximal and distal segments with one or more screws or bolts placed through holes in the nail. Locking the device to the main fracture fragments imparts resistance to axial compression and rotation, although care has to be taken when selecting a nail that the screw holes themselves do not become weak points in the system. If a screw hole is located at the fracture site the nail's AMI will be significantly reduced; the AMI of an 8 mm nail will be more than 2.5 times less at a 3.5 mm screw hole, for a bending force in the plane of the screw hole. Furthermore, the nail's resistance to axial compression and rotation will be entirely dependent on the strength of the nail–screw interface. Early nail designs relied on cortical screws, which have a relatively small AMI. Screw failure was occasionally seen with these systems. More recent designs have addressed this weakness by using solid bolts. These have a large unthreaded shaft and thus have a much larger AMI than a similarly sized cortical screw.

External skeletal fixation

Linear external skeletal fixation

ESF is a very versatile technique that can be used to create constructs of variable rigidity. A common feature of all ESF constructs is that transcutaneous fixation pins placed in the proximal and distal fracture fragments are rigidly linked via a connecting bar external to the skin. All ESF constructs therefore impart resistance to axial compression, bending and rotation, but to what extent will depend on the frame configuration and the ESF system used. All pins must engage both cortices of the bone. Half pins exit the skin on one side and are connected to a single connecting bar. Full pins exit the skin on both sides of the bone and are connected to two connecting bars.

There are numerous different ESF systems available, each with different biomechanical properties; these are specifically discussed in Chapter 10. The mechanical principles of ESF use are important to understand and are relevant to all systems.

ESF pins: For an ESF construct to provide stability, the frame itself must be sufficiently strong but there must also be a stable and secure interface between the fixation pins and the bone. When a bone–ESF construct is loaded (during weight bearing), a great deal of stress is applied at the pin–bone interface (PBI). Repeated stresses can result in micromotion at the PBI, bone resorption around the pin and subsequent pin loosening. The PBI is thus a potential weak point in any ESF construct. One of the goals of creating an ESF construct is to reduce the PBI stresses such that pin loosening does not occur. Using threaded pins is one way to enhance the PBI (Figure 4.5).

4.5 Types of pins for external fixators. **A:** Smooth pins rely on friction with the bone or bracing against other pins in the frame. **B:** Negative-profile threaded pins engage the bone more securely but are susceptible to failure at the shaft–thread junction. **C:** Ellis pins have a small length of negative-profile thread, designed to engage only one cortex. The weak point of the pin is protected from bending forces. **D:** Positive-profile threaded pins have a larger major diameter, so holding strength is increased. Because the shaft diameter is not reduced at the start of the thread, they are better able to resist the cyclic bending forces associated with weight bearing.

The increased pin–bone surface area that the threaded pin provides conveys two benefits over smooth pins: stresses at the PBI are dissipated over a larger area and the pull-out strength of the pin is greatly enhanced. The easiest (and cheapest) way to create a threaded pin is to take a solid pin and cut a thread into one end; this is called a negative-profile threaded pin. The AMI of the threaded section will be considerably less than the AMI of the solid shaft, since the core of the threaded section is smaller than the shaft. The abrupt transition from the strong shaft to the weaker thread creates a weak point in the pin known as a **stress riser**; bending forces applied to the pin will result in stresses being concentrated at this point, making it susceptible to failure. Using negative-profile threaded pins in an ESF construct can therefore enhance the PBI but at the expense of introducing a weakness into the frame itself. One strategy to avoid pin failure is to place the stress riser within the medullary cavity of the bone where it is protected from bending forces by the cortex between it and the ESF clamp. This is a compromise that requires a very short end-thread and means that only one of the cortices engaged by the pin has the benefit of a threaded PBI. Such pins are known as Ellis pins. A better solution is to use a positive-profile threaded pin in which the thread is built up on to the shaft of the pin rather than being cut into it. The core of the thread section is therefore the same size as the shaft section and there is a negligible change in AMI at the thread-shaft section and so no stress riser. Positive-profile threaded pins also have much greater pull-out resistance than negative-profile threaded pins with the same shaft diameter. An alternative strategy is to use a negative-profile pin with a **tapered run-out**, where the transition from the threaded to non-threaded portions of the pin occurs gradually, avoiding the formation of a stress riser (see Chapter 10).

Increasing the number of fixation pins in a fracture segment is another way to reduce the stresses at an individual PBI and to increase the strength of an ESF construct. A minimum of two pins per main bone segment is necessary to provide two-point fixation and avoid the potential for rotation about the axis of the pin. However, increasing the number of pins to three or four per main segment is considered ideal. There is no significant mechanical advantage to having more than four pins per segment. Spreading pins evenly along the length of the fracture fragment will also improve construct rigidity.

Axial compression will result in a bending force on half pins if there is a fracture gap present. The pins will act as cantilever beams and will be subjected to a bending moment about the clamp: the larger the working length of the pin, the larger the moment. Using the shortest pin length possible will therefore enhance the mechanics of the ESF construct, although clinically this will be limited by the soft tissues surrounding the bone and by the anticipated postoperative swelling: it is important to avoid the morbidity associated with clamps that rub on the skin. Some ESF clamps grip the fixation pin eccentrically relative to the connecting bar. These clamps should be arranged such that the grip-point is on the bone side of the connecting bar, thus reducing the working length of the pin.

Increasing the diameter of fixation pins will of course increase their AMI and the strength of the construct as a whole. The size of the pin must, however, be balanced against the size of the bone. Generally, pin diameter is limited to approximately 30% of the diameter of the bone in the plane that the pin is placed, to avoid excessively weakening the bone with large drill holes. For an elliptical bone, such as the radius, larger pins can be placed with less risk in the craniomedial–caudolateral or craniolateral–caudomedial planes, rather than in the medial–lateral plane.

There are no limitations to the size of connecting bars that can be used; this is an area where modern ESF systems differ from older systems. The connecting bar is susceptible to bending forces when used as part of a unilateral ESF construct. A larger connecting bar with a greatly increased bending resistance will therefore make a big difference to the overall strength of unilateral constructs; such constructs can now be used to safely stabilize fractures that historically would have required more complex bilateral frames. Clearly a large stainless steel connecting bar could be excessively heavy for some patients, so many systems employ materials such as carbon fibre and titanium to provide strong, stiff and yet light connecting bars.

ESF frames: ESF frame design plays a large part in the mechanics of an ESF construct (Figure 4.6). In general terms, as the complexity of the frame increases, so does its stiffness (White *et al.*, 2003). The simplest frame, known as

a type 1a frame (unilateral, uniplanar frame), consists of half pins and a single connecting bar. A type 1b frame (unilateral, biplanar frame) comprises two unilateral frames placed an angle to each other. A type 1b frame provides a moderate increase in axial compressive, torsional and mediolateral stiffness compared to a type 1a frame but, since it has an additional connecting bar and pins in the craniocaudal plane, it has a large increase in craniocaudal stiffness. The stiffness of a type 1b frame can be further enhanced by adding one or more diagonal connecting bars between the two unilateral frames (Lauer *et al.*, 1999). By incorporating full pins into an ESF construct, clamped to connecting bars on either side of the bone, bending forces are significantly reduced in the plane of the fixator. Such a frame (a bilateral, uniplanar frame) is known as a type 2 frame (or type 2a frame) if all the pins are full pins, or a modified type 2 frame (or type 2b frame) if there is only one full pin in each of the main fragments and the remaining pins are half pins. The more full pins that are used, the greater the compressive, torsional and bending stiffness of the construct. However, these frames are limited to fixation

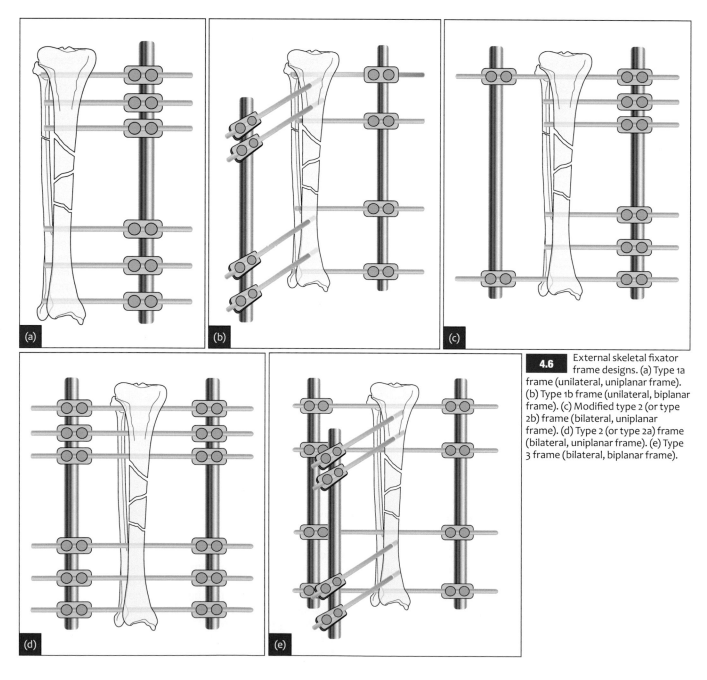

4.6 External skeletal fixator frame designs. (a) Type 1a frame (unilateral, uniplanar frame). (b) Type 1b frame (unilateral, biplanar frame). (c) Modified type 2 (or type 2b) frame (bilateral, uniplanar frame). (d) Type 2 (or type 2a) frame (bilateral, uniplanar frame). (e) Type 3 frame (bilateral, biplanar frame).

pins and connecting bars in the mediolateral plane; a type 1b frame is more resistant to craniocaudal bending than a modified type 2 frame, and is approximately equivalent to a full type 2 frame. Craniocaudal bending stiffness of a type 2 frame is enhanced by adding a cranial unilateral component, creating a type 3 frame (or bilateral, biplanar frame). A type 3 frame is approximately equivalent to a full type 2 frame in axial compression and torsion but is usually weaker in mediolateral bending since there are often fewer pins in the mediolateral plane than with a type 2 frame. Full type 2 or type 3 frames are rarely used; their rigidity may prevent beneficial axial micromotion at the fracture site and contribute to delayed bone healing.

ESF of upper limb fractures

The upper limb provides a mechanically unsound environment for ESF. Large muscle masses dictate that long pins have to be employed and, since fixation pins must avoid these muscles, pins must be clustered at the ends of the bone rather than being spread along the length of the bone. Furthermore, the proximity of the trunk limits the use of bilateral pins. A unilateral ESF construct with relatively long pins that are clustered proximally and distally will be exposed to large bending forces. The bending forces can be significantly reduced by incorporating an intramedullary pin into the repair. Adding a pin alone will result in a stronger and stiffer construct, and by leaving the pin long proximally and connecting it into the ESF construct ('tied-in'), strength is increased even further (Aron et al., 1991). Although bilateral pins cannot be used proximally, they can be used distally across the humeral and femoral condyles. This allows curved connecting bars to be incorporated into the ESF construct, passing cranially from proximolateral to distomedial, enhancing resistance to axial compressive loading.

Circular external skeletal fixation

Circular external skeletal fixation (CESF) uses small wires rather than large pins to transfix bone fragments. Each end of the wire is anchored to clamps attached to a ring that circles the limb. The wires can be tensioned to improve their mechanical characteristics; the greater the tension the stiffer the construct. The rings are connected by large threaded rods. As the frame is arranged around the circumference of the limb, bending forces are distributed evenly regardless of the plane of bending, and torsional forces are well resisted. The rods and rings create a very rigid structure but the use of wires rather than large pins allows for a degree of micromovement in the axial plane (perpendicular to the rings) that may be beneficial for bone healing. Unlike with a unilateral ESF construct, in a fracture gap model the wires self-tension with loading and impart non-linear stiffness properties to a CESF–bone construct. At low loads axial micromotion is present, but as loads increase there is an increase in stiffness and reduced micromotion. Numerous features of the frame will affect the mechanics of the construct with increasing number of rings, use of smaller diameter rings, increasing number and diameter of wires, greater wire tension and use of additional half pins on posts all tending to increase the stiffness of the bone–CESF construct (Lewis et al., 1998).

Plate and screw fixation

There are two general types of bone plate: locking and non-locking.

Non-locking plates

Non-locking plates such as the dynamic compression plate (DCP) or limited contact dynamic compression plate (LC-DCP) are anchored to bone with screws that pass through screw holes in the plate but which do not rigidly interface with the screw hole. The rigidity of these systems results from the compression that the screw head imparts on the plate when the screw is tightened, which compresses the plate on to the surface of the bone and creates a large frictional force between the plate and the bone. The system is therefore dependent on the screw being able to provide an axial compressive force when it is tightened. This force is a function of the interaction between the screw threads and the bone; the force that the screw head imparts on the plate must be countered by the resistance of the bone to screw pull-out. Screw pull-out strength is a function of the screw thread's profile and pitch (see Chapter 10), the length of the screw in bone, and of bone density. Pull-out strength is much greater in adult cortical bone than it is in cancellous bone or in the bone of very young patients. Screw thread profiles may be optimized to improve function in different types of bone. A 4 mm cancellous screw has a deeper thread profile than the 3.5 mm cortical screw (Figure 4.7). Increased screw pull-out resistance comes at the cost of a reduced AMI, and therefore weaker bending strength, due to the smaller size of the core of the 4 mm screw. It is therefore advisable to avoid the use of the 4 mm screw when it is likely to be subjected to bending forces, and cortical screws are often preferred even in cancellous bone. Since the stability of the plate–bone construct is dependent on the frictional force between the plate and the bone, the plate must be accurately contoured to the bone's surface. As well as reduced frictional force, poor contouring may also cause bone fragments to shift in position as screws are tightened; this is known as primary loss of reduction.

A larger cortical screw will of course have greater pull-out resistance than a smaller cortical screw. The size of the bone will govern the largest size of screw that can be safely employed; it is recommended that screw size does not exceed 25% of the bone diameter to avoid excessively weakening the bone. Since most plates are designed to be used with a single screw size, measuring the bone diameter from radiographs and calculating the maximum safe screw size will dictate plate size. The number of screws employed in the plate will clearly impact on the strength of the system; having at least three bicortical

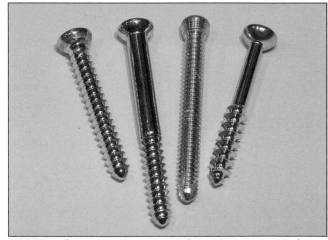

4.7 Different screw types. From left to right: 3.5 mm cortical screw; 3.5 mm shaft screw; 3.5 mm locking screw; 4 mm partially threaded cancellous screw.

screws in each main fragment is optimal. The length of the plate is also important; the longer the plate the greater the bending force that will be required to cause screw pull-out. Therefore, from a mechanical perspective it is preferable to use a plate that is long enough to span the length of the bone. Studies of screw position have demonstrated that bending strength is greatest when screws are widely spaced in a fracture segment rather than clustered at one end, and in a fracture gap model, placing some screws as close to the gap as possible minimizes plate strain over the fracture gap (Tornkvist *et al.*, 1996; Ellis *et al.*, 2001). Torsional strength is independent of screw position and relates solely to the number of screws employed in a fracture segment (Tornkvist *et al.*, 1996).

Plates can be used as compression plates, neutralization plates and bridging plates (Figure 4.8).

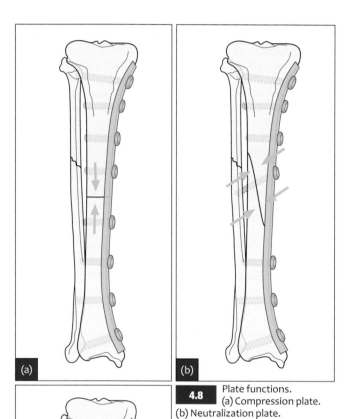

4.8 Plate functions.
(a) Compression plate.
(b) Neutralization plate.
(c) Bridging plate.

Compression plates: Compression plates are used on transverse and short oblique fractures. Since the reconstructed bone column will be able to resist compression but not tension, the plate should be positioned on the tension aspect of the bone. As long as the compression cortex is reduced, this allows the bone to load share with the plate and reduces bending stress on the plate. The plate should be over-contoured slightly, or 'pre-stressed', to ensure compression of the far (trans) cortex. If there is a defect at the compression cortex, the AMI of the plate–bone construct will be reduced and there will be much greater stress on the plate (Figure 4.9).

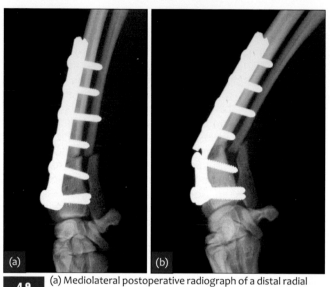

4.9 (a) Mediolateral postoperative radiograph of a distal radial fracture in a Maltese stabilized with a cranial T-plate. (b) The caudal cortex was not compressed, increasing the stress on the plate, which resulted in fatigue failure of the plate in the postoperative period.

Neutralization plates: Lag screws are used to compress oblique fracture surfaces. It is important to realize that any screw can be used as a lag screw; a lag screw is a way of employing a screw rather than a physical description of the screw itself. The near cortex is over-drilled to the outer diameter of the screw. This is called the glide hole and the screw's threads should move freely within it without engaging. The far cortex is drilled and tapped as normal. When the screw is tightened the head of the screw will compress the two cortices together. Some screws are optimized to be used as lag screws. The partially threaded 4 mm cancellous screw and the shaft screw (see Figure 4.7) both have non-threaded sections. Since these screws have no threads to interfere with the sides of the glide hole, they offer enhanced compression compared to a fully threaded screw used as a lag screw. Lag screws provide excellent compression of fracture fragments, which allows load sharing between the fixation and the bone, but they will typically be exposed to large bending and torsional forces. By using a plate alongside the lag screws these forces are neutralized; the plate in this situation is thus described as a neutralization plate.

Bridging plates: A plate that is used to span a non-reconstructed comminuted fracture is known as a bridging plate. Since there is no load sharing between the bone and the plate, a bridging plate is exposed to greater stresses than a compression or neutralization plate and a surgeon must consider this when selecting implants. Greater plate stress could lead to fatigue failure of the plate prior to fracture union.

The AMI of a DCP is greatest between screw holes and reduces considerably at each screw hole. Failure of plates typically occurs at a screw hole since this is where stresses are concentrated (see Chapter 29). The LC-DCP was designed so that its AMI would be similar along its length. This is achieved by having scalloped undercuts between screw holes. The LC-DCP is therefore weaker and less stiff than a comparable DCP (although the difference is less as plate size increases), but should distribute stresses more evenly along its length, potentially improving fatigue life of the implant (Little *et al.*, 2001). Although stresses are more evenly distributed, the reduced strength of the LC-DCP compared to a DCP would be a concern when using it on its own as a bridging plate. A lengthening plate has a solid midsection with no screw holes: there is thus a uniform stress distribution and the middle section of the plate is very strong. However, since fracture gaps vary in size, a lengthening plate of the correct size may not always be available. In some situations using a larger plate may be an option. The 3.5 mm DCP comes in standard and broad forms. The broad plate is thicker and wider and thus has an enhanced AMI compared to the narrow plate.

Another very effective strategy to reduce bridging plate stress is to augment the plate with an intramedullary pin: the so-called 'plate–rod' or 'pin–plate' technique. The pin protects the plate from bending stresses and will significantly reduce plate strain. The larger the pin, the larger the reduction in plate strain. Reducing plate strain increases the fatigue life of the implant (Hulse *et al.*, 1997). Using a pin that is too large may result in an excessively stiff construct that impairs fracture healing. Many factors other than pin size will affect fracture gap strain, including the size of plate, the size of the fracture gap and the size and activity of the patient postoperatively. In general, a pin size of 35–40% of the femoral canal size is advised to provide a balance between reducing plate strain and yet not being excessively stiff (Hulse *et al.*, 2000).

An important factor in avoiding fatigue failure of bridging plates is the time to fracture healing, and preserving the soft tissue envelope at the fracture site will encourage early bone healing. This can be achieved by minimally invasive plate osteosynthesis (MIPO) techniques (see Chapter 15). MIPO also favours the use of long bone plates to distribute screws better, since their use does not involve any additional soft tissue trauma. If an open approach is used manipulation of the intermediate fracture fragments should be avoided ('open but do not touch' approach).

Locking plates

Unlike a conventional plate, the screws of a locking plate rigidly interface with the plate's screw holes. This is typically by threads on the screw head and in the screw hole, or by a conical morse taper. The screw–plate interface can be considered equivalent to an ESF clamp, and the locking plate–screw construct mechanically behaves like an ESF construct rather than a conventional plate. Therefore, they are often referred to as internal fixators. Since the locking plate construct is not dependent on the screw creating an axially compressive force to compress the plate on to the bone surface, screw pull-out is much less of a concern. Failure of locking screws requires failure of a large section of bone around the screw, rather than screw pull-out. Locking plates are therefore ideally suited for use in weak bone such as osteoporotic bone. For the same reasons, locking plate screws do not need as deep a thread profile, which means that a locking screw can have a much greater core diameter, and thus AMI, than an equivalent-sized cortical screw. This is important because the screws of locking plate constructs subjected to axial loads will be subjected to greater bending loads than screws in a conventional plating system, due to the fixed-angle nature of the locking construct. This is a potential concern for locking systems such as the string-of-pearls (SOP) plate, which are designed around standard cortical screws with a relatively small AMI. Since locking plates act as fixed-angle constructs, they do not need to be contoured precisely to the bone's surface because tightening screws will not cause fragments to shift in position. However, locking plates should still be contoured to approximate the bone's surface; just as longer pins will reduce ESF rigidity, so will longer screws in a locking plate construct. Some systems, such as the locking compression plate (LCP), allow non-locking and locking screws to be used. If the surgeon chooses to use different types of screw in the same fracture fragment then the plate should be accurately contoured and the non-locking screws should be applied first to anchor the plate to the bone's surface. Only then should locking screws be inserted.

Kirschner wires

Kirschner wires are small diameter pins ranging from 0.6–2 mm in diameter. They may be used to stabilize small bone fragments and as part of a tension-band wire. They are often used to stabilize non-articular (Salter–Harris types I and II) physeal fractures. The bone is relatively wide at the physis and this increases the AMI of the K-wire–bone construct. Non-articular physeal fractures are also typically resistant to axial compression and there may be some degree of resistance to rotational forces from the topography of the physis, such as in the distal femur where the physis consists of peaks and valleys that interdigitate. Forces acting at the neighbouring joint will also have a short lever arm, and thus reduced bending moment, compared to a diaphyseal fracture. All of these features, along with the rapid healing which is expected with a physeal fracture, often allow K-wires to be used as the sole fixation despite their relative weakness. At least two K-wires should be used to provide rotational stability of the repair. K-wires are most commonly employed as 'crossed K-wires' (at an angle to one another and crossing). Where the joint surface is in line with the diaphysis (e.g. distal femur), this allows the wires to be introduced alongside the joint without interfering with the articular surface. The K-wires cross the fracture and engage the opposite cortex for added stability. Stability is enhanced by ensuring that the wires are as widely separated as possible at the level of the fracture; the wires should therefore 'cross' on the metaphyseal side of the physis. Fractures of the femoral capital physis are managed slightly differently: here, K-wires can be placed from distal to proximal. By orienting two or three K-wires parallel to one another, resistance to rotational and bending forces is ensured and axial compression during weight-bearing is converted into fracture site compression, which enhances the stability of the repair.

Orthopaedic wire
Cerclage wires

A cerclage wire is an orthopaedic wire that is passed around the circumference of the diaphysis and tightened. Cerclage wires may be placed to compress long oblique fractures or to prevent fissures from propagating. A correctly implemented cerclage wire can create good compression between long oblique fracture fragments but alone is not sufficient to withstand weight-bearing forces. Cerclage wires are therefore often used in conjunction with intramedullary pins. Cerclage wires are only effective at providing stability if they are placed very tightly, and remain tight, around a column of bone that is perfectly reduced. At least two wires should always be placed, at least 10 mm apart and at least 10 mm from the fracture ends. This is to avoid a single cerclage wire acting as a fulcrum for bending forces, and dictates that the pin–cerclage technique should only be used for long oblique fractures.

Achieving and maintaining a tight cerclage wire is critical and is dependent both on the tightening method and avoiding movement of the wire. The most commonly used tightening method, but also the weakest, is the twist method. A proper twist is achieved by twisting and tensioning the wire ends simultaneously, with equal tension applied to each end, so that the ends wrap around each other. This method can create moderate tension in the cerclage loop but this tension is reduced if the twist is wiggled during cutting and it is almost completely eliminated if the twist is folded over after it is cut, unless it is folded over whilst continuing to twist the wire. More secure fixation is achieved with a loop cerclage and even better fixation is achieved with a double loop cerclage (Figure 4.10) (Roe, 2002). These methods require a wire tightener with one (for single loop only) or two (for single or double loop) tightening cranks.

Regardless of the method of securing the cerclage wire, it will lose its tension, and therefore become ineffective, if the column of bone it is secured around becomes smaller. This may happen if the fracture fragments shift and collapse or if the wire moves along the diaphysis to an area with a slightly smaller circumference. Cerclage wires should, therefore, never be used on tapering areas of the bone such as at the metaphyses. All cerclage wires will become loose if the column they are supporting reduces in diameter by more than 1% (Roe, 1997). Although an enticing technique for inexperienced surgeons to use, the limitations of pin–cerclage wire fixation mean it is a common cause of fracture complications and more reliable techniques such as plate fixation, ESF or interlocking nails should be employed where possible.

Tension-band wires

A tension-band wire is used to stabilize avulsion fractures or osteotomies created during an approach to a joint, where the bone fragment is subjected to a tensile force from the tendons or ligaments that attach to it. The fragment can be reduced with one or two K-wires but these will be exposed to a large bending force if used alone. By adding a figure-of-eight tension-band wire the bending force on the K-wires is resisted. The resulting force vector creates compression at the fracture/osteotomy site (Figure 4.11). In order to allow compression if two K-wires are used they should ideally be parallel to each other and perpendicular to the fracture or osteotomy line, although the K-wire orientation is also governed by regional anatomical constraints.

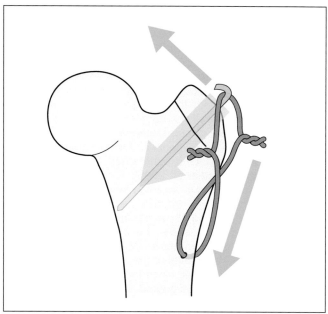

4.11 Tension-band wire. The pull of the gluteal muscles is resisted by the tension-band wire. The two forces combined result in a compressive force at the fracture (large pale arrow).

4.10 Cerclage wire tightening methods.
A: Twist method.
B: Single loop method.
C: Double loop method.

A

B

C

References and further reading

Aron DN, Foutz TL, Keller WG and Brown J (1991) Experimental and clinical experience with an IM pin external skeletal fixator tie-in configuration. *Veterinary and Comparative Orthopaedics and Traumatology* **4**, 86–94

Ellis T, Bourgeault CA and Kyle RF (2001) Screw position affects dynamic compression plate strain in an *in vitro* fracture model. *Journal Of Orthopaedic Trauma* **15**, 333–337

Hulse D, Ferry K, Fawcett A *et al.* (2000) Effect of intramedullary pin size on reducing bone plate strain. *Veterinary and Comparative Orthopaedics and Traumatology* **13**,185–190

Hulse D, Hyman W, Nori M and Slater M (1997) Reduction in plate strain by addition of an intramedullary pin. *Veterinary Surgery* **26**, 451–459

Lauer SK, Aron DN and Evans MD (1999) Finite element method evaluation: articulations and diagonals in an 8-pin type 1B external skeletal fixator. *Veterinary Surgery* **29**, 28–37

Lewis DD, Bronson DG, Samchukov ML, Welch RD and Stallings JT (1998) Biomechanics of circular external skeletal fixation. *Veterinary Surgery* **27**, 454–464

Little FM, Hill CM, Kageyama T, Conzemius MG and Smith GK (2001) Bending properties of stainless steel dynamic compression plates and limited contact dynamic compression plates. *Veterinary and Comparative Orthopaedics and Traumatology* **14**, 64–68

Muir P, Johnson KA and Markel MD (1995) Area moment of inertia for comparison of implant cross-sectional geometry and bending stiffness. *Veterinary and Comparative Orthopaedics and Traumatology* **8**, 146–52

O'Keefe R, Jacobs JJ, Chu CR and Einhorn TA (2013) *Orthopaedic Basic Science: Foundations of Clinical Practice, 4th edn.* American Academy of Orthopaedic Surgeons, Rosemont, Illinois

Perren SM (1979) Physical and biological aspects of fracture healing with special reference to internal fixation. *Clinical Orthopaedics and Related Research* **138**, 175–196

Roe SC (2002) Evaluation of tension obtained by use of three knots for tying cerclage wires by surgeons of various abilities and experience. *Journal of the American Veterinary Medical Association* **220**, 334–336

Roe SC (1997) Mechanical characteristics and comparisons of cerclage wires: introduction of the double-wrap and loop/twist tying methods. *Veterinary Surgery* **26**, 310–316

Tornkvist H, Hearn TC and Schatzker J (1996) The strength of plate fixation in relation to the number and spacing of bone screws. *Journal of Orthopaedic Trauma* **10**, 204–208

White DT, Bronson DG and Welch RD (2003) A mechanical comparison of veterinary linear external fixation systems. *Veterinary Surgery* **32**, 507–514

Chapter 5

Fracture healing

John Houlton

Bone healing is unusual because the repair tissue is similar to the original tissue: bone rather than scar tissue is formed. *Regeneration* may be a better term than repair. Accordingly, any tissue other than bone within a fracture gap represents incomplete healing (Schiller, 1988). Most fractures will heal without intervention, but it is important to look beyond bone healing and the restoration of normal bony anatomy when assessing the outcome of fracture treatment. The bone may heal well but the limb, or the whole patient, remains functionally poor due to subsequent deformity (malunion), soft tissue contracture and adhesions, or the development of secondary osteoarthritis.

Bone is strongest in compression and fractures as a result of pure compression are rare. They generally occur in cancellous bone with thin cortices, such as the metaphyses or vertebral bodies. In contrast, fractures seen in tubular bones are generally transverse, oblique or spiral. Spiral fractures result from primarily torsional forces, whereas transverse and oblique fractures are due to bending forces (see Chapter 4).

Comminuted fractures are generally the result of a mixture of forces, with the degree of comminution depending upon the energy absorbed into the bone up to the point of mechanical overload. The magnitude of energy released influences not only the degree of fragmentation but also the associated soft tissue damage and thus, indirectly, the vascularity of the bone.

If adequate vascularity is present, the pattern of fracture healing is dictated by the stability of the fracture. Stable fractures heal either by **contact healing** or **gap healing**. In contact healing bone union and remodelling occur simultaneously, whilst in gap healing they occur sequentially. Both are characterized by the lack of callus, a phenomenon termed primary bone union or **direct healing**. In contrast, unstable fractures heal with the formation of callus prior to the production of bone, so-called **indirect healing**.

Strain theory and bone healing

Strain is defined as the change in length of a fracture gap divided by its original length (see Chapter 4). In indirect healing, the sequence of development of the different tissue types in the fracture gap is dictated by the degree of interfragmentary strain. In conditions of high strain only flexible tissue such as granulation tissue can exist. In contrast, bone can only exist in conditions of less than 2% strain. Intermediate tissue such as fibrocartilage may exist in approximately 10–15% strain conditions.

Small fracture gaps experience conditions of high strain whilst large gaps, for the same amount of instability, have lower strain (Figure 5.1). Thus, imperfectly reduced fractures with small gaps may actually take longer to heal than comminuted fractures, where strain conditions are lower because the fracture gaps are larger.

The aim of fracture treatment should be to reduce not only fracture gaps, but also interfragmentary strain.

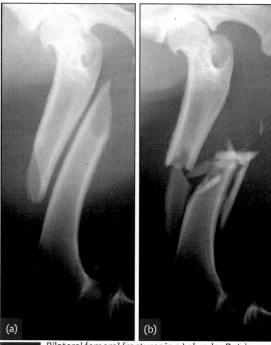

5.1 Bilateral femoral fractures in a Labrador Retriever. (a) Left leg. (b) Right leg. When the major fracture fragments have been realigned, the oblique fracture has higher strain conditions than the comminuted fracture due to the shorter length of its fracture gap.

Direct bone healing

Direct (or primary) bone union occurs under the stable conditions provided by interfragmentary compression. Such conditions are created by lag screw fixation, with or without the addition of a neutralization plate, or by an axially loaded dynamic compression plate. Danis (1949) was the first to observe that two bone fragments immobilized with a rigid plate healed without the formation of periosteal or endosteal callus. Later, Schenk and Willenegger

BSAVA Manual of Canine and Feline Fracture Repair and Management, 2nd edition. Edited by Toby Gemmill and Dylan Clements. ©BSAVA 2016

(1963) demonstrated that this healing occurred by direct osteonal proliferation.

Even when two bone fragments are compressed, there is never full congruency between their two surfaces. In some areas there are points of contact whilst in others there are micro-gaps between these points.

Contact healing

When the defect between the bone ends is less than 0.01 mm and interfragmentary strain is less than 2%, contact healing occurs. Primary osteonal reconstruction results in the direct formation of lamellar bone. A cutting cone of osteoclasts lining the end of the osteon nearest to the fracture plane removes dead bone whilst osteoblasts immediately behind these cells lay down new bone, thereby recreating the Haversian system (Figures 5.2 and 5.3). Cutting cones advance from one fragment to another at a rate of 50–100 µm/day, creating longitudinally oriented cavities that are simultaneously filled with osteoid. The newly formed lamellar bone is therefore parallel to the long axis of the bone. Radiographically, the fracture line gradually becomes indistinct.

As Haversian remodelling is a normal process in cortical bone, it is difficult to be sure when direct bone healing is complete, but fractures undergoing primary bone healing are initially weaker than those that heal by callus. It may take mature cortical bone 18 months to regain its normal internal architecture such that the fracture line is no longer identifiable and has been completely replaced by remodelled bone (Schatzker, 2000). This clearly has implications when considering implant removal.

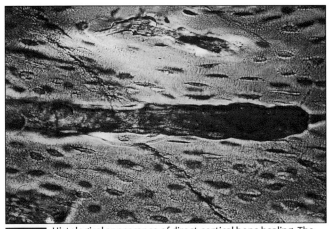

5.2 Histological appearance of direct cortical bone healing. The areas of dead and damaged bone are replaced internally by Haversian remodelling. The fracture line has been graphically enhanced.
(Reproduced from Perren and Claes (2000) with permission from the publisher)

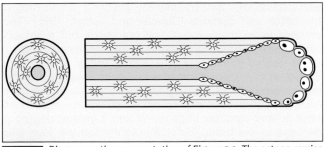

5.3 Diagrammatic representation of Figure 5.2. The osteon carries at its tip a group of osteoclasts that drill a tunnel into the dead bone. Behind the tip, osteoblasts form new bone.

Gap healing

Gap healing typically occurs in gaps of less than 0.8 mm to 1 mm and conditions of less than 2% strain. The fracture site fills by intramembranous bone formation with the newly formed lamellar bone oriented perpendicular to the long axis of the bone, rather than the parallel orientation of contact healing. Due to its perpendicular orientation, the newly formed bone is poorly anchored to the adjacent intact cortex. Consequently, the repair is inherently weak and the lamellar bone has to undergo secondary osteonal remodelling.

Secondary osteonal remodelling starts around 3 to 8 weeks later, with cutting cones arising from the surrounding intact bone as well as those formed from within the fracture gap. Eventually, the resultant resorption cavities mature into longitudinally oriented lamellar bone and the cortices are reformed. In a clinical situation, where a fracture has been well reduced and stabilized sufficiently to permit direct bone union, this always occurs through a combination of contact and gap healing.

Indirect bone healing

Healing of unstable fractures is characterized by the formation of callus prior to bone formation. Fracture resorption by osteoclastic removal of dead bone at the fractured ends occurs during the first few weeks. This effectively widens the fracture gap, increasing the interfragmentary distance (the denominator of the strain equation) and reducing strain conditions. This allows granulation tissue, capable of existing in relatively high strain conditions, to form in the fracture gap.

Indirect healing of a long bone fracture is classically described in three phases: the inflammatory phase; the reparative phase; and the remodelling phase. However, it is important to remember that this series of events is based on the description of a low-energy fracture with a well preserved soft tissue envelope.

Inflammatory phase

The inflammatory phase commences immediately following a fracture, when bleeding from ruptured blood vessels results in haematoma formation and the associated release of tissue growth factors. Neutrophils and, subsequently, macrophages migrate into the haematoma. These inflammatory cells begin phagocytosis of necrotic material and release further cytokines and growth factors, which in turn stimulate angiogenesis and bone formation. Angiogenesis occurs by the outgrowth of new capillaries from existing vessels. This depends on two factors: well vascularized tissue on either side of the fracture gap, and sufficient mechanical stability to allow the new capillaries to survive.

Activated platelets and macrophages appear to be especially important in this phase, releasing platelet-derived growth factor (PDGF) and transforming growth factor beta 1 (TGF-β1), both of which stimulate bone production (Lieberman et al., 2002). Vascular endothelial growth factor (VEGF), local acidity and cytokines contained in the haematoma mediate angiogenesis (Street et al., 2000), supported by inflammatory mediators such as prostaglandins E1 and E2. The subsequent cytokine cascade may also induce osteoclastic activity and the recruitment and proliferation of osteoprogenitor cells derived from mesenchymal stem cells in other tissues, such as muscle and bone marrow, into the fracture gap (Millis, 1999).

Fracture of the bone is frequently associated with disruption of the medullary vessels but, within hours, a transient extraosseous vascular supply is established from the surrounding soft tissues. The role of this extraosseous supply is crucial to successful fracture healing and has been the stimulus for the development of minimally invasive osteosynthesis. Both the extraosseous supply and the mechanical environment need to be considered when planning surgical stabilization of a fracture. Plating impairs periosteal blood supply, particularly when plates that rely on bone–plate friction for stability are employed. Conversely, locking plates that are not compressed against the bone have a less detrimental effect on vascularity. Intramedullary fixation impairs medullary blood supply, reducing cortical blood flow by 60–70% in the short term. In contrast, external fixation has the least effect on blood supply, especially if circular fixators with fine, tensioned transfixation wires are used and these are applied in a minimally invasive fashion.

Reparative phase

A decrease in soft tissue swelling heralds the end of the inflammatory phase and the commencement of the reparative phase, which is characterized initially by the formation of soft callus whilst hard callus develops later.

Early transformation of the haematoma into granulation tissue occurs, angiogenesis continues, and new tissue is formed within days of the initial injury. Subsequently, more mature connective tissue containing collagen fibres develops. Initially collagen types I, II and III form, but gradually type I (the primary structural protein of bone) becomes more common (Remedios, 1999). Throughout this period, the tensile strength of the tissue increases, aided by the diagonal formation of the fibres.

TGF-β and bone morphogenic proteins (BMPs) play a major role in the transformation of fibrous tissue into cartilage. Chondrocytes, formed from mesenchymal stem cells within the bone and adjacent soft tissues, create a soft callus that is able to resist compression but whose tensile strength is similar to the fibrous tissue it replaced (Mann and Payne, 1989). The callus is composed of external callus, formed from the periosteum and whose vascular supply is the extraosseous vessels, and internal callus, developed from the endosteum and vascularized by the medullary arterioles (Binnington, 1990).

External callus production is particularly evident in the healing of unstable fractures in young animals with marked osteogenic potential (Figure 5.4). As the diameter of the bone increases due to callus production, so does the resistance to bending and torsional forces. This is because rigidity increases by the fourth power of the radius of the bone: the distance from the neutral axis of the bone to the outer surface (see Chapter 4).

The strength of the soft callus is further reinforced by mineralization and the subsequent formation of hard callus. Mineralization proceeds from the fracture ends towards the centre of the site and, eventually, calcified fibrocartilage becomes woven bone by endochondral ossification. Woven bone may also be formed directly from osteoblasts within mesenchymal tissue by intramembranous ossification, provided the strain environment is sufficiently low. Osteoblasts can form woven bone rapidly, but, as it is randomly arranged, it is mechanically weak. Nevertheless, bridging of a fracture by woven bone is deemed to represent clinical union.

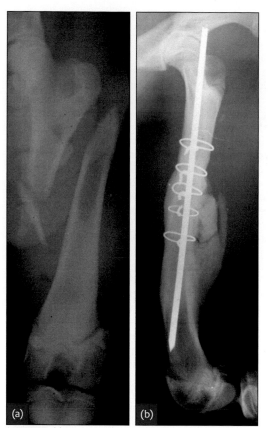

5.4 (a) Preoperative and (b) 6-week postoperative radiographs of a 6-month-old Boxer puppy. Despite the use of an intramedullary pin and cerclage wires, technical errors result in fracture instability. As the diameter of the bone increases due to callus production, so does the resistance to bending forces.

Remodelling phase

Although bone union is achieved at the end of the repair phase, healing is far from complete. Woven bone has to be replaced by cortical bone by the orchestrated action of osteoclastic bone resorption and osteoblastic bone formation, and the medullary cavity must be recreated. The process is governed by Wolff's law, which states that bone in a healthy animal will adapt to the loads under which it is placed. The remodelling is achieved via mechanotransduction, a process through which forces or other mechanical signals are converted to biochemical signals via piezoelectricity. As a piezoelectric substance, bone tissue induces a small electric potential when it deforms. Compression and bending of a tubular bone creates an electropositive environment on its convex side and an electronegative effect on its concave side. Electropositivity is associated with osteoclastic activity whilst electronegativity is associated with osteoblastic activity, thereby effecting remodelling of the callus and cortices (Duncan and Turner, 1995). This process takes many months, if not years, but eventually allows the injured bone to regain its optimal morphology.

As stated previously, the above series of events is based on the description of a low-energy fracture with a well preserved soft tissue envelope. Bones and their surrounding soft tissues damaged by high-energy injuries will have greater vascular impairment and a greater degree of damage to the bone. Surgical intervention will also alter both the mechanical environment and the soft tissue damage. Accordingly, fracture gap bridging can occur by three routes:

1. **Intercortical new bone formation or primary cortical union**. The fracture gap is obliterated by normal cortical remodelling. This only occurs when interfragmentary compression is employed and is the aim in rigid fixation (Müller, 1963).
2. **External bridging callus**. New bone arises from the periosteum and the soft tissues adjacent to the fracture. Small degrees of movement at the fracture stimulate external callus formation (McKibbin, 1978).
3. **Intramedullary bridging by endosteal callus**. This may occur early in the healing process in undisplaced fractures (Rhinelander, 1974) or in stable fractures where intramedullary blood vessel bridging can occur. If there is movement, endosteal callus can only form after periosteal callus has reduced the magnitude of the strain allowing capillary and bony bridging in the centre at a later stage.

Mechanical manipulation of fracture healing

Micromotion

Bone cells are responsive to strain in the matrix (Skerry et al., 1989) and interfragmentary movement has been shown to stimulate more rapid progression of indirect healing than totally rigid fixation (Goodship and Kenwright, 1985). However, motion at a fracture site encourages fracture healing only if it is within a permissible range known as **micromotion**. Micromotion has been shown to stimulate blood flow at the fracture site (Wallace et al., 1994) and to promote osteogenesis by stimulating periosteal callus, thereby speeding up union (Kenwright et al., 1986; Sarmiento and Latta, 2006). However, micromotion does not appear to stimulate endosteal callus.

Outside the range of micromotion, either increased or reduced movement will be deleterious to the healing process. Decreased loading will delay healing, whilst excessive motion will hamper osseous consolidation and result in delayed or non-union. Decreased loading is most commonly due to using excessively large bone plates or unduly stiff external fixators, especially in smaller patients. In contrast, excessive interfragmentary movement prevents the establishment of fragile new capillaries across the gap and can lead to fibrous encapsulation and implant loosening. Thus, in a clinical situation, the surgeon should strive for adequate stability to permit fracture healing, but sufficient flexibility to permit beneficial micromotion at the fracture site. There has been a shift in emphasis in recent years from the previous Arbeitsgemeinschaft für Osteosynthesefragen (AO) philosophy of demanding absolute rigidity to one of creating relative stability. The current generally accepted aim is to control interfragmentary strain to a level which optimizes the chosen method of healing rather than abolishing strain completely.

Dynamization

The term dynamization was originally used by De Bastiani (1984) to describe the transfer of a progressive load to a fracture site at a given point during the healing process by cyclic micromovement. Free axial movement was allowed whilst other forces were controlled. Subsequently, it has become apparent that different kinds of applied movement are of specific benefit at different stages of healing and

that the term dynamization should embrace all of these. The term should therefore describe cyclic micromovement, induced axial micromotion and 'staging-down'.

Cyclic micromovement is produced by early weight-bearing when a spring-loaded external fixator is locked. Weight-bearing causes mild flexion of the screw shafts, which immediately return to their unflexed state as soon as weight is taken off the frame, encouraging collapse and the subsequent recreation of the fracture gap under weight-bearing forces. Unlocking the column will cause progressive closure of the fracture gap and a corresponding reduction in cyclic movements. Locking and unlocking columns to permit linear movement is only possible on purpose-designed external fixators that are often prohibitively expensive for use in veterinary medicine.

In a tibial gap model in dogs, using an external fixator that could be rigidly locked or set to allow free axial movement whilst preventing bending and shear forces, early axial dynamization 1 week postoperatively appeared to accelerate callus formation and remodelling, and provided higher mechanical stiffness during the early stages of bone healing (Larsson et al., 2001). Dynamized ovine metatarsal diaphyseal osteotomies showed significantly greater callus formation and 45% greater tensile strength compared to those that were rigidly fixed. Histological analysis suggested the effect of dynamization occurred mainly after the 5th week (Claes et al., 1995). Late dynamization also enhanced fracture healing in a rat diaphyseal femoral osteotomy model, compared with a constant rigid or constant flexible fixation (Claes et al., 2011). These results indicate that once bony bridging has occurred dynamization may accelerate bone remodelling processes.

Locking and unlocking columns should not be confused with 'staging-down' an external fixator. This is also referred to as dynamization but staging-down involves the staged removal of elements of an external fixator construct when callus strength allows the stiffness of the fixator to be reduced. Staging-down is usually performed around 6 weeks following surgery and allows the gradual transfer of more load to the callus. This increase in functional loading increases the strength of the callus, reducing the time necessary for fracture immobilization but, because of the existing callus, micromotion is not measurably increased.

As well as being produced by weight-bearing forces, axial micromovement may also be induced by activating linear motors that are incorporated into external fixator frames. This has been shown to improve healing both experimentally in ovine models (Goodship and Kenwright, 1985; Claes et al., 1995) and in a clinical study involving patients with tibial fractures (Noordeen et al., 1995).

The optimal pattern of loading for a given stage of healing is still to be defined. In general, cyclic micromovement appears to be important in the initial stages of fracture repair, encouraging callus formation in the early weeks of healing. At a later stage, progressive loading will increase stability and compression of the callus and may be more appropriate during callus maturation to create conditions that are conducive to consolidation.

The use of fewer implants, particularly the use of fewer screws in bone plate fixation, may also stimulate callus formation and remodelling. In a cadaveric ulnar osteotomy model, stripped of soft tissue and subjected to four-point mechanical testing to failure in both tension and medial–lateral bending modes, the number of screws was shown to be less important than the length of the plate in providing bending strength to the construct (Sanders et al., 2002). The use of fewer implants spawned an alternative method of dynamizing bone: the selective removal of screws from a bone plate. This was initially proposed to counteract osteopenia following internal fixation employing dynamic compression plates. Using a bone plate model, Tornkvist (1996) showed removal of 25–50% of the total number of screws increased strain per load with a resultant increase in elastic deformation of the bone–plate construct. These results are the basis of staged selective screw removal at various time points during fracture healing to maintain bone mass but in practice this is rarely done as it necessitates additional surgical procedures.

Summary

The rational basis for fracture treatment is the interaction between three elements: the cell biology of bone regeneration, the revascularization of injured bone by the surrounding soft tissues, and the mechanical environment of the fracture. The surgeon should be aware of, and consider, the interaction between these elements when choosing the optimal treatment of a clinical patient.

References and further reading

Binnington AG (1990) Bone remodelling and transplantation. In: *Canine Orthopaedics 2nd edn*, ed. WG Whittick, pp. 166–189, Lea and Febiger, Philadelphia

Claes L, Blakytny R, Besse J *et al.* (2011) Late dynamization by reduced fixation stiffness enhances fracture healing in a rat femoral osteotomy model. *Journal of Orthopaedic Trauma* **25**, 169–174

Claes LE, Wilke HJ, Augat P *et al.* (1995) Effect of dynamization on gap healing of diaphyseal fractures under external fixation. *Clinical Biomechanics* **10**, 227–234

Danis R (1949) *Theorie et Pratique de l'Osteosynthese*. Masson, Paris

De Bastiani G, Aldegheri R and Renzi Brivio L (1984) The treatment of fractures with a dynamic axial fixator. *Journal of Bone and Joint Surgery (British Volume)* **66-B**, 538–545

Duncan RL and Turner CH (1995) Mechanotransduction and the functional response of bone to mechanical strain. *Calcified Tissue International* **57**, 344–358

Goodship AE and Kenwright J (1985) The influence of induced micromovement upon the healing of experimental tibial fractures. *Journal of Bone and Joint Surgery (British Volume)* **67-B**, 650–655

Kenwright J, Goodship AE, Kelly DJ *et al.* (1986) Effect of controlled axial micromovement on healing of tibial fractures. *Lancet* **328**, 1185–1187

Larsson S, Kim W, Caja VL *et al.* (2001) Effect of early axial dynamization on tibial bone healing: a study in dogs. *Clinical Orthopaedics and Related Research* **388**, 240–251

Lieberman JR, Daluiski A and Einhorn TA (2002) The role of growth factors in the repair of bone. *Journal of Bone and Joint Surgery (American Volume)* **84-A**, 1032–1044

Mann FA and Payne JT (1989) Bone Healing. *Seminars in Veterinary Medicine and Surgery (Small Animal)* **4**, 312–321

McKibbin B (1978) The biology of fracture healing in long bones. *Journal of Bone and Joint Surgery (British Volume)* **60-B**, 150–162

Millis DL (1999) Bone- and non-bone-derived growth factors and effects on bone healing. *Veterinary Clinics of North America: Small Animal Practice* **29**, 1221–1246

Müller ME (1963) Internal fixation for fresh fractures and nonunion. *Proceedings of the Royal Society of Medicine* **56**, 455–460

Noordeen MH, Lavy CB, Shergill NS *et al.* (1995) Cyclical micromovement and fracture healing. *Journal of Bone and Joint Surgery (British Volume)* **77-B**, 645–648

Perren SM and Claes L (2000) Biology and biomechanics in bone healing. In: *AO Principles of Fracture Management*, eds. TP Ruedi and WM Murphy, pp. 9–32. Thieme Medical Publishers, Stuttgart

Remedios A (1999) Bone and bone healing. *Veterinary Clinics of North America Small Animal Practice* **29**, 1029–1044

Rhinelander FW (1974) Tibial blood supply in relation to fracture healing. *Clinical Orthopaedics and Related Research* **105**, 34–81

Sanders R, Haidukewych GJ, Milne T *et al.* (2002) Minimal *versus* maximal plate fixation techniques of the ulna: the biomechanical effect of number of screws and plate length. *Journal of Orthopaedic Trauma* **16**, 166–171

Sarmiento A and Latta L (2006) The evolution of functional bracing of fractures. *Journal of Bone and Joint Surgery (British Volume)* **88-B**, 141–148

Schatzker J (updated by Houlton JEF) (2000) Concepts of fracture stabilization. In: *Bone in Clinical Orthopaedics, 2nd edn*, ed. G Sumner-Smith, pp. 327–347. Thieme, Stuttgart

Schenk RK and Willenegger H (1963) On the histolological picture of so-called primary healing of pressure osteosynthesis in experimental osteotomies in the dog. *Experentia* **19**, 593–596

Schiller AL (1988) Bones and Joints. In: *Pathology*, ed. E Rubin and JL Farber, pp. 1304–1393. Lippincott, Philadelphia

Skerry TM, Bitensky L, Chayen *et al.* (1989) Early strain-related changes in enzyme activity in osteocytes following bone loading *in vivo*. *Journal of Bone and Mineral Research* **4**, 783–788

Street J, Winter D, Wang JH *et al.* (2000) Is human fracture haematoma inherently angiogenic? *Clinical Orthopaedics and Related Research* **378**, 224–237

Tornkvist H, Hearn TC and Schatzker J (1996) The strength of plate fixation in relation to the number and spacing of bone screws. *Journal of Orthopaedic Trauma* **10**, 204–208

Wallace AL, Draper ER, Strachan RK *et al.* (1994) The vascular response to fracture micromovement. *Clinical Orthopaedics and Related Research* **301**, 281–290

Chapter 6

Imaging of fractures

Gawain Hammond

Diagnostic imaging is a vital component in the diagnosis and management of fractures. At initial presentation fractures can be identified and classified to permit planning of optimal treatment. Subsequently, fractures can be monitored to assess healing and identify developing complications.

Imaging modalities

Diagnostic imaging modalities for investigation of fractures include radiography, magnetic resonance imaging, ultrasonograpy and nuclear scintigraphy.

Diagnostic radiography

This remains the most commonly used modality, due to both its widespread availability and the excellent bone imaging it provides. For optimal bone imaging, a radiographic facility should have a combination of general and high detail (extremity) radiographic plates available, as well as a grid for use in larger patients. A selection of sandbags and foam positioning wedges are also useful. It should be remembered that radiography does not allow assessment of the articular cartilage and only allows limited assessment of the soft tissues around the fracture. In addition, radiographic detection of a loss of bone mineral requires at least a 30% reduction in the mineral density; thus small changes in bone opacity (either through lysis or new bone formation) can take 7–10 days to become radiographically apparent. This can hamper the diagnosis of acute undisplaced (or incomplete) fractures, and may delay the diagnosis of some complications of fracture repair. Principles for radiography of fractures are given in Figure 6.1.

- Obtain at least two orthogonal radiographs of the fracture site
- Include joints proximal and distal to the fracture (for long bones)
  - Assess for rotation of the fracture fragments
  - Check for articular extension of the fracture
- Radiograph contralateral limb for comparison
- For trauma cases, image thorax and abdomen for concurrent problems
- Consider horizontal beam radiography when patient movement needs to be minimized (e.g. vertebral fractures)
- Use stressed radiographs to assess joint laxity, if suspected
- Sedation or anaesthesia is usually required for adequate radiographic quality

6.1 Principles of radiography of fractures.

Computed tomography

Although the availability of computed tomography (CT) scans is generally limited to larger referral hospitals, it can provide excellent assessment of fractures due to its high resolution and lack of superimposition. It is particularly valuable for skull, spinal and pelvic fractures, as well as injuries to the carpus and tarsus. In addition, three-dimensional models of the bone can be generated, which can allow therapeutic planning (e.g. complex pelvic fractures) (Figure 6.2).

Magnetic resonance imaging

Magnetic resonance imaging (MRI) is largely limited to referral hospitals and, whilst it can be used to image fractured bones (e.g. in the vertebral column), its use for appendicular fractures is limited.

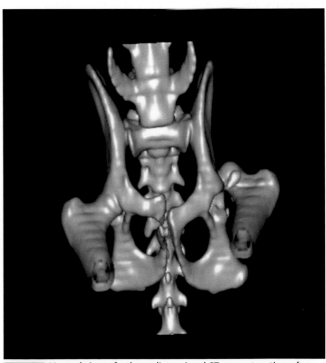

6.2 Ventral view of a three-dimensional CT reconstruction of a complex pelvic fracture, sacroiliac luxation and hip luxation allowing clear visualization of the spatial relationships between the fragments and articulations.
(Courtesy of T Liuti)

Ultrasonography

Ultrasonography generally provides poor skeletal imaging, so its use in the assessment of fractures is largely limited to the assessment of associated soft tissue pathologies (e.g. tendon ruptures) and the detection of remote concurrent disease (e.g. urinary bladder rupture) associated with trauma. Ultrasonography will allow visualization of the surface of the bone and may allow visualization of callus formation and vascularization at the fracture site (Risselada et al., 2005; Risselada et al., 2006). However, the lack of spatial orientation on the ultrasound image and inability to image below the surface of the bone precludes complete assessment of the initial injury and the subsequent healing process.

Nuclear scintigraphy

Whilst nuclear scintigraphy is sensitive for the increased bone activity associated with fractures, the anatomical resolution is generally insufficient to allow assessment of the fracture for treatment planning. This, coupled with radiation safety implications, limit its use. However, it can be very useful in equine orthopaedics for the detection of early, undisplaced stress fractures, which can be difficult to identify by other means; this has also been reported in Greyhounds (Tobin et al., 2003).

Fracture identification

When obtaining radiographs to diagnose a fracture, the area to be imaged is usually determined by the clinical signs of the patient and the results of clinical and orthopaedic examinations. As a rule, at least two orthogonal radiographs of the fracture area should be obtained to allow full assessment. The typical radiographic findings in a traumatic fracture are:

- Altered shape of the bone
- Disruption or discontinuity of the cortex and medulla with radiolucent lines crossing the bone (Figure 6.3).

Where an undisplaced fracture is present, careful scrutiny of the radiograph may be required to identify the fracture line. In some cases where acute incomplete fracture is suspected but cannot be visualized, it may be necessary to wait 7–10 days and repeat radiographs. This will allow some remodelling of the fracture margins and hence widen the fracture gap, making it more apparent.

Where fracture fragments have overridden (or a folding fracture is present) there will be an area of apparent increased bony opacity. The orthogonal radiograph should confirm the relative position of the bone fragments (Figure 6.4).

The radiolucent line associated with a fracture can be mimicked by overlying fascial planes or skin folds, by the normal nutrient foramen and by the Mach line effect (an optical illusion creating the appearance of a dark line where two bones overlap; see Figure 6.17). Care should be taken to exclude these artefacts before diagnosing a fracture (none of these will result in an altered bone shape). In addition, small fracture fragments can be mimicked by sesamoid bones (which can occasionally be multipartite), separate centres of ossification (in immature animals), dirt on the coat or contaminants in the soft tissue (e.g. associated with a soft tissue wound). Where radiographs are

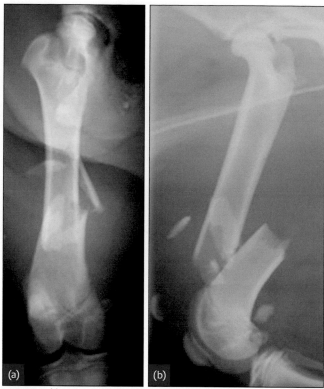

6.3 (a) Craniocaudal and (b) mediolateral radiographs of the femur of a dog with a comminuted fracture of the distal diaphysis. There is complete interruption of the cortex of the bone with displacement of the distal fragments. Note how both orthogonal radiographs are required to fully assess the number and position of the fragments.

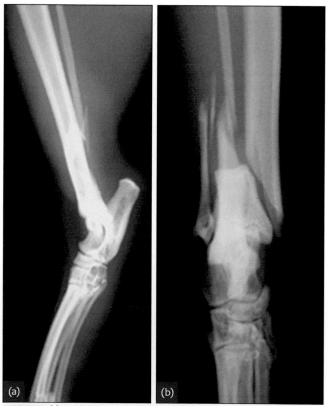

6.4 (a) Mediolateral and (b) caudocranial radiographs of the distal tibia and fibula of a dog with an oblique distal diaphyseal fracture of the tibia and a comminuted fracture of the distal diaphysis of the fibula. Note on the mediolateral view that there is an area of increased opacity resembling sclerosis of the distal diaphysis of the tibia – this is due to superimposition of the proximally displaced distal fragment as can be seen on the caudocranial view.

obtained using a digital radiography system, it is recommended to include a scaler of known size (either a commercially-available scaler or a metal object, such as a coin) at the level of the bone in relation to the radiographic plate, so that it appears on the radiograph and allows accurate assessment of the necessary implant sizes.

Radiographic description of fractures

When a fracture is identified on a radiograph, various features of the fractured bone and surrounding soft tissue should be considered to maximize the information regarding the fracture and ensure the correct treatment protocol is initiated.

How old is the fracture?

In the majority of cases this will be indicated by the history, but this is occasionally uncertain. Recent fractures will show sharply defined margins to the fracture fragments and will not show evidence of bone remodelling or periosteal new bone. Older fractures (greater than 7–10 days) will show less clearly defined fracture margins due to bone resorption, and may also show some early evidence of periosteal new bone around the fracture site as the bone starts to produce callus (Figure 6.5).

Is the fracture pathological?

The ends of the bone fragments at the fracture site (as well as any other skeletal structures on the radiograph) should be examined for decreased bone density, decreased cortical thickness, pre-existing periosteal reactions, changes in the trabecular pattern, unusual fracture configurations or locations and areas of lysis. These changes may indicate an underlying weakness to the bone due to metabolic (e.g. nutritional or renal hyperparathyroidism) or neoplastic disease (e.g. osteosarcoma) (Figure 6.6; see Chapter 13). Folding fractures are often pathological (Figure 6.7).

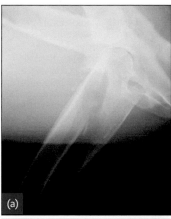

6.6 (a) Mediolateral radiograph of the proximal femur of a dog with acute non-weight-bearing lameness, showing a complete oblique fracture of the proximal diaphysis. (b) On close inspection of the fracture site, a periosteal reaction on the cranial cortex (arrowhead) and patchy lysis of the caudal cortex (arrowed) were noted, indicating pre-existing disease and suggesting a pathological fracture (in this case due to a bone tumour).

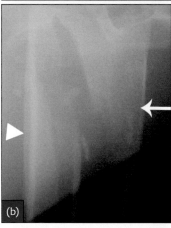

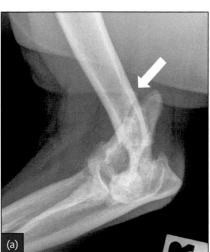

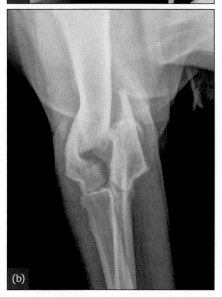

6.5 (a) Mediolateral and (b) craniocaudal radiographs of the elbow of a dog with an old medial condylar fracture of the elbow. Note the rounding and loss of sharpness of the fragment margins and some early callus formation (periosteal new bone) on the caudal aspect of the humerus proximal to the fracture site (arrowed).

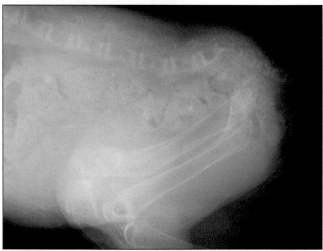

6.7 Lateral radiograph of the hindquarters of a kitten with nutritional secondary hyperparathyroidism. Note the generalized decrease in bone density with associated distortion of the vertebral column, and the folding fracture in the mid-diaphysis of the more cranial femur (indicated by the split cortical lines).

Could the fracture be open?

Diagnosis of an open fracture is often achieved through clinical examination, but the radiograph should be examined for evidence of gas within the soft tissues around the fracture site, suggesting a cutaneous wound allowing communication with the fracture site (Figure 6.8).

Is the fracture complete or incomplete?

Complete fractures will extend across the entire bone, whereas incomplete or greenstick fractures will only cross one cortex (Figure 6.9). However, if a greenstick fracture is present, there may still be some alteration of bone shape.

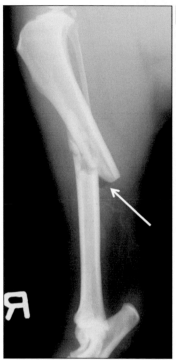

6.8 Mediolateral radiograph of the tibia of a dog with an open mid-diaphyseal fracture. Note the area of gas opacity (arrowed) distal to the proximal fragment, indicating the presence of gas in the soft tissues.

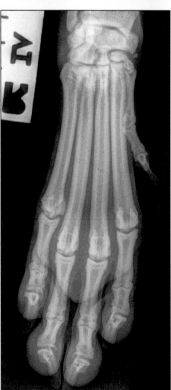

6.9 Dorsopalmar radiograph of the manus of a dog, with an incomplete fracture of the third metacarpal bone. A faint lucent line can be seen crossing the lateral cortex of the mid-diaphysis of the third metacarpal bone; it does not extend across the medial cortex and no significant displacement of the fracture is present.

How many fragments are present?

The fracture may be simple (single fracture line), multiple (several non-connecting fracture lines) or comminuted (multiple bone fragments at a single fracture site).

In what direction do the fracture lines travel?

The fracture may be transverse, oblique, longitudinal, spiral or comminuted. This may affect the method of stabil-ization used, as a transverse fracture has greater inherent stability (resistance to compression) and may only require fixation to resist rotation and angulation, whereas an oblique or spiral fracture, which is more likely to be unstable, will require stabilization to maintain the bone length.

Is there articular involvement?

An articular fracture will extend within the limits of the joint capsule, although it may not actually cross the joint surface (Figure 6.10). In addition, is there evidence of luxation or subluxation associated with the fracture (e.g. hip luxation associated with a pelvic fracture)?

Is the patient immature?

If the patient is immature, is there growth plate involvement (a Salter–Harris fracture)?

Is there evidence of avulsion?

Some periarticular fractures (e.g. tibial tuberosity, olecranon) can be displaced by the pull of the associated tendons or ligaments (Figure 6.11).

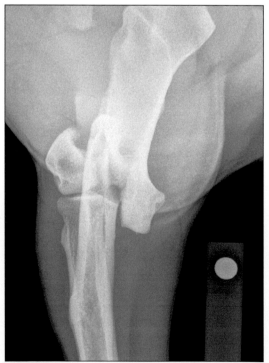

6.10 Craniocaudal radiograph of the elbow of a dog with an articular lateral humeral condylar fracture: the articular surface of the humerus is clearly disrupted.

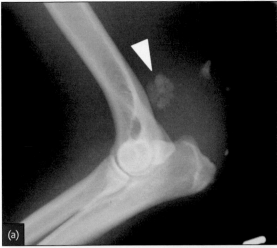

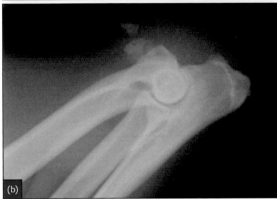

6.11 Mediolateral (a) neutral and (b) flexed radiographs of the elbow of a dog with triceps tendon avulsion associated with an avulsion fracture of the olecranon. An irregular mineralized opacity is seen caudal to the distal humerus on both radiographs (arrowhead): this is calcinosis cutis. Caudal to this is a triangular mineralized opacity which remains in a stable position when the elbow is flexed: this is the proximally displaced avulsion fragment from the olecranon. Note the extensive soft tissue swelling surrounding the olecranon and distal triceps area.

Is there compression or overriding of the fracture ends?

This will result in an apparent shortening of the bone, often accompanied by an increase in bone opacity. This can be of particular importance when assessing vertebral fractures.

What associated soft tissue changes are present?

In the majority of limb fractures, there will be some soft tissue swelling surrounding the fracture; with articular fractures this may include a joint effusion.

Further considerations for imaging fractures in different areas of the skeleton are given below:

Long bone fractures

The location of the fracture within the bone (proximal epiphyseal or metaphyseal, diaphyseal, distal metaphyseal or epiphyseal) should be described, along with any articular involvement and physeal involvement in immature animals. With multiple or comminuted fractures, the presence of butterfly fragments should be identified; these may

be seen on only one radiographic view. In addition, fissures may extend proximally or distally from a diaphyseal fracture, and care should be taken to identify these as they may affect the nature of the implants used for stabilization

Articular fractures

If the fracture line enters the joint capsule, and in particular if it crosses the subchondral bone of the articular surface, care should be taken to identify a step in the subchondral bone – inaccurate reduction and apposition of articular fractures is likely to result in increased degenerative joint disease postoperatively.

Carpus/tarsus

The complex nature of these joints can make identifying fractures of specific bones difficult, particularly if minimal displacement is seen, and a thorough knowledge of the anatomy of these joints is necessary. As well as the standard mediolateral and dorsopalmar/plantar views, oblique views and radiographs with the joints in flexion and extension may assist in diagnosis. In addition, where trauma to these joints is suspected, stressed views to assess for instability (e.g. collateral ligament damage) may be beneficial. If available, a CT scan can be extremely useful in assessing the carpal and tarsal joints, although even this may miss small fractures (Figure 6.12) (Hercock *et al.*, 2011).

Distal limb fractures

Superimposition of the metacarpals/metatarsals and phalanges (particularly on mediolateral radiographs) can make identification of fractures and/or luxations of the paw difficult, and may require oblique or 'splayed' radiographs of the digits, often through placing cotton wool wedges between the digits or using tape to separate the digits to minimize superimposition.

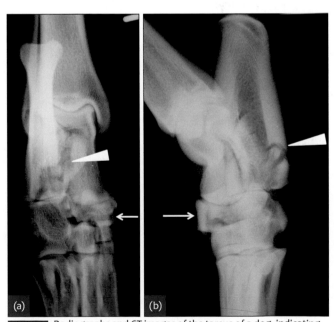

6.12 Radiographs and CT images of the tarsus of a dog, indicating the additional information that can be obtained from advanced imaging. (a) Dorsoplantar and (b) mediolateral radiographs. Irregular lucent lines can be seen crossing the calcaneus (arrowhead) and the central tarsal bone has an altered shape with cranial displacement of the cranial cortex (arrowed). (continues). ▶

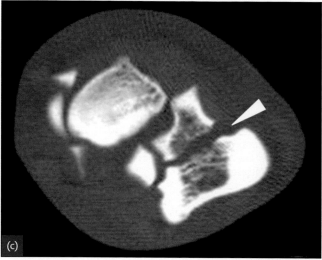

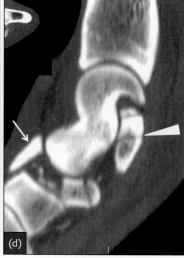

6.12 (continued) Radiographs and CT images of the tarsus of a dog, indicating the additional information that can be obtained from advanced imaging. (c) Transverse and (d) reconstructed sagittal CT images. The fractures of the calcaneus (arrowhead) and the central tarsal bone can be seen to be markedly comminuted (arrowed).

Pelvis

Pelvic fractures are usually multiple (at least two fractures and/or luxations are usually present) and radiographic assessment can be challenging. A minimum of a lateral and a ventrodorsal (VD) radiograph of the pelvis is indicated when pelvic injury is suspected; in particular, fractures of the body of the ilium may be overlooked on a VD view whilst being clearly seen on the lateral view. Where articular (acetabular) involvement is suspected, both frog-legged and extended VD radiographs will allow full assessment of the cranial and caudal extents of the acetabular rim. Whilst the margin of the dorsal rim can be seen on standard VD radiographs, additional assessment can be made using a skyline craniocaudal view of the pelvis obtained with the patient in sternal recumbency with the hindlimbs drawn cranially (Slocum and Devine, 1990); however, routine views should be obtained initially to check for obvious instability of the pelvis. If available, CT scanning is often extremely useful in assessment of pelvic fractures, particularly for minimally displaced acetabular fractures (Draffan *et al.*, 2009). Luxations of the sacroiliac joints are most easily identified on a VD view.

Vertebral column

If a spinal fracture (or luxation) is suspected, extreme care should be used when moving the patient and horizontal beam radiography should be considered to obtain orthogonal views in preference to repositioning the patient (Figure 6.13). Due to superimposition, vertebral fractures can be difficult to identify on radiographs, particularly in the thoracic spine where the proximal aspects of the ribs are also present. Advanced imaging (CT scanning or MRI) is often required to fully assess these injuries. Luxations of the vertebral column can be subtle (although dramatic clinical signs may be present) and careful assessment of the alignment of the vertebral column is indicated. Stressed views can be considered, but these must be performed with great caution to avoid further trauma to the spinal cord. Definitive identification of spinal cord compression will require myelography or MRI, but must be balanced with the risks these techniques pose to further displacing the fracture during positioning of the patient. In many cases myelography or MRI adds little to information gleaned from high quality radiography and careful clinical assessment of the patient.

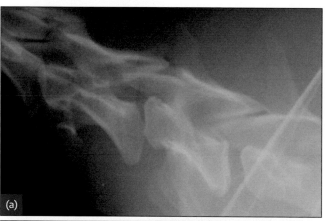

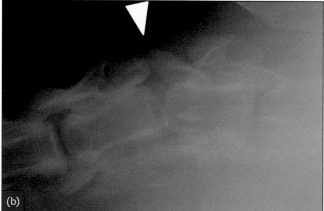

6.13 Radiographs of the cervical spine of a dog presenting with acute tetraplegia following collision with a tree. (a) On the lateral view there is dorsal displacement of the body of the sixth cervical vertebra relative to the fifth, with an associated fracture of an articular facet. (b) Without moving the patient, the horizontal beam VD view allows the complete luxation of one of the vertebral synovial joints (arrowhead) to be identified.

Skull

The complex anatomy and the superimposition of different areas of the skull on conventional radiographs can easily mask mildly displaced fractures, particularly depression fractures of the calvarial or maxillary areas. Assessment for mandibular fractures will often require lateral oblique and VD (intraoral) views as well as standard dorsoventral

(DV) and lateral radiographs, whilst maxillary fractures may be identified using a DV (intraoral) technique. The skull is another area where CT and MRI are significantly superior to conventional radiography for assessment for fractures, as well as allow assessment of the calvarium for intracranial haemorrhage (Figure 6.14).

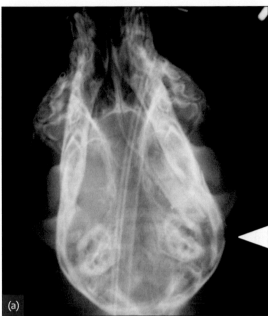

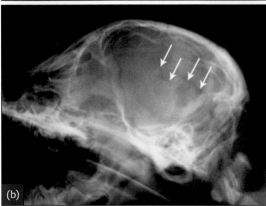

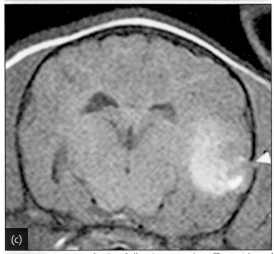

6.14 Images of a dog following a road-traffic accident. (a) A DV radiograph of the skull shows a breach in the cortex of the left calvarium (arrowhead). (b) In the lateral view an irregular lucent line can be seen crossing the calvarium (arrowed). (c) Transverse T1-weighted MR image. As well as the left calvarial fracture (arrowhead), hyperintensity within the parenchyma of the brain, consistent with intracranial haemorrhage, can also be identified.

Fracture healing

Following diagnosis and treatment of the fracture, imaging (in particular radiography) is used to assess the progression of healing and to identify complications associated with the fracture or the healing process.

At least two orthogonal radiographs should be obtained immediately after treatment of the fracture (whether conservative or surgical) to assess the reduction, apposition and alignment of the fracture fragments – this will allow malposition of fracture fragments to be immediately corrected and reduce the risk of malunion. If implants have been placed, then factors to assess include:

- The size of the implant relative to the fracture, bone and patient – is the implant likely to have sufficient strength?
- The placement of screws or pins – is there sufficient cortical engagement above and below the fracture to give fracture site stability?
- Do the implants enter a joint space? – if so, this may need immediate correction
- Have any joint (sub)luxations been reduced (and, if necessary, stabilized)?
- Will the position of the implant allow long-term normal use of the limb?

A useful mnemonic for assessing radiographs of fractures is the 'Four As' system; this is described in Figure 6.15.

Apposition	Apposition or reduction of the fracture fragments
Alignment	Alignment of the bone and adjacent joints
Apparatus	Apparatus or implants used; size, number, accuracy of placement and implant integrity should be assessed
Activity	Activity of the bone; radiographs should be assessed for evidence of healing as well as pathological processes such as osteomyelitis

6.15 The 'Four As' system for assessment of postoperative radiographs.

The timing of subsequent radiographic examinations will vary depending on the age of the patient and the nature of the fracture. In general, radiographs should be obtained if they will influence clinical decisions regarding case management. In immature animals, radiographs every 2 to 3 weeks may be indicated (particularly if premature closure of a growth plate or development of an angular limb deformity is possible). In mature animals, radiographs every 6 to 8 weeks are usually sufficient if healing appears to be progressing normally. When repeating radiographs, the same views as the initial postoperative radiographs should be obtained, as this will allow more straightforward comparison of changes. An example of the radiographic progression of fracture healing over time is shown in Figure 6.16.

PRACTICAL TIP

As soft tissue swelling (which can be severe immediately following trauma and surgery) resolves, the exposure factors may need to be reduced to avoid overexposure

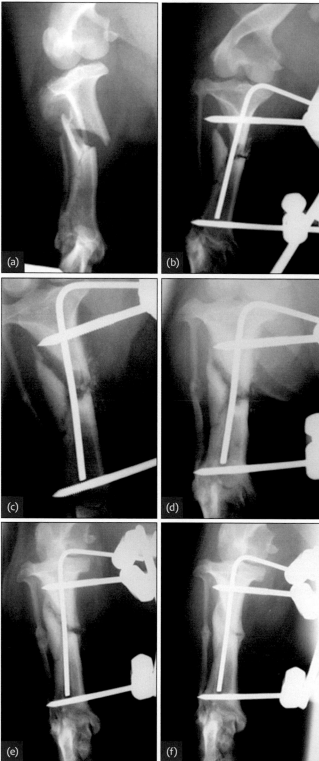

On follow-up radiographs, as well as assessing the position of the fracture fragments, the implants should be examined for evidence of instability (e.g. peri-implant lucent halos, movement, implant fractures). The amount of periosteal callus and remodelling, and bridging of the fracture ends, should be examined and related to the anticipated stage of fracture healing.

The general bone density should also be assessed: when there is disuse of the limb, there may be a general decrease in bone density due to disuse osteopenia (often accompanied by a reduction in muscle bulk).

Radiographic artefacts associated with fracture assessment

There are a number of common artefacts and faults that can compromise interpretation of any radiograph. These can include under- or overexposure, under- or overdevelopment, poor positioning, grid lines and poor labelling. There are some further artefacts that are more specific to orthopaedic radiography and should be noted. The **Mach line effect** is noted above as a possible cause of an apparent fracture line. Another common problem is the fracture site being obscured by the implants, thereby making the healing of the fracture difficult to assess. With the more common implants this can often be overcome with orthogonal radiographs or by obtaining a deliberately oblique view, but occasionally (particularly with the more complex circumferential external fixation systems) obtaining a clear view of the fracture site can be almost impossible. Where digital radiography is used, the presence of implants can cause an edge enhancement effect called the **Uberschwinger effect**. This results in the presence of a dark halo around the edges of implants which can be difficult to differentiate from the genuine lucency caused by implant loosening or infection (Figure 6.17).

6.16 Sequential craniocaudal radiographs of the tibia/fibula of a dog following fracture, showing a normal fracture healing sequence. (a) Initial preoperative radiograph showing a multiple fracture of the mid-diaphysis of the tibia and associated fibular fracture. (b) Immediate postoperative radiograph showing placement of an intramedullary pin and external fixator to reduce and stabilize the fracture. (c) 2 weeks postoperatively: note the loss of sharpness of the fracture margins and early development of irregular periosteal new bone around the fracture site. (d) 4 weeks postoperatively there is increased remodelling of the fracture ends and some closure of the fracture space associated with bridging of the fracture gap. (e) 8 weeks postoperatively there is increased infilling of the fracture gap, with smoother periosteal reaction forming a continuous callus around both tibial and fibular fractures. (f) 12 weeks postoperatively there is continued remodelling of the callus and almost complete healing and bridging of the tibial and fibular fractures.

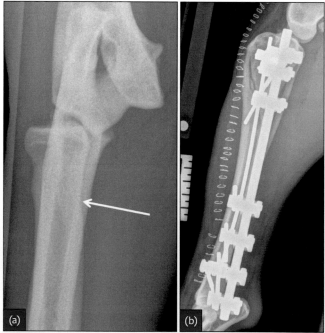

6.17 Examples of radiographic artefacts. (a) Craniocaudal radiograph of a dog with a lateral elbow luxation. The apparent lucent line (arrowed) across the medial aspect of the proximal ulna is a Mach line resulting from superimposition of the radial head. (b) Mediolateral postoperative radiograph of a tibial fracture repaired with external fixation. There is marked superimposition of the implants on the fracture site, making assessment difficult – this is significantly easier on (c) the caudocranial view. (continues) ▶

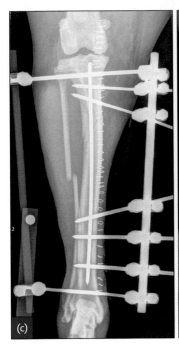

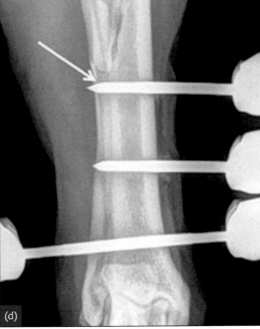

6.17 (continued) Examples of radiographic artefacts. (c) Caudocranial postoperative radiograph of a tibial fracture repaired with external fixation. On (b) the mediolateral view there is marked superimposition of the implants on the fracture site, making assessment difficult – this is significantly easier on this view. (d) Uberschwinger artefact on an immediate postoperative radiograph of a tibial fracture repair. A faint lucent line is seen around the implants (arrowed) and could be mistaken for early implant loosening.

Complications of fracture repair

Whilst many complications of fracture repair may be strongly suggested by the clinical presentation and examination of the patient at follow-up examination, diagnostic imaging is critical to identify these changes and allow an appropriate plan of action to be developed. The diagnosis and management of these complications are described in more detail in Chapters 28 to 31.

Delayed union

This refers to a fracture that has not healed within the expected timeframe. This timeframe can be somewhat subjective; factors such as the age and breed of the patient as well as the location and complexity of the fracture may influence normal progression of healing.

Radiographically, a delayed union will be seen as persistence of a visible fracture line with open ends to the adjacent medullary cavities. Continued evidence of healing progression is usually (but not always; Figure 6.18) seen, such as development of callus or remodelling of fracture ends.

Non-union

Non-union can be diagnosed when there is evidence that the process of fracture healing has ceased without union of the fracture ends. It is unlikely that a non-union can confidently be diagnosed until at least 12 weeks following the fracture, although a lack of progression of fracture healing on consecutive radiographic studies will raise concern. Other radiographic changes suggestive of a non-union can include smooth rounded fracture ends with closure of the medullary cavity (see Chapter 31). Cases of non-union can be broadly divided into two subtypes: biologically active (viable) non-union and biologically inactive (non-viable) non-union.

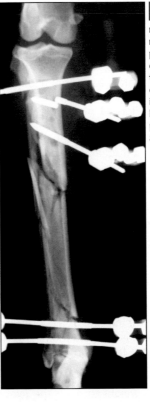

6.18 Delayed union of a tibial fracture. Craniocaudal radiograph of the tibia of a dog with multiple fractures taken 7 weeks postoperatively. There is no evidence of callus formation or remodelling of the fracture margins, indicating a lack of healing activity. Note the fractured implant and areas of increased lucency around the external fixator pins: this suggests implant loosening and possible infection.

Biologically active (viable) non-union

In these cases, the non-union most commonly arises from instability at the fracture site preventing bridging of the fracture gap. Many cases will show hypertrophic non-union (Figure 6.19), with significant periosteal proliferation either side of, but not crossing, the fracture gap, giving an 'elephant's foot' appearance to the fracture ends. Less marked periosteal proliferation can produce a more 'horse's foot' appearance. Some viable non-unions will not show obvious periosteal new bone. These are known as

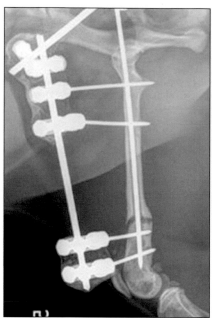

6.19 Mediolateral radiograph of the femur of a cat 10 weeks following stabilization of a femoral fracture of the distal diaphysis. Note the increased lucency around the two distal pins and the widening of the distal end of the proximal fracture fragment with a failure of callus to bridge the fracture site: this is consistent with a hypertrophic non-union due to instability.

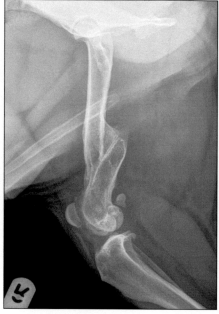

6.20 Mediolateral radiograph of the femur of a dog, showing malunion of a previous mid-diaphyseal fracture. The distal fragment has fused to the proximal fragment in a caudoproximal location.

oligotrophic non-unions, and may be seen with some unstable fractures with an avulsion component, or where there is systemic disease such as hyperadrenocorticism.

Biologically inactive (non-viable) non-union

Common causes include:

- An excessive gap between viable areas of bone (defect non-union)
- Interposition of a partially devitalized intermediate fragment (dystrophic non-union)
- Interposition of avascular necrotic bone fragments associated with a comminuted fracture (necrotic non-union)
- Atrophic non-union. This is most commonly seen in antebrachial fractures in toy breeds, and radiographs will show tapering fracture ends with no evidence of callus formation. If the non-union affects the ulna but not the radius it may be of limited clinical significance.

Malunion

Malunion occurs when the fracture ends fuse in an anatomically incorrect alignment, and may result in a combination of angular or rotational deformity of the limb or a shortening of the limb. A mild degree of malunion is common in many fractures, particularly where there has been a multiple or comminuted fracture. However, the clinical significance of the malunion will depend on the effect on the angulation of the limb and the transfer of weight through the joints either side of the fractured bone: abnormal loading will lead to the development of degenerative joint disease. Full assessment requires at least two orthogonal radiographs or a CT scan, including the joints above and below the fracture, to allow evaluation of the degree of deformity, as well as the likely impact on joint function (Figure 6.20).

Implant failure

Implant failure can result from fracture of the implants themselves or from loosening of the implant from the bone (see Chapter 29).

Implant fracture

This may occasionally occur due to failure of the metal of the implant. This can be due to acute overload (rare in companion animals due to the relatively small body mass), an inherent implant defect (unlikely given the rigorous quality control of implant manufacturers) or, more commonly, due to cyclic fatigue failure.

Radiographic evidence of implant failure will include a broken or deformed implant (see Figure 6.18) or altered angle of different components of the repair. Comparison to previous radiographs can be invaluable in detecting this.

Implant loosening and movement

Implants can lose their anchor point in the bone for various reasons:

- Infection
- Bone necrosis due to thermal damage during surgery
- Stress and subsequent micromotion at the implant–bone interface
- Fracture site instability leading to implant migration (Figure 6.21).

Radiographic evidence of implant loosening will be a lucent halo (often of irregular thickness) developing around one or more of the implants placed into the bone (either within the medullary cavity or through the cortex). Care needs to be taken with digital radiography systems not to mistake the Uberschwinger effect for genuine bone lysis (see above).

Infection

Osteomyelitis will often be suspected on clinical examination, with common radiographic findings including:

- Soft tissue swelling (especially in acute cases)
- Lysis of bone (particularly around implants; see above)
- Irregular periosteal reaction (Figure 6.22), often with slightly ill-defined margins (indicating active bone turnover) and extending some distance away from the fracture site. It should be remembered that, depending

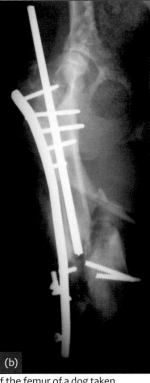
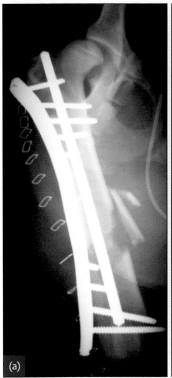

on the radiographic view, periosteal reaction may not be seen at the bone margins, but may instead be seen as an area of increased bone density
- Sequestrum/involucrum formation.

It should be remembered that acute osteomyelitis may not be radiologically detectable due to the time lag before bone lysis and periosteal reaction is radiologically visible, and it is critical that the clinical presentation in combination with the radiographic appearance should be considered when deciding on a treatment plan (see Chapter 30). In addition, the radiological changes of resolving osteomyelitis can lag behind the pattern of clinical improvement.

Stress protection

Where an over-large implant is used, there may be insufficient weight transfer through the healing bone (stress protection). This will result in a degree of atrophy or poor healing at the fracture site (seen as a reduced bone density).

Disuse osteopenia

In cases where the limb is not used following the fracture, there can be a general decrease in bone density which can be seen on radiographs (particularly in the distal limb) as a diffuse loss of bone opacity. In these cases, there will be an increased risk of pathological fracture when weight is returned to the limb.

Sequestrum/involucrum formation

A bone fragment that loses its vascular supply and becomes devitalized as a result may remain within the fracture site, potentially impeding normal fracture healing or providing a nidus for infection. Radiographically this will be seen as a fragment of bone with persistently sharply defined margins (the sequestrum) lying in a radiolucent space which often contains pus (Figure 6.23). Surrounding this lucent space is likely to be a sclerotic border in the vital bone (the involucrum), which represents the bone's attempt to wall off the sequestrum. Occasionally, the infection centred on the sequestrum may cause a sinus tract breaching the skin surface. If a sequestrum is identified, surgical removal is usually indicated.

6.21 Craniocaudal radiographs of the femur of a dog taken (a) immediately and (b) 4 weeks postoperatively following stabilization of a fracture with a plate and intramedullary pin. On the follow-up radiograph, there is marked proximal migration of the intramedullary pin, with multiple screw fractures distally and separation of the distal end of the femur from the plate.

6.22 Mediolateral radiograph of the tibia of a dog with osteomyelitis following stabilization of a tibial fracture (part of the external fixator frame had been removed prior to this radiograph being obtained). There is an irregular periosteal reaction along both cranial and caudal aspects of the tibia and lucency around the single external fixator pin remaining in the distal tibia; the tracks of the removed pins are also unusually wide. The exuberant irregular periosteal reaction raises a strong concern for osteomyelitis.

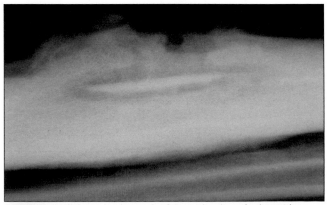

6.23 Mediolateral radiograph of the mid-radius of a dog with a sequestrum/involucrum. Note the well defined linear area of bone with increased opacity (the sequestrum) surrounded by a zone of lucency, itself surrounded by a sclerotic margin (the involucrum). In addition, there is extensive surrounding periosteal reaction associated with chronic osteomyelitis.

Excessive callus formation or ossification of elevated periosteum

Excess callus (associated with instability, infection or bone grafts) or ossification of elevated and/or stripped areas of periosteum can result in a significant bony protuberance at the fracture site. In the majority of cases this will be clinically insignificant but, theoretically, these changes could cause interference with normal limb function if present close to joints.

Soft tissue atrophy

Atrophy of the muscles may be seen where there is poor use of the limb following treatment of the fracture. Whilst this may be appreciated on physical examination, marked muscle atrophy should be considered when radiographing the limb as it will require a reduction in exposure factors to avoid overexposing the skeletal components and thereby compromising assessment of the fracture site.

Fracture-associated neoplasia

Rarely, bone tumours, usually osteosarcoma, may develop at a fracture site. In the majority of reported cases, there is a history of complications in fracture healing, such as instability or infection.

References and further reading

Butterworth SJ (2006) Long bones – fractures. In: *BSAVA Manual of Canine and Feline Musculoskeletal Imaging*, ed. F Barr and R Kirberger, pp 49–70. BSAVA Publications, Gloucester

Dennis R, Kirberger RM, Barr F and Wrigley RH (2010) Skeletal system: general. In: *Handbook of Small Animal Radiology and Ultrasound, 2nd edn*, pp. 1–37. Saunders Elsevier, Philadelphia

Draffan D, Clements D, Farrell M *et al.* (2009) The role of computed tomography in the classification and management of pelvic fractures. *Veterinary Comparative Orthopaedics and Traumatology* **22**, 190–197

Hammond G and McConnell F (2013) Radiology of the appendicular skeleton. In: *BSAVA Manual of Canine and Feline Radiography and Radiology*, ed. A Holloway and F McConnell, pp. 240–301. BSAVA Publications, Gloucester

Henry GA (2013) Fracture healing and complications. In: *Textbook of Veterinary Diagnostic Radiology, 6th edn*, ed. DE Thrall, pp. 283–306. Elsevier, St Louis

Hercock CA, Innes JF, McConnell F *et al.* (2011) Observer variation in the evaluation and classification of severe central tarsal bone fractures in racing greyhounds. *Veterinary Comparative Orthopaedics and Traumatology* **24**, 215–222

Papageorges M and Sande RD (1990) The Mach phenomenon. *Veterinary Radiology* **31**, 191–195

Risselada M, Kramer M, de Rooster H *et al.* (2005) Ultrasonographic and radiographic assessment of uncomplicated secondary fracture healing of long bones in dogs and cats. *Veterinary Surgery* **34**, 99–107

Risselada M, Kramer M, Saunders JH, Verleyen P and Van Bree H (2006) Power Doppler assessment of the neovascularization during uncomplicated fracture healing of long bones in dogs and cats. *Veterinary Radiology and Ultrasound* **47**, 301–306

Sande R (1999) Radiography of orthopaedic trauma and fracture repair. *Veterinary Clinics of North America: Small Animal Practice* **29**, 1247–1260

Slocum B and Devine T (1990) Dorsal acetabular rim radiographic view for evaluation of the canine hip. *Journal of the American Animal Hospital Association* **26**, 289–296

Tobin E, Weaver M, Skelly C and McAllister H (2003) The use of scintigraphy in the investigation of occult lameness in 19 racing Greyhounds. *Scientific Proceedings of the 46th Annual Congress of the British Small Animal Veterinary Association*, p. 588

Chapter 7

Preoperative assessment of the fracture patient

Ralph Abercromby

Fracture management can be an exciting and rewarding veterinary discipline. However, because unrelated tissues are frequently damaged and may be of greater clinical concern, the entire patient must be suitably assessed and preoccupation with an obvious fracture, at the expense of other injuries, must be avoided. Investigations, injuries and treatments require prioritization based on clinical significance; definitive fracture management may need to be delayed in some patients.

Patient assessment proceeds in phases:

- Telephone advice
- Initial patient examination
- Detailed examination of body systems
- Plans for definitive treatment or further investigation.

Telephone advice

Evaluation and management begin at first contact and decisions have to be made from information provided by personnel who are likely to be untrained. Decisions will be required as to the advisability of moving the patient and advice should be given for potentially life-saving first aid (e.g. maintenance of airway, control of haemorrhage) and general patient care (e.g. methods to move/transport, covering/temporary stabilization of injured regions).

Initial patient examination

A rapid but thorough initial examination must be performed and a detailed history taken. Priority is given to any life-threatening injuries; the first few minutes after arrival are pivotal to survival of the severely traumatized patient. Once the 'ABCDE' of emergency medicine has been managed (airway, breathing, circulation, disability, exposure), further more detailed examination and assessment are pursued (see the *BSAVA Manual of Canine and Feline Emergency and Critical Care* for more information).

Detailed examination of body systems

A more thorough examination, perhaps facilitated by analgesic administration, is performed following management of any life-threatening injuries. A memorable, comprehensive protocol (system/organ-based or region-based) should be established to ensure all body systems are assessed.

Full examination requires a variety of skills and equipment. In the early stages, experience and well trained senses can be more valuable than expensive monitoring or diagnostic equipment. Observation and regular repeat assessments are paramount. Essential equipment includes stethoscope, torch, percussion hammer or similar and sterile needles, catheters and syringes (for detection of free fluid or air in the thorax or abdomen).

Thoracic and abdominal examinations

Thoracic and abdominal injuries frequently accompany fractures of unrelated regions. For each, plain radiography and occasionally ultrasonography are indicated. In addition, needle thoraco/abdominocentesis is easily performed and can provide rapid confirmation of clinical suspicions of the presence of free material such as air or blood, or the presence of a ruptured viscus. Ultrasonography may be more reliable for the identification of these conditions.

Potential differential diagnoses for thoracic injuries include:

- Pneumothorax
- Pneumomediastinum
- Haemothorax
- Pulmonary parenchymal haemorrhage
- Rib fractures
- Diaphragmatic rupture
- Haemopericardium
- Neurogenic pulmonary oedema
- Traumatic myocarditis.

Traumatic myocarditis (blunt trauma to the heart producing cardiac contusion ± myocardial infarction) can result in arrhythmias and even death. Therefore this should always be considered and would justify sequential electrocardiograms on the day of admission and occasionally thereafter if it is suspected.

The ability to void urine or faeces does not exclude injury to associated organs and further investigations, such as contrast radiography or ultrasonography, may be indicated in selected cases.

Orthopaedic examination

In many cases the presence and location of a fracture is obvious from the clinical examination. This, however, may not always be the case; fractures can sometimes be difficult to detect where only one of a pair or group of bones is injured (e.g. radius/ulna, tarsal or carpal bones) or where fractures are incomplete (e.g. greenstick fracture) and adjacent structures can afford a degree of support. In such cases more subtle signs have to be relied on, such as localized swelling or skin discoloration, or exquisite pain on direct palpation. Forced or stress manoeuvres of bones and joints can be considered to assist exclusion of fractures when no other signs have been identified.

Having identified or excluded grossly unstable fractures, the remainder of the musculoskeletal system, as far as is practical, should be examined. It is essential to exclude additional injuries in cases when an obvious fracture has been detected. Ranges of motion of all joints, deep palpation of bones and soft tissues and assessment of integrity of all structures – not just bone – should be performed. Where concurrent injuries allow, the patient should be examined at rest, on rising and at various forms of exercise. Multiple long bone fractures are likely to preclude such an examination but an undisplaced fracture may only become evident on more critical evaluation following observation of a relatively mild lameness at exercise.

The integrity of both neural and vascular structures should be confirmed. Excellent fracture repair is of little value if the distal limb is avascular or acceptable limb function is not possible because of spinal or peripheral nerve injury. Uncertainties of tissue viability or future function may be important to an owner's decision whether or not to pursue treatment.

Should the distal limb be warm and soft tissues bleed when pricked with a needle, the blood supply to the limb is generally assumed to be adequate. Shock and peripheral vasoconstriction, however, reduce the value of such tests. Correction of circulating blood volume and treatment of shock may make assessment more reliable but uncertainty as to tissue viability may persist. Further investigation with contrast studies, Doppler ultrasonography or scintigraphy may assist detection of blood supply to a specific part of a limb.

An increase in pressure within anatomically restricted regions (compartment syndrome), if untreated, may result in vascular or neural damage. If suspected, compartment syndrome can be treated with a fasciotomy; however, the condition appears to be considerably less prevalent in veterinary patients than in humans.

Regular and repeated re-examinations are essential to assess progression or resolution of any problems.

Neurological examination

Critical evaluation of the neurological system is vital since injuries to the neurological system may present with signs suggestive of musculoskeletal injury and *vice versa*. However, neurological examination can be difficult to perform in the severely traumatized patient. Although diagnosis of specific lesions is often challenging, it is usually possible to localize and grade the severity of any problem. Assessment of mental status, cranial nerve reflexes, gait, posture, proprioception and local spinal reflexes typically enables identification or exclusion of neurological problems, and classification as lower or upper motor neuron.

Sensory fields of the limbs should be assessed, as a loss of pain perception can indicate a severe neurological lesion. The area affected may be localized to a general region (e.g. to the brain or specific spinal cord segments) or to a more specific site (e.g. a peroneal nerve injury). Ophthalmic examination is usually performed in conjunction with the neurological examination.

For a more detailed description of the neurological examination the reader is referred to other texts such as the *BSAVA Manual of Canine and Feline Neurology.*

> **PRACTICAL TIP**
>
> Abnormal signs may be transient, reflecting swelling or contusion rather than anatomical disruption, or may be static or progressive. **Repeat examinations at regular intervals are therefore essential**

Some injuries, such as those causing increased intracranial pressure, may require immediate investigation and management. Others, such as nerve root avulsion or peripheral nerve transection, may significantly affect the prognosis for return to acceptable post-treatment quality of life. Careful assessment is required to identify such injuries and prevent inappropriate treatment of less critical injuries.

Clinical findings may suggest more extensive examination is required, such as myelography or magnetic resonance imaging (MRI). Electrodiagnostics such as electromyography can be useful to document denervation of specific regions, but valid conclusions may require a delay of, or retesting after, 3–7 days.

Fractures of the skull and spine are discussed in Chapters 17 and 18, respectively.

Imaging the fracture region

High quality radiographs in at least two orthogonal planes are essential to confirm and further evaluate the extent of fractures. Radiographs should include adjacent joints, and it is often helpful to obtain images of the contralateral limb as well. The radiographs provide vital information allowing formation of primary and secondary treatment plans. They can also assist in providing an accurate prognosis with respect to expected return to function and estimation of the possible costs of therapy. Further information on imaging of fractures can be found in Chapter 6.

General anaesthesia is usually necessary to produce the quality of radiographs required for treatment planning without causing unnecessary pain or additional soft tissue damage, and is of little concern when the intention is to proceed with definitive treatment under the same anaesthetic. However, if surgery is to be delayed to allow treatment of life-threatening injuries, anaesthesia for the purpose of radiography alone cannot be justified, especially if any information gleaned is unlikely to alter the immediate management of the situation. In such cases, radiographs obtained with the patient conscious or lightly sedated can be considered to allow an interim diagnosis to be confirmed. Following patient stabilization, higher quality radiographs can then be obtained to allow detailed planning of treatment.

When available, the use of computed tomography (CT) may provide additional information and also allows three-dimensional reconstruction that can assist in fracture planning; this is especially useful for assessment of craniomaxillofacial, spinal and pelvic fractures (Figure 7.1),

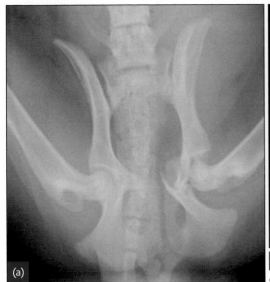

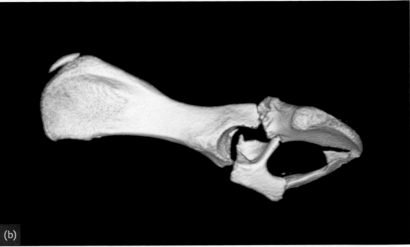

7.1 (a) A ventrodorsal radiograph and (b) a reconstructed three-dimensional CT image showing a comminuted acetabular fracture in an 8-month-old Border Terrier. It is easier to appreciate the extent of the comminution on the reconstructed CT image.

as well as those involving the carpus or tarsus. CT and MRI may also be of use where pathological fracture is considered possible; MRI in particular can provide details relating to soft tissue structures that radiography cannot. Three-dimensional modelling based on CT or MR images can also help surgeons plan or even rehearse surgical procedures, especially those which may be challenging or with which they are unfamiliar.

Fracture Patient Assessment Score

When managing fractures, care should be taken to avoid simply matching to a similar looking fracture pattern in a textbook and slavishly attempting to recreate the treatment pattern chosen in that case. To do so would be to ignore the multiple variables that cannot be included in the illustration but which could have a profound influence on outcome.

Following thorough clinical examination, stabilization of more critical injuries and detailed radiography, the preoperative data should be assessed and evaluated. A useful systematic approach is to apportion information to one of three main categories: *mechanical, biological* and *clinical*. This ensures all relevant information is considered, and can be used to create a **Fracture Patient Assessment Score (FPAS)** (Figure 7.2). This score can subsequently be used to help determine an appropriate fracture treatment plan. This should include theatre organization, surgical approaches, reduction techniques, tissue management priorities, implant choices and postoperative care regimes.

In simplistic terms, **mechanical** factors relate to the anticipated forces on the implants and determine the required strength and stability of the selected fixation technique. **Biological** factors, which relate to both local soft tissue damage at the fracture site and the patient's systemic health, provide an indication as to how quickly bone healing will progress and therefore how long implants are required to function. **Clinical** factors such as patient and owner compliance also affect implant choice; internal fixation may be preferable to the use of an external skeletal fixator for the stabilization of a fracture in an aggressive dog, and more robust fixation may be

necessary in an animal that the owner admits cannot be adequately confined.

Categories are assigned a score on a scale from 1 to 10; 10 being most favourable and 1 being least favourable. In practice, subcategories are frequently allocated to high (8–10), medium (4–7) or low (1–3) status, where high tends to indicate better outcome with fewer complications likely and low indicates a greater risk of poor outcome and of more complications developing.

Mechanical factors

- Patient size and weight.
- Number of limbs affected.
- Pre-existing musculoskeletal, neurological or generalized disease.
- Ability to achieve load sharing between implants and reconstructed bone fragments.

In a large heavy patient there are larger loads at the fracture site compared to a smaller animal. However, obesity in a smaller animal may also introduce a high risk value, due to poorer gait and mobility. The greater the number of limbs injured, the greater the loading of any repair technique. Concurrent unrelated conditions such as pre-existing degenerative joint disease, neurological dysfunction, or amputation of another limb are likely to increase loading of the implants.

The extent of fracture reconstruction achieved affects implant loading. The lower the proportion of load borne by bone, the greater the load on implants and the greater the concern regarding cyclic fatigue and failure (see Chapter 4). A simple transverse fracture can be reconstructed to facilitate significant load transfer directly between bone fragments, protecting the implants. On the other hand, the management of a comminuted non-reducible fracture will result in no load sharing by bone; the load will all borne by implants and consequently there is a higher risk of implant failure.

Biological factors

Biological factors give an indication of the rate of healing and, therefore, the duration over which the repair technique must function.

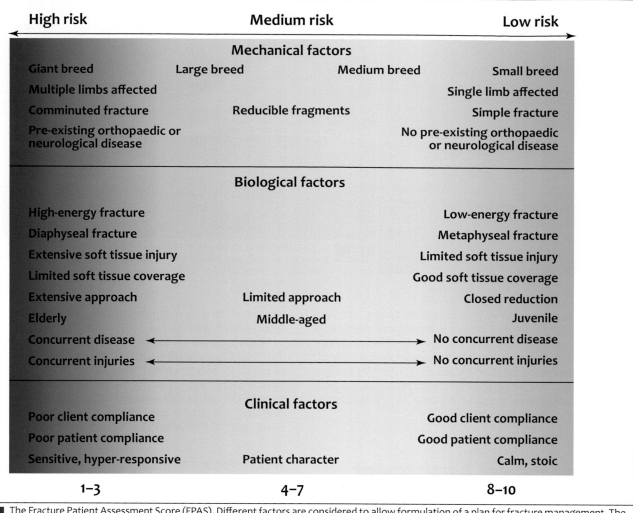

	High risk	Medium risk	Low risk
Mechanical factors			
	Giant breed	Large breed	Medium breed	Small breed
	Multiple limbs affected			Single limb affected
	Comminuted fracture	Reducible fragments		Simple fracture
	Pre-existing orthopaedic or neurological disease			No pre-existing orthopaedic or neurological disease
Biological factors			
	High-energy fracture			Low-energy fracture
	Diaphyseal fracture			Metaphyseal fracture
	Extensive soft tissue injury			Limited soft tissue injury
	Limited soft tissue coverage			Good soft tissue coverage
	Extensive approach	Limited approach		Closed reduction
	Elderly	Middle-aged		Juvenile
	Concurrent disease ←		→	No concurrent disease
	Concurrent injuries ←		→	No concurrent injuries
Clinical factors			
	Poor client compliance			Good client compliance
	Poor patient compliance			Good patient compliance
	Sensitive, hyper-responsive	Patient character		Calm, stoic
	1–3	**4–7**		**8–10**

7.2 The Fracture Patient Assessment Score (FPAS). Different factors are considered to allow formulation of a plan for fracture management. The risk of complications is shown at the top and the FPAS is shown at the bottom of the figure.

Local factors at the fracture site include:

- Quality of soft tissue envelope
- Extent of soft tissue damage
- High- or low-energy fracture
- Region of bone fractured
- Surgical approach.

Systemic factors include:

- Age
- General health
- Concurrent disease
- Concurrent injuries.

The soft tissue envelope around the fracture is critical to healing, providing vascularity, cells and growth factors to the fracture site. The soft tissue envelope tends to be of better quality over the proximal limb (e.g. humeral and femoral fractures) compared to the distal limb (e.g. carpal, tarsal and paw fractures). Injury to the soft tissue envelope will adversely affect healing. High-energy, open, highly comminuted fractures with denuded, devitalized and contaminated bone fragments are at considerably greater risk of delayed and/or complicated healing than are closed, low-energy, incomplete or relatively undisplaced fractures. Similarly, the detrimental biological effect of any surgery must be considered. An open approach will usually be more traumatic than closed, whilst aggressive fragment manipulation can cause further soft tissue damage.

Epiphyseal and metaphyseal fractures will typically heal more quickly than those in cortical regions due to the former's greater blood supply, number of osteogenic cells present, surface area on which to lay down new bone and inherent mechanical stability. Areas of limited soft tissue attachment will heal more slowly than those where it is greater.

For fractures of similar type, immature patients are likely to heal significantly more quickly than mature patients. In addition, concurrent generalized disease such as hyperadrenocorticism, diabetes mellitus, renal failure or neoplasia is likely to adversely affect healing.

Clinical factors

- Anticipated client compliance with postoperative instructions.
- Anticipated patient compliance and behaviour.
- Home environment.

Clinical factors relate to postoperative effects of anticipated patient behaviour, owner compliance and environment on fracture healing and management. Most clinical factors relate indirectly to mechanical forces at the fracture site but other issues, such as anticipated patient tolerance of technique used (e.g. external skeletal fixation (ESF) or coaptation), are also considered.

Most clinical factors will not be determined on direct patient examination or radiography but rather from historical features as well as from a degree of clinical intuition. A thorough discussion of the various management options available and postoperative care requirements must be performed *before* embarking on a management plan.

The more active a patient is, the greater the demands on the repair and the greater the risk of soft tissue complications should coaptation or ESF management be applied. In these patients, use of stable internal fixation without the need for any external support may improve comfort, improve limb use and improve fracture healing whilst minimizing complications.

A patient's home environment also affects management choices. Avoidance of stairs may not be feasible, leading to increased loading of the repair technique. Similarly, a client may be unable or unwilling to enforce controlled lead only activity or the presence of additional pets or young children in the house may increase demand on the fixation.

Application of the FPAS

The FPAS attempts to produce individual subcategory scores and an overall numerical score. It is, however, generally utilizing subjective criteria and therefore care should be taken to avoid rigid dependence on individual numbers. The core value of the FPAS is enforcing careful systematic assessment and interpretation of a variety of important factors.

FPAS high score with general agreement across the categories

A patient with such a score would typically be a small or medium-sized young animal with a reducible two-part relatively transverse fracture. Implants would not need to be of extreme strength or stiffness, nor be expected to function for extended periods. Management options such as intramedullary devices, simple ESF or relatively small plates and bone screws may be considered.

FPAS low score with general agreement across the categories

A patient with such a score may well be elderly with irreducible fractures, considerable soft tissue injury, additional health issues and an owner or environment likely to place undesirable pressures on the repair technique. Techniques used must be strong and must be able to retain stability and integrity for extended periods. Pin–plate, bone lengthening plates, interlocking nails or more complex type 2 or 3 external fixators may be considered.

Conflicting scores across the categories

Where there is obvious discrepancy between categories the surgeon has to assess carefully the likely effect of each on healing. More emphasis is typically placed on the category with the low score. An immature patient (good biological score) with an irreducible fracture (poor mechanical score), or an elderly patient (poor biological score) with a reducible transverse fracture (good mechanical score) have conflicting criteria. The former requires a robust repair technique but which should be redundant within a relatively short period (e.g. pin and type 1 external skeletal fixator), whilst the latter will demand a technique that will remain stable and intact for a considerably longer period (e.g. bone plate or interlocking nail).

Forming a treatment plan

A treatment plan follows full clinical and radiographic evaluation of the patient. Repair technique decisions should not be delayed until fragments are exposed at surgery; neither should surgery be commenced with only one planned procedure. Complications may be encountered that will require modification of Plan A, or indeed a change to Plan B, C or D. Potential complicating factors or situations should be considered and management thereof planned for. At surgery, they should not be encountered unexpectedly but merely require application of an already prepared treatment plan.

Mental translation of the fracture pattern seen on two-dimensional radiographs into the three-dimensional intraoperative situation can be difficult. Images of the intact contralateral bone allow assessment of bone size (length, diameter, medullary diameter at various sites), but not necessarily relationship to fragment size and fracture lines.

Where radiographic film is used, all major fragments from both orthogonal views can be traced on to separate sheets of clear acetate to allow reconstruction of the bone. Having done so, implant templates can then be used to ascertain the size and number of implants required. Care should be taken to ensure implants do not interfere with each other and that fissure lines and proximity of adjacent joint surfaces are considered. A similar technique can be applied to digital radiographs using appropriate software, though care must be taken to account for any magnification. Although not likely to be available to many at present, three-dimensional reconstruction of digital imaging information can improve accuracy in determining implant size, position and direction.

When planning repair, attention must be paid to the relative importance of biological and mechanical aspects of repair and healing (application of the FPAS). This is especially relevant when deciding whether to reconstruct a fracture or whether to apply bridging fixation across a more comminuted fracture; the surgeon must consider whether any mechanical advantage of reconstruction outweighs the biological disadvantage of fragment manipulation, or *vice versa*.

Accurate reduction and stable fixation of all fragments produces a construct that will, to a large extent, protect implants. However, if this is to the detriment of the blood supply and soft tissue envelope, healing time will be increased considerably and, therefore, the risk of late-stage implant failure will be increased. Conversely, failure to adequately control strains and stresses that might reasonably be anticipated could result in premature implant failure at a fracture site otherwise thought to have excellent biological healing potential.

The surgeon has some control over the mechanical properties of repair but has limited influence on biology, beyond attempting to mitigate any iatrogenic deterioration, and attempting to enhance it with the use of bone grafts. With simple fractures or those with a single large intermediate fragment, anatomical reconstruction of the fracture(s) can significantly improve stability with relatively little biological cost. Conversely, with more comminuted fractures, the mechanical gains from reconstruction are modest, whereas significant biological damage could be incurred by extensive fragment manipulation; these fractures are more appropriately managed using minimally invasive reduction and application of bridging fixation (see Chapter 8).

The relative pros and cons of the variety of fixation techniques being considered for repair (see Chapter 10) and of the multiplicity of implants available for each must be appreciated and understood when formulating a plan. Appropriate attention to all factors of the FPAS must be given. Failure of fracture fixation, even after the patient has been discharged, is likely to indicate that an inadequate assessment of mechanical, biological and clinical factors has been made and an inappropriate treatment plan selected.

PRACTICAL TIP

A careful, systematic approach to patient and fracture assessment and its application to produce a considered plan of management will minimize complications and maximize the chance of a successful outcome

---

Acknowledgements

The author would like to acknowledge the work of Ann Johnson, which has been important in producing the Fracture Patient Assessment Score.

References and further reading

Fossum TW (2013) *Small Animal Surgery Textbook, 4th edn*. Elsevier Mosby, Missouri

King LG and Boag A (2007) *BSAVA Manual of Canine and Feline Emergency and Critical Care, 2nd edn*. BSAVA Publications, Gloucester

Platt S and Olby N (2013) *BSAVA Manual of Canine and Feline Neurology, 4th edn*. BSAVA Publications, Gloucester

Chapter 8

Principles of fracture fixation

Rob Pettitt

It is now more than 100 years since Dr William Halsted devised a list of surgical principles to guide surgeons on improving their surgical technique, but they still remain valid today (Figure 8.1). Failure to apply these principles increases the risk of complications associated with any surgical procedure and thus risks poor outcomes; this applies as much to fracture surgery as any other operation. Alongside these principles, those proposed by the Arbeitsgemeinschaft für Osteosynthesefragen (AO) group were detailed in 1958 for fracture fixation (Figure 8.2). Their main intention was to implement effective and rational management of injured osseous and soft tissue structures to promote rapid restoration of function. These original aims were centred on restoration of anatomy and establishment of stability, whilst preserving the adjacent blood supply. In recent years there has been an appreciation of the benefits of less invasive approaches to fracture fixation, but the original AO principles are still valid in this evolving context.

Halsted's principles of surgery
• Atraumatic tissue handling
• Adequate haemostasis
• Strict aseptic technique
• Preservation of blood supply
• Elimination of dead space
• Accurate apposition of tissues
• Minimal tension on tissues

8.1 Halsted's principles of surgery.

AO principles of fracture fixation
• Accurate anatomical reduction
• Rigid stabilization appropriate to the requirements of the fracture
• Preservation of the blood supply to soft tissues and bone
• Early and safe mobilization of the limb and patient

8.2 AO principles of fracture fixation.

Aims of fracture surgery

The primary aims of fracture treatment are to alleviate pain, achieve fracture healing and restore function to as near normal a level as possible. Most fractures will eventually heal without surgery; however, the functional use of the limb may be severely impaired if the fractures are not treated appropriately, because of resultant poor limb alignment (malunion) or secondary soft tissue contractures.

With most diaphyseal fractures the patient can be expected to return to full function, whereas those with articular fractures are predisposed to the development of osteoarthritis which may lead to poor function in the long term (Anderson *et al.*, 1990). Animals presented with appendicular fractures often have other soft tissue injuries that may be urgent or life-threatening. Animals should be thoroughly assessed for signs of other injuries, such as thoracic or abdominal trauma or shock. Once the patient is haemodynamically stable, a careful examination of the whole animal is essential to avoid overlooking more subtle lesions (see Chapter 7). High quality radiographs can then be obtained to allow precise characterization of the fracture. Information from the history, clinical assessment, laboratory results and radiographs is then assessed to allow a rational plan for management of the case to be formulated (see Chapter 7).

Importance of the soft tissue envelope

In long bones the vascular supply is derived predominantly from the diaphyseal nutrient artery, which enters at the nutrient foramen and divides into ascending and descending branches. These branches supply the axial two-thirds of the cortex and the medullary canal. Vessels from the periosteum supply the abaxial third of the cortex. Metaphyseal and epiphyseal arteries supply the ends of the long bones and the physes (in juvenile animals). The nutrient veins pursue the reverse course to the arteries and provide the efferent drainage from the bone marrow. However, the majority of the blood supply to the bone itself is not returned via the nutrient vein. After passing through capillary beds, the blood flows in a centrifugal fashion to the periosteal vessels and ultimately enters larger veins at the extremities of the bones adjacent to the articular surfaces. Following fracture of a bone, the nutrient vessels are inevitably disrupted, which results in a relatively hypoxic state (Brighton and Krebs, 1972). The intrinsic bone vasculature has a relatively poor ability to sustain the healing process; a temporary extraosseous supply derived from the surrounding soft tissue envelope is created and maintained until the primary supply is fully restored. Preservation of this extraosseous supply to the bone is critical for healing.

Surgical approaches, tissue handling and placement of implants have a significant effect on the integrity of the soft tissues, which will have already been significantly disrupted by the trauma. Elevation of the periosteum may occasionally be required to place a bone plate, especially in immature animals. Any periosteal elevation should be limited to the minimum area necessary to apply the plate, rather than wide margins to increase observation. Manipulation of intermediate fragments should be performed with great caution as this will disrupt their blood supply. In most cases there is no justification for using cerclage wires or suture material to hold the fragments in some form of apposition unless the intention is full reconstruction of the fracture.

Application of AO principles

Whilst the principles of the reduction of fragments and the application of implants to achieve stability seem obvious, both the AO and Halsted principles make particular reference to the preservation of the blood supply. The tendency of the surgeon is to elevate soft tissues from the bone to improve exposure and aid the visualization and reduction of the fracture; however, dissection must be minimized to avoid damaging the extraosseous vascular supply. During planning, the surgeon needs to consider whether to reconstruct a fracture or whether to leave intermediate fragments undisturbed and apply bridging fixation.

Simple fractures

As a general rule, simple fractures, or those with only one large intermediate fragment, are amenable to reconstruction without significant soft tissue trauma, and reconstruction can give significant mechanical advantages as load sharing between the implants and bone can be achieved. Whilst minimizing soft tissue trauma, the fracture is completely reduced and then rigidly stabilized using an appropriate fixation method such as plates, lag screws and cerclage wires (Figure 8.3). Provided the fracture gap is less than 0.1 mm and absolute stability is achieved, direct healing can occur (see Chapter 5). This takes longer than indirect healing, but the mechanical loading on the implant is reduced so the risk of implant failure is decreased. Furthermore, a smaller implant can be used; this is especially important in areas where soft tissue coverage is minimal, such as distal tibial fractures in cats. In addition, patients are generally very comfortable following accurate reconstruction and rigid stabilization of a fracture, and therefore early mobilization of the limb is possible, which reduces the risk of fracture disease (see Chapter 28).

Comminuted fractures

Experimental work and clinical trials in humans and dogs have concluded that with comminuted fractures, where fragment reduction can be difficult, **biological osteosynthesis** can offer significant reductions in surgical and healing times without increasing complication rates (Claes *et al.*, 1999; Horstman *et al.*, 2004; Guiot and Déjardin, 2011; Pozzi *et al.*, 2012). Using this approach, the AO principles of fracture treatment are still applied, but preservation of fracture biology is emphasized at the expense of individual fragment reduction.

In general, reconstruction is less desirable if there are more than one or two intermediate fragments. The mechanical advantages of reconstruction are modest,

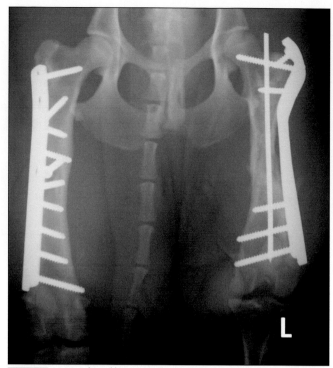

8.3 Ventrodorsal hip-extended radiograph of a dog with bilateral femoral fractures, stabilized 8 weeks earlier. The right femur had a simple oblique fracture which was reconstructed and stabilized using lag screws and a neutralization plate. This fracture healed directly with the resultant lack of callus. A more comminuted fracture was present on the left. This was reduced indirectly and stabilized using a pin and plate applied as bridging fixation. Secondary (callus) healing has occurred.

whereas the biological cost of manipulation tends to be greater as reduction is more challenging. Therefore, the biological cost of manipulation and reconstruction may outweigh any mechanical advantage; the net effect will be detrimental to healing. These non-reconstructable fractures are usually better treated using bridging fixation.

In these cases, indirect reduction is performed without direct manipulation at the fracture site. The principal proximal and distal fragments are aligned, restoring overall bone length and alignment of adjacent joints. Bridging fixation is applied across the fracture site. The haematoma, containing essential growth factors which initiate healing, should be left undisturbed; no attempt is made to manipulate intermediate fragments. Partial reconstruction will add little to the overall stability of the bone and should not be attempted. When reconstruction is not performed the implants will be required to bear proportionally more load in the early stages of fracture healing. Therefore, a stronger method of fixation should be selected (Figure 8.3). However, excessively rigid constructs should be avoided to optimize the strain environment at the fracture site (see Chapter 5).

The reduction of a comminuted fracture using an open approach whilst avoiding manipulation of intermediate fragments and the fracture site haematoma is termed 'open but do not touch'. In an attempt to further reduce biological disruption at the fracture site, **minimally invasive osteosynthesis** (MIO) has been developed (Perren, 2002). Fractures are reduced indirectly in a closed fashion, then applied through small incisions made away from the fracture site. MIO has been shown to reduce healing times and to minimize complications in humans, and has recently been applied successfully to small animal patients (see Chapter 15).

PRACTICAL TIP

For comminuted fractures, individual fragments should not be manipulated unless the mechanical advantage of manipulation and reconstruction outweighs the biological cost of the manipulation

In practice, biology and mechanics must be considered in all fracture patients, along with all other principles. For each fracture, the surgeon must decide how much emphasis to place on different principles, especially when balancing preservation of biology with fragment reconstruction.

Reduction of fractures

As previously mentioned, preservation of the soft tissue envelope is essential to maximize the potential for a successful outcome. When reducing fractures, the fragments should be firmly grasped using appropriate instrumentation and excessive soft tissue disruption avoided. Fractures attended to a few days after occurrence will be affected by muscle contraction; this will make fracture reduction harder and fatiguing these muscles will facilitate easier manipulation. Reduction can be achieved in a number of ways (see Chapter 11), but caution needs to be exercised to avoid worsening the fracture configuration during the reduction process, especially where fissures are present. The use of muscle relaxants to aid reduction of fractures has been described; however, clinically, these agents are rarely beneficial.

Once the fracture has been reduced it can be held in place using fragment forceps. Alternatively, a temporary Kirschner (K) wire can be placed across the fracture. This technique is sometimes more suitable than forceps as the K-wire is relatively small and is less likely to interfere with placement of definitive implants such as bone plates. The pin can then be removed once the fracture is stabilized with the definitive technique. Intramedullary pins can also be used to assist with temporary stabilization.

Decision making in fracture stabilization

WARNING

Most failures in orthopaedic surgery are due to poor decision making by the surgeon

There is now a bewildering plethora of implants and techniques available to the orthopaedic surgeon to manage fractures in cats and dogs (see Chapters 10 and 11). Many implants were designed for one specific purpose but can be adapted to fit other clinical situations. For most fractures, there are frequently multiple perfectly suitable ways to achieve stabilization. Experienced surgeons often have favoured techniques, which are usually based around previous successes, but to the novice orthopaedic surgeon the decision-making process is often daunting. A systematic approach to fracture assessment and planning is obligatory (see Chapter 7). It is always wise to have back-up plans when managing fractures in the event that the primary plan proves to be ineffective. For inexperienced surgeons, or for more complex fractures, referral to more experienced colleagues at the outset should be considered.

PRACTICAL TIP

The most effective and cheapest fracture repair is the one that is successful first time without complications

Asepsis

The act of implanting any foreign material, including orthopaedic implants, increases the risk of infection so strict attention must be paid to aseptic techniques. Predisposing factors to postoperative infections include:

- Avascular tissues
- Presence of foreign material
- Increased surgical times
- Loose implants
- Poor theatre practice
- Contamination from hair/skin of animal.

Ideally, a clean surgical environment is required for fracture surgery. A dedicated theatre suite for orthopaedic surgery is not practical in most first-opinion practices, but there are a few general measures that should be achieved.

- To minimize the risk of airborne bacterial contamination, the operating room should not have a general thoroughfare.
- All staff in the theatre should wear dedicated surgical clothing. Operating staff should wear sterile operating attire (e.g. gloves and gowns).
- The clipping and preparation of the animal should be performed outside theatre with a final scrub after transfer of the patient to the operating table.
- If required, placement of a purse-string suture and/or evacuation of the patient's bladder should be performed prior to transfer into theatre.
- Consideration should be given to the organization of the theatre; surgical checklists are very useful to ensure important aspects of theatre set-up are not overlooked (see Chapter 11).

Surgical equipment

All instruments should be sterilized; autoclave sterilization is generally suitable. Drills and other electrical devices (burrs and saws) may not be suitable for autoclave sterilization so alternative methods are necessary, such as gas sterilization by ethylene oxide. Covering a non-sterile device with a specific instrument surgical drape is another alternative (Figure 8.4); however, this is not an ideal compromise as contamination of the surgical site can occur (see Chapter 9). Instruments with sharp points should have the tips protected with small autoclavable plastic covers to prevent inadvertent penetration through the sterile bags. All instruments should be double wrapped. Large instruments, and some orthopaedic instrument sets, will not fit into a standard autoclave so some form of external sterilizing service may have to be sought. Sterilization of orthopaedic equipment by soaking in sterilizing solutions is not always effective and is not advisable (Rutala and Weber, 2008).

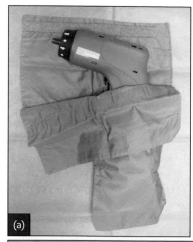

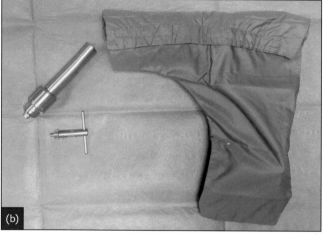

8.4 (a) Non-sterile orthopaedic drill inside a sterile drill shroud (a drape designed specifically for the instrument). (b) Sterile chuck and key prior to attachment to the drill inside the sterile drape.
(Courtesy of R Hewitt and H McCrorie)

Orthopaedic equipment should be kept in a dedicated store. This should not be overloaded or accidental damage to the sterilized instrument bags could occur. Instruments should be handed aseptically to the surgeon and placed on a fully draped trolley. The trolley should be sited close to the surgeon, ideally with no gap between trolley and surgical table.

Draping

A wide surgical margin should be clipped for all fracture surgeries. In practice, for most fractures, this usually means clipping the entire limb from the dorsal and ventral midline to just proximal to the paw. For fractures of the manus and pes, the clip should start proximal to the elbow or stifle joints respectively, and should be sufficiently distal to allow adequate draping. If necessary, complete clipping of the paw should be performed. The limb should be surgically scrubbed and prepared before the patient is moved to theatre. Before moving the patient, the scrubbed area should be covered with a sterile drape which is removed once the animal is positioned. A final preparation should be performed in theatre.

It is important to have an impermeable layer when draping, to prevent wicking of bacteria from underneath the drapes into the surgical site. Cloth drapes can be used as the primary layer but then a disposable impermeable layer should be used superficially. Alternatively, disposable drapes can be used for both layers. The limb should be draped in a four-quartered manner to allow all around access (Figure 8.5). The paw should be protected with a cohesive bandage; this is then further draped by the surgeon with a sterile impermeable layer and covered with

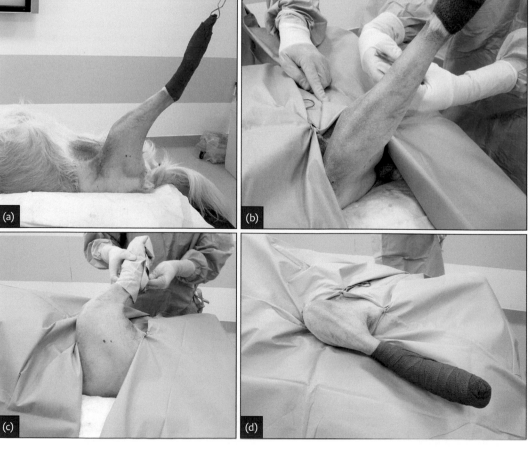

8.5 Four-quarter draping of the limb to allow all around access. (a) The paw is protected with a cohesive dressing and the limb is suspended. (b) After complete or partial four-quarter draping, (c) the paw can be grasped by the surgeon in an aseptic fashion using an impermeable drape. (d) A final layer of sterile cohesive bandage material is applied and the final quarter drape applied if this has not already been done.

a final layer of sterile cohesive bandage. It is advantageous to then apply a second large impermeable drape to cover the four-quarter draping (Figure 8.6). The use of adhesive incise drapes has not been demonstrated to significantly reduce contamination of the surgical wound in dogs undergoing ovariohysterectomy or stifle arthrotomy (Owen et al., 2009). However, adhesive drapes may have a place in procedures such as total joint replacement where any infection could lead to catastrophic complications. If adhesive drapes are used, iodine-impregnated drapes are preferred. They can be further attached to the edges of the surgical wound using staples or continuous sutures to prevent loss of adherence during surgery.

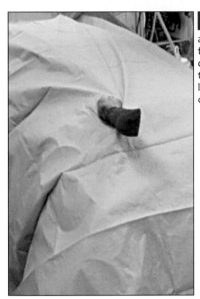

8.6 After four-quarter draping of the limb and draping of the paw, a further large impermeable drape can be placed to cover the entire surgical field. The limb is pulled through a hole cut in the drape.

Antibiotics

Antibiotics should not be used to justify poor aseptic technique, traumatic tissue handling or inadequate haemostasis. Most fractures are closed and so, at surgery, are classified as clean wounds. Reported infection rates for surgeries on clean wounds are 2–4.8% (Brown et al., 1997). Fracture surgeries justify the use of perioperative antibiotics because they tend to be prolonged, tissues are often traumatized and implants are placed during the surgery. These all result in a reduction in the host's defence mechanisms and increase the risk of infection. The use of perioperative antibiotics for orthopaedic procedures has been shown to be beneficial clinically (Whittem et al., 1999), but postoperative antibiotic therapy is more controversial. It may be more justifiable in those patients that have an increased risk of infection due to concomitant disease (e.g. hyperadrenocorticism), or in those cases where the risk of infection could be catastrophic, such as joint replacements. For general orthopaedic surgery the evidence supporting the use of prophylactic postoperative antibiotics is poor. The current recommendation is that postoperative antibiotics are not required in most elective orthopaedic cases, unless a breakdown of asepsis is noted at surgery. However, Fitzpatrick and Solano (2010) evaluated 1000 consecutive tibial plateau levelling osteotomy (TPLO) surgeries and found a significant reduction in infection rates in patients prescribed 14 days of post-operative antibiotics. Another recent prospective study of 93 dogs undergoing routine plate application

demonstrated a protective benefit from a 7-day course of antibiotics (either cephalosporin or potentiated amoxicillin) compared to no antibiotics at all (Pratesi et al., 2012). Further work is needed to confirm these findings in other groups of patients, but these studies suggest there may be an indication for prophylactic postoperative antibiotics for some small animal orthopaedic surgeries.

It is important that the clinician chooses appropriate antibiotics based on the likely infectious agents and ensures the drug will be present at the surgical site before the first incision. The most common source of contamination is from the patient's skin; expected bacteria are likely to be Gram-positive commensals, especially *Staphylococcus* species. When selecting an antibiotic it is important to consider a number of factors:

- Spectrum of activity – a wide spectrum is preferable
- Pharmacokinetics of the drug
- Availability
- Route of administration – intravenous is preferred for perioperative use
- Toxicity
- Compliance with the cascade system for prescribing non-licensed drugs.

Beta-lactam groups of antibiotics such as cephalosporins (e.g. cefuroxime) and potentiated amoxicillin are the most appropriate. The aim is to have maximum concentrations at the surgical site for the duration of surgery, so the drug should be administered intravenously 30–60 minutes before the first incision (Weese and Halling, 2006) and repeated every 90–120 minutes throughout surgery. Doses are 10–15 mg/kg for cephalosporins and 20 mg/kg for potentiated amoxicillin. The variable rate of uptake into the plasma that occurs with depot preparations makes these unsuitable for perioperative use. The continuation of antibiotics post-surgery, if required, should utilize a drug of a similar class to that given during surgery. If a surgical site infection is present, a sample should be taken for bacteriological culture and sensitivity immediately before commencing broad-spectrum antibiotics as described above. The therapy should be tailored depending upon the results of the culture. In the absence of culture results, administration of multiple antibiotics should be avoided as this will select for resistant bacterial populations.

Analgesia

Fractures are inherently painful and appropriate analgesia before, during and following surgery is essential. A balanced multimodal approach is preferable.

Stabilization of the fracture will significantly reduce the associated pain. Distal limb fractures (below the elbow and stifle) are very amenable to a well applied bandage, which can be utilized prior to any surgery. For fractures of the humerus or femur, there is a risk a bandage may slip below the fracture site and increase instability by acting as a pendulum; this could increase discomfort and soft tissue trauma. Therefore, for most proximal limb fractures, bandaging is not routinely recommended.

Perioperative phase

Pain should be managed with a licensed mu opioid agonist analgesic such as methadone or pethidine (see the *BSAVA Manual of Canine and Feline Anaesthesia and Analgesia*).

If these are not available then other mu opioid agonists, such as morphine, can be considered. Partial opioid agonists, such as buprenorphine, are less suitable for perioperative use in fracture patients. Studies have shown that methadone is superior to buprenorphine in dogs undergoing orthopaedic surgeries (Hunt *et al.*, 2013); in cats it has been shown that both methadone and morphine are suitable analgesics (Steagall *et al.*, 2006). Partial agonists will competitively inhibit the action of pure agonists. For further information readers are directed to the *BSAVA Manual of Canine and Feline Anaesthesia and Analgesia*.

Non-steroidal anti-inflammatory drugs (NSAIDs) should be incorporated into a balanced approach to analgesia provided there is no pre-existing renal impairment or intolerance to the medication. Care should be taken in the perioperative period as anaesthesia may result in a decrease in blood pressure. Supportive treatments, such as intravenous fluid therapy, will help maintain blood pressure and reduce the risks associated with decreased renal perfusion. There are a multitude of NSAIDs available for dogs. At the time of publication only three NSAIDs are licensed in cats, one of which (meloxicam) is licensed for long-term use.

In patients with unremitting pain who fail to respond to routine analgesia, other adjunctive techniques using drugs of different analgesic classes can be considered, for example constant rate intravenous infusions of morphine-lidocaine-ketamine or medetomidine. Longer-acting preparations, such as transdermal fentanyl patches or solution, are also available. Finally, perioperative local analgesia in the form of epidurals and nerve blocks can be very effective (see the *BSAVA Manual of Canine and Feline Anaesthesia and Analgesia*).

Postoperative phase

Opioid analgesia should be continued for as long as necessary post-surgery. A flexible, pre-emptive approach to analgesia should be adopted, with regular examinations to assess the efficacy of the pain management. There are various pain scoring systems available (e.g. the Glasgow Composite Pain Score, www.gla.ac.uk) that offer clinicians a reliable, albeit somewhat subjective, assessment of their patients. Patients should not be discharged until they are comfortable and adequate analgesia can be provided using oral medication only.

NSAIDs are generally continued in the immediate postoperative period. It is well documented that NSAIDs can prevent heterotrophic ossification in humans but controversy remains regarding the clinical effects of NSAIDs on fracture healing. Only a handful of prospective studies exist in humans and most show no effect (Barry, 2010). Research using rodents and rabbits has indicated that NSAIDs can negatively affect bone healing but whether these effects are clinically significant in dogs and cats remains controversial and unproven. It should be borne in mind that early patient mobilization is facilitated by appropriate analgesia, and the benefits of mobilization are likely to outweigh any hypothetical negative effects of NSAIDs on bone healing.

NSAIDs can be supplemented with other analgesics, although their use may be off license. In dogs, the author's preference is to add a short course of paracetamol and codeine (Pardale-V®) at a paracetamol dose of 10 mg/kg twice daily. Paracetamol should never be used in cats due to its high toxicity in this species. Tramadol is popular amongst veterinary surgeons (veterinarians) although there is little evidence of its efficacy and the drug is not licensed for use in dogs or cats in the United Kingdom. Tramadol itself is metabolized into eight substrates of which only one is active in the dog, and that is only for a short (1- to 2-hour) period.

The duration of postoperative analgesia required is case-dependent, but in most patients should not be more than 2 to 4 weeks. Animals exhibiting significant signs of pain beyond this timeframe should be carefully reassessed.

Open fractures

Open fractures vary in their severity and can represent true orthopaedic emergencies. Consideration must be given to immediate emergency treatment, management of the wound and management of the fracture itself. The surgeon must be aware of the intricate interactions between management of the wound and the fracture. Further details on the management of open fractures are given in Chapter 12.

Articular fractures

Unlike diaphyseal fractures, where restoration of limb length and alignment of adjacent joints are the important factors, articular fractures need careful anatomical reconstruction and rigid internal fixation. Care needs to be taken to align the joint surface as accurately as possible. Step malalignment of the articular surface can be especially detrimental and can lead to severe post-traumatic osteoarthritis. However, even with accurately aligned articular fractures, osteoarthritis is an inevitable sequel in many cases (Gordon *et al.*, 2003). The prognosis for a return to normal function for most articular fractures is good in the short term at least, but osteoarthritis will progress in the long term. The clinical effect of this can vary depending upon the affected joint but will often require long-term medical management. If osteoarthritis is especially severe, salvage surgical procedures such as arthrodesis or total joint replacements can be considered at a later date (see the *BSAVA Manual of Canine and Feline Musculoskeletal Disorders*).

For some articular fractures, acute reduction and stabilization is not possible and an alternative treatment technique is required. For small chip fractures fragment excision may be appropriate. Non-reconstructable or chronic fractures of the articular surfaces may require early arthrodesis rather than an attempt at primary repair, such as radiocarpal bone fractures in Boxers (Li *et al.*, 2000).

In certain cases, such as non-reconstructable comminuted acetabular fractures, it may be appropriate to manage conservatively in the first instance. If lameness persists in these cases, salvage surgery, such as total hip replacement or femoral head and neck excision, can be considered in the future.

Fractures in juvenile animals

Fractures in skeletally immature animals present unique challenges to the surgeon, because the bone is in a state of growth. Fractures in juveniles heal rapidly and so non-unions are very uncommon; conversely, malunions are more likely if prompt intervention is not performed. The production of excessive callus is common, which allows for rapid healing, but may make implant removal more challenging. In contrast to fractures in skeletally mature animals, diaphyseal fractures in juvenile patients are commonly minimally displaced and often caused by relatively low impact trauma. The periosteum in the growing animal is much thicker and stronger so has a tendency to partially stabilize these fractures, which allows for a more conservative approach to treatment in many cases. The other important feature of juvenile bones is the presence of physes (growth plates) (Figure 8.7). These are relatively weak sections in the bone and fractures through the physes (termed Salter–Harris fractures) are common.

Bone	Average closure time (months)	
	Dog	Cat
Scapula: • Tuber scapulae	6	4
Hemipelvis: • Multiple junction (acetabulum) • Tuber ischia (secondary)	3.6 10	– –
Femur: • Femoral head • Greater trochanter • Distal	10.5 10.5 11	8 7.5 15
Fibula: • Proximal • Distal	10 9.5	13 12
Humerus: • Proximal • Lateral/medial condyle • Lateral epicondyle	12.5 6 7	21 3 3
Metacarpals/tarsals: • Distal epiphysis II–V	7	9
Phalanges: • Proximal II–V	6	4.5
Radius: • Proximal • Distal	8.5 10.5	7 16.5
Tibia: • Proximal • Tibial crest • Distal • Medial malleolus	11 8 10.5 4.5	15 15 10.5 –
Ulna: • Proximal • Distal	10 8.5	10 18
Carpus: • Carpal bones • Accessory	3.5 4.5	– 4
Tarsus: • Tarsal bones • Fibular tarsal	5 3	– 9
Skull: • Individual bones, formed by intramembranous ossification, are joined at birth by fibrous sutures. These remain functionally open until 11–14 months of age, after which they may become fused by calcification		
Vertebrae: • The primary centres have fused to form a complete neural arch at birth. The epiphyseal plates stay open for varying periods up to 11 months		

8.7 Average time of radiographic growth plate closure in the dog and cat. There is considerable variation in these times between different breeds and sizes of animals.

Special considerations for juvenile patients

With all fractures a prompt and accurate assessment is essential in order to maximize outcomes. In juveniles this is even more important as the extremely rapid healing process means that reduction of fractures can be very challenging after only a few days. Radiographic interpretation is often complicated by the presence of the growth plates and incompletely calcified bones, combined with the potential for minimally displaced fractures.

The periosteum can allow increased stability of a fracture as well as restricting the displacement of any fragments. It is, however, very easily stripped from the bone so care must be taken when manipulating bone fragments during surgery. This has to be balanced against breaking down any callus already produced in order to accurately reduce the fracture. To avoid excessive soft tissue dissection, or when attempting closed reduction, an imperfect reduction may be more acceptable for diaphyseal fractures as long as limb length and appropriate alignment of adjacent joints are acceptable.

Bone healing is rapid, and the generally smaller size of the juvenile patient mean that relatively less robust fixation is required. In addition, juvenile bones have been hypothesized to be prone to stress protection osteopenia, therefore less rigid implants may be preferable (Cabassu, 2001), although this needs to be appreciated in the context of the fracture (e.g. an articular fracture will always benefit from a rigid method of stabilization). The converse, however, is that the bone is often softer so less resistant to implants pulling out, and careful consideration should be given to implant selection; cancellous screws may be preferable to cortical screws in some patients. It should also be borne in mind that younger patients are often more active and can be difficult to confine in the postoperative period.

The growing skeleton of juvenile animals has a relatively high demand for calcium and animals that are in a poor state of nutrition may have a relative deficiency. Secondary hyperparathyroidism due to poor nutrition, and less commonly renal disease, may result in multiple folding fractures as a result of a poorly mineralized skeleton (Figure 8.8). These pathological fractures are usually managed conservatively unless significant displacement has occurred (see Chapter 13).

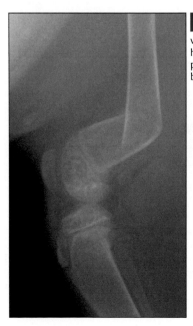

8.8 A folding fracture of the femur in a cat with nutritional secondary hyperparathyroidism. Note the poor definition between the bone and soft tissues.

Non-displaced fractures of the distal limb may be more amenable to non-surgical management using casts or splints (see Chapter 16), especially if the periosteum remains intact. However, managing casts in juveniles may be challenging; repeated cast changes are often necessary and can prove expensive. These fractures can often be managed effectively with a type 1a external skeletal fixation (ESF) construct. Internal fixation is often unnecessary for these fractures and can necessitate excessive periosteal disruption to apply the implants.

Traction epiphyseal fractures

Muscles often insert on small tuberosities of bone adjacent to physes. Avulsion fractures of these tuberosities are common and occur as a direct result of the traction forces applied by tendons at their insertions. This is because the cartilage layer is relatively weak compared to the stronger attachment of the musculotendinous unit to the adjacent apophysis. There are a number of sites where avulsion fractures are encountered (Figure 8.9); the most common are the tibial tuberosity (see Chapter 24) and the greater trochanter (see Chapter 23). The challenge with these fractures is to neutralize the large avulsion forces acting on relatively small pieces of bone. Surgical intervention is necessary in most cases unless there is only mild displacement, but the small fragments make implant placement difficult. The fragments are usually stabilized with a tension-band technique (see Chapter 11).

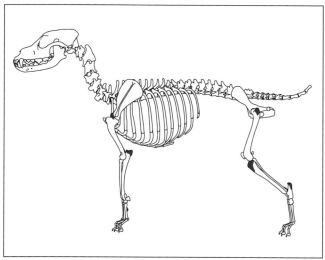

Location of the common sites of avulsion fractures at traction epiphyses.

Salter–Harris (growth plate) fractures

There are six categories of Salter–Harris fractures (see Chapter 2); these are used for classification but, in contrast to humans, have no known prognostic value in small animals. In reality, careful monitoring of these fractures post-healing is needed as the majority of these growth plates are damaged at the time of the original injury resulting in premature complete or partial closure.

Premature closure can result in loss of bone growth. For single non-paired bones, such as the humerus and femur, compensatory overgrowth from the physis at the opposite end of the affected bone may be sufficient to prevent a significant shortening of the limb. Premature closure of distal limb physes has also been shown to

induce a relative overgrowth of the more proximal bones in the same limb (Clements *et al.*, 2004), again helping to maintain overall limb length. Compensatory mechanisms, such as a relative flexion or extension of the joints, may also help to minimize the clinical effect of any shortening. In paired bones, or cases of partial physeal closure, angular deformities may occur; these can have a more clinically significant effect. For paired bones, such as the radius and ulna, the non-affected bone attempts to grow normally but this growth is restricted asymmetrically by the prematurely retarded bone. This results in a deviation of the limb. For the tibia and fibula this is less marked than the antebrachium as the amount of growth is approximately equal from the physes at either end of the crus. In the antebrachium, 85% of the growth of the ulna comes from the distal growth plate so premature closure of this physis can be very significant, especially in very young patients where there is a significant amount of potential growth remaining. The conical shape of the distal ulnar growth plate is unique (Figure 8.10); laterally applied forces, which result in a shear force across other physes, are readily converted to compressive forces resulting in damage to the germinal layer and predisposing it to premature closure (a Salter–Harris type V injury). For fractures of the distal radius and ulna, premature closure of the distal ulnar growth plate is common even if radiographically the fracture does not appear to involve the physis. The clinician needs to monitor such patients carefully post-surgery and it is always prudent to warn owners from the outset of the risk of a deformity.

In addition to the considerations for juvenile diaphyseal fractures previously described, a number of additional considerations apply for physeal fractures. Surgical intervention is usually indicated but the epiphyseal fragment must be very carefully manipulated in order to preserve the germinal layer in the physis. Various stabilization techniques can be employed. Historically, Rush pins were

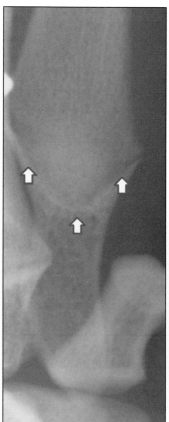

Craniocaudal radiograph of the distal ulna in a dog showing the unique conical shape of the physis (arrowed). Lateral forces applied to the ulna result in compression of the physis which can lead to damage to the germinal chondrocytes (a Salter–Harris type V injury).

thought to allow continued longitudinal bone growth whilst offering sufficient stabilization for the fracture to heal. In addition, recommendations were often made to remove implants early enough to allow physeal growth to continue. However, in practice, continued growth rarely occurs because the physis usually closes secondary to the original trauma or the stability of the fixation applied. The potential for remaining growth is determined by the age of the animal in relation to the anticipated time for normal physeal closure (see Figure 8.7).

Physeal fractures involving the articular surface should be managed as described previously; accurate articular surface reconstruction and rigid fixation are mandatory in these cases.

Postoperative management of fracture patients

Postoperative management is guided by the same factors that are considered during the preoperative decision-making process and thus must be considered on an individual basis. Analgesia and antibiotic therapy have been described earlier in this section, and specific recommendations are made at the end of each operative techniques section.

Following surgery of the distal limb, an appropriately placed modified Robert Jones bandage can be used to minimize postoperative swelling and soiling of the surgical site and to provide support. The wound itself should be covered with a light protective dressing immediately following surgery. The bandage should be maintained until any significant postoperative swelling has subsided; this can range from 2–3 days up to 1–2 weeks in some cases. Bandages are not generally helpful for fractures proximal to the elbow or stifle.

Animals should be hospitalized until any pain is under control and manageable with oral medication. Most patients should be weight-bearing within a few days; if not, then it may be necessary to repeat radiographs to check for implant failure. In some cases it can be helpful to place a sling under the thorax or abdomen to assist with ambulation. The patient does not always need to be fully supported by this sling; rather it is there to prevent any slipping which might overload the fixation.

Management at home is case-dependent but some general rules apply. For dogs, exercise should be restricted to short lead walks. The duration of these can be gradually increased depending on clinical progress, but unrestricted activity should be avoided. In between walks, the management is dependent upon the nature of the patient. Cage rest is prudent if the animal will tolerate it; if cage rest is not possible then the patient should be kept in as small an area as is practical and prevented from undertaking vigorous activities. Feline patients are best managed by cage confinement. If an external skeletal fixator has been applied, caution is needed to prevent entanglement of the cage and the frame.

Physiotherapy is an essential part of the postoperative rehabilitation in humans. The evidence for the benefit of canine physiotherapy is less clear, with little objective evidence to support its use, although it is an evolving field. Readers are referred to the *BSAVA Manual of Canine and Feline Rehabilitation, Supportive and Palliative Care* for further information.

If external coaptation has been applied then owners need to be carefully briefed regarding its care. Limbs can be comfortably maintained in a cast for 4–6 weeks if necessary but the cast will need regular monitoring and changing during this period. It is advisable that owners are given clear instruction for daily checks, and weekly checks should be performed by a veterinary surgeon. Complications due to an incorrectly placed or maintained cast can progress rapidly and early intervention is essential in order to prevent catastrophic consequences (Anderson and White, 2000).

Postoperative follow-up radiography should be obtained at an appropriate time after surgery. The exact timing of this will vary according to the age of the patient and the type of fracture, but would typically be between 3 to 4 weeks following surgery for juvenile patients and 6 to 8 weeks following surgery for skeletally mature patients (see Chapter 6). As a rule, radiographs should be obtained when the results of imaging will influence clinical management of the case. The purpose of these radiographs is to document implant stability and healing of the fracture thereby allowing an increase in exercise and, if appropriate, removal of any implants.

References and further reading

Anderson DM and White RAS (2000) Ischemic bandage injuries: a case series and review of the literature. *Veterinary Surgery* **29**, 488–498

Anderson TJ, Carmichael S and Miller A (1990) Intercondylar humeral fracture in the dog – a review of 20 cases. *Journal of Small Animal Practice* **31**, 437–442

Barry S (2010) Non-steroidal anti-inflammatory drugs inhibit bone healing: a review. *Veterinary and Comparative Orthopaedics and Traumatology* **23**, 385–392

Borrelli J, Prickett W, Song E, Becker D and Ricci W (2002) Extraosseous blood supply of the tibia and the effects of different plating techniques: a human cadaveric study. *Journal of Orthopaedic Trauma* **16**, 691–695

Brighton CT and Krebs AG (1972) Oxygen tension of healing fractures in the rabbit. *Journal of Bone and Joint Surgery (American Volume)* **54A**, 323–332

Brown DC, Conzemius MG, Shofer F and Swann H (1997) Epidemiologic evaluation of postoperative wound infections in dogs and cats. *Journal of the American Veterinary Medical Association* **210**, 1302–1306

Cabassu JP (2001) Elastic plate osteosynthesis of femoral shaft fractures in young dogs. *Veterinary and Comparative Orthopaedics and Traumatology* **14**, 40–45

Claes L, Heitemeyer U, Krischak G, Braun H and Hierholzer G (1999) Fixation technique influences osteogenesis of comminuted fractures. *Clinical Orthopaedics and Related Research* **365**, 221–229

Clements DN, Gemmill TJ, Clarke SP, Bennett D and Carmichael S (2004) Compensatory humeral overgrowth associated with antebrachial shortening in six dogs. *Veterinary Record* **154**, 531–532

Farouk O, Krettek C, Miclau T, Schandelmaier P and Tscherne H (1998) Effects of percutaneous and conventional plating techniques on the blood supply to the femur. *Archives of Orthopaedic and Trauma Surgery* **117**, 438–441

Field JR and Tornkvist H (2001) Biological fracture fixation: a perspective. *Veterinary and Comparative Orthopaedics and Traumatology* **14**, 169–178

Fitzpatrick N and Solano MA (2010) Predictive variables for complications after TPLO with stifle inspection by arthrotomy in 1000 consecutive dogs. *Veterinary Surgery* **39**, 460–474

Gordon WJ, Besancon MF, Conzemius MG et al. (2003) Frequency of post-traumatic osteoarthritis in dogs after repair of a humeral condylar fracture. *Veterinary and Comparative Orthopaedics and Traumatology* **16**, 1–5

Guiot LP and Déjardin LM (2011) Prospective evaluation of minimally invasive plate osteosynthesis in 36 nonarticular tibial fractures in dogs and cats. *Veterinary Surgery* **40**, 171–182

Horstman CL, Beale BS, Conzemius MG and Evans R (2004) Biological osteosynthesis *versus* traditional anatomic reconstruction of 20 long-bone fractures using an interlocking nail: 1994–2001. *Veterinary Surgery* **33**, 232–237

Houlton J, Cook J, Innes J and Langley-Hobbs S (2006) *BSAVA Manual of Canine and Feline Musculoskeletal Disorders*. BSAVA Publications, Gloucester

Hunt JR, Attenburrow PM, Slingsby LS and Murrell JC (2013) Comparison of premedication with buprenorphine or methadone with meloxicam for postoperative analgesia in dogs undergoing orthopaedic surgery. *Journal of Small Animal Practice* **54**, 418–424

Li A, Bennett D, Gibbs C et al. (2000) Radial carpal bone fractures in 15 dogs. *Journal of Small Animal Practice* **41**, 74–79

Lindley S and Watson P (2010) *BSAVA Manual of Canine and Feline Rehabilitation, Supportive and Palliative Care: Case Studies in Patient Management*. BSAVA Publications, Gloucester

Owen LJ, Gines JA, Knowles TG and Holt PE (2009) Efficacy of adhesive incise drapes in preventing bacterial contamination of clean canine surgical wounds. *Veterinary Surgery* **38**, 732–737

Perren SM (2002) Evolution of the internal fixation of long bone fractures - the scientific basis of biological internal fixation: Choosing a new balance between stability and biology. *Journal of Bone and Joint Surgery (British Volume)* **84B**, 1093–1110

Pozzi A, Risselada M and Winter MD (2012) Assessment of fracture healing after minimally invasive plate osteosynthesis or open reduction and internal fixation of coexisting radius and ulna fractures in dogs via ultrasonography and radiography. *Journal of the American Veterinary Medical Association* **241**, 744–753

Pratesi A, Grierson J, Downes C and Moores AP (2012) Long term results of the efficacy of postoperative antibiotic prophylaxis in clean orthopaedic surgery: a prospective randomised study in 93 dogs. *Veterinary Surgery* **41**, E7

Rutala W and Weber D (2008) *Guideline for disinfection and sterilization in healthcare facilities.* Centers for Disease Control and Prevention, Augusta

Seymour C and Duke-Novakovski T (2007) *BSAVA Manual of Canine and Feline Anaesthesia and Analgesia, 2nd edn.* BSAVA Publications, Gloucester

Steagall PVM, Carnicelli P, Taylor PM *et al.* (2006) Effects of subcutaneous methadone, morphine, buprenorphine or saline on thermal and pressure thresholds in cats. *Journal of Veterinary Pharmacology and Therapeutics* **29**, 531–537

Weese JS and Halling KB (2006) Perioperative administration of antimicrobials associated with elective surgery for cranial cruciate ligament rupture in dogs: 83 cases (2003–2005). *Journal of the American Veterinary Medical Association* **229**, 92–95

Whittem TL, Johnson AL, Smith CW *et al.* (1999) Effect of perioperative prophylactic antimicrobial treatment in dogs undergoing elective orthopedic surgery. *Journal of the American Veterinary Medical Association* **215**, 212–216

Chapter 9

Orthopaedic instrumentation

Jonathan Pink

Surgical instruments made from a variety of metals, including copper, bronze and brass, date back at least as far as ancient Greek civilization. The addition of carbon to iron to produce steel resulted in alloys that could be hardened, and these were used by the Romans to manufacture surgical instruments (Milne, 1907). Whilst steel manufacture developed substantially during the 19th century, corrosion became less problematic after the discovery of stainless steel in the early 20th century. The first power drills and saws were introduced towards the end of the 19th century and sterilizable pneumatic instruments and, more recently, electrically powered instruments have become widely used over the last 40–50 years.

Materials

'Stainless steel' refers to a family of steels that contain at least 10.5% chromium (Cobb, 2010). The chromium produces a very thin boundary or passive layer that resists corrosion and is self-repairing by oxidation if the metal is abraded during use. Depending on its microscopic structure, stainless steels may be defined as being martensitic, austenitic, ferritic or duplex. These are subdivided into different grades depending on the proportions of different elements such as iron, carbon, chromium, nickel, copper, manganese, sulphur, silicon and molybdenum. Whilst a number of different classification systems exist, grades are commonly referred to according to their ISO (International Organization for Standardization) numbers or AISI (American Iron and Steel Institute) grades. In contrast to surgical implants, which must sustain long-term exposure to a warm saline environment and for which specific surgical forms of AISI 316 austenitic steel are used, most surgical instruments are manufactured from commercial AISI 420 martensitic steel, which can be hardened and tempered by heat treatment to create the specific mechanical properties required (Newson, 2002).

While the majority of surgical instruments are manufactured from stainless steel, other materials may be used. Tungsten carbide inserts may be soldered or welded to stainless steel to increase the durability of forceps and cutting instruments. Soldered (unlike welded) inserts can be replaced when worn. Aluminium, being malleable, is used for templating guides to aid bone plate contouring; in addition, its light weight makes it appropriate for some instrument parts and cases. Screwdriver and tap handles are often made from phenolics.

Instrument manufacture

The first stage of instrument manufacture involves the production of blanks from stainless steel bar stock which is heated to a high temperature and shaped under pressure, although some components are shaped from cold stock. The blanks are milled to refine their basic shape and the components are then assembled and ground to their final form. For high-quality instruments, this is a skilled process and is performed by hand. The instrument is then tempered to create the physical properties required. Tempering involves heating the instrument to a high temperature followed by rapid cooling until the instrument reaches the correct hardness (measured in Rockwell hardness or HR scales). Too hard an instrument will be brittle and may break too easily, while too soft an instrument will deform or lose its cutting edge prematurely. The final stage of manufacture involves removal of any undesirable sharp edges, sharpening of cutting edges and adjustment of blades and locks before final polishing. Instruments may be left with a highly polished or, alternatively, a matt finish if avoidance of glare is important.

Orthopaedic instrumentation

Basic surgical instrumentation is described in the *BSAVA Manual of Canine and Feline Surgical Principles*. Whilst most orthopaedic instruments are only used for specific types of procedure, periosteal elevators are used routinely and should be added to the basic surgical kit.

Retractors

Surgical retractors can be self-retaining or hand-held. Hand-held retractors can have smooth blades or a sharp rake or claw and can be single- or double-ended (Figure 9.1). Hand-held retractors obviously necessitate a scrubbed assistant, and they are particularly useful for careful retraction of vulnerable tissues, such as retraction of the biceps femoris muscle to expose the proximal femur whilst minimizing the risk of trauma to the sciatic nerve.

Self-retaining retractors for orthopaedic surgery usually have a ratchet lock and are available with either single tips, as with the Gelpi, or an array of rake tips (West or Weitlaner). Tips may be either sharp or blunt; sharp tips are less likely to slip if embedded in collagenous tissue such as joint capsule, whilst blunt tips are less likely to traumatize muscle and blood vessels. Care must always be taken to ensure that the retractors do not exert pressure directly on to nerves or blood vessels. A selection of Gelpi retractors offers versatility for most orthopaedic procedures. Gelpi retractors are available in a variety of sizes (mini, small and standard) and with varying limb length depending on the depth of tissue to be retracted (Figure 9.2).

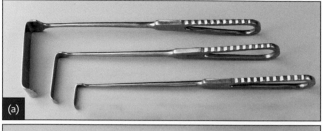

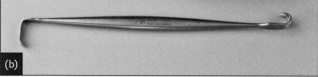

9.1 (a) Large, medium and small Langenbeck retractors. (b) Senn retractor with a sharp claw at one end and a smooth blade at the other.

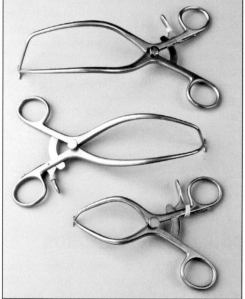

9.2 Gelpi retractors.

Periosteal elevators

Periosteal elevators are designed to separate muscle from bone either by elevation of the periosteum, or by severing muscle fibres at their attachment to bone. It is important that the sharp edge of the elevator is used in the direction of the acute angle between the muscle fibres and bone to minimize soft tissue trauma. There are many different designs of elevator, but the Arbeitsgemeinschaft für Osteosynthesefragen (AO) design is a good general purpose elevator for use in most sizes of dog and the Freer elevator is a finer instrument that is useful for cats, toy breed dogs or for more delicate dissection (Figure 9.3).

Power tools

An ever-increasing range of power tools is available for performing a range of drilling and cutting tasks. Whilst

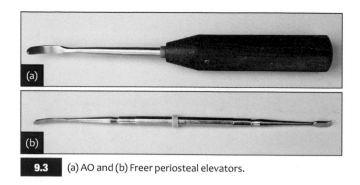

9.3 (a) AO and (b) Freer periosteal elevators.

top-of-the-range power tools from the human orthopaedic market are inevitably expensive to purchase, second-hand reconditioned ex-hospital equipment or even modified construction tools can offer a cheaper alternative.

Drills

Any attempt at surgical fracture management, with the exception perhaps of pin and cerclage techniques, will necessitate an orthopaedic drill. Whilst hand drills were originally used, a power drill is faster and causes less 'wobble', which enlarges the hole and reduces implant security. Power drills may be pneumatic or electrically powered with corded and battery options available. Pneumatic drills are robust and easy to control, although they are constrained by the air hose and require a regulated medical air source. Unless the air driving the turbine is exhausted remotely from the hand piece, a sterile air supply should be used. Pneumatic drills and hoses can be autoclaved.

Electrically powered drills tend to operate at higher speed than pneumatic units (3000–4000 rpm compared to 900–1000 rpm). Corded micromotor electric drills have small low-voltage motors in the hand piece and so only require thin power leads. Whilst they operate at high speed and have good torque levels, they have largely been superseded by battery units. Surgical drill batteries tend to use nickel cadmium (NiCad) or occasionally nickel metal hydride (NiMh) or lithium ion (Li-ion) chemistry. Nickel cadmium and nickel metal hydride batteries are prone to memory effect (the reduction in usable capacity resulting from repeated recharging before the battery is fully discharged). Careful adherence to the manufacturer's recommendations is therefore necessary to maximize the useful life of the batteries; a drill where the battery has poor capacity and loses power during surgery is far from ideal. Whilst the hand pieces (but *not* the batteries) of modern battery drills can be autoclaved, older battery or corded units may require gas sterilization.

The cheapest option is to use a modified construction drill. Several companies providing veterinary orthopaedic equipment offer a 7.2V NiCad Makita® drill that has had its original chuck replaced with a long stainless steel surgical chuck (Figure 9.4). This is a relatively low-speed drill (maximum 600 rpm) that has a far higher torque than other drills designed specifically for surgical use. It is also more bulky and cumbersome than dedicated surgical units, but nonetheless offers an affordable entry option for veterinary orthopaedics. These drills do not survive autoclaving and therefore must be either gas sterilized or covered with a sterile shroud; the surgeon should be aware that use of a shroud carries a risk of strike-through. In addition, ethylene oxide may not penetrate the lubricants used inside the drill and, since cooling of the drill relies on a flow of air

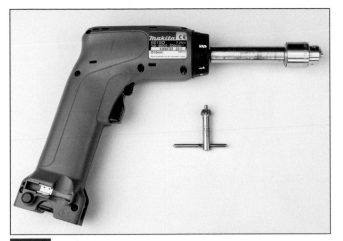

9.4 Makita® battery drill modified for orthopaedic use.

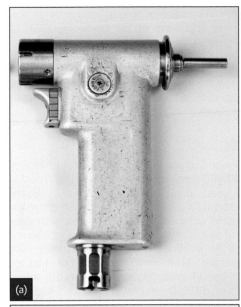

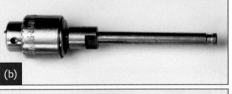

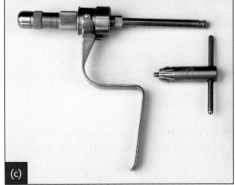

9.6 (a) Hall® Mini-Driver™ pneumatic hand piece with different attachments: (b) chuck and (c) pin driver (with chuck key).

in and out of the vent holes over the motor, this could represent a source of contamination of the surgical site.

Orthopaedic drill bits are manufactured from surgical stainless steel and generally have a 'slow spiral' design (few revolutions of the helix per unit length) (Figure 9.5). Drill bit flutes are consequently prone to clogging with moist bone/blood/fat debris, which will reduce their efficiency (Natali *et al.*, 1996). Blunt or clogged drill bits generate more heat, and bone necrosis occurs above 47–50°C (Bonfield and Li, 1968; Augustin *et al.*, 2012). Furthermore, greater pressure tends to be applied when drilling with a blunt or clogged drill bit, which increases the risk of breakage or 'plunging', whereby there is excessive penetration of the soft tissues beyond the bone (Alajmo *et al.*, 2012; Gaspar *et al.*, 2013). Conventional drill bits can tend to 'walk' when drilling on curved bone surfaces and drill bits with spurred or pointed tips have been produced to aid stability as the hole is started (Figure 9.5b). The use of appropriate drill guides will also help to stabilize the drill bit on the bone.

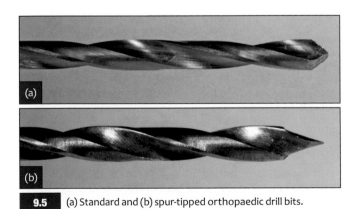

9.5 (a) Standard and (b) spur-tipped orthopaedic drill bits.

Modular power tools

Whilst stand-alone drills and saws are available, modular units offer great versatility and potential value for money. These units comprise an electric or pneumatic hand piece with a variety of attachments (Figure 9.6). The most commonly used attachments include the drill chuck, sagittal saw and pin driver, although quick-couple attachments for drills, taps and screwdrivers, reamers and even radiolucent attachments for use with fluoroscopy are available.

Saws

Sagittal saws use a flat blade that oscillates at 90 degrees to the axis of the hand piece (Figure 9.7). These are versatile tools that can be used to create osteotomies to treat deformities, aid exposure (e.g. trochanteric or acromion osteotomies), or less commonly to resect fracture ends in the management of non-unions. Blades vary in length, width, kerf (thickness) and tooth size and design. A variety of blade sizes is useful, remembering that blades with a smaller kerf will remove less bone and so should cut more

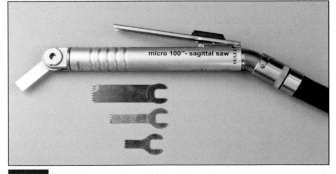

9.7 Hall® Micro 100™ sagittal oscillating saw.

easily and generate less heat. However, clogging of the teeth will reduce the efficiency of the blade resulting in greater friction and heat generation. Lavage and regular cleaning of the blade during use will reduce the risk of thermal necrosis. Whilst sagittal saw attachments are usually coupled to modular units, more precise osteotomies can be performed with a dedicated unit with a small 'pencil' style hand piece.

High-speed drills

These are stand-alone units that operate at far higher speed (90,000–100,000 rpm) and lower torque than modular units and are used to drive burrs (Figure 9.8). Burrs must always be used with a burr guard that both provides support and protects adjacent soft tissues. As with saw blades, clogging of the burr will reduce cutting efficiency and increase heat generation. Remote motor drills with flexible drive shafts are sometimes used with burrs as an alternative to high-speed drills. However, these are lower speed, higher torque, difficult to shroud and are tiring due to the weight of the flexible shaft.

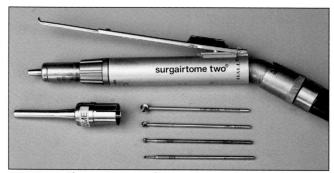

9.8 Hall® Surgairtome Two® high-speed pneumatic drill, long burr guard and a selection of burrs.

With a wide range of different power options available, the following criteria should be considered when deciding what to purchase:

- Cost
- Reliability and durability
- Power
- Comfort
- Flexibility – range of attachments and ease of changing
- Ease of maintenance, cleaning and sterilization.

Forceps

Orthopaedic forceps are used for manipulating bone fragments, maintaining fracture reduction and for holding bone plates in position prior to screw placement. Most have a standard hinged design and are locked with either a spin lock or ratchet mechanism. Spin locks are easier to untighten with the non-dominant hand and tend to be more robust than ratchets, though are more expensive. A wide range of forceps are available which vary in size and in the shape and conformation of their tips, which may be pointed or serrated (Figure 9.9). A selection of different designs and sizes are required if fracture reduction and plate stabilization are to be attempted.

Plate-holding forceps may have one tip that is designed to fit over the plate or into a screw hole or, as in the Lowman clamp, have a sliding rather than a hinge mechanism. Self-centring forceps have an elongated hinge hole that allows limited sliding to maintain alignment of the jaws (Figure 9.10).

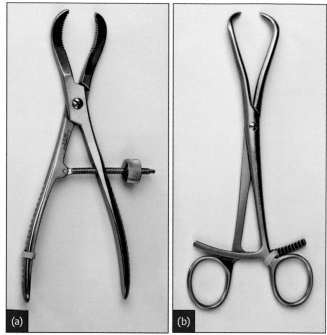

9.9 (a) Serrated bone-holding forceps with speedlock. (b) Pointed reduction forceps with ratchet.

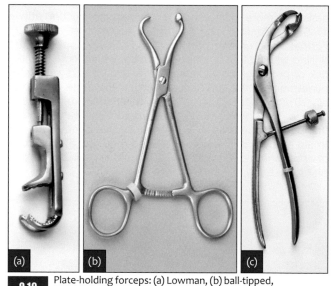

9.10 Plate-holding forceps: (a) Lowman, (b) ball-tipped, (c) self-centring.

Non-powered cutting instruments

A variety of non-powered cutting instruments are available. Curettes have a cupped or open end with a sharp edge and can be single- or double-ended, straight or angled (Figure 9.11a). They are used most frequently for resection of articular cartilage during arthrodesis and for the harvesting of cancellous bone grafts. Rongeurs are effectively forceps with curette-like tips that are used for resecting small quantities of bone or fibrous/collagenous soft tissues, for example the teres ligament from the acetabular fossa. Double-action rongeurs have two hinges that provide increased mechanical advantage, reducing the amount of effort required (Figure 9.11b).

Osteotomes, chisels and gouges are all designed to be struck with a mallet (Figure 9.12). Osteotomes have bevels on both sides of the blade, whereas a chisel has a bevel on only one side. Osteotomes are perhaps easier to control,

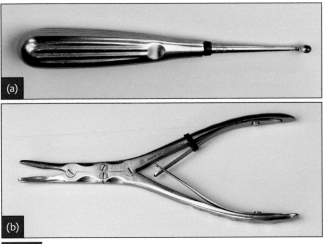

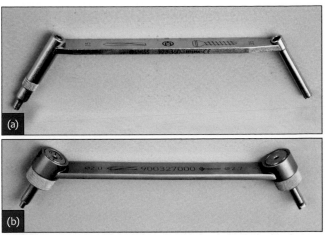

9.11 (a) Single-ended curette. (b) Double-action rongeurs.

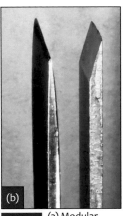

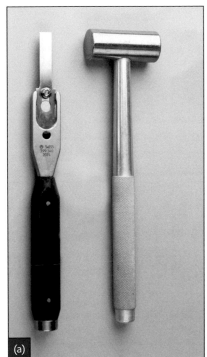

9.12 (a) Modular osteotome (left) and mallet (right). (b) The tips of an osteotome (left) and a chisel (right). Different sized osteotome blades can be attached to the hand piece.

9.13 Drill guides. (a) A combined spring-loaded universal and tubular guide. (b) A dynamic compression plate (DCP) load-neutral guide.

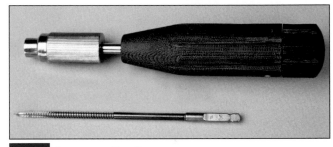

9.14 Bone tap and handle.

It is almost always necessary to contour bone plates, although substantially less precision is required if a locking system is used (see Chapter 10). Hand-held bending irons are simple, robust and usually sufficient, although hand-held pliers or a bench bone press may be necessary for larger plates (Figure 9.15).

Orthopaedic screwdrivers most commonly have a hexagonal head, the size of which is dependent on the size of screw. Slotted, cruciform and star-drive screwdrivers are

although less robust than chisels. In fracture management they may be used to create osteotomies for improved surgical access if an oscillating saw is not available. The blade of a gouge is curved and they are sometimes used to shape areas of bone or to create an opening in the proximal humerus or distal femur for harvesting bone graft. These tools should be kept sharp if they are to be used effectively and in a controlled manner.

Plate and screw placement

Screw holes should normally be drilled through a drill guide to help position and stabilize the drill bit and protect adjacent soft tissues (Figure 9.13). Drill guides can have a simple tubular design, or have a spring-loaded or oval tip to facilitate placement of loaded or neutral screws in compression plates (see Chapters 10 and 11). Taps are used to cut threads in bone and generally have an AO-style quick-couple design whereby they are inserted into a tap handle that may be cylindrical or T-shaped (Figure 9.14). The clearance flutes of taps should be kept clean.

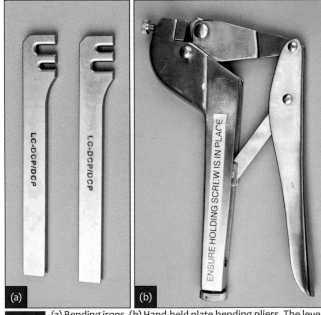

9.15 (a) Bending irons. (b) Hand-held plate bending pliers. The lever inherent to the pliers allow significantly more force to be generated, which aids contouring of larger plates. (continues) ▶

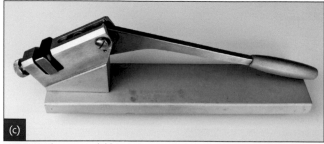

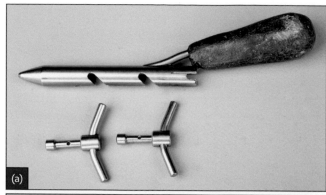

9.15 (continued) (c) Bench-mounted press. The lever inherent to the bench-mounted press allow significantly more force to be generated, which aids contouring of larger plates.

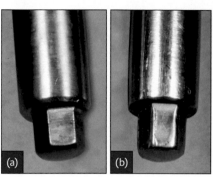

9.16 (a) New and (b) worn hexagonal screwdriver tips.

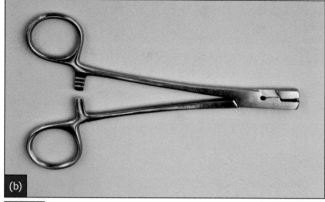

used for specific screw designs. As the tips of screwdrivers become worn, they are more likely to slip and damage the screw recess and should be replaced (Figure 9.16).

9.18 (a) Double loop cerclage tensioning device. (b) Wire twisters.

Pin and wire placement

Pin cutters generally have tungsten carbide inserts that are sufficiently hard to allow cutting of surgical steel pins and wires. Exceeding the recommended limit of the instrument by attempting to cut too large an implant is likely to damage the blade tips (Figure 9.17).

Orthopaedic wire should be twisted with wire twisters, ensuring both strands twist symmetrically. Tensioning devices are available for using with single or double loop cerclage (Figure 9.18) (see Chapters 10 and 11).

Jacobs chucks are hand-held chucks, used primarily for inserting intramedullary pins (Figure 9.19). An extension tube should be fitted to the handle to minimize the risk of self-trauma if the pin slips in the chuck during insertion.

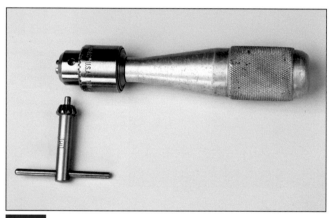

9.19 Jacobs chuck and chuck key.

Instrument care

Instrument life can be maximized by careful use, cleaning and storage. Inappropriate use (e.g. cutting too large a pin with small pin cutters or twisting orthopaedic wire with needle holders) is usually the result of impatience rather than ignorance and can wreck good-quality instruments. Organic material must be removed after use to minimize corrosion and a surgical lubricant (usually an oil-in-water emulsion) should be applied to moving parts. Power tools should be lubricated according to the manufacturer's instructions. Instruments should be dried and inspected for defects prior to sterilization. Loose packaging of drill bits, taps, osteotomes and chisels may damage their cutting edges and these items should be packaged appropriately.

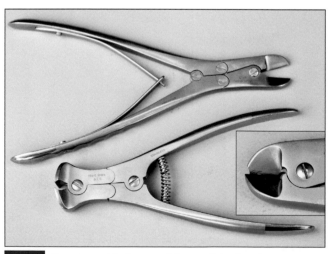

9.17 Pin cutters with close-up of damaged tips (inset).

References and further reading

Alajmo G, Schlegel U, Gueorguiev B, Matthys R and Gautier E (2012) Plunging when drilling: effect of using blunt drill bits. *Journal of Orthopaedics and Trauma* **26**, 482–487

Augustin G, Zigman T, Davila S *et al.* (2012) Cortical bone drilling and thermal osteonecrosis. *Clinical Biomechanics* **27**, 313–325

Baines S, Lipscomb V and Hutchinson T (2012) *BSAVA Manual of Canine and Feline Surgical Principles: A Foundation Manual*. BSAVA, Gloucester

Bonfield W and Li CH (1968) The temperature dependence of the deformation of bone. *Journal of Biomechanics* **1**, 323–329

Cobb HM (2010) *The History of Stainless Steel*. ASM International, Ohio

Gaspar J, Borrecho G, Oliveira P, Salvado F and Martins dos Santos J (2013) Osteotomy at low-speed drilling without irrigation *versus* high-speed drilling with irrigation: an experimental study. *Acta Médica Portuguesa* **26**, 231–236

Milne JS (1907) *Surgical Instruments in Greek and Roman Times*. Clarendon Press, Oxford

Natali C, Ingle P and Dowell J (1996) Orthopaedic bone drills – can they be improved? Temperature changes near the drilling face. *Journal of Bone and Joint Surgery (British Volume)* **78**, 357–362

Newson T (2002) *Stainless Steel – A Family of Medical Device Materials*. BSSA, Sheffield

Chapter 10

Orthopaedic implants

Mike Farrell

An orthopaedic implant is a device designed to either restore the structural integrity of a damaged bone or to replace an absent bone or joint. In the field of fracture repair, selection of the most appropriate fixation is influenced by a wide range of mechanical, biological and clinical factors (see Chapters 4 to 8). The guiding principles for fracture fixation were defined in 1958 by the Arbeitsgemeinschaft für Osteosynthesefragen (AO). The original principles (Figure 10.1) are still applied today, although the relative importance of different principles can vary according to the environment of each individual fracture. The recent trend towards 'biological' stabilization of comminuted long bone fractures emphasizes the principle of atraumatic surgical technique at the expense of anatomical reduction. Using this approach, restoration of normal spatial limb alignment is achieved using bridging fixation of the fracture, with minimal manipulation of fracture fragments (see Chapter 8).

Implant	Disruptive force			
	Bending	Rotation	Axial (shear)	Avulsion
Intramedullary pin	++	–	–	–
Intramedullary pin and cerclage wire	++	+	+	–
Interlocking nail	++	+	+	–
Bone plate and screws	+	++	++	++
External skeletal fixator	++	++	++	+
Pin and tension-band wire	–	–	–	++

10.2 Comparison of the ability of different implants to resist disruptive forces. ++ = good; + = acceptable; – = poor.

AO principles of fracture fixation

- Accurate anatomical reduction
- Rigid stabilization appropriate to the requirements of the fracture
- Preservation of blood supply to soft tissues and bone
- Early and safe mobilization of the limb and patient

10.1 AO principles of fracture fixation.

The ability of an implant to resist the disruptive forces acting on a fractured bone depends on the implant's material properties, its structure and the location of the implant relative to the bone. In clinical cases, a combination of disruptive forces usually exists (see Figure 4.3) and all these forces must be neutralized by the chosen fixation technique. Importantly, the mechanics of the entire bone–implant construct must be considered (see Chapter 4).

If an important disruptive force is not neutralized, this will frequently result in delayed union, non-union or malunion of a fracture. The best example of this problem is the use of intramedullary pins (which only neutralize bending forces) as the sole fixation in diaphyseal femoral fractures that are also subjected to important rotational and shear forces. The ability of individual fixation constructs to resist the various disruptive forces is summarized in Figure 10.2. As no single implant is able to resist all disruptive forces, veterinary surgeons (veterinarians) often use a combination of implants, especially for comminuted fractures.

Implant materials

The mechanical properties of implant materials are described in terms of the deformation (also known as strain) produced by an applied stress (see Chapter 4). Such behaviour can be plotted on a stress–strain diagram. Load–deformation diagrams are similar to stress–strain diagrams but load–deformation diagrams are affected by the dimensions and shape of an implant as well as its material properties. Thus, a 2 mm stainless steel cortical screw has the same stress–strain curve as the equivalent 3.5 mm screw, but their load–deformation curves are different.

The manufacturers of implants specify the properties and the purity of the metallic raw materials within narrow limits. The prefix ISO is used to describe metallic biomaterials that have been standardized within these narrow limits by the International Organization for Standardization. The most important materials used in implants for internal fixation are wrought stainless steel (ISO 5832-1), unalloyed titanium (ISO 5832-2) and wrought titanium-aluminium-vanadium alloy (ISO 5832-3).

Stainless steel

The primary stainless steel used for orthopaedic implants is an alloy standardized by the American Iron and Steel Institute (AISI) as type 316L. This medical grade stainless steel is derived from the common 18/8 stainless steel alloy (18% chromium, 8% nickel) used in tableware. Addition of molybdenum (3%) and reduction of carbon content (maximum 0.03%) optimizes 316L stainless steel's corrosion resistance (Black, 1980). Nickel content is also increased to 12% in order to maintain the microstructural stability. Implant materials containing iron must be in the austenitic condition (Smith, 1985). Austenitic stainless steel is not sensitive to external magnetic fields (e.g. those used in magnetic resonance imaging (MRI)). In contrast, materials in the ferritic state react dramatically to external magnetic fields, which may lead to displacement of the implant. Although cast stainless steel alloy is available, the vast majority of modern stainless steel implants are manufactured from the wrought alloy because of its improved mechanical properties and reduced impurity content. Wrought stainless steel is steel that has been heated and worked to produce its shape and form, whilst cast steel has been melted and poured into a mould to produce the desired shape. Various treatments can significantly impact the mechanical properties of wrought stainless steel. For example, annealing (heating to temperatures of 1010–1020°C) and cold working can produce two- to three-fold increases in yield strength (Black, 1980).

Titanium

Two forms of titanium are commonly used in the manufacture of orthopaedic implants: commercially pure titanium and the titanium alloy Ti-6Al-4V, containing 6% aluminium and 4% vanadium (Black, 1980). The alloy Ti-6Al-7Nb, containing 6% aluminium and 7% niobium, is also occasionally used for some implants in human orthopaedics. The mechanical properties of pure titanium vary according to its impurity content. Higher impurity content produces stronger but less ductile titanium. Pure titanium is more expensive to manufacture than stainless steel; however, the additional cost is offset by benefits including lighter weight, excellent corrosion resistance and improved biocompatibility. In comparison to stainless steel, pure titanium has a lower Young's modulus (approximately half that of stainless steel; see Chapter 4), lower shear strength and lower abrasion resistance. In veterinary surgery, commercially pure titanium implants are most commonly used in tibial tuberosity advancement surgery.

The titanium alloys Ti-6Al-4V and Ti-6Al-7Nb have mechanical properties similar to cold-worked stainless steel. In comparison to stainless steel, titanium alloy has superior fatigue and corrosion resistance; however, titanium-based alloys have not yet found widespread use in veterinary surgery due primarily to their relatively higher cost.

Adverse effects related to orthopaedic implants

The most important non-mechanical requirement of an orthopaedic implant is inertness. Although medical grade biomaterials are considered biocompatible, entirely inert biomaterials do not exist. In humans, it is estimated that 6% of the population has a hypersensitivity to one or more of the constituents of stainless steel, most commonly nickel (Deutman et al., 1977). In veterinary medicine, hypersensitivity reactions to alloy constituents appear to be very rare. Adverse reactions to implants typically present with evidence of local infection (pain, inflammation, oedema, fluid accumulation or draining sinuses) and are frequently the result of gradual implant loosening (Smith, 1983). Chronically infected implants are often coated with a thin layer of microorganisms within an adherent organic polymeric film known as a biofilm (Costerton, 2005). Removal of the implant(s) and the associated biofilm usually effects prompt relief of the clinical signs.

Other concerns exist regarding the potential for metallic implants to incite bone tumour formation at the site of implantation. The relationship between metal implants and primary bone tumours is particularly controversial in the vicinity of implants used in the proximal tibia for tibial plateau levelling osteotomy (TPLO). Currently, the argument against a causal relationship is compelling: the incidence of osteosarcoma is very low relative to the number of animals receiving TPLO implants. Furthermore, TPLOs tend to be performed more commonly in breeds at higher risk of this tumour. An annual incidence of 0.007% was reported in a population of 30,636 TPLO patients surveyed more than 1 year after surgery (Slocum, 2005). In comparison, the incidence of naturally occurring, primary malignant proximal tibial bone neoplasia within the general canine population is approximately 0.0015% per year (Dernell et al., 2007; Egenvall et al., 2007).

Orthopaedic wire

Orthopaedic wire is manufactured from 316L stainless steel. In comparison to other implants, orthopaedic wire is more ductile, allowing it to be easily contoured and secured using twist knots. The main clinical indications for orthopaedic wire are cerclage wiring and tension-band fixation. In addition, interfragmentary wiring is occasionally used for management of certain fractures of the mandible and maxilla (see Chapter 17).

Cerclage wiring

A cerclage wire fully encircles a bone to appose long oblique fragments and produce a limited amount of interfragmentary compression. Provided that the principles for application of cerclage wires (Figure 10.3) are strictly adhered to, there should be no detrimental effect on osseous healing (Wilson, 1987). A loose cerclage wire, however,

Principles for the application of cerclage wires
• Cerclage wires are inappropriate for sole fixation of fractures – they are commonly used to provide interfragmentary compression as a supplement to intramedullary pins or nails
• The fracture should be two-piece and fully reconstructable. Use of cerclage wires should be avoided for comminuted fractures
• Two-piece fractures should be oblique or spiral with a fracture length at least double the diameter of the bone
• At least two cerclage wires should be used
• Wires must not be less than 10 mm apart and must be at least 5 mm from the end of the fracture fragment
• All wires must be tight. To avoid loosening, the wire should be fixed perpendicular to the long axis of the bone. Cerclage wire application should be avoided on wedge-shaped (metaphyseal) bones
• Wire diameter must be sufficient for the size of the bone it is applied to. Tensile strength of the wire is related to its cross-sectional area. For dogs weighing 20 kg or more the minimum diameter should be 1 mm (18 G). The minimum size for smaller dogs and cats is 0.8 mm (20 G)
• Entrapment of soft tissues must be avoided

10.3 Principles for the application of cerclage wires.

will move up and down the bone and disrupt the extra-osseous blood supply and, as well as doing nothing to stabilize the fracture, will lead to avascular bone fragments and delayed union or non-union. Due to the strict selection criteria, the indications for cerclage wire application are limited. In reality, cerclage wires are most useful as temporary fixation devices for maintenance of anatomical reduction of oblique and spiral fractures prior to application of a bone plate and screws. This technique is particularly useful when lag screws are being placed through the plate. If necessary, the cerclage wires can be removed after the contoured plate and first few screws have been placed.

The three most common methods for tightening and securing cerclage wires are twist, single loop and double loop knots (see Chapter 11).

Tension-band wiring

Tension-band fixation is applied to neutralize the avulsion force applied to fracture (or osteotomy) fragments by attached tendons or ligaments. The tension-band wire is generally used in conjunction with 0.9–2 mm diameter Kirschner (K) wires or pins. The tension-band wire provides a force equal and opposite to the distracting force. The resultant force vector results in compression across the fracture or osteotomy site (Figure 10.4). Tension-band wires can be used wherever a distractive force from a ligament or tendon attachment exists (Figure 10.5).

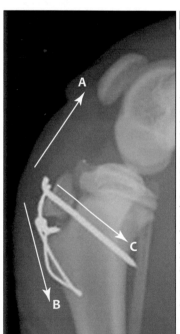

10.4 Tension-band wiring. The tension-band converts a distractive force to compression. One or two bicortical K-wires are inserted perpendicular to the fracture line. The tension-band wire is then applied in a figure-of-eight configuration; symmetrical twists in both portions of the wire are recommended to ensure even wire tension. The selected tension-band wire diameter should be relatively large, as the wire functions to oppose the major distractive force of the attached tendon or ligament, in this example, from the quadriceps muscle. This force is converted to a compressive force oriented approximately parallel to the K-wire. A = distractive force; B = distractive force; C = compressive force.

Specific indications for tension-band wires	
Forelimb	Hindlimb
Acromial fracture	Greater trochanter (femur) fracture
Supraglenoid tubercle fracture	Patella fracture
Greater tubercle (humerus) fracture	Tibial tuberosity avulsion
Olecranon fracture	Malleolar fracture
Styloid process fracture (radius/ulna)	Calcaneal fracture

10.5 Specific indications for tension-band wires.

Wires used for pinning
K-wires

K-wires are 316L stainless steel pins of 0.9–2 mm diameter. They are available with trocar or bayonet tips. Arthrodesis wires are the most useful type of K-wire, having a trocar tip at each end. By convention, pins with a diameter larger than 2 mm are known as Steinmann pins. These have a diameter of 2.4–6.4 mm, a length of 300 mm and a three-faced trocar tip design. The resistance of a pin or wire against applied bending forces is governed by its area moment of inertia (AMI) (see Chapter 4). AMI varies by the fourth power of the pin's radius; therefore, small increases in pin diameter manifest as large increases in bending resistance. For example, if a 4 mm pin is chosen instead of a 3 mm pin, the AMI increases over three-fold. K-wires are used for the repair of juxta-articular fractures as crossed pins, as parallel pins (see Chapter 23), as a component of tension-band fixation of avulsion fractures, and as intramedullary devices in small bones. They can also be used for the temporary fixation of fracture fragments prior to application of interfragmentary compression using lag screws.

Rush pins

Rush pins are modified pins that are usually used in pairs to stabilize physeal fractures, almost exclusively of the distal femur (see Chapter 23). When applied appropriately, Rush pins provide three-point fixation under spring-loaded tension. Rush pins are commercially available for human use, but are most commonly made as required for individual use, using appropriately sized K-wires or small Steinmann pins (Figure 10.6).

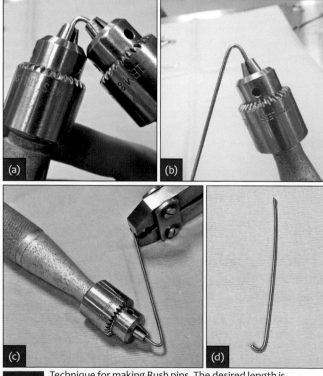

10.6 Technique for making Rush pins. The desired length is calculated to be a minimum of three times the height of the physeal fragment. (a) The pin is secured between two chucks which are used to create a hooked end (b) at one end of the pin that can be trimmed to length. (c) The sledged end is created by cutting obliquely using a dedicated pin cutter. (d) A gentle bend is created along the remaining length of the pin. (continues) ▶

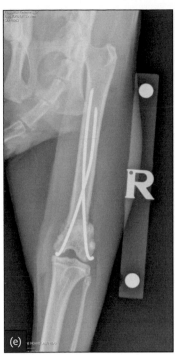

10.6 (continued) Technique for making Rush pins. (e) Postoperative craniocaudal radiograph showing correct application of Rush pins in a mildly comminuted feline supracondylar femoral fracture.

Principles of intramedullary pin fixation

- Smooth intramedullary pins only neutralize bending forces – the position of the pins in the neutral axis of the bone confers excellent bending resistance, but smooth pins cannot effectively resist rotational forces or axial collapse
- Use is best reserved for diaphyseal fractures in straight bones – stability requires significant purchase in both main fracture fragments
- Significant protrusion of pins from the bone should be avoided – this is particularly important in the proximal femur, in which a malpositioned pin with a protruding tip can cause irreversible trauma to the sciatic nerve (see Chapter 28). This problem is best avoided by placing pins in a normograde fashion (see Chapter 23) and by countersinking the pin tip or leaving the pin protruding through the skin so that it can be tied to an external skeletal fixator (Figure 10.8b)
- Medullary canal fill should be maximized – if pins are used with cerclage wires, fill should be at least 70–80% of the diameter of the medullary cavity at its narrowest point (Roe, 2003)

10.7 Principles of intramedullary pin fixation.

reconstructable diaphyseal fractures, this force can be neutralized using multiple cerclage wires, although this fixation is somewhat tenuous. If the fracture is not amenable to cerclage reconstruction, secondary fixation (Figure 10.8) should be applied.

Rush pins have several important advantages compared to crossed pins when they are applied to physeal fractures:

- Biomechanical superiority – Rush pins cross each other relatively proximal to the fracture compared to crossed pins, leading to improved neutralization of rotational forces and caudal bending forces
- Improved potential for continued growth – the bone can theoretically continue to grow along the Rush pins, which are not rigidly anchored in the proximal fragment. In reality, this rarely occurs
- Potential for more rapid healing – the spring-loaded elastic fixation allows dynamic impact load compression, which means that controlled axial forces act on the fracture with every step.

Despite these biomechanical advantages, in comparison to the more commonly selected crossed pins, Rush pins are more challenging to insert and require additional planning and preparation.

Intramedullary devices

Intramedullary pins

The most frequently chosen implant for intramedullary application is the Steinmann pin. This implant can be used with good results provided that the principles of application are followed (Figure 10.7). The most essential of these principles is that a smooth intramedullary pin is only able to neutralize bending forces and cannot resist rotation or axial collapse. Historically, there have been some simple design alterations to Steinmann pins intended to improve the rotational resistance of intramedullary pins. For example, the Trilam nail has three lamellae running down its length to improve endosteal purchase. These variations do not, however, address the important problem of axial collapse in oblique or comminuted fractures. In oblique

Interlocking nails

Interlocking nails are 316L stainless steel or commercially pure titanium intramedullary pins containing a variable number of transverse cannulations through which implants can be placed, usually through the use of a temporary jig that is removed after implant placement. The advantage of this implant system is that rotation, axial collapse and nail migration are prevented, and the location of the nail close to the neutral axis is a biomechanically advantageous

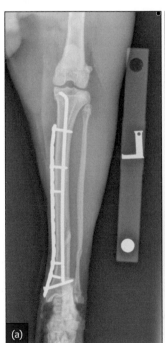
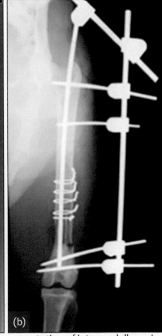

10.8 Techniques available for augmentation of intramedullary pin fixation of diaphyseal fractures. (a) Addition of a plate is known as 'pin–plate' or 'plate–rod' fixation. The pin diameter is usually reduced to 35–40% of the medullary canal diameter to allow purchase of at least four cortices in each fragment by the screws in the plate-and-screw construct. (b) A similar principle is followed using a tied-in external skeletal fixator. Morbidity is often significantly greater using this technique compared with pin–plate fixation.

position with excellent resistance to bending. This effect is magnified when anatomical reconstruction is not possible. Interlocking nails are the implants of choice in humans for the fixation of femoral, tibial and humeral fractures. They have been used in cats and dogs for the stabilization of femoral, humeral and tibial fractures. However, their application is limited by the size of the bone affected and the nature of the fracture. Suitable fractures are diaphyseal, comminuted fractures in straight bones. Commercially available interlocking nail systems include:

- VIN: Numédic Company, France
- INN: Mizuho Ikakogyo, Japan
- The Orginal Interlocking Nail System™: Innovative Animal Products, USA
- I-Loc®: BioMedtrix, USA
- 3.5 mm titanium ILN: Freelance Veterinary, UK (Figure 10.9a).

The Original Interlocking Nail System™ is the most commonly applied interlocking nail used in veterinary practice. Nail sizes include 10, 8, 6, 4.7, 4 and 3.5 mm diameter with variable lengths from 120 to 230 mm. They have three to four pre-placed holes per nail, 11 mm or 22 mm apart (Figure 10.9b). The 10 mm and 8 mm nail systems accept 3.5 mm cortical screws, 6 mm nails accept 2.7 mm screws, and 3.5–4.7 mm nails accept 2 mm screws.

To reduce the incidence of screw breakage, 2 mm, 2.7 mm and 3.5 mm locking bolts have been developed to replace the corresponding screws. These bolts have self-tapping threads below the head of the bolt that engage in the cis (near) cortex. They also have a significantly higher AMI than the corresponding screws and are cut to length, which eliminates the need to keep a large

bolt inventory. The recently introduced I-Loc® nail incorporates a Morse taper coupling system between the interlocking bolt and the nail. This feature confers a superior rotational stability compared to all other available models for veterinary use.

Bone screws

Screws are differentiated by the manner in which they are inserted into bone, their function, their size and the type of bone they are intended for. They are divided broadly into self-tapping and non-self-tapping screws, cortical and cancellous screws, and there is now a subcategory of locking screws intended for use with locking plates. The terminology used to describe variations in screw morphology is described in Figure 10.10.

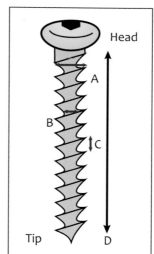

10.10 Glossary of screw morphology. Head = the design of the recess within the screw head varies. Screws may have a slot or a cruciate, hexagonal or star-shaped recess. Tip = self-tapping screws (shown here) have a thread-cutting tip. Thread diameter (A) = the widest diameter of the screw; this is the diameter that defines the screw size (e.g. 3.5 mm, 2.7 mm). Core diameter (B) = the difference between the thread diameter and core diameter is the thread height. Pitch (C) = the distance between adjacent threads. Screw working distance (D) = the length of bone traversed by the screw.

Screw sizing

Screw holding power diminishes significantly as the diameter of the screw approaches 40% of the diameter of the bone, and the bone itself can be weakened. For these reasons, it is recommended that the screw size should be 25% of the diameter of the bone, although slightly larger screws (up to 33% of bone diameter) can be used, in exceptional circumstances. There are a number of different screws available to enable fixation of bones of different diameters (Figure 10.11). Each screw size has a corresponding drill bit and tap. Screw working distance, defined as the length of bone traversed by a screw, is not the same as screw length because screw length

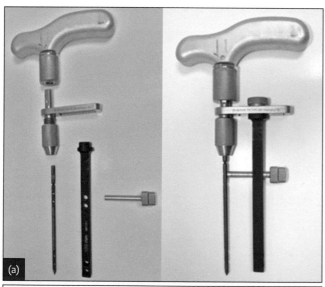

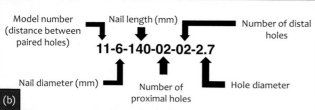

Model number (distance between paired holes) → Nail length (mm) → → Number of distal holes

11-6-140-02-02-2.7

Nail diameter (mm) → Number of proximal holes → Hole diameter

10.9 (a) The 3.5 mm titanium ILN pre-assembly (left) and post-assembly (right). A drilling guide is attached via a coupling system to the proximal end of the nail, which allows the drill guide to be perfectly matched to the cannulations in the nail. (b) Interlocking nail coding system.

Cortical screws		Cancellous screws	
Thread (mm)	Core (mm)	Thread (mm)	Core (mm)
1.5	1.1	4.0	1.9
2.0	1.4	6.5	3.0
2.4	1.7		
2.7	1.9		
3.5	2.4		
4.5	3.2		
5.5	3.9		

10.11 Summary of the available cortical and cancellous screws and their thread and core diameters.

includes the head of the screw and the tip of the screw, which should protrude through the trans (far) cortex. Commercial screw racks contain a device for measuring screw length (Figure 10.12). Screws are inventoried according to the screw length rather than the screw working distance. In order to ensure the correct working distance, after measuring the depth of the screw hole with a depth gauge, at least 2 mm must be added to the measured depth.

Cortical and cancellous screws

Cortical screws are fully threaded. They have a relatively larger core diameter than cancellous screws (see Figure 10.11). As the AMI of a screw varies by the fourth power of the core diameter, these screws have significantly greater bending resistance (see Chapter 4). Cancellous bone screws have a relatively thin core and a wide and deep thread (Figure 10.13). This increases holding power in fine trabecular bone, which is found in metaphyseal and epiphyseal areas. Cancellous bone screws are available with either a full or partial thread. Fully threaded screws can be used for fixing plates in metaphyseal and epiphyseal bone; partially threaded screws can be used as lag screws. In reality, the improved holding power of cancellous screws is rarely considered clinically important, whereas their narrow core diameter often results in screw fracture; therefore, in practice, cortical screws are routinely used in fine trabecular bone as well as cortical bone.

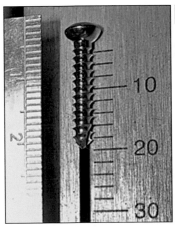

10.12 Screw length measurement. This 2.7 mm diameter 20 mm screw is measured from the head to the tip. The threads on the tip will not engage the trans cortex. If the head of the screw is countersunk into the bone, this screw will have a working distance of approximately 18 mm.

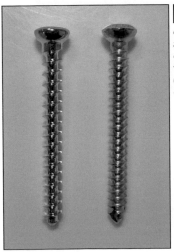

10.13 A non-self-tapping 4 mm diameter cancellous bone screw (left) and a self-tapping 3.5 mm diameter cortical bone screw (right). Note the relatively larger core diameter (at the expense of thread height) of the cortical screw.

Non-self-tapping and self-tapping screws

Non-self-tapping screws have a rounded tip. They require the use of a tap (which corresponds exactly to the profile of the screw thread) to cut a thread in the bone prior to their insertion. The screws can be removed and reinserted with ease without fear of inadvertently cutting a new channel, because it is difficult for a screw alone to cut a channel in cortical bone. In contrast, self-tapping screws have a cutting tip. They are designed so that once a pilot hole has been drilled into the bone they can be inserted by simply screwing them in. If self-tapping screws are reinserted and inadvertently angled relative to the original pilot hole and thread, they will cut a new path and destroy the thread that has already been cut.

Lag screw technique

Apposition of major bone fragments without application of compression will inevitably result in small gaps at the fracture site. This results in high interfragmentary strain (see Chapter 4) and very high loads being transmitted to the fixation device. A very effective way of reducing interfragmentary strain is to produce compression between the main fracture fragments. This permits direct transfer of load from one fragment of bone to the other, which diminishes the load borne by the fixation device and increases the stability of the fixation. The most effective way to achieve compression between bone fragments is by means of a lag screw. A lag screw is any screw whose threads purchase only in the trans cortex. This is achieved either by drilling a hole in the cis cortex that is equal in diameter to the screw thread diameter, or by using a partially threaded cancellous screw, which has a smooth screw shank (see Chapter 11).

Positional screws

In rare instances, the adjacent surfaces of oblique fractures will not abut one another when a compressive force is applied to them. Application of lag screws or cerclage wires would be inappropriate in these instances because a compressive force would cause the fragments to collapse. Reconstruction of these fractures can be achieved using positional screws. Thread holes are drilled in both the near cis and trans cortices so the relative position of the two fragments is maintained when the positional screw is inserted (see Chapter 11).

Plate screws

Plate screws are used to attach plates to bones. Their function varies according to whether the bone plate employs a locking or non-locking mode of load transfer (see below).

Bone plates

Bone plates are internal implants that are differentiated either by their function or by the system of coupling between the bone plate and screw. They can be used in neutralization, compression, bridging or buttress modes (Figure 10.14).

* Neutralization – when a fracture has been anatomically reconstructed using lag screws or cerclage wires, this fixation alone would be unable to withstand the normal disruptive forces. Compressed fragments are therefore spanned with a plate and screws to neutralize these disruptive forces; the plate is in neutralization mode.

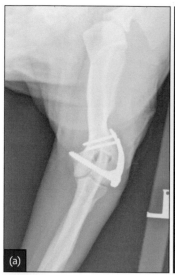
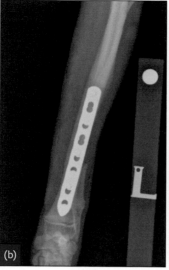
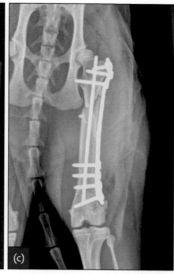
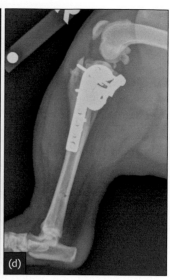

10.14 Bone plate function. (a) Neutralization. (b) Dynamic compression. (c) Bridging. (d) Buttress.

- Dynamic compression – dynamic compression plates (DCPs) and locking compression plates (LCPs) have a specific screw hole geometry that allows axial compression to be applied across transverse or short oblique fractures.
- Bridging – when anatomical fracture reconstruction is deemed inappropriate the fracture can be spanned by the fixation device. This is termed bridging function. As the plate is positioned eccentrically with respect to the neutral axis of the bone, bending forces are generated in the plate which can lead to cyclic fatigue. Therefore bridging plates are usually paired with intramedullary devices.
- Buttress – buttress function refers to the use of a plate and screws to hold collapsed juxta-articular fragments in position after they have been reduced ('shoring up' the collapsed fragment).

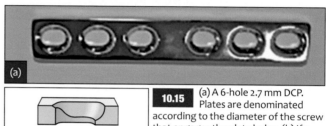

10.15 (a) A 6-hole 2.7 mm DCP. Plates are denominated according to the diameter of the screw that engages the plate holes. (b) If a screw is placed eccentrically, the screw head can move along the hole during tightening, causing compression at the fracture site.

Types of bone plate

Dynamic compression plates

Despite the misleading name, DCPs achieve *static* compression due to the interaction between the screw hole geometry and eccentric placement of a screw into the hole. The screw hole permits simultaneous downward and horizontal movement of the screw head during tightening (Figure 10.15).

Historically, placing a DCP required the use of two drill guides; a neutral guide (labelled green) with a central hole for the drill bit and a load guide (labelled yellow) with an eccentric drill hole oriented away from the fracture (Figure 10.16). Recently, a universal drill guide was introduced that allows insertion of a neutral screw or compression screw according to the amount of pressure applied to the guide (Figure 10.17).

The DCP has an extended middle segment without holes. The holes on either side of the middle segment only allow compression to be applied towards the centre of the plate. The geometry of the DCP hole allows longitudinal angulation of screws of up to 25 degrees, and transverse angulation of up to 7 degrees. This can produce a challenge if a lag screw is being placed through the plate or if a screw must be aimed away from a fracture line.

The amount of compression depends on the plate and screw size: 3.5 mm DCP plate and screw constructs

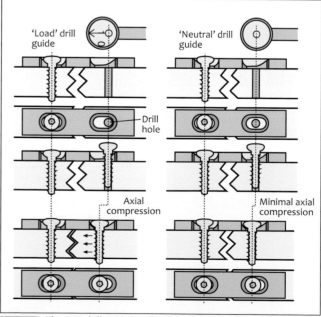

10.16 The DCP drill guide has 'load' and 'neutral' functions. Using the load guide, the screw is placed eccentrically in the hole; tightening the screws causes compression at the fracture site. Using the neutral guide, the screw is placed in the centre of the hole, and minimal compression is generated.

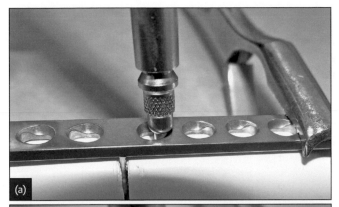

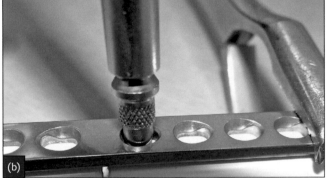

10.17 Use of the universal drill guide to produce compression in a DCP. (a) Dynamic compression. The universal guide is placed eccentrically (away from the fracture) without exerting pressure. (b) Neutral insertion. When the universal guide is pressed into the plate hole, it centres itself and allows neutral pre-drilling.

can produce 1 mm of compression for the first eccentric screw, with diminished compression for each subsequent screw. There is no additional advantage of placing more than two screws in compression on either side of the fracture. In addition, excessive compression can lead to fissure formation and must be avoided.

Limited contact dynamic compression plates

The limited contact dynamic compression plate (LC-DCP) is a modification of the DCP with several beneficial features:

- Grooves in the undersurface of the plate between the screw holes – the sculpted undersurface of the LC-DCP confers a more even stiffness profile compared to the DCP, where stress is concentrated at each screw hole (see Chapter 29). The smaller footprint of the LC-DCP results in significantly improved periosteal blood supply to the plated bony segments (Brinker *et al.*, 1984). The plate footprint is further reduced by giving the LC-DCP a trapezoid cross-section with the smaller surface contacting the bone
- The plate holes allow increased screw angulation – screws can be angled 40 degrees in the longitudinal plane
- Uniform screw hole spacing – the screw hole has been redesigned so that compression can be produced in both directions.

Other non-locking plates

A huge variety of other non-locking plates are available. In addition, custom implants can be manufactured to order for specific indications.

Reconstruction plates: Reconstruction plates are DCP-style plates available in 2.7 or 3.5 mm sizes with notches between the screw holes to allow three-dimensional contouring (Figure 10.18). Reconstruction plates have a low stiffness and strength and should only be used in situations where disruptive forces are small and other plates cannot be easily contoured to fit, for example acetabular fractures (Dyce and Houlton, 1993).

Veterinary cuttable plates (VCPs): These are semi-tubular, round-hole plates that are available in multiple sizes (Figure 10.19). They are purchased as long plates and cut to the desired length. High screw density is useful when bone stock is limited, for example juxta-articular fractures. VCPs can be stacked on top of one another to increase stiffness and strength (McLaughlin *et al.*, 1992).

Veterinary T-plates: Multiple shapes and sizes of T-plate, from 1 mm to 4.5 mm, are available with round holes in the expanded T-section and round or DCP holes in the long arm of the plate (Figure 10.20). T-plates are used when there is a small juxta-articular fragment, such as distal radial (Hamilton and Langley-Hobbs, 2005) and ilial (von Pfeil, 2008) fractures. T-plates are also available as locking plates.

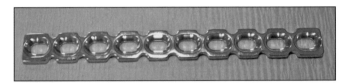

10.18 A 2.7 mm reconstruction plate.

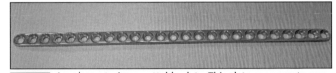

10.19 A 2.0/2.7 veterinary cuttable plate. This plate can accept 2 mm or 2.7 mm screws.

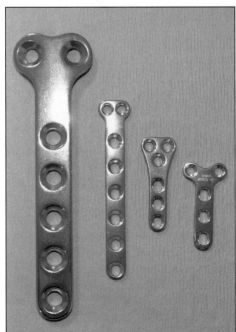

10.20

Various veterinary T-plates. From left to right: 3.5 mm 7-hole round-hole T-plate, 2 mm 8-hole DCP-type T-plate, 2 mm 6-hole DCP-type T-plate and 2 mm 5-hole DCP-type T-plate.

Acetabular plates: Acetabular plates are round-hole plates that are pre-contoured to the shape of the canine acetabulum (Figure 10.21). Relatively small plates are sufficient in this location because they are applied on the tension surface of the bone (see Chapter 22). Acetabular plates can also be applied in other regions in which contouring of standard plates is challenging (Chase and Farrell, 2010).

Supracondylar plates: Supracondylar plates are DCP-style plates that are pre-contoured to the complex shape of the lateral surface of the canine distal femur (Figure 10.22). These plates have been used to stabilize distal femoral corrective osteotomies (Roch and Gemmill, 2008) and are also available as locking plates.

Carpal/tarsal arthrodesis plates: Pancarpal and pantarsal arthrodesis plates are both available in 2, 2.7 and 3.5 mm sizes (Figure 10.23). The plates allow the use of larger screws proximally and smaller screws distally in the metacarpal or metatarsal bones. These plates are thinner and tapered at the distal end to minimize problems with soft tissue cover. The pancarpal arthrodesis plates provide 10 degrees of carpal extension without further contouring. These plates can also be applied to fractures in tapered bones such as the canine ulna.

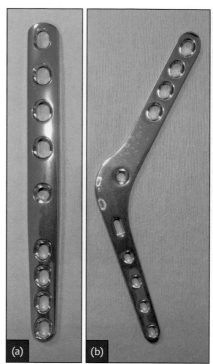

10.23
(a) A 3.5/2.7 mm 9-hole hybrid pancarpal arthrodesis plate.
(b) A 2.7/2 mm left 10-hole pantarsal arthrodesis plate.

(a)   (b)

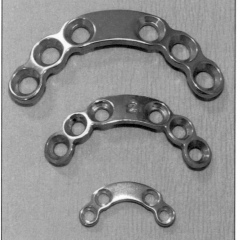

10.21
Acetabular plates. From top to bottom: 3.5 mm 6-hole, 2.7 mm 6-hole and 2 mm 4-hole acetabular plates.

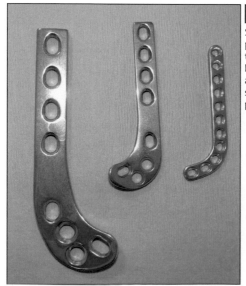

10.22
Supracondylar plates. From left to right: 3.5 mm left, 2.7 mm right and 2 mm right supracondylar plates.

Locking plates

Non-locking plate and screw constructs rely on frictional transfer of load between the bone and the plate. The frictional force generated must exceed the disruptive forces for the construct to be stable. Locking plate and screw constructs do not rely on plate–bone compression to maintain stability. This feature confers a number of important advantages to locking plate and screw constructs.

Locking plate advantages:

- Elimination of screw toggling – construct failure by toggling is not possible because the entire plate and screw construct acts as a single unit. Screw toggling is a mechanism of construct failure in which plate screws pivot within the plate holes as a consequence of axial load being applied to the construct
- Improved periosteal vascularity – there is no requirement for compression of the plate against the bone
- Simpler plate contouring – the construct acts as an internal fixator. Accurate contouring of the plate to the bone surface is not required
- Monocortical screw fixation – unicortical placement of conventional screws can be unstable because the screw is fixed at a single point only, making it susceptible to toggling. Locking screws are fixed to the plate as well as the cis cortex, making the screw much more stable.

Locking plate disadvantages:

- Fixed screw angles – many locking plate systems do not allow screws to be angled. Lag screws cannot be placed through these plates and screws cannot be directed away from joints or fracture lines
- Increased cost – locking head screws are more expensive to manufacture and are significantly more expensive than conventional screws
- Pre-contoured plates cannot be used to reduce fractures – when locking plates are applied to bones as

internal fixators, the bone fragments must already be reduced or spatially aligned. Their position will be fixed as the locking screws are tightened because locking screws cannot draw bone fragments against the plate.

Different locking plate systems have different coupling mechanisms between the screw head and the plate hole. Regardless of the system, these constructs incorporate a rigid interaction between the screw head and plate (Figure 10.24).

Locking compression plate (LCP): The LCP has the unique feature of merging locking screw technology with conventional plating techniques. LCPs have combination locking and compression holes (Combi hole™). This allows placement of standard cortical or cancellous bone screws on one side or threaded conical locking screws on the opposite side of each hole (Figure 10.24). Holes are oriented so that the compression component of the hole is directed towards the middle of the plate. The LCP is available in stainless steel or titanium. Sets used for small animal internal fixation include the 2, 2.4, 2.7 and 3.5 mm systems (Figure 10.25).

String-of-pearls (SOP) plate: SOP plates are available in 2, 2.7 or 3.5 mm sizes (Figure 10.26). The two main advantages are the ability to contour the SOP with six degrees of freedom and the ability to use standard cortical screws that are significantly less expensive than the locking screws used in other systems. Disadvantages include the tendency of the screw holes to deform during contouring and the relatively weaker shear strength of cortical screws compared to locking head screws (see Figure 10.24).

Polyaxial locking plates: The locking plate systems listed above are known as 'fixed angle' locking systems because the screw and its head must be positioned exactly perpendicular to the screw hole so that the screw threads and the threads in the plate engage perfectly. Recently, several systems have been introduced that have an incomplete thread in the screw hole, which allows a limited degree of

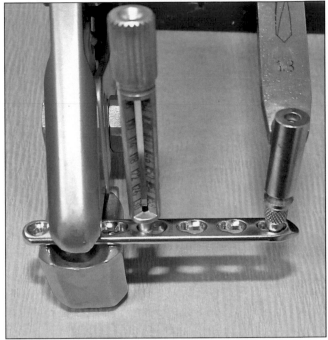

10.25 A 7-hole 2.7 mm LCP with a bending press (left). The locking drill guide (centre) ensures that the 2.0 mm drill bit is positioned perpendicular to the threaded section of the Combi hole™. Use of a threaded guide is important in fixed angle locking plates to ensure that the plate and screw threads match perfectly. The universal guide (right) can be used for preparation of non-locking screws. Non-locking screws must always be placed before locking screws because the non-locking screws would be unable to compress the plate against the bone after locking screw application.

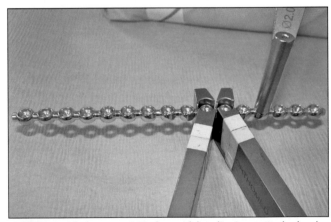

10.26 A 16-hole 2.7 mm SOP plate with bending irons attached and a guide for a 2.0 mm drill bit. Although the drill guide is not threaded, it can only couple perpendicularly with the screw hole.

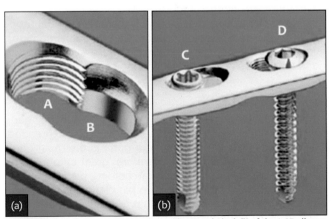

10.24 Locking screw technology. The Combi hole™ of the LCP allows cortical screws to be inserted on one side of the hole in either a neutral or compression mode, and threaded conical locking screws to be inserted on the other side of the hole. (a) A = threaded plate hole for locking screws; B = dynamic compression unit (DCU) for standard screws. (b) C = locking screw in the threaded side of the Combi hole™; D = cortical screw in the compression side of the Combi hole™. Note that the locking screw has a shallow thread profile because it does not need to generate a large frictional force between the plate and the bone. This allows a larger core diameter, which provides greater bending strength. (© DePuy Synthes UK)

screw angling (Figure 10.27). This is useful in the repair of juxta-articular fractures as screws can be angled away from a joint. Most of these systems are fabricated from commercially pure titanium.

Fixin: The Fixin system uses a 'Morse taper' effect rather than threads to lock the screw head to the plate (Figure 10.28). A removable threaded 'bushing' couples with the plate and the shape of the screw hole in the centre of the bushing is slightly less tapered than the cylinder of the screw head. The Morse fit produces permanent cold welding between the screw and plate so screw removal requires unscrewing of the bushing from the plate.

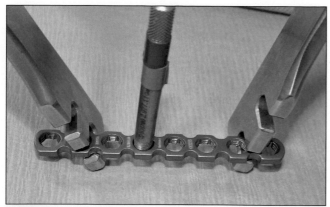

10.27 An 8-hole 2.7 mm VetLox plate with bending irons attached. The threaded locking screw guide that is shown in this image can be replaced with a non-locking guide allowing up to 30 degrees screw angulation in all directions.

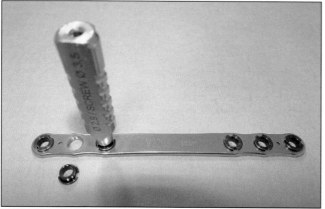

10.28 A 6-hole 3.5 mm Fixin plate with the second threaded bushing removed. The attached 2.9 mm drill guide has a Morse taper coupling system which ensures that the screw hole is drilled perpendicular to the plate.

Advanced locking plate system (ALPS): The ALPS is manufactured from commercially pure titanium and titanium alloys. All holes accept either standard or locking screws and a compression drill sleeve is available that allows dynamic fracture compression to be applied using cortical screws. The plate has a reconstruction design allowing contouring in multiple planes (Figure 10.29) and has a sculpted surface in contact with the bone that produces point contact only. This minimizes vascular damage to the underlying bone.

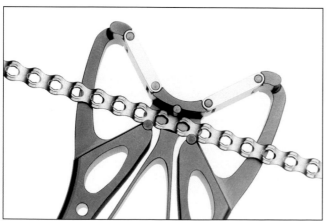

10.29 A dedicated bending press is available to facilitate contouring of the ALPS plate in multiple planes.
(© KYON AG)

Biodegradable plates and screws

Over the past 30 years, there have been significant advances in the development of biodegradable materials. The principle advantage proposed for the use of biodegradable internal fixation implants is the potential to engineer implants that are degraded at a rate matching new tissue formation, which would eliminate the need for a second surgery to remove the implants. In addition to the provision of structural support, biodegradable materials can provide a substrate upon which stem cells can be seeded that can facilitate new tissue formation at the site of injury. The most common biodegradable implant material is polylactide, which has been used in the manufacture of pins, staples, suture anchors, screws and plates. Although biodegradable implants have not yet gained widespread use in veterinary medicine, the successful use of polylactide plates was reported for the repair of radial fractures in a population of toy breed dogs (Saikku-Backstrom *et al.*, 2005).

External skeletal fixation

External skeletal fixators consist of a series of percutaneous transfixation pins that penetrate both cortices of the bone to which they are applied and are connected by some form of external bar(s). The transfixation pins connected to an individual external bar either penetrate the bone from one side only (uniplanar, type 1) or continue through the soft tissues and skin deep to the trans cortex where they are fixed to a second bar. This latter biplanar fixation is referred to as a type 2 configuration when it is part of a linear external skeletal fixation (ESF) construct. Circular ESF uses transfixing wires that produce multiplanar fixation. The various external skeletal fixator configurations are illustrated in Figure 10.30.

ESF systems are popular in general practice because they are very versatile and are perceived to be relatively easy to apply compared with plates and screws. They can effectively neutralize all disruptive forces and are amenable to a wide variety of simple and complex fractures. Their indications, contraindications, advantages and disadvantages are listed in Figure 10.31.

The principle factor governing the biomechanical properties of external skeletal fixators is the frame configuration; in addition the transfixation pins, clamps and connecting bars also have an influence (see Chapter 4).

Transfixation pins

Transfixation pins (see Figures 10.32 to 10.34) are made from 316L stainless steel and may be smooth or threaded. The interface between the pin and bone is the most common site of construct failure; therefore, great care must be taken to maximize transfixation pin holding power. In order to prevent thermal necrosis during pin placement, pre-drilling is recommended with a bit that is 0.1 mm smaller than the narrowest core diameter of the pin. If pins are inserted using a drill rather than a Jacobs chuck, the torque should be low and speeds should be less than 150 rpm. Pins should be selected with a thread diameter that is no more than 33% of the bone diameter. Where possible, threaded pins should be selected in preference to smooth pins because they dissipate applied forces across a larger area within the transfixed bone, resulting in a significant improvement in holding power. When smooth pins are used, they should be angled to maximize fixator stiffness.

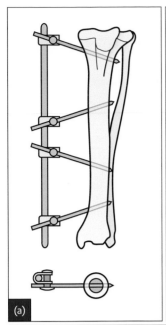

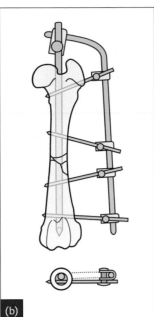

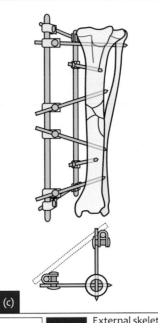

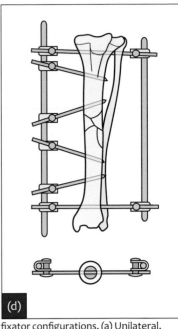

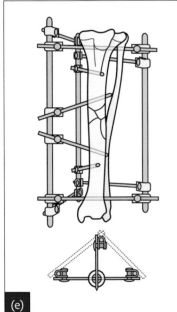

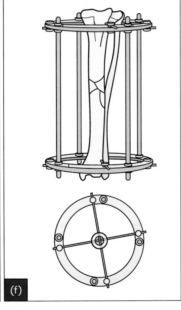

10.30 External skeletal fixator configurations. (a) Unilateral, uniplanar (type 1a). (b) Unilateral, uniplanar with intramedullary pin tie-in. (c) Unilateral, biplanar (type 1b). (d) Modified bilateral, uniplanar (type 2b). (e) Bilateral, biplanar (type 3). (f) Ilizarov ring.

Indications	Contraindications
• Diaphyseal fractures • Metaphyseal fractures (circular ESF system or hybrid circular–linear ESF system) • Comminuted (non-reconstructable) fractures • Mandibular and maxillary fractures • Contaminated and high-grade open fractures • Stabilization after corrective osteotomy • Transarticular immobilization	• Lack of availability of safe soft tissue corridors (best applied to injuries distal to the elbow and stifle joints) • Not suitable if rigid fixation is required (e.g. anatomically reconstructed fractures, articular fractures) • Low clinical fracture patient assessment scores (FPAS) (see Chapter 7)
Advantages	**Disadvantages**
• Effective neutralization of bending, rotational and axial forces • Configuration stiffness can be varied • Facilitates preservation of fracture site biology • Facilitates open wound management • Minimal instrumentation is required • Simple to combine with other fixation systems • Clinical and radiographic assessment of fracture healing is straightforward • Implants can be readily removed • Allows linear and angular traction allowing progressive correction of limb deformities	• High morbidity if safe corridors are not respected during transfixation pin placement • Relatively fast rate of cyclic construct fatigue at the pin–bone interface (do not use in fractures with low biological FPAS scores) • The perception of ESF as a panacea of fracture fixation has led to inappropriate use

10.31 Indications, contraindications, advantages and disadvantages for ESF.

Negative-profile threaded pins

Negative-profile threaded pins have a thread cut into the shaft. They are easy to manufacture and therefore relatively inexpensive. Standard negative threaded pins suffer the disadvantage of a 'stress riser' where the stiffer shaft of the pin meets the weaker threaded portion (see Chapter 4). This stress riser is prone to failure if it is positioned outside the bone. This disadvantage has been mitigated by the use of end threaded (Ellis) pins (Figure 10.32) that protect the stress riser within the medullary cavity of the transfixed bone. Alternatively, DuraFace® pins have been designed with a gradually tapering fully threaded tip and a relatively larger shaft. These features produce relatively stiffer pins with stress being dissipated over a larger area.

Positive-profile threaded pins

Positive-profile threaded pins are stronger than negative end threaded pins because their core diameter at the threaded portion is the same size as the shaft diameter (Figure 10.33). They are more expensive than negative threaded pins. Positive end threaded pins are commonly referred to as InterFace® pins.

Positive-profile pins are also available with threads in the central portion of the pin. These pins are available in the same sizes as InterFace® pins and are commonly referred to as CenterFace® pins (Figure 10.34). Centrally threaded pins are used in biplanar ESF configurations. Although there is a thread-cutting facility similar to that employed in self-tapping screws, there can still be

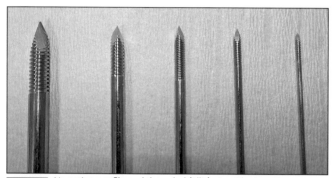

10.32 Negative-profile end threaded (Ellis) pins. The junction between the shaft and the threaded portion is a 'stress riser'. The pins are designed so that this point is placed inside the medullary cavity with the negative thread seated in the far cortex. If this junction is outside the near cortex of the bone, there is a high risk of pin fracture at this site.

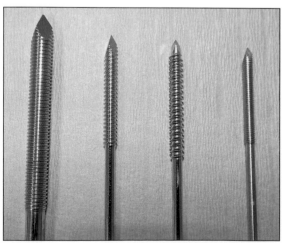

10.33 Positive-profile end threaded pins are available with diameters from 0.9 mm to 4 mm.

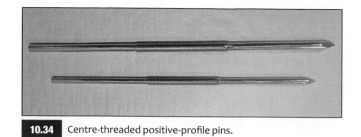

10.34 Centre-threaded positive-profile pins.

significant heat generation during pin insertion. Pre-drilling is mandatory for these pins, and use of the equiv-alent end threaded pin to cut the thread is recommended before inserting the centrally threaded pins.

Connecting clamps

Connecting clamps are used to connect the transfixation pins to the connecting bar, or to link connecting bars to one another. There are a wide variety of clamps available.

Kirschner–Ehmer clamp

The Kirschner–Ehmer clamp is the oldest clamp available for veterinary use (Figure 10.35). There is only one securing nut that applies friction to the transfixation pin and con-necting bar simultaneously. This system suffers the disad-vantage of not allowing additional clamps to be secured to the middle section of a connecting bar after the ESF construct has been assembled. The available sizes are:

- Small – <5 kg animals, 3.2 mm connecting bar, 2.4 mm maximum pin diameter
- Medium – 5–30 kg animals, 4.8 mm connecting bar, 3.2 mm maximum pin diameter
- Large – >30 kg animals, 8 mm connecting bar, 4 mm maximum pin diameter.

SK™ system

Modern clamps have been developed with separate fix-ation bolts for the transfixation pin and connecting bar (Figure 10.36). Other clamps are available that have been manufactured using similar principles. The primary advan-tage is the ability to add and remove clamps to the middle section of a connecting bar after the ESF construct has been partially assembled. Transfixation pin sizes are equivalent to those used in Kirschner–Ehmer constructs. Connecting bars are sized differently:

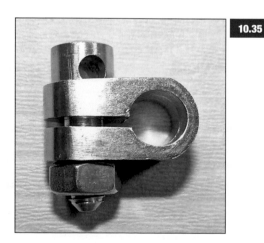

10.35 Kirschner–Ehmer clamp.

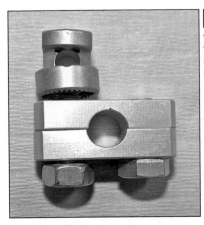

10.36 SK™ clamp. The primary bolt on the left is used to secure the transfixation pin; the secondary bolt on the right secures the connecting bar.

- Mini – 3.2 mm stainless steel connecting bar
- Small – 6.3 mm titanium or carbon fibre connecting bar
- Large – 9.5 mm carbon fibre connecting bar.

Connecting bars

Connecting bars can either be rods (to which the transfixation pins are connected using clamps) or acrylic resin. Rods are available in various diameters depending on the clamp size. Construct biomechanics are also affected by the material properties of the connecting bar(s).

Stainless steel

A 316L stainless steel Steinmann pin can be used as a connecting bar. These are usually used in the minisystems where they have the advantage of being easy to contour and cut to length.

Carbon fibre

Carbon fibre is particularly anisotropic, which means it neutralizes axial forces very well, but is less able to resist large bending forces. Carbon fibre rods have the advantage of being radiolucent, making radiographic interpretation of fracture healing easier (Figure 10.37).

Titanium

Titanium connecting bars are available for use with the small and large SK™ systems (Figure 10.37). Titanium is stiffer than carbon fibre and lighter than stainless steel and is better able to resist large bending forces.

Acrylic resin and ESF putty

Free-form ESF constructs can be made using acrylic or ESF putty to replace the connecting clamps and bars (Figure 10.38). The latter is moulded by hand and sets in 2 to 3 minutes.

Partially threaded connecting bars

Partially threaded titanium connecting bars allow the attachment of linear ESF connecting bars to a ring in order to construct a hybrid ESF device (Figure 10.39).

Hinges

In linear ESF constructs, hinges are either bonded to the connecting bars using ESF putty or are screwed on to partially threaded connecting bars (Figure 10.40). Hinged linear ESF constructs are used most commonly to temporarily support tarsal joints where collateral ligament insufficiency is present. The hinges in these transarticular constructs must be perfectly centred over the centre of rotation of the tibiotarsal joint.

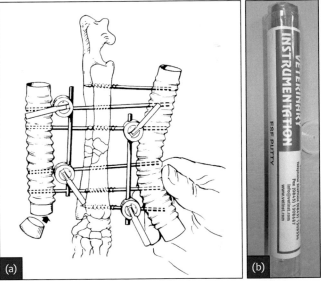

10.38 (a) Temporary fracture stabilization using removable clamps and steel bars. Plastic tubing is pushed over pin ends following fracture reduction and bottom-plugged. Acrylic is mixed in self-contained packets and poured into tubing while still in the liquid phase. The steel clamps and bars are removed once the acrylic has set. (b) ESF putty.
(a, Courtesy of JP Lapish)

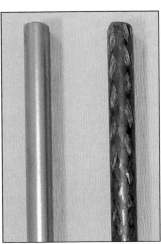

10.37 Titanium (left) and carbon fibre (right) 6.3 mm connecting bars for use with the small SK™ system.

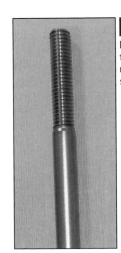

10.39 A partially threaded 6.3 mm connecting bar. One or more of these bars is used to attach a circular external skeletal fixator ring to a small SK™ linear ESF construct resulting in a hybrid linear–circular external skeletal fixator.

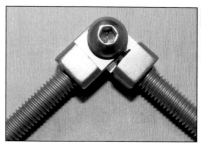

10.40 A 6.3 mm SK™ hinge. One or more hinges can be incorporated into either linear or circular ESF constructs.

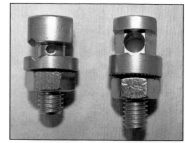

10.42 A wire clamp (left) and a small transfixation pin clamp (right).

Circular external skeletal fixation

Circular external skeletal fixation (CESF) constructs are most frequently used in the correction of angular limb deformities.

- The thin wires employed for bone fixation are able to transfix very small juxta-articular bone fragments.
- Threaded connecting bars allow motors to be attached between the fixation rings on the major bone fragments. Daily turning of the motors produces a distractive force across an osteotomy. As the bone fragments are distracted, new bone forms in the defect by a process called 'distraction osteogenesis'.
- Hinges can be incorporated into the CESF constructs allowing gradual correction of angular limb deformities.

CESF and hybrid linear–CESF are versatile techniques that can also be applied to long bone fracture repair and temporary transarticular stabilization.

CESF transfixation wires

Smooth wires are available in longer lengths than K-wires (125–200 mm) to allow them to be inserted as part of CESF configurations and tensioned using a specific wire tensioner. Application of tension to the wires significantly increases their stiffness. These wires are available with stoppers ('olive' wires) (Figure 10.41) or without. The wires incorporate single-facet cutting tips that effectively prevent skipping of the pin tip on the bone fragment during drilling. The stopper is used when fragments can only be fixed in a single plane. When stopper wires are driven in opposing directions, translation of the bone fragment along the smooth wires is prevented.

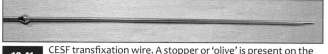

10.41 CESF transfixation wire. A stopper or 'olive' is present on the wire.

CESF connecting clamps

Transfixation wires are attached to CESF rings using dedicated wire clamps. If a wire that has been driven through a bone does not intersect a ring hole on the opposite side of the limb, the eccentric slot can be used to fix the wire (Figure 10.42). If a bilateral wire cannot be placed because of a lack of availability of a safe corridor on both sides of the transfixed limb, a pin clamp can be used to fix a unilateral transfixation pin (Figure 10.42).

CESF rings and arches

A large inventory of full rings, incomplete (sector) rings, stretch rings and arches are available for mounting of the CESF clamps (Figure 10.43).

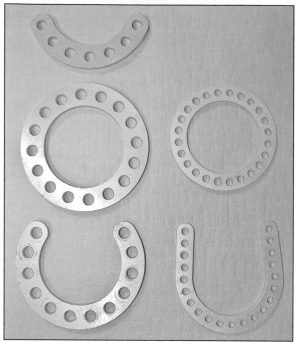

10.43 Various styles and sizes of rings serve as the basic structural element of CESF and hybrid ESF frames. These include full rings (right and left centre), sector rings (three-quarter) (bottom left), stretch rings (bottom right) and spinal arches (top left).

Threaded connecting bars

Fully threaded connecting bars (Figure 10.44) are used to attach adjacent rings to one another in CESF constructs. These threaded bars allow the rings to be adjusted in the axial plane to produce distraction across an osteotomy or compression across a fracture. Partially threaded bars (see Figure 10.39) are used to attach rings to linear ESF components to produce hybrid linear–CESF constructs.

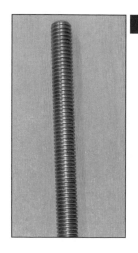

10.44 Fully threaded 6.3 mm connecting bar.

References and further reading

Black J (1980) Biomaterials for internal fixation. In: *Fracture Treatment and Healing*, ed. B Heppenstall, pp. 113–123 . WB Saunders, Philadelphia

Brinker WO, Hohn RB and Prieur WD (1984) Basic aspects of internal fixation. In: *Manual of Internal Fixation in Small Animals*, pp. 3–8. Springer-Verlag, Berlin

Chase D and Farrell M (2010) Fracture of the lateral trochlear ridge after surgical stabilization of medial patellar luxation. *Veterinary and Comparative Orthopaedics and Traumatology* **23**, 203–208

Costerton JW, Montanaro L and Arciola CR (2005) Biofilm in implant infections: its production and regulation. *International Journal of Artificial Organs* **28**, 1062–1068

Dernell WS, Ehrhart NP and Straw RC (2007) Tumors of the skeletal system. In: *Withrow and MacEwen's Small Animal Clinical Oncology, 4th edn*, ed. SJ Withrow and DM Vail, pp. 540–582. WB Saunders, St Louis

Deutman R, Mulder TJ, Brian R (1977) Metal sensitivity before and after total hip arthroplasty. *Journal of Bone and Joint Surgery (American Volume)* **59-A**, 862–865

Dyce J and Houlton JEF (1993) Use of reconstruction plates for repair of acetabular fractures in 16 dogs. *Journal of Small Animal Practice* **34**, 547–553

Egenvall A, Nodtvedt A and von Euler H (2007) Bone tumors in a population of 400 000 insured Swedish dogs up to 10 years of age: incidence and survival. *Canadian Journal of Veterinary Research* **71**, 292–299

Hamilton MH and Langley-Hobbs SJ (2005) Use of the AO veterinary mini T-plate for stabilization of distal radius and ulna fractures in toy breed dogs. *Veterinary and Comparative Orthopaedics and Traumatology* **18**, 18–25

McLaughlin RM, Cockshutt JR and Kuzma AB (1992) Stacked veterinary cuttable plates for treatment of comminuted diaphyseal fractures in cats. *Veterinary and Comparative Orthopaedics and Traumatology* **5**, 22–25

Roch SP and Gemmill TJ (2008) Treatment of medial patellar luxation by femoral closing wedge ostectomy using a distal femoral plate in four dogs. *Journal of Small Animal Practice* **49**, 152–158

Roe SC (2003) Internal fracture fixation. In: *Textbook of Small Animal Surgery, 3rd edn*, ed. D Slatter, pp. 1798–1818. WB Saunders, Philadelphia

Rooks RL, Tarvin GB, Pijanowski GJ and Daly WB (1982) *In vitro* cerclage wiring analysis. *Veterinary Surgery* **11**, 39–43

Saikku-Backstrom A, Ralha JE, Vallmaa T and Tulamo R-M (2005) Repair of radial fractures in toy breed dogs with self-reinforced biodegradable bone plates, metal screws, and light-weight external coaptation. *Veterinary Surgery* **34**, 11–17

Slocum TD (2005) Incidence of neoplasia with TPLO surgery and Slocum implant. In: *Proceedings of the 32nd Veterinary Orthopaedic Congress*, Veterinary Orthopedic Society, 5–12 March 2005, Snowmass, Colorado, USA

Smith GK (1983) Systemic aspects of metallic implant degradation. In: *Biomaterials in Reconstructive Surgery*, ed. L Rubin, pp. 229–236. CV Mosby, St Louis

Smith GK (1985) Orthopaedic biomaterials. In: *Textbook of Small Animal Orthopaedics*, ed. CD Newton and DM Nunamaker, pp. 127–131. JB Lippincott, Philadelphia

von Pfeil DJF (2008) The use of stacked T-plating in dogs. *Veterinary and Comparative Orthopaedics and Traumatology* **4**, 260–265

Wilson JW (1987) Effect of cerclage wires on periosteal bone in growing dogs. *Veterinary Surgery* **16**, 299–302

Chapter 11

Basic surgical techniques

James Grierson

This chapter aims to outline the general organizational approach to the surgical fixation of fractures, along with describing some of the basic surgical techniques involved in fracture reduction and fixation. It is not designed to be an exhaustive or detailed review of techniques, but rather an overview of the main principles.

It must be remembered that fracture surgeries are not routine operations. They are often demanding in terms of technical skill needed, equipment requirements, time and also concentration by the surgeon. Fractures are not surgeries to be rushed through theatre and preparation is vital for all aspects of the operation.

> *'By failing to prepare, you are preparing to fail.'*
> **– Benjamin Franklin**

There are many aspects of preparation required, some of which have been discussed already such as having more than one plan for the stabilizing fracture (see Chapter 7) and adherence to good surgical techniques (see Chapter 8).

For information on theatre cleaning, patient preparation and preparation of the surgical team, readers are referred to other texts, such as the *BSAVA Manual of Canine and Feline Surgical Principles*.

Surgical planning and safety checklists

In June 2008, the World Health Organization (WHO) launched a second Global Patient Safety Challenge known as 'Safe Surgery Saves Lives' to reduce the number of surgical deaths across the world. This included improving anaesthetic safety practices, ensuring the correct site of surgery, avoiding surgical site infections and improving communication within the team. A core set of safety checks were identified in the form of a WHO Surgical Safety Checklist for use in any operating theatre environment.

The checklist identifies three phases of an operation: before the induction of anaesthesia ('sign in'), before the incision of the skin ('time out') and before the patient leaves the operating room ('sign out'). In each phase, a checklist coordinator (normally a nurse) must confirm that the surgery team has completed the listed tasks before they proceed with the operation. The complexity of the list may vary depending on the type of surgery being performed; for example, neurosurgery would have a very different checklist to colorectal surgery.

This checklist can be adapted for use in veterinary practice to reduce the chances of mistakes and complications occurring (Figure 11.1).

Theatre set-up and organization

Making a preoperative plan and sharing it with the nursing team should ensure that all equipment is available.

- Make a list of all equipment that will be required for the surgery and include any extras that may be needed should the plan change.
- Check that the equipment is available and in a good state of repair.
- Check all sterile packets for their integrity and, if there is any doubt, re-sterilize.
- Almost all orthopaedic surgery will involve the use of some form of power tool. The availability of compressed air for air-powered equipment should be checked; for any battery-powered equipment, charging levels should be checked along with the availability of additional batteries should they be required.
- Check whether any specific implants required for the surgery are available.
- Ensure that the operating theatre has been set up to facilitate optimal patient positioning.
- Check whether a scrubbed assistant will be required.
- Make sure that there is adequate and unimpeded access to the surgical site. In cases of surgery to the head, neck or thoracic limb there can sometimes be 'clashing' with the anaesthetist. Use of extension lines and longer tubing, as well as consideration of surgeon position, will minimize any problems.
- Distractions should be kept to a minimum and interruptions to surgery should only be made if essential.

Patient set-up and positioning

Prior to starting any surgery a number of patient and positioning checks should be performed.

- Patient positioning in theatre is critical. Depending on the area of the fracture and the surgical approach the

Surgery Planning and Safety Checklist

Patient details

Name:...

Age:.. Sex:..

Breed:.. Case number:...

Procedure(s)

Surgical site   LF ☐   RF ☐   LH ☐   RH ☐   Abdo ☐   Thorax ☐   Head ☐   Neck ☐   Perineal ☐

Lead surgeon: .... Date of procedure:................................

Pre-surgery

Diagnosis: ....

....

Weight:..

Other health issues: ....

....

....

Anaesthesia concerns: ....

Current medication: ....

Surgery plan

Premedication: ACP   Methadone

                              0.005 0.01 0.02 mg/kg   0.1 0.2 0.3 mg/kg

Other:..

Preoperative imaging: XR ☐   CT ☐   US ☐   MRI ☐

Other procedures: ....

....

Epidural: No ☐   Morphine ☐   Local ☐

Local block?..

Preoperative meds: Intravenous antibiotic 20 mins before surgery? Yes ☐ No ☐

                       NSAID?...

Patient safety checklist *(To be confirmed verbally with the team before starting surgery. Tick boxes.)*

Preoperative:	
Confirm patient name	
Confirm procedure	
Confirm limb/surgical site	
Kit/implants available, sterile and checked for tears?	
Intravenous antibiotics given?	

Postoperative:	
Procedure logged	
Is swab count complete (or not applicable)?	
Have any specimens that have been taken been appropriately labelled?	
Have any equipment problems been identified that need to be addressed?	
Purse-string removed?	
Bladder emptied?	

Other comments:...

....

....

11.1   A surgical safety checklist to be used when performing orthopaedic surgery.

position of the patient will need to differ. What position will the animal need to be in: lateral, sternal or dorsal recumbency? Is there a requirement to have the leg suspended so that it can then be draped out and manipulated during the procedure? Is access for a bone graft going to be needed and can this can be easily accessed with the patient in the current position and draped?

- Are appropriate aids available for patient positioning, for example, sandbags and/or ties?
- Is the lighting appropriate? If surgical lighting is used the position of the 'elbow' of the gantry often dictates direction and angulation of the light; addressing this once sterile can be difficult and approximate lighting position should be set and adjusted prior to surgery.
- Is appropriate preoperative imaging available and clearly visible?
- If surgical plans and measurements have been made to guide the surgery, are they available and clearly visible?

Trolley set-up

Having an organized trolley is an important starting point in any procedure. Much time can be wasted rummaging around under a pile of instruments for that elusive retractor. Whilst the exact organization of the trolley is based on surgeon preference, a few general rules can be applied.

- Before accepting individual instruments or kits first check that the item is required. Has the package integrity been maintained? Is a sterilization indicator present, and has it been checked? Has the kit exceeded its expiry date?
- All kits should be checked to confirm that the internal sterilization indicator has changed before they are placed on the trolley.
- All sharps should be placed on a metal or solid plastic surface to avoid penetration of the drapes.
- All sharp pointed instruments (e.g. pointed reduction forceps, Gelpi retractors, towel clips) should be placed on the trolley with the points up.
- When moving boxes containing kit around the instrument trolley, they should be lifted and not pushed/dragged to avoid damage to the drapes.

- Instruments should be returned to their place of origin on the trolley; excessively bloody instruments should be cleaned with a sterile swab before returning to the trolley.
- Kits containing multiple instruments should be opened and organized before starting surgery to ensure that all instruments are present.
- Only necessary instruments from kits should be removed and placed in an accessible area on the trolley.
- Dirty instruments should not be returned to clean kit boxes.
- The kit and instrument trolley should be positioned in such a way as to avoid walking around or excessive movement to acquire kit; use of an assistant facilitates this.
- When requesting implants of a particular size (e.g. drill bits, taps, screws) it is important to confirm the size verbally prior to use to avoid problems or complications.

The final point is a reminder that, as these are not routine surgeries, caution should always be exercised. Fracture repairs can be unforgiving and a small mistake in theatre could result in major postoperative complications later down the line. Preoperative preparation and organization of the theatre does not take much time to do. In almost all cases better organization will facilitate theatre flow as well as reduce surgical time.

References and further reading

Baines S, Lipscomb V and Hutchinson T (2012) *BSAVA Manual of Canine and Feline Surgical Principles: A Foundation Manual.* BSAVA Publications, Gloucester

Johnson AL, Houlton JEF and Vannini R (2005) *AO Principles of Fracture Management in the Dog and Cat.* AO Publishing, Switzerland

Marti JM and Miller A (1994a) Delimitation of safe corridors for the insertion of external fixator pins in the dog 1: Hindlimb. *Journal of Small Animal Practice* **35**, 16–23

Marti JM and Miller A (1994b) Delimitation of safe corridors for the insertion of external fixator pins in the dog 2: Forelimb. *Journal of Small Animal Practice* **35**, 78–85

Piermattei DL, Flo GL and DeCamp CE (2006) *Brinker, Piermattei, and Flo's Handbook of Small Animal Orthopedics and Fracture Repair, 4th edn.* Elsevier, St Louis

Piermattei DL and Johnson K (2004) *An Atlas of Surgical Approaches to the Bones and Joints of the Dog and Cat, 4th edn.* Saunders Elsevier, St Louis

World Health Organization (2009) *Surgical Safety Checklist.* www.who.int/patientsafety/safesurgery/en/

OPERATIVE TECHNIQUE 11.1

Fracture reduction

EQUIPMENT EXTRAS

Gelpi retractors; periosteal elevator; Hohmann retractors; pointed reduction forceps; bone-holding forceps.

SURGICAL TECHNIQUES

Approach

Appropriate for bone involved.

Reduction techniques

A number of different techniques can be employed with a view to reducing the fracture fragments to their original anatomical position.

Countertraction

Traction is applied distal to the fracture whilst countertraction is applied proximal to the fracture (Figure 11.2a) and the limb manipulated until the fracture is reduced (Figure 11.2b). Slow application of force is often more effective. Additionally, holding the fracture in traction for a few minutes at a time helps to fatigue the muscles and any local tissue contraction and further facilitates reduction. Countertraction can be performed via an open or closed approach. If performed via an open approach, direct force can be applied to the bones using bone-holding forceps. When positioning the patient prior to surgery, the possible use of countertraction during surgery should be considered and the patient secured appropriately to the operating table.

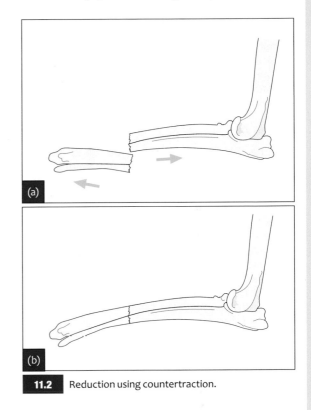

11.2 Reduction using countertraction.

Toggling

Using traction alone to reduce fractures accurately is often very difficult. In toggling, the bone fragments are angled to form a V shape to allow the bone ends to be brought into contact (Figures 11.3ab); the ends are kept in contact whilst the bone is forcefully reduced by pressure at each end of the bone (Figure 11.3c). In some cases maintenance of pressure will fatigue the muscles and allow reduction. Great care must be taken to avoid propagating any fissures. Control of the bone fragments is most easily achieved with serrated reduction forceps.

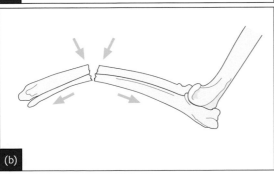

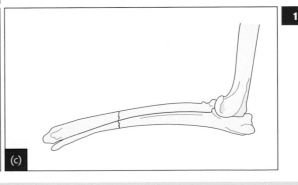

11.3 Toggling technique.

➡

→ **OPERATIVE TECHNIQUE 11.1 CONTINUED**

Levering

This reduction technique involves the use of an instrument, such as a Hohmann retractor, that is slipped between the two fracture segments and used to lever the bones apart (Figure 11.4a) before allowing reduction (Figure 11.4b).

Pointed forceps

In some cases the final reduction can be difficult to achieve due to overriding muscle forces. Appropriate use of pointed reduction forceps can achieve the last small amount of distraction of oblique fractures. The pointed reduction forceps are applied across a partially reduced oblique fracture with finger pressure and then rotated to force the bone fragments into the reduced position (Figure 11.5).

Pusher pin

A large Steinmann pin can be used to distract the fracture. The pin is placed in the medullary canal and driven across the fracture site and into the metaphysis of the distal fragment (Figure 11.6a). Continued pressure allows distraction of the limb and aids in alignment of other fragments (Figure 11.6b). Ancillary fixation, such as a plate, is needed to maintain the reduction. The pin can either be left *in situ* as part of the fixation technique or removed following stabilization. If a narrow pin is used (relative to the bone diameter), the sharp tip can be cut off to reduce the risk of the pin penetrating an adjacent joint as it is advanced into the bone.

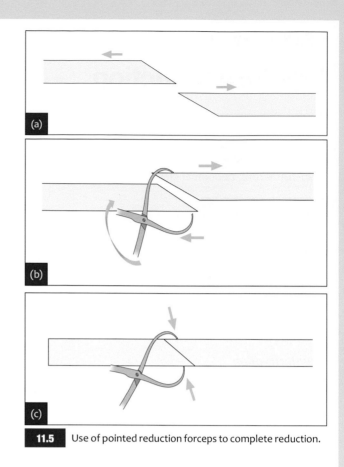

11.5 Use of pointed reduction forceps to complete reduction.

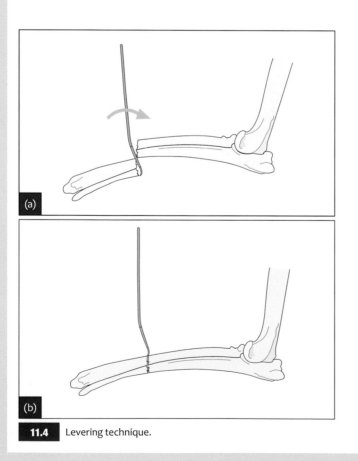

11.4 Levering technique.

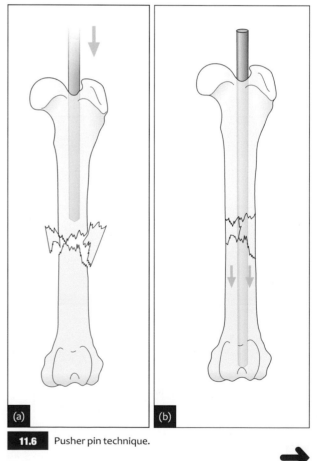

11.6 Pusher pin technique.

→

→ **OPERATIVE TECHNIQUE 11.1 CONTINUED**

Reduction devices

The use of an orthopaedic distractor can aid reduction in difficult to reduce fractures. Transfixation pins are applied through both cortices proximal and distal to the fracture (Figure 11.7a) and then attached to the distractor using wing nuts (Figure 11.7b). The wing nuts sit on a threaded rod that allows the fracture to be slowly distracted until reduction has been achieved (Figure 11.7c). These are rarely used in small animal orthopaedics; however, modified external skeletal fixator devices can be used in a similar fashion.

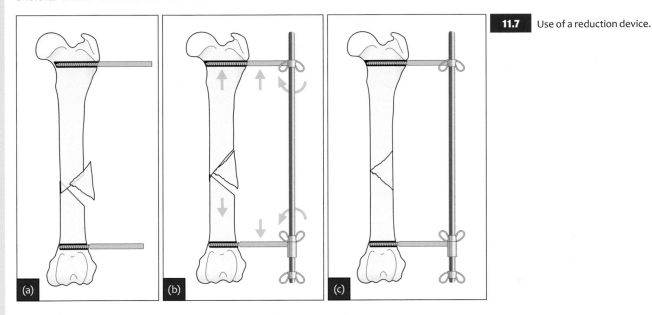

11.7 Use of a reduction device.

> **WARNING**
>
> Care should always be taken with handling of bone fragments. In skeletally immature animals the amount of force applied should be tempered to avoid damaging the bone

---

OPERATIVE TECHNIQUE 11.2

Insertion of intramedullary pins

EQUIPMENT EXTRAS

Gelpi retractors; bone-holding forceps; pointed reduction forceps; Jacobs chuck or appropriate drill; small and large pin cutters; appropriate pin(s).

SURGICAL TECHNIQUES

Approach

Appropriate for bone involved.

Selection of pin size

- Depends on the technique being performed with additional fixation external to the medullary canal (e.g. cerclage wire or plate): 30–50% of canal diameter for pin–plate combinations (usually 35–40%), or if used as the primary fixation with additional cerclage wire, 70–80% of medullary canal diameter at its narrowest point.
- The length of the pin can be determined from radiographs of contralateral limb. Aim for the tip to impact in the distal metaphysis. It is prudent to have another pin of the same length available during surgery, which can help when visually estimating how far a pin has been driven into the bone. ➡

→ **OPERATIVE TECHNIQUE 11.2 CONTINUED**

- The pin can be cut to an appropriate length preoperatively or alternatively it can be notched and broken *in situ* or cut following insertion (robust, sharp pin cutters are required; a hacksaw is inappropriate if the pin in fully seated as it will traumatize the adjacent soft tissue structures).

Reduction and fixation

The fracture is exposed if required and the fragment ends examined for fissuring. Assessment of the appropriateness of the selected pin diameter can also be performed at this stage. If possible and appropriate, fissures can be protected using cerclage wires.

Normograde pin insertion

The pin is driven into the medullary canal from the end of the bone and advanced along it, traversing the fracture site and then impacting into the metaphysis of the opposing fragment (Figure 11.8a). The pin is then cut. In some cases of simple fractures it may be possible to perform closed normograde insertion; however, this is rarely achieved unless intraoperative imaging is available.
    Landmarks for normograde pinning:

- Humerus – greater tubercle proximally
- Femur – intertrochanteric fossa, immediately medial to greater trochanter
- Tibia – craniomedial aspect, immediately caudomedial to insertion of straight patellar ligament. NB minimal pin should be left protruding here to avoid damage to the stifle joint.

Retrograde pin insertion

The pin is inserted into the medullary canal at the fracture site and driven through it until it exits the bone at a distant site (Figure 11.8b). The chuck is reversed and the pin is drawn out until only the tip is visible at the fracture site. The fracture is reduced and the pin is driven across the fracture site and impacted in the metaphysis of the opposing fragment. The use of double-pointed pins can be advantageous.

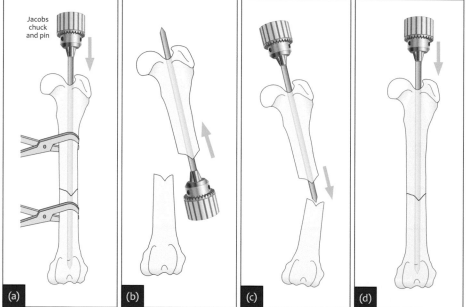

Jacobs chuck and pin

(a) (b) (c) (d)

11.8 (a) Normograde pin insertion. (b) Retrograde pin insertion. (c) Fracture is reduced and pin driven across the fracture site. (d) Pin is impacted into the distal metaphysis, taking care not to penetrate the joint.

PRACTICAL TIPS

- Remember to allow for radiographic magnification (usually 10–15%) when selecting pin sizes. A small increase in pin diameter confers a large increase in strength
- The tibia should only be pinned normograde due to the risk of iatrogenic damage to the stifle joint when pins are inserted retrograde
- Removing the tip of the pin following insertion through the first fragment and before insertion into the distal fragment reduces the chances of driving the pin through the metaphysis and out of the bone

WARNING

Intramedullary pins should never be applied to the radius

OPERATIVE TECHNIQUE 11.3

Insertion of interlocking nail

EQUIPMENT EXTRAS

Reamers to prepare medullary cavity; interlocking nail and extension piece; appropriate drill, drill bits, guides and tap; screws or bolts (all appropriately sized for the bone and patient).

SURGICAL TECHNIQUES

Approach

Appropriate for bone involved.

Selection of nail size

The largest size that will fit into the medullary cavity ensuring two screws/bolts per fragment.

Reduction and fixation

1   The medullary canal is opened in either a normograde or retrograde manner and a reamer used to achieve the correct size for the nail.

2   The nail must be passed normograde (Figure 11.9a); this is often done using an insertion tool.

3   The fracture is then reduced; a limited surgical approach can be used.

4   The nail is then driven across the fracture site and into the metaphysis in a similar manner to placement of an intramedullary pin.

5   With the nail in its final position, a drilling jig is applied so that the drill holes are accurately aligned to the holes in the nail (Figure 11.9b).

6   The distal fragment is locked first by placing the distal screws through the bone and nail. Any rotational alignment is then corrected before locking the proximal fragment (Figure 11.9c).

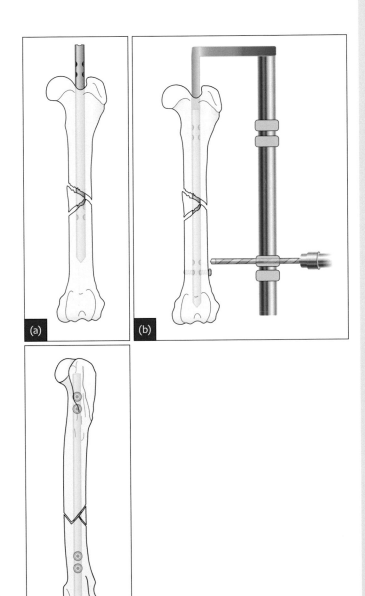

(a) (b) (c)

11.9 Application of an interlocking nail.

PRACTICAL TIPS

- Suitable for selected fractures of the humerus, femur and tibia
- Accurate measuring for nail length is critical for placement and success in this procedure
- Avoid application of forces to the jig (with instruments or tissues) as this may cause malalignment of the drill holes and nail holes

OPERATIVE TECHNIQUE 11.4

Application of cerclage wire

Gelpi retractors; bone-holding forceps; pointed reduction forceps; parallel pliers and wire cutters or combined cutter/twisters; assorted sizes of wire; wire passer; double loop cerclage wire tightener.

SURGICAL TECHNIQUES

Approach

Appropriate for bone involved.

Reduction and fixation

Application of cerclage wire

For full cerclage (Figure 11.10a), the wire is passed around the bone avoiding soft tissue entrapment (a wire passer can be helpful); for hemicerclage the wire is passed through a bone tunnel (Figure 11.10b). At least two cerclage wires should be applied.

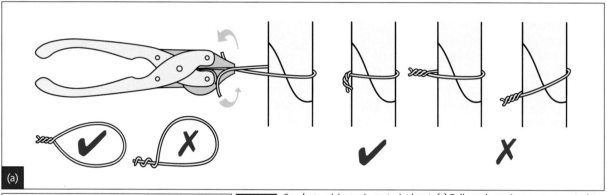

(a)

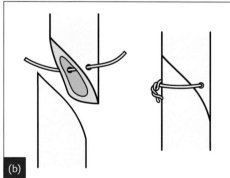

(b)

11.10 Cerclage wiring using a twist knot. (a) Full cerclage. A secure, even twist knot is created. This is usually bent over whilst continuing to twist the wire, to maintain tension, and is then cut short. The wire must be fully tightened and should be perpendicular to the bone. (b) Hemicerclage. The wire is applied through a bone tunnel.

The wire can then be secured in one of three ways.

- Twist – the wire is pulled tight and the first twists started by hand; excess wire is then removed. The wire ends are then twisted around each other using needle pliers or twisters; firm tension is required to ensure the twist remains tight and secure. The end is then cut short leaving three twists (Figure 11.10a). The twist knot only generates 50% of the static tension produced by a loop knot of equivalent diameter.
- Single loop – formed using a length of wire with an eye at one end (Figure 11.11a). The free end of the wire is passed around the bone and through the eye (Figure 11.11b) and then inserted into a wire tightener and the crank tightened (Figure 11.11c). The cerclage is tightened further by turning the crank (Figure 11.11d). The wire tightener is then bent over so that the free end of the wire is folded back on itself (Figure 11.11e). The crank is loosened a little to allow folding to be completed and the wire to be cut leaving 5–10 mm exposed (Figure 11.11fg).

→

→ **OPERATIVE TECHNIQUE 11.4 CONTINUED**

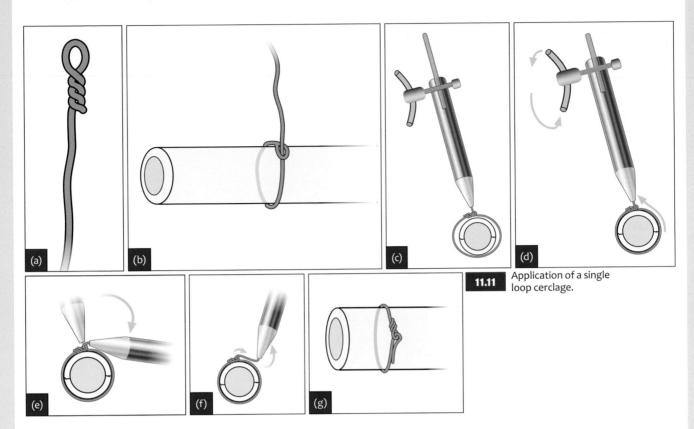

11.11 Application of a single loop cerclage.

- Double loop – formed using a straight length of wire folded in the middle with the folded end passed around the bone (Figure 11.12a). The two free ends are then passed through the formed loop and secured in the two cranks of a double loop wire tightener. The cerclage is tightened further by turning the cranks. The wire tightener is then bent over so that the free ends of the wires are folded back on themselves. The crank is loosened a little to allow folding to be completed and the wire to be cut leaving 5–10 mm exposed (Figure 11.12b).

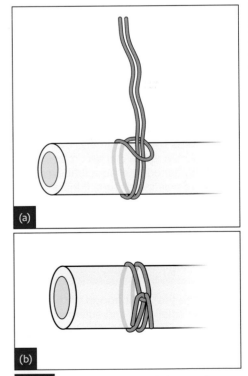

11.12 Application of a double loop cerclage.

PRACTICAL TIPS

- If twists need to be bent over then this should be done at the same time as twisting to maintain tension. Bending of a twisted knot can be done to reduce soft tissue irritation but it reduces static tension by 30–70%, although this can be reduced by continuing to twist as the knot is bent
- A minimum of three twists is required on a twist knot to maintain tension
- Double loops have superior strength compared to twists or single loops, but can be more challenging to apply
- Wires must be applied perfectly perpendicular to the long axis of the bone

WARNING

If the bony column cannot be reconstructed then cerclage wire should not be used. Cerclage wires are always used with additional fixation such as an intramedullary pin, external fixator or plate

OPERATIVE TECHNIQUE 11.5

Application of tension-band wiring

Pointed reduction forceps; Jacobs chuck or motorized pin driver; parallel pliers and wire cutters or combined cutter/ twisters; assorted sizes of wire; assorted pin sizes; pin cutters.

SURGICAL TECHNIQUES

Approach

Appropriate for bone involved.

Reduction and fixation

A transosseous tunnel is drilled distant from the fracture site in the main fragment (distance should be approximately the same distance below the fracture line as the pins are above it) (Figure 11.13).

- A piece of wire is passed through this bone tunnel and the ends crossed over. This is best done first as once the pins are placed it can be hard to place this wire.
- The fracture or osteotomy is reduced using one or two small pins such as Kirschner wires or arthrodesis wires. Accounting for anatomical constraints, the pins should ideally be placed perpendicular to the fracture line and parallel to one another (Figure 11.13a).
- A second piece of wire is passed around the ends of the pins (care is taken to avoid unnecessary entrapment of important soft tissue structures, e.g. tendons) or through a bone tunnel adjacent to the pins (Figure 11.13b).
- The ends of the pins are bent over and the wires twisted tight and evenly (tension must be placed on the wire as it is tightened to ensure that even and secure twisting occurs) (Figure 11.13c).
- The wires are cut short and the ends are bent down flat to the bone (Figure 11.13d).

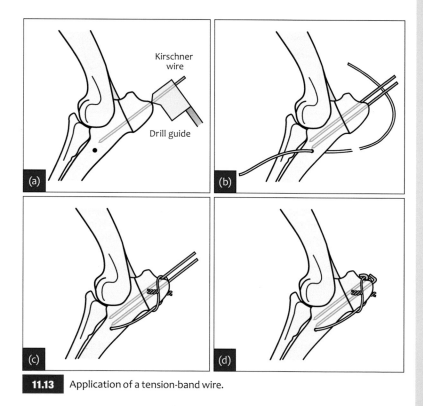

11.13 Application of a tension-band wire.

PRACTICAL TIPS

- Place the wire through the bone tunnel before placing the pins
- Use small pins and suitably large gauge tension-band wire; it is the tension-band wire that will resist disruptive forces. Ensure the wire tension-band is of adequate length

WARNING

Always use two pieces of wire to get even tension in the tension-band wire

OPERATIVE TECHNIQUE 11.6

Placement of external skeletal fixators

EQUIPMENT EXTRAS

Appropriate retractors and bone-holding forceps if an open reduction is used; motorized pin driver (such as a drill); small and large pin cutters; appropriate drill, drill bits, transfixation pins, clamps and connecting bars; two spanners for tightening clamps.

SURGICAL TECHNIQUES

Approach

Detailed knowledge of safe corridors is needed for successful application of external skeletal fixation (ESF) constructs (Marti and Miller, 1994ab).

Reduction and fixation

The fracture is reduced. Reduction may be open or closed and may involve ancillary fixation such as intramedullary pins. An appropriate sized ESF system is selected based on patient and bone size and fracture configuration.

Pin placement

- Transfixation pins should not exceed 33% of the diameter of the narrowest part of the bone. They should not be placed through existing wounds or surgical approaches unless absolutely necessary.
- For each pin, a stab incision is made through the skin, ensuring that pins can be placed without interfering with adjacent joints or vital soft tissue structures.
- The incision should be large enough (5–10 mm) to avoid tension on the skin after pin placement.
- All holes should be pre-drilled using a drill bit slightly smaller than the diameter of the transfixation pin.
- Threaded pins can be placed perpendicular to the bone axis (preferable), whereas smooth pins should be placed at 60–70 degrees to the bone axis to reduce the chance of their pulling out. In practice, smooth transfixation pins are rarely used because of the mechanical advantages afforded by threaded pins (see Chapter 10).
- All pins must penetrate both cortices of the bone.
- Pin placement should be performed using a motorized pin driver to reduce wobble associated with insertion.

Frame construction

- The proximal and distal transfixation pins are inserted first (Figure 11.14a).
- The connecting bar is attached using clamps to connect it to the transfixation pins; a gap of around 10 mm is left between the clamp and the skin (Figures 11.14b).
- Fracture reduction is checked and then additional transfixation pins are placed, as above, using clamps connected to the bar as a guide to ensure proper alignment (Figure 11.14c).

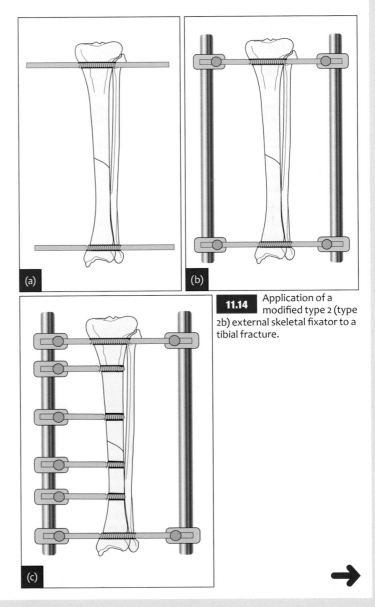

11.14 Application of a modified type 2 (type 2b) external skeletal fixator to a tibial fracture.

→ **OPERATIVE TECHNIQUE 11.6 CONTINUED**

- All transfixation pins should be inserted at target points on the bone fragment that will optimize the mechanical stability of the ESF construct. For most fractures, a 'far–near–near–far' configuration is used, with pins placed to span the length of each major bone segment. Transfixation pins should ideally be kept at a distance equal to three times the implant diameter or half the bone diameter from the fracture edge or fissure.
- The remaining clamps are tightened and fracture alignment checked again.
- Insert (ideally) three or four transfixation pins into each major bone fragment – two per fragment is considered the minimum requirement.

POSTOPERATIVE MANAGEMENT

Following surgery, a soft absorbent padded dressing is cut and placed around the individual pins to absorb any discharge. Sterile sponges or swabs can then be placed between the skin and fixator clamps and also between the skin and connecting bars. The whole limb can then be wrapped in a padded dressing. This may help to reduce postoperative swelling and improves patient comfort. This dressing is normally changed daily for the first 2–3 days; sedation is rarely needed.

Following this, the padded bandage and dressings are generally removed. The frame clamps and pin ends are wrapped with a cohesive bandage to prevent clamp interference as well as minimize damage to adjacent skin and furniture!

The ESF pins do not require cleaning unless any discharge is excessive. The insertion sites are left alone to heal; generally a crust has formed within 24–48 hours and this provides a natural barrier to infection.

Ideally frames should be checked once a week. At each check the pin insertion sites should be examined for evidence of discharge and infection. All clamps should be checked and tightened as appropriate.

OPERATIVE TECHNIQUE 11.7

Insertion of positional screw

EQUIPMENT EXTRAS

Appropriate retractors and bone-holding instruments; appropriate drill, drill bits, guides and taps; screws of appropriate sizes.

SURGICAL TECHNIQUES

Reduction and fixation

- Sometimes it is not appropriate to produce compression across the fracture site as it may cause collapse of the fracture; in these cases a positional screw is used.
- The fracture is reduced and stabilized temporarily using pointed reduction forceps.
- A hole the same diameter as the screw core is drilled through both the cis (near) and trans (far) cortices of the bone.
- The appropriate length of screw is measured using a depth gauge. Both the cis and trans cortices of the bone are tapped and the screw is inserted. Depending on the depth of gauge used, it may be necessary to select a screw approximately 2 mm longer than the measured depth to ensure that there is adequate thread contact in the trans cortex (Figure 11.15).
- Tightening the screw does not generate any axial compression as both cortices are engaged by the threads and the positions of the two fragments are maintained.

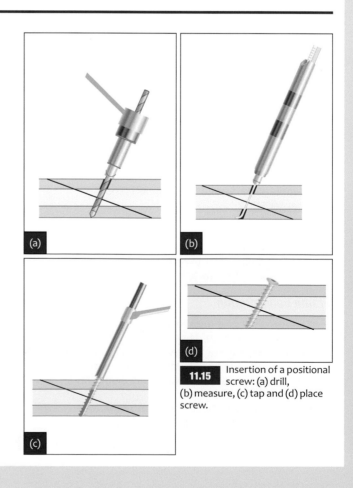

11.15 Insertion of a positional screw: (a) drill, (b) measure, (c) tap and (d) place screw.

OPERATIVE TECHNIQUE 11.8

Application of lag screw

EQUIPMENT EXTRAS

Appropriate retractors and bone-holding instruments; appropriate drill, drill bits, guides and taps; screws of appropriate sizes.

SURGICAL TECHNIQUES

Reduction and fixation

The fracture is reduced and stabilized temporarily using pointed reduction forceps. A hole the same diameter as the screw threads is drilled in the cis cortex (gliding hole) and an insert guide is passed through this (Figure 11.16). A drill the same diameter as the screw core is inserted through this guide to ensure central placement and a hole is drilled in the trans cortex (thread hole). The hole in the cis cortex should be countersunk if necessary, although this should be done cautiously in the very thin cortices of canine and feline bone.

The appropriate length of screw is measured using a depth gauge. The trans cortex only is tapped and the screw is inserted. Depending on the depth of the gauge used, it may be necessary to select a screw approximately 2 mm longer than the measured depth to ensure there is adequate thread in the trans cortex.

Tightening the screw generates axial compression along its length and compresses the trans cortex towards the screw head, where it engages the cis cortex. For optimal function the screw should be inserted midway between the perpendicular to the fracture line and the perpendicular to the longitudinal axis of the bone. A lag effect can be created by using a partially threaded cancellous screw or a shaft screw, although it may be difficult to ensure that the threaded portion of the screw is of an appropriate length.

A lag screw can be inserted through a plate hole if desired, in which case the plate rather than the screw head engages the cis cortex.

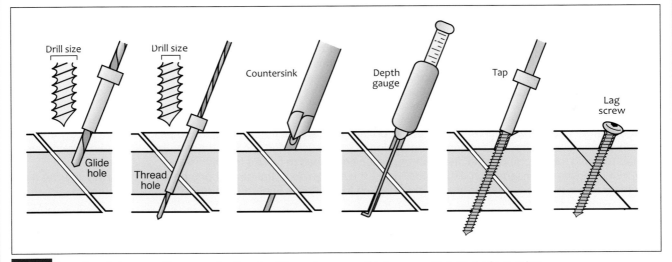

11.16   Insertion of a lag screw. The screw direction should be as close as possible to perpendicular to the fracture line.

OPERATIVE TECHNIQUE 11.9

Application of dynamic compression plate

Gelpi retractors; bone-holding forceps; pointed reduction forceps; appropriate drill, drill bits and taps; plate and screws of appropriate sizes.

SURGICAL TECHNIQUES

Approach

Appropriate for bone involved.

Reduction and fixation

The fracture and most or all of the length of the bone involved is exposed. Great care is taken to avoid excessive dissection around the bone which could compromise its vascularity. Bone ends are carefully examined for evidence of fissuring that would preclude compression being applied across the fracture site.

The fracture is reduced and reduction can be maintained using bone-holding forceps, temporary Kirschner wires or the hands of an assistant.

The plate is contoured to fit the bone. A small gap of around 2 mm should be left between the plate and bone over the fracture to produce compression of the trans cortex; this is known as 'pre-stressing' the plate (Figure 11.17). With the plate held on the bone, an appropriately sized thread hole is then drilled close to one fracture end using the drill guide in the neutral position (Figure 11.18a). The hole is measured through the plate and the thread is tapped. The plate is applied to the bone and the screw is inserted and tightened (Figure 11.18b).

Using the drill guide in the compression position, the screw hole on the opposite side of the fracture is drilled, ensuring that the plate is aligned with the bone, in particular at its most proximal and distal aspects (Figure 11.18c). This hole is measured and tapped as before. The screw is inserted and fully tightened, compressing the fracture (Figure 11.18d). After insertion of the compression screw, it is possible to insert a second screw with compression function if desired. Before this screw is tightened, the screw on the same side of the fracture has to be loosened to allow the plate to slide on the bone. After the second compression screw is tightened the loose screw is retightened. Great care is needed to avoid 'over-compressing' the fracture, which could lead to fissure formation.

Further screws are inserted on either side, using the drill guide in the neutral position, progressively moving away from the fracture (Figure 11.18e). All screws are checked for tightness prior to closure.

11.17 Application of a pre-stressed plate. (a) Exact contouring of a plate to a bone can result in a narrow gap in the trans cortex after screw tightening. (b) The plate can be pre-stressed to create a slight curve in the plate over the fracture line. (c) Following screw tightening the trans cortex is compressed.

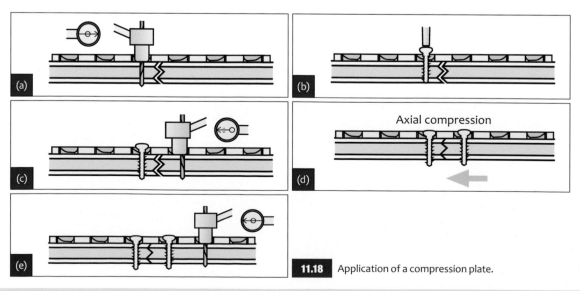

11.18 Application of a compression plate.

OPERATIVE TECHNIQUE 11.10

Application of neutralization plate

EQUIPMENT EXTRAS

Gelpi retractors; bone-holding forceps; pointed reduction forceps; appropriate drill, drill bits and taps; plate and screws of appropriate sizes.

SURGICAL TECHNIQUES

Approach

Appropriate for bone involved.

Reduction and fixation

The fracture and most or all of the length of the bone involved is exposed. Great care is taken to avoid excessive dissection around the bone which could compromise its vascularity.

The fracture is reduced by reconstructing the fragments. Reduction can be maintained using bone-holding forceps, temporary Kirschner wires, positional screws, lag screws or the hands of an assistant.

Interfragmentary compression is achieved using lag screws and the fracture is rebuilt until only two main fragments remain (Figure 11.19). These are reduced with care and stabilized using one or more additional lag screws. Consideration must be given to the location of the lag screw heads in relation to the final position of the plate; lag screws may be inserted through the plate if required. The plate is contoured to the bone without any pre-stressing.

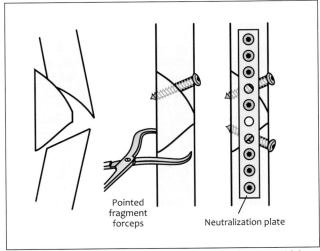

Pointed fragment forceps

Neutralization plate

11.19 Application of a neutralization plate in conjunction with lag screws.

Plate screws are inserted using the drill guide in the neutral position following the steps detailed in Operative Technique 11.9. The order of the screw insertion is not critical; it may be advantageous to insert the terminal plate screws first to ensure that the ends of the plate are located over bone. Not all screw holes need to be filled, but the surgeon should aim to engage at least six cortices above and below the fracture if possible. All screws are tightened prior to closure.

The function of the plate is to neutralize all rotational, bending and shearing forces once the fracture has been reconstructed using lag screws.

OPERATIVE TECHNIQUE 11.11

Application of bridging plate

EQUIPMENT EXTRAS

Gelpi retractors; bone-holding forceps; pointed reduction forceps; appropriate drill, drill bits and taps; plate and screws of appropriate sizes.

SURGICAL TECHNIQUES

Approach

Appropriate for bone involved.

Reduction and fixation

The fracture and most or all of the length of the bone involved is exposed. Great care is taken to avoid excessive dissection around the bone which could compromise its vascularity.

Little or no attempt is made to reconstruct the fracture fragments, although the overall bone length and anatomical orientation of adjacent bones must be restored.

A pre-contoured plate (see Figure 11.17) is applied to the major proximal and distal fragments to maintain normal bone length and alignment. At least three screws (six cortices) should be achieved in each fragment (Figure 11.20). The drill guide is used in the neutral position.

The function of the plate is to act as a splint to maintain the correct length of the bone and normal spatial alignment of the joints proximal and distal to the fracture.

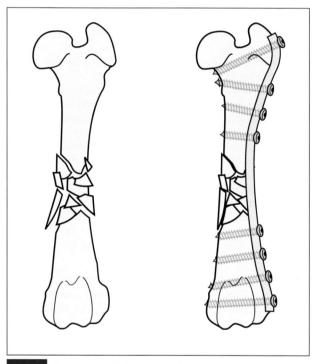

11.20 Application of a bridging plate.

WARNING

Use a longer and stronger plate as a bridging plate since it is subjected to significant bending forces during weight-bearing

PRACTICAL TIP

Because of concerns regarding further biological damage, no attempt should be made to reconstruct individual fracture fragments if reconstruction will not contribute significantly to the mechanical stability of the fracture

OPERATIVE TECHNIQUE 11.12
Pin–plate stabilization

EQUIPMENT EXTRAS

Gelpi retractors; bone-holding forceps; pointed reduction forceps; appropriate drill, drill bits and taps; plate and screws of appropriate sizes; large pin cutters; appropriate sized pins.

SURGICAL TECHNIQUES

Approach

Appropriate for bone involved.

Reduction and fixation

Exposure is limited to that needed to apply the plate and place the intramedullary pin. In order to preserve the biology of the fracture site, little or no attempt is made to reconstruct the fracture.

An intramedullary pin is placed as previously described (see Operative Technique 11.2). The pin can be 30–50% of the medullary canal diameter, although 35–40% is considered optimal (Figure 11.21ab). The bone length and the orientation of adjacent joints is checked.

A pre-contoured plate is applied to the major proximal and distal fragments to maintain normal bone length and alignment. As long a plate as possible is used to reduce any lever arm on the fixation. At least two screws (four cortices) should be placed in each fragment, four if possible (Figure 11.21c). The drill guide should be used in the neutral position. Screws will need to be angled to avoid hitting the pin and in some cases will be monocortical. Locking plate/screw systems can be considered as these confer more stability to monocortical screws compared to conventional systems. In complex fractures the screws should be away from the fracture site; in more simple fractures the far-near-near-far rule can be applied.

The function of the plate is to act as a splint to maintain the correct length of the bone and normal spatial alignment of the joints proximal and distal to the fracture whilst resisting compression and rotational forces. The pin is effective in protecting the fracture from bending forces. In addition, the use of the pin simplifies the surgical technique by maintaining alignment of the bone during plate application.

A similar technique can be used for a pin/ESF combination; this can be especially useful in cats.

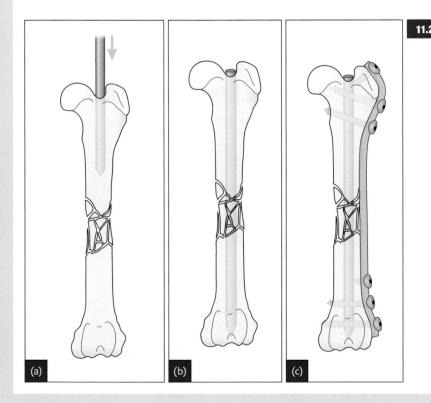

11.21 Application of a pin–plate construct.

(a) (b) (c)

Chapter 12

Open fractures

Steve Bright

An open fracture is diagnosed where there is communication between the fracture fragments and the external environment. These fractures occur when sharp bone fragments penetrate the skin or when a traumatic injury causes damage to the skin and soft tissues resulting in exposure of the fracture site. Open fractures frequently affect the distal limbs as there is little soft tissue coverage of the bones in these regions. Fractures involving body cavities such as the nasal cavity or sinuses are also types of open fracture. An open wound is inevitably contaminated, but the degree of contamination varies depending on the size of the wound, source of the trauma that caused the injury and whether foreign material is present within the wound.

Although open wounds are contaminated, it is important to differentiate between wound contamination and infection. Whether infection develops after contamination is dependent on several factors including:

- The amount of bacterial contamination – microscopic contamination or the presence of gross foreign material
- Time between contamination and treatment – treatment should commence as soon as possible to prevent infection
- Patient factors, such as age and concurrent disease
- Type of wound – crush injuries can lead to major soft tissue trauma and thus cause devascularization.

Open fractures can be classified according to the type of soft tissue injury associated with the fracture. Several classification systems have been developed. Historically in small animal orthopaedics, open fractures have been graded as:

- Grade I – a small wound created by the fracture fragment (inside to outside). The fragment returns to within the soft tissue envelope leaving no bone protruding
- Grade II – the wound is created from external trauma (outside to inside). There is more soft tissue damage with contusion of the skin and reversible muscle damage. There is minimal tissue loss
- Grade III – a more severe wound created from external trauma (outside to inside). There is loss of skin, soft tissue and bone, which may be severe. This grade can be further subdivided by the extent of the soft tissue, periosteal and vascular injury.

In human medicine, this has been expanded and the Gustilo and Anderson grading of open fractures is now widely used and relatively simple (Figure 12.1). This system

Grade	Definition
I	Open fracture; clean wound; wound <1 cm in length
II	Open fracture; wound >1 cm in length without extensive soft tissue damage
III	Open fracture with extensive soft tissue laceration, damage or loss or an open segmental fracture; also includes open fractures requiring vascular repair, or fractures that have been open for 8 hours prior to treatment
IIIa	Type III fracture with adequate periosteal coverage of the fractured bone, despite extensive soft tissue laceration or damage
IIIb	Type III fracture with extensive soft tissue loss and periosteal stripping and bone damage; usually associated with massive contamination; will often need further soft tissue coverage procedure (i.e. free or rotational flap)
IIIc	Type III fracture associated with an arterial injury requiring repair, irrespective of degree of soft tissue injury

12.1 The Gustilo and Anderson grading scheme for open fractures.

has been used to develop treatment plans and also to provide prognostic information for open fractures in humans (Evans *et al.*, 2010).

Open fracture management

The aims of open fracture management are:

- To prevent contamination progressing to infection
- To stabilize the bone and provide optimal wound management
- To achieve osseous union and promote early return of limb function.

It is useful to consider the management of open fractures in four different stages:

- First aid
- The rational use of antibiotics
- Wound management
- Fracture management.

First aid

Open fractures are often associated with significant trauma and, therefore, assessment of the patient for concomitant, potentially life-threatening, disease is mandatory. Triage is an important method of prioritizing the patient's problem list and any life-threatening disease should be managed as a primary concern. Triage is a complex area; detailed descriptions on how to perform this can be found in other texts (Brown and Drobatz, 2007).

The hospital environment is a significant source of bacteria that could lead to infection of open wounds (Patzakis *et al.*, 2000). Antibiotic resistance is a growing concern in both human and veterinary medicine, and infection with multi-resistant bacteria can prove incredibly challenging to treat successfully. Open wounds must be covered with sterile dressings to prevent further contamination whilst the patient is stabilized.

External bleeding can be addressed with direct pressure or bandaging until such time that the bleeding can be definitively controlled. The emergency use of tourniquets is infrequent in small animal surgery but could be considered in patients with life-threatening haemorrhage.

Do:

- Cover the wound with a sterile dressing to prevent further contamination
- Provide support to the fracture until definitive treatment can be pursued; consider using a Robert Jones dressing or a gutter splint
- Obtain diagnostic radiographs as early as possible, once any life-threatening injuries have been addressed and the patient is stable.

Do not:

- Leave the wound open for any length of time; consider using an adhesive sterile dressing if a support dressing is removed in radiography
- Probe or manipulate the fracture unnecessarily.

> **WARNING**
>
> When applying a dressing to an open fracture, take care not to apply the dressing too tightly. After trauma, the tissue will swell, which may cause further neurovascular compromise in its own right. This can be exacerbated with an overtight dressing

Use of antibiotics

Which microbial contaminants will develop into infection is difficult to predict. Historically, samples have been taken from contaminated wounds and submitted for bacterial culture and sensitivity. The usefulness of these data is poorly documented in the veterinary literature, but in the human field blood cultures and swabs taken from contaminated tissues before debridement have not been found to provide useful information on the bacterial populations likely to cause a clinical problem. Cultures taken after debridement can be more accurate in predicting infection but isolation of the infecting organism is successful in less than 50% of cultures; commensal skin flora are cultured more commonly (Lee, 1997). Thus, in human medicine, culture taken after debridement from contaminated tissues at the outset of treatment is therefore deemed unnecessary.

The use of prophylactic antibiosis is highly controversial in both veterinary and human orthopaedics. There is evidence in favour of the use of perioperative antibiotic therapy in elective canine orthopaedic procedures (Whittem *et al.*, 1999), but there is very little information on the use of antibiotics in fracture management, particularly in open fracture management. In human orthopaedics,

meta-analysis of publications evaluating antibiotic usage in patients with open fractures revealed that they reduced the risk of infection developing, but the optimum type and duration of antibiotic therapy was unclear (Gosselin *et al.*, 2004). Information on the optimum choice of antibiotic and the optimum duration of therapy is also lacking in veterinary orthopaedics. In the UK, the British Association of Plastic, Reconstructive and Aesthetic Surgeons and the British Orthopaedic Association have endorsed specific advice on the use of antibiotics for the management of open fractures of the lower limb. Their recommendations are that antibiotics should be given as soon as possible after injury, ideally within the first 3 hours, generally using a first generation cephalosporin or amoxicillin/clavulanate (co-amoxiclav). The antibiotics can be continued for up to 72 hours postoperatively. Gentamicin can be added at the time of surgery, but should not be continued postoperatively (Griffin *et al.*, 2012). Given the lack of literature pertaining to canine and feline patients, it is reasonable to apply the same recommendations in veterinary practice. The typical causative agents of post-traumatic osteomyelitis are aerobic bacteria, especially staphylococcal species, although many other organisms such as pyogenic streptococci, *Escherichia coli*, *Pseudomonas* spp., *Proteus* spp. and *Klebsiella* spp. are also commonly isolated (Soontornvipart *et al.*, 2003).

> **WARNING**
>
> The use of prophylactic antibiotic therapy is not a substitute for meticulous surgical technique and optimal theatre protocols

As some of our veterinary patients, particularly cats, can go missing following injury, gross infection at the fracture site is often present due to the time elapsed between injury and presentation at the clinic. If a purulent exudate is present, this indicates infection and treatment should be instigated. In these cases, bacterial culture samples *should* be taken from deep tissues following initial debridement to ensure skin commensals are avoided. Empirical treatment with amoxicillin/clavulanate or a first generation cephalosporin is instigated whilst awaiting culture and sensitivity results. Antibiotic therapy is altered if necessary on the basis of these results.

Wound management

Historically, the first 6–8 hours after contamination has been regarded as a 'golden window' of opportunity in the management of open wounds. Management within this window was considered to reduce the risk of postoperative infection. There is, however, no strong evidence to support this. Nonetheless, the main focus of treatment should still be decisive management as soon as possible to decontaminate the wound and to prevent further contamination.

After first aid to prevent further wound contamination, definitive treatment of the wound and fracture is pursued. If there is only a small wound with minimal tissue devitalization, wound management and definitive fracture fixation may be performed simultaneously. Alternatively, if there is gross contamination it is likely that open wound management will be required. The period of wound management will vary depending on the size and type of wound. In some cases open wound management may be required over several days prior to definitive fixation of the fracture. External skeletal fixation (ESF) can be used as a temporary measure to stabilize the tissues and allow wound management and healing, obviating the need for implant placement at the site of contamination and helping to maintain the bandage or dressing materials used at the site. In some cases ESF can also be used as a definitive method of fracture stabilization.

Debridement is essential in the management of open wounds. Initial decontamination can be performed using gentle lavage and physical removal of gross foreign material. Lavage with large volumes of sterile isotonic fluid (saline or lactated Ringer's solution) is optimal. Hypotonic solutions, such as tap water, are not ideal lavage fluids as they can cause cellular necrosis to occur over time; therefore use of these fluids should be avoided if possible.

Once the patient is fit for anaesthesia, definitive wound management can be performed in an aseptic area. This should be carried out using meticulous surgical technique to preserve all viable tissue. Care should also be taken to identify and maintain neurovascular structures. Any devitalized tissue should be debrided and the wound lavaged with sterile isotonic fluid. It is essential to remove all devitalized tissue to reduce the risk of leaving a nidus for infection, which may delay wound and bone healing. Obviously devascularized bone fragments without soft tissue attachments should be removed as these are unlikely to contribute to bone healing and may have an adverse effect. Areas of devitalized skin or soft tissue may not be evident initially. If there is any question regarding soft tissue viability, open wound management can be undertaken and over the first few days a line of demarcation should develop between vascularized and necrotic tissue.

During debridement, lavage of the wound is important to maintain tissue hydration and to remove microscopic contaminants. This can be performed using specially designed instruments but, more commonly in veterinary medicine, an intravenous fluid set-up, 3-way tap, 18 G needle and 20 ml syringe are used to deliver approximately 8 psi of pressure (Figure 12.2). If the pressure is too low, the contaminants will not be removed; if it is too high, the contaminants can be forced into the tissues and become more challenging to remove.

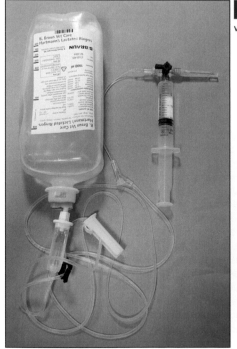

12.2 Fluid set-up for wound lavage.

Wound closure

If there is minimal contamination, it may be possible for the wound to undergo primary closure. If there is considerable dead space, the use of passive or closed suction drains could be considered although there is little evidence that they improve postoperative outcomes and therefore should be used with caution (Chandratreya *et al.*, 1998; Gaines and Dunbar, 2008).

With more severely traumatized wounds, open wound management is instigated rather than primary wound closure. Details on best practice for open wound management are described in other texts (Anderson, 2009). Once satisfactory granulation tissue has started to form, definitive wound management should be planned. This may involve delayed primary wound closure or complete healing by second intention. For large defects secondary procedures such as skin grafts or axial pattern skin flaps may be required (Moores, 2009; White, 2009).

> **PRACTICAL TIP**
>
> If in doubt, leave the wound open initially and consider definitive closure following formation of granulation tissue

Fracture management

The primary aim of fracture management is to provide a stable environment to allow the bone to heal. Inadequate stability will lead to delayed or non-union. Reduced stability will also compromise wound healing and will predispose to higher rates of surgical site infection.

In cases where contamination and soft tissue damage are minimal, definitive treatment can be pursued as if the fracture were closed. For instance, in a type I fracture where the bone fragment has penetrated the skin, often in an area where the bone is already close to the skin surface, the wound may be extended to form part of the approach. The wound edges may require minimal debridement or excision and the wound is lavaged with copious volumes of sterile saline or lactated Ringer's solution. Type I fractures are associated with lower levels of soft tissue injury and are often a result of low impact trauma. These fractures therefore tend to be reconstructable and internal fixation can be considered. Plate and screw fixation, either as a compression or neutralization fixation, applied using appropriate techniques, will lead to a very stable fracture environment, which should lead to early limb use and return to function. Although there is research demonstrating that skeletal implants can be associated with increased rates of infection (Petty *et al.*, 1985), inadequate fixation and persistent instability is likely to be a far more significant factor in the development of persistent infection in open fractures.

Internal fixation should be considered where there is/ are:

- A lower risk of infection
- An articular fracture which requires rigid fixation
- Multiple orthopaedic injuries requiring early patient mobilization
- Fractures in which ESF is impractical
- Fractures in patients with poor healing potential, where ESF is not advisable.

With modern developments in internal fixation, more rigid fixation can be achieved with fewer implants. This is particularly true in view of the number of commercially available locking implant systems (see Chapter 10).

When fractures are comminuted and non-reconstructable, bridging fixation is required. Several options for bridging fixation are available including:

- Bridging plating (see Operative Technique 11.11)
- Pin–plate fixation (see Operative Technique 11.12)
- Interlocking nail (see Operative Technique 11.3)
- ESF (see Operative Technique 11.6).

An 'open but do not touch' or 'biological healing' approach to fracture management aims at preserving the fracture haematoma and the soft tissue envelope around the fracture. In the case of an open fracture, this haematoma is contaminated. However, if contamination is minimal, the superficial areas can be decontaminated by gentle lavage in an attempt to try to preserve the remaining haematoma. Percutaneous or minimally invasive osteosynthesis (MIO) can also be considered in these cases.

ESF can be applied at a site distant from the fracture, thus preserving the surrounding soft tissues and fracture haematoma (Figure 12.3). Good outcomes can be achieved with comminuted fractures in small animals (Johnson *et al.*, 1996; Dudley *et al.*, 1997; Whittem *et al.*, 1999). External

skeletal fixation also allows access for continued open wound management if required. Conversely, ESF can be associated with complications such as pin loosening (see Figure 12.3b), which can lead to fracture instability, and this can predispose to development of infection. Since maintenance of stability at the fracture site is obligatory in these cases, internal fixation is often preferred, even for comminuted fractures. Clients should be warned that, should infection develop, implant removal may be required once the fracture has healed.

With high level trauma, the blood supply to the bone can be significantly compromised and detachment of fragments from the surrounding soft tissues can occur. Care should be taken when assessing blood supply to the fracture site and to the bone fragments. The aim is to retain all viable fracture fragments but, if there is complete detachment of soft tissue and where there is significant contamination, it may be necessary to remove some devitalized fragments (Figure 12.4). Fragments without a significant blood supply represent a risk of forming a sequestrum. If there is significant loss of periosteal attachment to a major fracture fragment, devitalization and subsequent sequestration can also develop (Figure 12.5).

If there is concern regarding the healing potential of a fracture, a bone graft should be considered. Cancellous autograft can be placed safely in a contaminated wound (Millard and Towle, 2012). However, as bone grafts are avascular, there are risks with their early use and acute grafting should be pursued with caution. In some cases, delayed bone grafting can be considered 2–3 weeks after the original surgery when decontamination has occurred and a granulation tissue bed exists to encourage survival of the graft.

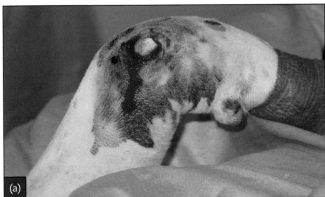

(a)

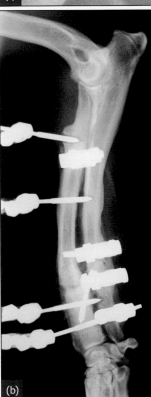

(b)

12.3 (a) Preoperative preparation of an open fracture of the left radius and ulna in a 4-year-old Springer Spaniel. The fracture was stabilized with a seven-pin type 1b external skeletal fixator. (b) Radiograph of the same patient 8 weeks postoperatively, showing satisfactory callus formation at the radial and ulnar fracture sites. Note the bone lucency around the most proximal fixation pin, indicating loosening of the pin.

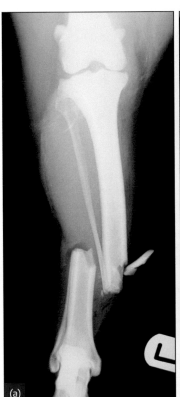

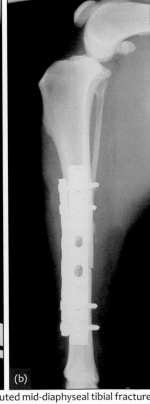

(a)   (b)

12.4 (a) Radiograph of a comminuted mid-diaphyseal tibial fracture in a 6-year-old Border Collie. Note the proximal tibial diaphysis protruding through the soft tissue envelope. The bone fragment was completely denuded of soft tissue attachment. (b) Immediate postoperative radiograph of the fracture managed with fragment removal and orthogonal dynamic compression plate and screw fixation.

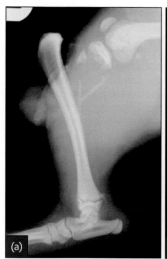

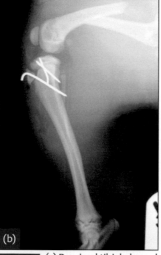

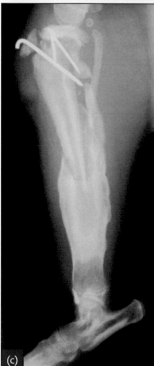

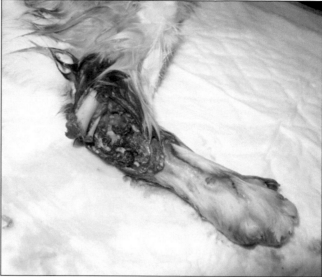

12.5 (a) Proximal tibial physeal fracture in a 10-week-old Border Terrier that had been kicked by a horse. There was denuding of the metaphyseal and proximal diaphyseal periosteum and cranial tibial muscle avulsion.
(b) Postoperative radiograph showing reduction and stabilization with multiple Kirschner wires. Note the concomitant femoral diaphyseal fracture. (c) Radiograph taken 6 weeks postoperatively showing sequestration of the entire proximal tibia. The discontinuity of the cortices in the mid-diaphyseal region of the tibia resulted from the lack of blood supply (rather than trauma). The distal end of the sequestrum was not originally fractured.
(Courtesy of E Maddock)

12.6 Open distal tibial physeal fracture with concurrent tarsocrural luxation. This patient had a concomitant distal femoral physeal fracture. Flystrike is also present. Due to devascularization of the distal tibial epiphysis, amputation was considered the most appropriate treatment option.

- Type III fracture where there is significant neurovascular compromise
- When owners do not want to put their animal through complicated fracture and wound management, opting for a quicker return to pet lifestyle and reduced morbidity
- When there are financial constraints.

> **PRACTICAL TIP**
>
> It is very important that owners are made aware not only of the treatment options available but also the financial implications of such treatment and complication risks

If the degree of tissue damage or loss involving a joint is severe, concerns should be raised regarding long-term joint function. In these cases, arthrodesis can be considered as a limb-sparing salvage surgery, but amputation may also need to be considered. When indicated, arthrodesis can be performed as a delayed procedure following assessment of limb function but it may also be considered in the early phases of treatment, particularly if the prognosis for acceptable joint function is considered poor from the outset.

> **PRACTICAL TIP**
>
> Arthrodesis is an end-stage salvage procedure; if in doubt it can always be performed at a later date

Early assessment of neurovascular function in patients with open fractures is mandatory as very severe trauma may lead to limb- or even life-threatening injuries. In some situations early amputation may be considered the most appropriate treatment option (Figure 12.6). Situations where early amputation may be considered include:

Shearing injuries

These are specific open wounds, most commonly occurring in the distal limb, and are frequently a result of vehicular trauma. The tarsus is the most common site affected, and medial injuries are more common than lateral (Harasen, 2000). These injuries can be associated with soft tissue and bone loss (Figure 12.7). Shearing injuries are usually associated with joint instability, which in the tarsus can be a result of malleolar fractures or damage to the collateral ligaments, and in the carpus is frequently due to damage to the collateral ligaments. Incomplete rupture of the collateral ligaments may result in minimal or no instability of the joint. However, if the ligaments are completely ruptured or have been traumatically removed, instability can be severe.

Malleolar fractures can be stabilized to improve joint stability using various techniques including Kirschner wires, tension-band wires and lag screws (see Chapter 26). Transarticular ESF is often used to immobilize the joint to allow management of soft tissues injuries and augment fracture repair (see Chapter 25). If the carpal or tarsal collateral ligaments are significantly damaged, management

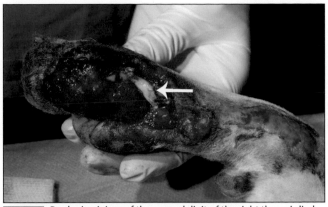

12.7 Degloving injury of the second digit of the right thoracic limb (in the same patient as in Figure 12.3). There was luxation of the metacarpophalangeal joint with concurrent soft tissue and bone loss exposing the first phalanx (arrowed) and the base of the second phalanx. The injury was managed as an open wound, which led to healing by the development of a functional ankylosis of the metacarpophalangeal joint.

options include transarticular ESF or ligament prosthesis, which can lead to improved limb function. However, in over 20% of patients limb function is considered poor (Diamond *et al.*, 1999). Surgical salvage with arthrodesis may be required to improve limb function. In severe open fracture grade III injuries, arthrodesis can be performed as an acute, definitive procedure, which can lead to a good to excellent outcome (Benson and Boudrieau, 2002).

Prognosis

The prognosis for open fractures varies widely depending on several factors including the severity of injury, open fracture grade and fracture location.

Less severe injuries, such as grade I open fractures, should have a similar prognosis to closed fractures and, with appropriate fixation, the outcome for mid-diaphyseal fractures would be considered excellent in most cases. However, with increasing severity of soft tissue injury the prognosis becomes more guarded and slower bone healing rates are seen in higher grade open fractures (Henley *et al.*, 1998).

With rigid fixation most fractures would be expected to heal. Open wound management and stabilization of fractures with ESF can lead to satisfactory outcomes in patients with unstable fracture sites but, when complications develop, further surgery may be required to promote definitive bone healing (Ness, 2006). A major complication associated with open fracture management is the development of infection. Superficial surgical site infection may be managed with appropriate courses of antibiotics based on culture and sensitivity. If internal fixation is performed and deep surgical site infection develops, implant removal may be required to definitively manage the infection although this can only be performed when satisfactory fracture union has occurred. In cases with deep surgical site infection undergoing implant removal, the long-term outcome should not be significantly affected. If chronic

osteomyelitis develops then this is likely to require further management, which may have an adverse effect on long-term outcome (see Chapter 30).

References and further reading

Anderson D (2009) Management of open wounds. In: *BSAVA Manual of Canine and Feline Wound Management and Reconstruction, 2nd edn*, ed. JM Williams and A Moores, pp. 37–53. BSAVA Publications, Gloucester

Benson JA and Boudrieau RJ (2002) Severe carpal and tarsal shearing injuries treated with an immediate arthrodesis in seven dogs. *Journal of the American Animal Hospital Association* **38**, 370–380

Brown AJ and Drobatz KJ (2007) Triage of the emergency patient. In: *BSAVA Manual of Canine and Feline Emergency and Critical Care, 2nd edn*, ed. LJ King and A Boag, pp. 1–7. BSAVA Publications, Gloucester

Chandratreya A, Giannikas K and Livesley P (1998) To drain or not drain: literature *versus* practice. *Journal of the Royal College of Surgeons of Edinburgh* **43**, 404–406

Diamond DW, Besso J and Boudrieau RJ (1999) Evaluation of joint stabilization for treatment of shearing injuries of the tarsus in 20 dogs. *Journal of the American Animal Hospital Association* **35**, 147–153

Dudley M, Johnson AL and Olmstead M (1997) Open reduction and bone plate stabilization, compared with closed reduction and external fixation, for treatment of comminuted tibial fractures: 47 cases (1980–1995) in dogs. *Journal of the American Veterinary Medical Association* **211**, 1008–1012

Evans A, Agel J, DeSilva G *et al.* (2010) A new classification scheme for open fractures. *Journal of Orthopaedic Trauma* **24**, 457–464

Gaines RJ and Dunbar RP (2008) The use of surgical drains in orthopedics. *Orthopedics* **31**, 702–705

Gosselin RA, Roberts I and Gillespie WJ (2004) Antibiotics for preventing infection in open limb fractures. *Cochrane Database of Systematic Reviews*, CD003764

Griffin M, Malahias M, Khan W and Hindocha S (2012) Update on the management of open lower limb fractures. *The Open Orthopaedics Journal* **6** (Suppl 3), 571–577

Harasen GL (2000) Tarsal shearing injuries in the dog. *Canadian Veterinary Journal* **41**, 940–943

Henley MB, Chapman JR, Agel J *et al.* (1998) Treatment of type II, IIIA, and IIIB open fractures of the tibial shaft: a prospective comparison of unreamed interlocking intramedullary nails and half-pin external fixators. *Journal of Orthopaedic Trauma* **12**, 1–7

Johnson AL, Seitz SE, Smith CW, Johnson JM and Schaeffer DJ (1996) Closed reduction and type-II external fixation of comminuted fractures of the radius and tibia in dogs: 23 cases (1990–1994). *Journal of the American Veterinary Medical Association* **209**, 1445–1448

Lee J (1997) Efficacy of cultures in the management of open fractures. *Clinical Orthopaedics and Related Research* **339**, 71–75

Millard R and Towle H (2012) Open Fractures. In: *Veterinary Surgery: Small Animal, 1st edn*, ed. K Tobias and S Johnston, pp. 572–575. Elsevier Saunders, Missouri

Moores A (2009) Axial pattern flaps. In: *BSAVA Manual of Canine and Feline Wound Management and Reconstruction, 2nd edn*, ed. JM Williams and A Moores, pp 100–143. BSAVA Publications, Gloucester

Ness MG (2006) Treatment of inherently unstable open or infected fractures by open wound management and external skeletal fixation. *Journal of Small Animal Practice* **47**, 83–88

Patzakis MJ, Bains RS, Lee J *et al.* (2000) Prospective, randomized, double-blind study comparing single-agent antibiotic therapy, ciprofloxacin, to combination antibiotic therapy in open fracture wounds. *Journal of Orthopaedic Trauma* **14**, 529–533

Petty W, Spanier S, Shuster JJ and Silverthorne C (1985) The influence of skeletal implants on incidence of infection. Experiments in a canine model. *Journal of Bone and Joint Surgery (American Volume)* **67**, 1236–1244

Soontornvipart K, Nečas A, Dvořák M, Zatloukal J and Smola J (2003) Post-traumatic bacterial infections in extremities before and after osteosynthesis in small animals. *Acta Veterinaria Brno* **72**, 249–260

White RAS (2009) Free skin grafting. In: *BSAVA Manual of Canine and Feline Wound Management and Reconstruction, 2nd edn*, ed. JM Williams and A Moores, pp. 144–158. BSAVA Publications, Gloucester

Whittem TL, Johnson AL, Smith CW *et al.* (1999) Effect of perioperative prophylactic antimicrobial treatment in dogs undergoing elective orthopedic surgery. *Journal of the American Veterinary Medical Association* **215**, 212–216

Chapter 13

Pathological fractures

Ignacio Calvo

Pathological fractures occur because an underlying disease process has weakened the bone. Due to this weakness a pathological fracture develops, usually in association with normal activity rather than being associated with a major traumatic event. It is not uncommon for pathological fractures to be preceded by pain or lameness (termed **prodromal** lameness). Pathological fractures account for less than 3% of all fractures encountered in dogs in small animal practice (Boulay *et al.*, 1987).

The most common aetiologies underlying pathological fractures in dogs and cats include:

- Neoplasia
- Metabolic disease (e.g. hyperparathyroidism)
- Inflammatory disorders (e.g. bacterial or fungal osteomyelitis)
- Genetic disorders (e.g. osteogenesis imperfecta)
- Idiopathic (e.g. bone cysts)
- The stress riser effect (e.g. a fracture associated with an external skeletal fixation (ESF) pin or adjacent to the end of a plate)
- Following the failure of fusion of ossification centres (e.g. slipped femoral capital epiphysis).

A history of a fracture occurring spontaneously or following minor trauma should alert the clinician to a potential pathological origin, particularly if the fracture is complex in configuration or if multiple fractures have occurred. Failure to recognize the pathological nature of a fracture could lead to incorrect clinical decisions, such as inappropriate stabilization or unnecessary surgery. In addition, an incorrect prognosis may be given if the true aetiology of the fracture is not considered.

The prognosis and treatment of pathological fractures are ultimately defined by the primary disease process, and the location and relative severity of the fracture.

Neoplasia

Primary malignant bone neoplasia is the most common cause of pathological fractures in dogs and cats. Benign and metastatic bone neoplasia can also lead to pathological fractures (Figure 13.1), although these are less common.

Osteosarcoma (OSA) is the most common primary bone tumour in dogs, accounting for up to 85% of the malignant tumours originating from the skeleton. Primary OSA represents 5% of all canine tumours. Other

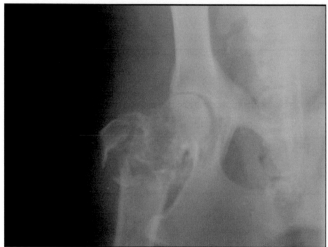

13.1 Craniocaudal radiograph of a pathological fracture of the proximal femur secondary to a primary bone tumour (osteosarcoma). Note the lysis of bone giving a 'moth-eaten' appearance, loss of trabecular detail and irregular cortical thinning adjacent to the fracture lines in the metaphyseal and femoral neck areas. A transverse fracture through the metaphyseal region extending to and causing lateral displacement of the greater trochanter is present. Ill-defined new bone is present at the level of the lesser trochanter; this may represent periosteal reaction or a fracture fragment.

primary neoplastic conditions affecting the skeleton can also be associated with pathological fractures (e.g. chondrosarcoma, fibrosarcoma, haemangiosarcoma). For further information regarding musculoskeletal neoplasia readers are referred to the *BSAVA Manual of Canine and Feline Oncology*.

Bone neoplasia in cats is uncommon. OSA usually affects older cats (mean age of 9 years). Tumours occurring in the long bones are twice as common as those occurring in the axial skeleton and, in contrast to dogs, feline OSA more commonly affects the hindlimbs and is more common in the diaphyseal rather than metaphyseal regions of long bones. OSA-associated metastatic disease in cats is also less common than in dogs (Watters and Cooley, 1998). The clinical signs associated with pathological fractures are similar to those in dogs.

The two major differential diagnoses for lesions with the same clinical and radiographic features as primary bone neoplasia are bacterial and fungal bone disease. Bacterial osteomyelitis is usually associated with previous surgery or penetrating injury, although haematogenous spread is also a possibility (Figure 13.2) (see Chapter 30).

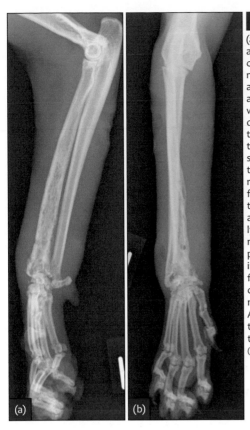

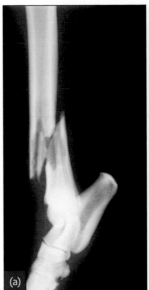

13.2
(a) Mediolateral and (b) craniocaudal radiographs of the antebrachium of an 8-year-old cat with bacterial osteomyelitis of the distal half of the radius and the styloid process of the ulna. The radiographic features (soft tissue swelling, aggressive bone lysis and irregular new bone production) are indistinguishable from those that characterize a neoplastic disease. A previous biopsy tract is apparent in the distal radius.
(Courtesy of T Gemmill)

Fungal osteomyelitis is extremely rare in the UK and is usually polyostotic (affecting several bones) although monostotic forms can be seen. Fungal osteomyelitis occurs more commonly in endemic areas such as the southern USA (see Chapter 30).

Clinical approach
Diagnostic work-up

When bone neoplasia is suspected in association with a fracture, radiographic assessment is warranted and orthogonal radiographic views should be obtained; if available, a computed tomography (CT) scan will provide a more accurate assessment of the extent of the affected bone. Radiographic changes associated with bone neoplasia are often quite striking (see Figure 13.1), although they can also be more subtle. When a pathological fracture is present radiographs usually show a primary osteolytic lesion, sometimes with minimal periosteal changes (Figure 13.3). The radiographic features associated with bone neoplasia may include:

- Destruction of cortical bone
- Growth of the tumour beyond the original confines of the bone
- Thinning of the cortices
- Loss of trabecular detail of metaphyseal bone
- Expansion into the surrounding soft tissues
- Pathological fracture
- Periosteal reaction causing palisading mineralization perpendicular to the bone shaft, giving rise to a 'sun-burst' effect
- Elevation of the periosteum with new bone formation (Codman's triangle)
- Destruction of the normal trabecular architecture with adjacent sclerosis and indistinct transitional zone between normal and neoplastic bone.

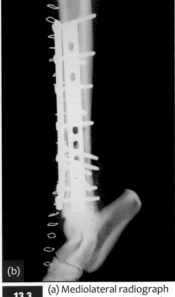

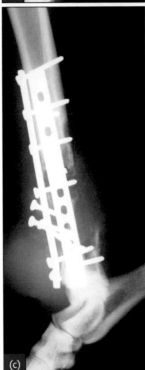

13.3
(a) Mediolateral radiograph of an oblique pathological fracture of the tibia in an 8-year-old Greyhound. Note the minimal periosteal changes and the reduced bone density at the fracture site. Lucency is present proximal to the butterfly fragment in the proximal fragment (tibia). Scalloped irregular thinning of the cortex is present at the cranial and caudal aspects of the tibia at the fracture level. There is also loss of definition of the fracture margins. (b) Mediolateral radiograph taken immediately postoperatively. Biaxial plating was performed due to a high suspicion of pathological fracture secondary to bone neoplasia, although a biopsy sample obtained at the time of surgery revealed only reactive bone. (c) Follow-up radiograph taken 5 months after surgery. Note the obvious bone lysis and soft tissue swelling at the site of the original fracture and screw loosening and displacement. Destruction of the cortical bone, growth of the tumour beyond the original confines of the bone, thinning of the cortex and an indistinct transitional zone between normal and neoplastic bone are also present.

Primary bone neoplasia seldom invades joint spaces or crosses the articular cartilage (North and Banks, 2009). A list of the differential clinical and radiographic features of the most common musculoskeletal tumours is provided in Figure 13.4.

Clinical staging

If bone neoplasia is suspected thoracic radiographs should be performed. Inflated left and right lateral and dorsoventral views should be obtained. Although only 10% of dogs are initially presented with radiographic evidence of pulmonary metastasis, approximately 98% of dogs will have microscopic pulmonary micrometastasis at the time of diagnosis. The rationale behind obtaining thoracic radiographs prior to treatment is that the survival of dogs with visible metastatic lesions (>1 cm in diameter) is unlikely to be prolonged by chemotherapy, and therefore an extremely guarded prognosis should be given (Ogilvie et al., 1993). CT is more sensitive in detecting

Tumour type	Clinical features	Radiographic features
Osteosarcoma (dog)	Appendicular skeleton in metaphyseal locations; also possible in axial skeleton	Lysis, unorganized periosteal response, osteoid production, cortical destruction
Osteosarcoma (cat)	Appendicular or axial skeleton, variable sites	Often juxtacortical or parosteal
Chondrosarcoma	Primarily flat bones (axial skeleton)	Blastic, with features of slower growth
Haemangiosarcoma	Appendicular skeleton, variable locations	Lysis
Fibrosarcoma	Appendicular skeleton	Lysis without osteoid production

13.4 Differential clinical and radiographic features of the most common musculoskeletal tumours.

pulmonary metastasis than radiographic evaluation; however, the clinical relevance of small lesions seen on CT is currently unclear. After the lungs, the most common metastatic site is bone, although regional bone metastasis is observed in less than 5% of dogs.

Abdominal ultrasonography, haematology, biochemistry and urinalysis should be performed since metastatic disease may also affect the kidneys, spleen, liver and gastrointestinal tract. Occasionally alkaline phosphatase (ALP) is elevated; this has been associated with poor prognosis. Dogs with high ALP before surgery have a shorter survival and disease-free interval, and failure of ALP to decrease after surgery is also correlated with shorter survival and disease-free interval (Ehrhart *et al.*, 1998).

Bone biopsy

When the signalment, history, physical examination and radiographic findings are consistent with primary bone neoplasia, it is not uncommon practice for the experienced clinician to proceed immediately with treatment, especially if a fracture is present. However, if there is any doubt over the diagnosis, histopathological examination of a biopsy sample should be performed prior to treatment. If a fracture is present, it can be stabilized pending the histology results, although the client should be advised of the possibility of underlying neoplasia. A sample should also be submitted for bacterial and fungal culture and sensitivity. The author recommends performing this routinely, as bone biopsy is not absolutely sensitive for obtaining a diagnosis of neoplasia where it exists. A negative culture allows more definitive exclusion of potential infectious causes of the pathology in the light of an equivocal pathology report, which gives the clinician a stronger indication to proceed with treatment given a high suspicion of neoplastic disease.

Bone biopsy samples can be obtained with a Michel's trephine (the author's preference), Jamshidi bone marrow biopsy needle, by surgical biopsy (wedge) or by fine-needle aspiration. The Michel's trephine allows sampling of a larger core maximizing the chance of diagnosis, although the caveat is that the larger deficit may predispose to pathological fracture, and sampling requires general anaesthesia. The Jamshidi collects a smaller core, which reduces the risk of fracture, but non-diagnostic samples are more common. The reported diagnostic accuracy of a Jamshidi needle is 83% (Powers *et al.*, 1988) *versus* 94% for the Michel's trephine (Wykes *et al.*, 1985).

Fine-needle aspiration and cytology can be performed before recourse to a more invasive bone biopsy. Aspiration of the intramedullary region is performed through areas of cortical lysis. In dogs, ultrasound-guided samples of aggressive lesions (in which cortical bone destruction must be present) have been associated with a sensitivity of 97% and specificity of 100% for confirmation of the presence of a sarcoma (Britt *et al.*, 2007).

At times, it may be necessary to obtain a rapid diagnosis of a pathological process during the surgical procedure. The surgeon may wish to know if the margins of resection for a malignant neoplasm are clear before closing, or an unexpected disease process may be encountered which requires a definite diagnosis to aid decision making. This can be obtained using a cryomicrotome or cryostat. The tissue sample (bone) is processed by freezing and is put on to the cryostat for sectioning. The tissue sections are placed on a glass slide, which are then ready for staining (Jaffar, 2006). The whole process takes about 5 to 10 minutes, plus the time taken by the pathologist to assess the slides.

Treatment

If a bone tumour is diagnosed (with or without concurrent pathological fracture), the treatment plan should focus on quality of life. This should be achieved by controlling pain (management of the bone lesion), and prolonging the survival time and disease-free interval using chemotherapy and potentially bisphosphonates.

Amputation is a palliative pain-relieving procedure for the treatment of primary bone neoplasia. It is cheap, relatively straightforward and has a low complication rate. Amputation is generally very well tolerated by dogs and owners; animals normally adjust rapidly to a three-legged gait. However, limb amputation results in significant changes in the percentage of bodyweight carried by the remaining limbs and will cause shifting of the dog's centre of gravity. These changes are more pronounced in dogs undergoing forelimb amputation. Therefore, an in-depth orthopaedic and neurological examination of all other limbs should be performed before surgery is performed. The median survival time for dogs with appendicular OSA, after amputation alone, is around 5 months and the 1-year survival is 11% (Spodnick *et al.*, 1992). Median survival time for dogs having adjunctive chemotherapy in addition to amputation is approximately 1 year regardless of the specific protocol used (Demell, 2011).

Limb-sparing surgery is a palliative pain-relieving procedure with a similar survival time to amputation; these patients can equally benefit from adjunctive chemotherapy. Historically, pathological fracture associated with a primary malignant bone tumour has been considered a contraindication to limb salvage surgery, as it has been hypothesized that fracture results in dissemination of tumour cells into adjacent tissue and damage to the microcirculation, facilitating metastasis. However, in humans, evidence has recently emerged to suggest that limb salvage surgery for pathological fractures provides a similar long-term prognosis to amputation (Covey *et al.*, 2014); this may also be the case in dogs and cats. Limb-sparing surgery may be considered in cases where amputation is refused, or in dogs which have significant concurrent orthopaedic or neurological disease. Suitable candidates should have the tumour confined to one site, with less than 50% of the length of the bone affected. Ideally magnetic resonance imaging, CT or scintigraphy should be performed to ascertain this. The less the tumour invades the surrounding soft tissues, the more likely resection will be complete and thus the chances of tumour seeding are reduced. Limb-sparing surgery normally consists of resection of the affected area and implantation and fixation of another material such as bone autograft or allograft or a metallic prosthesis (Figure 13.5). Limb-sparing surgery is a technically demanding procedure and should only be performed by surgeons with significant training and experience. If limb surgery is being considered, it is best for the surgeon performing the procedure to decide what type of preoperative biopsy is obtained (if any at all) to allow the biopsy tract to be excised at the time of definitive surgery.

Bisphosphonates are a group of drugs described as anti-osteoclastic because they inhibit bone resorption without inhibiting bone mineralization. They can be used as a palliative treatment in cases not suitable for other therapies. It has been shown that this medication can decrease bone pain and delay progression of bone lesions. The main side effect is nephrotoxicity; consequently, renal function should be assessed prior to and during treatment.

The use of bisphosphonates in animals that already have a pathological fracture remains controversial since there is a theoretical concern for retarded fracture healing secondary to bisphosphonate therapy. Very little evidence is available to support or refute its use when attempting to stabilize a pathological (neoplastic) fracture. Peter et al. (1996) conducted an experimental study in which a transverse fracture of the radius was surgically induced in healthy Beagles. In this experimental model, treatment with alendronate before or during fracture healing or both resulted in no delay to healing. Tomlin et al. (2000) successfully used alendronate 40 days after surgical stabilization of a pathological tibial fracture (secondary to OSA) in a dog to suppress bone remodelling and osteolysis; healing of the fracture was achieved during the treatment.

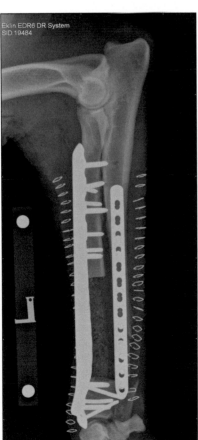

13.5 Limb-sparing surgery performed in an 11-year-old Pointer with a pathological fracture of the distal radius and ulna. The most distal screw in the ulna caused propagation of an undetected fissure. The gap left after resection of the area has been filled with an autologous cancellous graft, a coarse osteoallograft and bone morphogenic protein 2 (BMP-2) in a collagen sponge (TruScient®).
(Courtesy of T Sparrow)

Hyperparathyroidism

Parathyroid hormone (PTH) acts on bone to regulate the rate of bone formation and resorption so that the concentration of calcium in the extracellular fluid is maintained at a constant level (Figure 13.6) (see Chapter 3). Sustained release of excessive PTH stimulates the release of calcium and phosphate from bone mineral stores, resulting in osteopenia; subsequently, pathological fractures may occur.

Calcium and phosphate have a complex relationship that has a significant effect on calcium homeostasis. It is important to appreciate that, as calcium and phosphate exist in serum close to their saturation points, an increase in one causes a reciprocal decrease in the other through the formation of insoluble calcium phosphate complexes. Calcium is present in the serum in three definable fractions: free ionized calcium (50%), protein-bound (40%) and complex-bound (10%). Ionized calcium is the biologically active form and is subject to rigid homeostatic control.

There are three forms of hyperparathyroidism:

- Congenital hyperparathyroidism (also known as hereditary neonatal primary hyperparathyroidism)
- Primary hyperparathyroidism
- Secondary (renal or nutritional) hyperparathyroidism.

Hereditary neonatal primary hyperparathyroidism is extremely rare, having only been reported to date in two German Shepherd Dogs (Thompson et al., 1984). A possible autosomal recessive mode of inheritance was suggested.

Primary hyperparathyroidism

Primary hyperparathyroidism is associated with hyperplasia of the parathyroid glands and increased production of PTH in the absence of a known stimulus. It occurs rarely in middle-aged to older dogs and very rarely in cats. Hypercalcaemia is the hallmark abnormality, which commonly leads to polyuria, polydipsia and listlessness. Pathological fractures appear to be very rare (Gear et al., 2005). In severe cases, the mineral removed from the skeleton can be replaced by immature fibrous connective tissue, a process known as fibrous osteodystrophy. Although this can potentially be generalized throughout the skeleton, it is more commonly accentuated in local areas such as the cancellous bone of the skull. A clinical manifestation of this condition is 'rubber jaw', in which fibrous osteodystrophy of the mandible progresses to the point where it becomes flexible; the jaw can be rotated and bent without producing a fracture due to the lack of adequately mineralized bone matrix. The bone trabeculae and the laminae durae dente are no longer visible on radiographs of the mandible, which leads to the appearance that the teeth are 'floating' in soft tissue.

The diagnosis of primary hyperparathyroidism is made by demonstrating elevated calcium and an inappropriately high PTH concentration without azotaemia. However, the diagnosis can be complicated, especially if there is concurrent renal failure. If serum ionized calcium is high and phosphate is low, secondary hyperparathyroidism can be excluded. Urine specific gravity is not helpful in differentiating primary or secondary hyperparathyroidism, as calcium interferes with the responsiveness of the kidneys to antidiuretic hormone (Gear et al., 2005).

Secondary hyperparathyroidism

Secondary hyperparathyroidism (renal or nutritional) is more common than primary hyperparathyroidism.

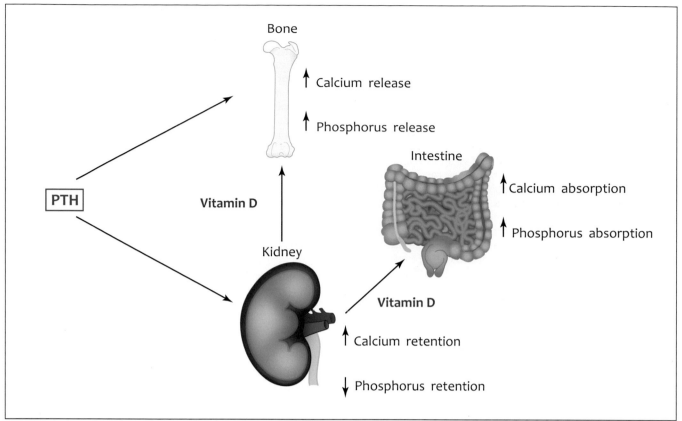

13.6 Actions of parathyroid hormone (PTH). PTH acts on kidney and bone to increase the serum concentration of calcium. Vitamin D acts on bone and intestine to increase the serum calcium concentration. In the kidney, PTH plays a crucial role in the formation of the most metabolically active form of vitamin D. A negative feedback system exists between PTH and the metabolically active form of vitamin D.

Renal secondary hyperparathyroidism

Hyperparathyroidism can be present in up to 85% of cats with chronic renal failure, although hypercalcaemia occurs in less than 10% of these cases. The primary aetiological factor for increased PTH secretion and parathyroid gland hyperplasia is phosphate retention due to the inability of the failing kidney to excrete sufficient phosphate, resulting in an increase in the formation of insoluble complexes of calcium and phosphate. This results in a decrease of ionized calcium and subsequent increase in PTH production. In the kidneys, PTH stimulates the production of 1,25-dihydroxyvitamin D_3 (1,25(OH)$_2$D$_3$), also called calcitriol, which is the most metabolically active form of vitamin D. The reduced number of functioning nephrons impairs the formation of 1,25(OH)$_2$D$_3$ (see Chapter 3); this lack of active vitamin D also reduces the negative feedback on PTH, thus contributing to an increase in its secretion. In severe cases fibrous osteodystrophy develops (Weller *et al.*, 1985).

Renal secondary hyperparathyroidism is diagnosed in an animal with a history of being fed a balanced diet by demonstrating increased serum PTH in the presence of normal or low values of total and ionized calcuim (to rule out primary hyperparathyroidism). The presence of abnormal kidney architecture on ultrasonography and presence of azotemia or isosthenuria can help in the diagnosis of kidney disease.

Nutritional secondary hyperparathyroidism

Nutritional secondary hyperparathyroidism may occur in young animals being fed diets low in calcium and high in phosphorus (e.g. a solely red meat diet) for prolonged periods of time. The consequent low level of ionized calcium causes chronic stimulation of the parathyroid glands, resulting in hyperplasia and increased secretion of PTH. These animals are rarely hypocalcaemic since the kidneys respond to the increased PTH by increasing calcium resorption. This form of hyperparathyroidism is more commonly associated with multiple pathological fractures, in particular folding or greenstick fractures where the bone is bent but only fractured on one side. Treatment in these cases consists of feeding a commercially available balanced puppy or kitten food, pain management and cage rest (Tomsa *et al.*, 1999). In other instances the fractures can be more severe and displaced and surgical intervention may be attempted as well as dietary change (Figure 13.7); however, owners should be made aware of the guarded prognosis. Locking rather than non-locking implants may be advantageous in these cases (see Chapter 10), because locking systems are more secure in soft, osteopenic bone and clinically the risk of failure of the screw–bone interface is decreased. Pathological fracture of the spine may occur, resulting in severe neurological deficits; the prognosis in these cases is extremely guarded.

Nutritional secondary hyperparathyroidism is diagnosed in an animal with a history of prolonged feeding of a nutritionally inappropriate diet, and by demonstrating increased serum PTH in the presence of normal values of total and ionized calcium (to rule out primary hyperparathyroidism). The presence of normal kidney architecture on ultrasonography and the absence of azotemia or isosthenuria should help to exclude renal secondary hyperparathyroidism.

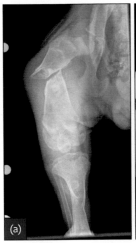
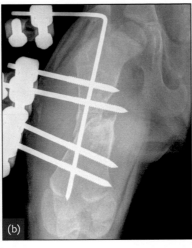
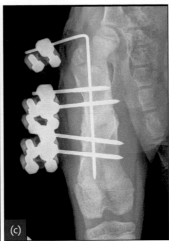

13.7 (a) Caudocranial radiograph of a displaced mid-diaphyseal pathological femoral fracture in a puppy with nutritional hyperparathyroidism. Note the generalized osteopenia and thin bone cortices. (b) Caudocranial radiograph taken immediately postoperatively following fracture stabilization with an intramedullary pin tied into an external skeletal fixator. (c) Caudocranial radiograph 4 weeks after surgery, which demonstrates healing at the fracture site and a subjective increase in the bone density following the feeding of a normal balanced diet in the postoperative period.

Osteogenesis imperfecta

Osteogenesis imperfecta (OI) is an inherited congenital disease usually caused by mutations in one of the two genes coding for type I collagen (*COL1*), which is the primary structural protein of bone, as well as being the most abundant structural component of the skin, cartilage, tendons and ligaments. Mutations causing OI have also been identified in genes coding for a peptidase involved in the biosynthesis of collagen (serpin peptidase inhibitor, clade H, member 1) and a genetic test is available to screen Dachshunds for this condition (Eckardt *et al.*, 2013). The mutations cause abnormalities in the structure and function of type I collagen leading to generalized osteopenia and fragile bones that can be affected by pathological fractures (Figure 13.8). As a result, OI-affected dogs tend to show clinical signs such as reduced agility and pain when handled. Dogs suffering from OI can also exhibit other signs such as dentinogenesis imperfecta, also known as glassy teeth (brittle and translucent teeth) or joint hyperlaxity (Eckardt *et al.*, 2013). Onset of clinical signs is most common in puppies and kittens between 10 and 18 weeks of age. Diagnosis is challenging and should begin by excluding other causes of pathological fractures. Cultured fibroblasts from skin biopsy specimens have been used successfully to diagnose OI in dogs, since mutations in the *COL1* genes are reflected in the structure of type I collagen synthesized by skin fibroblasts. The mutations result in a change in the electrophoretic mobility of the type 1 collagen, procollagen or both which can be detected by electrophoresis (Campbell *et al.*, 1997). Alternatively, the structure of the collagen fibrils in tissues or cell cultures can be assessed with electron microscopy and their appearance used to diagnose OI.

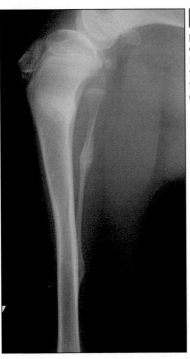

13.8 Mediolateral radiograph of a puppy diagnosed with osteogenesis imperfecta. Note the healed pathological fractures of the tibial and fibular diaphyses.
(Courtesy of N Fitzpatrick)

Bone cysts

Bone cysts are benign fluid-filled lesions of unknown aetiology. Radiographically, they are characterized by an expansile radiolucent area in the metaphysis near to, but usually not affecting, the physis or epiphysis. The cortex is usually thinned by the expanding cyst. Bone cysts may be asymptomatic, but in other cases can cause lameness or pathological fractures. Three forms of bone cysts have been reported in dogs:

* Simple bone cysts (most common type) – these can affect one bone (monostotic) or several bones at the same time (polyostotic). They are lined with fibrous connective tissue and are filled with serosanguineous fluid. Dobermanns are predisposed to polyostotic bone cysts. Large breeds are generally more affected and they tend to be diagnosed in young adulthood. On radiographs they appear as well marginated radiolucent expansile bone lesions with thin cortices and no visible periosteal reactivity (Stickle *et al.*, 1999)
* Aneurysmal bone cysts (rare) – these differ from the other types in that they are filled with large vascular sinusoids and are locally invasive osteolytic lesions. Malignant transformation has been reported with this type. Aneurysmal bone cysts have a distinctive radiographic appearance, comprising osteolytic expansile lesions with focal areas of lucency resembling 'soap bubbles' divided by bony septa and surrounded by a thin shell of periosteal new bone (Barnhart, 2002)
* Subchondral bone cysts (relatively common but very rarely of clinical significance) – associated with

osteochondritis dissicans lesions, these cysts are lined with synovial membrane and are filled with fibrous or serosanguinous fluid (Figure 13.9).

It can be challenging to distinguish between a benign bone cyst and early neoplasia, and therefore biopsy and clinical staging (as described for bone tumours) should be performed. The traditional treatment for bone cysts is curettage and cancellous bone grafting; however *en bloc* resection and replacement with a cortical allograft or metallic endoprosthesis has also been described.

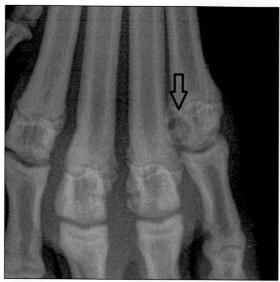

13.9 Suspected subchondral bone cyst (arrowed) in a 6-month-old Lakeland Terrier in the head of the 5th metacarpal.

Fracture-associated sarcoma

Fracture- or implant-associated neoplasia is a historically documented phenomenon. Fracture-associated sarcomas of dogs are very rare but, if present, tend to occur with a median lag phase of 6 years following initial fracture, and the original fracture usually occurs between 1 and 3 years of age (Stevenson *et al.*, 1982). It has been hypothesized that chronic inflammatory processes may lead to neoplastic transformation and that OSAs could potentially form as a sequel to altered cellular activity of osteoblasts and osteoclasts associated with fractures and/or metallic implants (Atherton and Arthurs, 2012). Neoplasia has also been documented in association with elective osteotomies (see Chapter 10). To date, the relationship between the fracture and the subsequent development of neoplasm has been purely associative, and no dependency between the two conditions has been identified. In the absence of rigorous epidemiological studies documenting the prevalence of implant- and non-implant-associated neoplasia, in populations of dogs with similar underlying genetic and environmental risks for the disease, the relationship between the fracture and the tumour must remain circumstantial.

Stress riser effect

When a plate is applied to bone, the plated section is stiffer than the rest of the bone and there is an abrupt transition from the plated to the non-plated bone. This is termed the 'stress riser' point, and can be associated with pathological fractures. Although not a common phenomenon, it can be seen in circumstances where there is a long lever arm acting at the stress riser point, such as following plate application for stifle arthrodesis or when the implant used is not spanning a sufficient length of bone. Metacarpal fractures have been associated with plates covering less than 50% of the metacarpal bones when performing pancarpal arthrodesis. The stress riser phenomenon can also be seen with ESF (Figure 13.10).

In some instances the weakening of the bone is caused by the surgeon, leading to fractures during normal activity. Examples of this include the occurrence of a radial fracture shortly after performing a proximal ulnar osteotomy, especially if the radius is not properly protected during surgery and is damaged with the oscillating saw; fractures through drill holes for oversized implants such as ESF pins or screws that are more than 50% of the bone diameter; or re-fracture after premature plate removal.

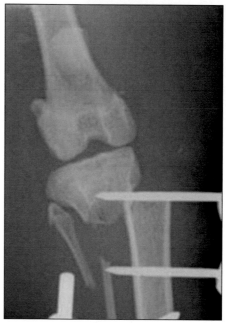

13.10 Stress fracture of the proximal tibia in a cat through an ESF pin tract.
(Courtesy of T Gemmill)

References and further reading

Atherton MJ and Arthurs G (2012) Osteosarcoma of the tibia 6 years after tibial plateau leveling osteotomy. *Journal of the American Animal Hospital Association* **48**, 188–193

Barnhart MD (2002) Malignant transformation of an aneurysmal bone cyst in a dog. *Veterinary Surgery* **31**, 519–524

Basher AWP, Doige CE and Presnell KR (1988) Subchondral bone cyst in a dog with osteochondrosis. *Journal of the American Animal Hospital Association* **24**, 321–326

Berg J, Gebhardt MC and Rand WM (1997) Effect of timing of postoperative chemotherapy on survival of dogs with osteosarcoma. *Cancer* **79**, 1343–1350

Boulay JP, Wallace LJ and Lipowitz AJ (1987) Pathological fracture of long bones in the dog. *Journal of the American Animal Hospital Association* **23**, 297–303

Britt T, Clifford C, Barger A *et al.* (2007) Diagnosing appendicular osteosarcoma with ultrasound-guided fine needle aspiration: 36 cases. *Journal of Small Animal Practice* **48**, 145–150

Campbell BG, Wootton JA, Krook L *et al.* (1997) Clinical signs and diagnosis of osteogenesis imperfecta in three dogs. *Journal of the American Veterinary Medical Association* **211**, 183–87

Covey JL, Farese JP and Bacon NJ (2014) Stereotactic radiosurgery and fracture fixation in 6 dogs with appendicular osteosarcoma. *Veterinary Surgery* **43**, 174–181

Dernell WS (2011) Tumours of the skeletal system. In: *BSAVA Manual of Canine and Feline Oncology, 3rd edn*, ed. JM Dobson and BDX Lascelles, pp. 159–178. BSAVA Publications, Gloucester

Eckardt J, Kluth S, Dierks C *et al.* (2013) Population screening for the mutation associated with osteogenesis imperfecta in Dachshunds. *Veterinary Record* **172**, 364

Ehrhart N, Dernell WS, Hoffmann WE *et al.* (1998) Prognostic importance of alkaline phosphatase activity in serum from dogs with appendicular osteosarcoma: 75 cases (1990–1996). *Journal of the American Veterinary Medical Association* **213**, 1002–1006

Gear RNA, Neiger R, Skelly BJS *et al.* (2005) Primary hyperparathyroidism in 29 dogs: diagnosis, treatment, outcome and associated renal failure. *Journal of Small Animal Practice* **46**, 10–16

Green EM, Adams WM and Forrest LJ (2002) Four fraction palliative radiotherapy for osteosarcoma in 24 dogs. *Journal of the American Animal Hospital Association* **38**, 445–451

Jaffar H (2006) Intra-operative frozen section consultation: concepts, applications and limitations. *The Malaysian Journal of Medical Sciences* **13**, 4–12

North S and Banks T (2009) Tumours of the skeletal system. In: *Small Animal Oncology, An Introduction*, ed. S North and T Banks, pp. 209–225. Saunders Elsevier, London

Ogilvie GK, Straw RC, Jameson *et al.* (1993) Evaluation of single-agent chemotherapy for the treatment of clinically evident osteosarcoma metastasis in dogs: 45 cases (1987–1991). *Journal of the American Veterinary Medical Association* **202**, 304–306

Peter CP, Cook WO, Nunamaker DM *et al.* (1996) Effect of alendronate on fracture healing and bone remodelling in dogs. *Journal of Orthopaedic Research* **14**, 74–79

Powers BE, LaRue SM, Withrow SJ *et al.* (1988) Jamshidi needle biopsy for diagnosis of bone lesions in small animals. *Journal of the American Veterinary Medical Association* **193**, 205–210

Ramirez O, Dodge RK, Page RL *et al.* (1999) Palliative radiotherapy of appendicular osteosarcoma in 95 dogs. *Veterinary Radiology and Ultrasound* **40**, 517–522

Spodnick GJ, Berg J, Rand WM *et al.* (1992) Prognosis for dogs with appendicular osteosarcoma treated by amputation: 162 cases (1978–1988). *Journal of the American Veterinary Medical Association* **200**, 995–999

Stevenson S, Hohn RB, Pohler OE *et al.* (1982) Fracture-associated sarcoma in the dog. *Journal of the American Veterinary Medical Association* **180**, 1189–1196

Stickle R, Flo G and Render J (1999) Radiographic diagnosis – benign bone cyst. *Veterinary Radiology and Ultrasound* **40**, 365–366

Thompson KG, Jones LP, Smylie WA *et al.* (1984) Primary hyperparathyroidism in German shepherd dogs: a disorder of probable genetic origin. *Veterinary Pathology* **21**, 370–376

Tomlin JL, Sturgeon C, Pead MJ *et al.* (2000) Use of the bisphosphonate drug alendronate for palliative management of osteosarcoma in two dogs. *Veterinary Record* **147**, 129–132

Tomsa K, Glaus T, Hauser B *et al.* (1999) Nutritional secondary hyperparathyroidism in six cats. *Journal of Small Animal Practice* **40**, 533–539

Watters DJ and Cooley DM (1998) Skeletal neoplasm. In: *Cancer in Dogs and Cats: Medical and Surgical Management*, ed. W Morrison, pp. 639. Teton NewMedia, Jackson

Weller RE, Cullen J and Dagle GE (1985) Hyperparathyroid disorders in the dog: primary, secondary and cancer-associated (pseudo). *Journal of Small Animal Practice* **26**, 329–341

Wykes PM, Withrow SJ and Powers BE (1985) Closed biopsy for diagnosis of long bone tumours: accuracy and results. *Journal of the American Animal Hospital Association* **21**, 489–494

Chapter 14

Bone grafts and alternatives

Gareth Arthurs

Bone grafting is the transplantation or implantation of bone or a bone substitute into a site to replace missing bone or to enhance bone healing. Indications for grafting include:

- Complex fractures
- Fractures with poor healing potential
- Filling of bone defects
- Arthrodesis
- Intervertebral fusion
- Treatment of delayed or non-union fractures.

In small animal orthopaedics, the most common applications of bone grafts are joint arthrodeses and treatment of fractures. Bone grafts can enhance healing by various mechanisms:

- **Osteoconduction** is the provision of a scaffold matrix that allows healing tissue to grow across it; this includes vascular, fibrous, cartilaginous and bone tissue phases
- **Osteoinduction** is the stimulation and activation of adjacent host mesenchymal cells to differentiate into cells involved in bone growth, including osteoblasts and osteoclasts. This is caused by growth factors released by the bone graft
- **Osteogenesis** is the formation of new bone by the graft itself. The graft needs to contain viable osteoblasts that deposit osteoid, or stem cells that are induced and differentiate into osteoblasts
- **Osteopromotion** is the enhancement of bone formation without being directly osteoinductive or osteoconductive. For example, enamel matrix derivative alone has no osteoinductive properties, but it can enhance the osteoinductive effect of demineralized bone matrix. Alternatively, creating a vascular and oxygen-rich environment allows bone healing to proceed
- **Osteointegration** is the process by which the graft material is integrated into the surrounding host bone.

Autografts

An autogenous bone graft is harvested from the recipient's own body; this is the most commonly used form of bone graft. Cancellous bone, cortical bone, or a mix of both, are used. Properties of bone autografts include:

- Osteogenesis – a fresh live autograft should include osteoblasts, osteoclasts and precursor stem cells, but only a fraction of the harvested live cells survive the transplantation process; this function of osteogenesis is almost unique to autografts
- Osteoconduction – the graft comprises cortical bone or trabecular cancellous bone; both contain hydroxyapatite and collagen, which are osteoconductive
- Osteoinduction – the autograft contains a number of beneficial osteoinductive growth factors
- Non-immunogenic, no risk of disease transmission or graft rejection.

An autogenous bone graft is arguably the optimal graft product. However, autogenous grafting is not without its disadvantages; these are associated with the procedure of harvesting from the patient and include:

- The requirement for a second surgical site, which increases surgical time, cost and morbidity
- Pain from the harvest site – this is a problem with human autografting but appears to be less significant in dogs and cats
- Potential risk of bone fracture at the harvest site
- Cosmetic damage (scarring of the harvest site); this is not a significant concern for most dogs and cats
- Graft yield can be of variable quantity and quality with respect to the volume of graft harvested and the proportion of cells that are biologically active. The comparative properties of different bone graft sites and cell survival following harvesting is poorly documented in dogs and cats. Conditions such as myelodysplasia or advanced age may significantly impact harvest yield.

Autogenous graft types include:

- Cancellous autograft – the graft is harvested by introducing a curette into the metaphysis of long bones; cancellous bone is then retrieved. This produces small quantities of particulate trabecular bone and blood. No processing is required and it is immediately ready for grafting (see Operative Technique 14.1)
- Cortical–cancellous autograft – a mix of cortical and cancellous bone. This can be harvested in different ways; an example would be application of a reamer to the lateral ilial wing; initially cortical and then cancellous bone is cut but the resultant graft is a mix of finely morsellized bone

BSAVA Manual of Canine and Feline Fracture Repair and Management, 2nd edition. Edited by Toby Gemmill and Dylan Clements. ©BSAVA 2016

- Non-vascularized cortical autograft – sections of resected cortical bone are harvested and grafted. For example, the use of non-vascularized ulnar and rib grafts into a mandibular non-union defect in dogs has been reported (Boudrieau *et al.*, 1994). Once the graft has revascularized osteointegration should occur, but this may be a slow process taking up to 1 year. One disadvantage is that, at the time of transplantation, the grafted section of bone is avascular and could potentially act as a nidus for infection
- Vascularized cortical bone graft – this is an intricate procedure that involves the transplantation of a bone segment including its vascular supply. An example would be the transplantation of a section of ulna, vascularized by preservation of the caudal interosseous artery and vein, into an adjacent radial ostectomy defect site created by excision of a distal radial bone tumour. The advantage is that the grafted bone retains its vascular supply and therefore all its biological properties. Implants may be attached and osteointegration should progress quickly; radiographic union within 20 weeks has been reported (Séguin *et al.*, 2003).

Cancellous bone has excellent osteoconductive properties, but provides no structural support. Cytokines and growth factors within the graft contribute to osteoinduction, including transforming growth factor beta 1 (TGF-β1), bone morphogenic proteins (BMPs), epidermal growth factor, platelet-derived growth factor, fibroblast growth factor and vascular endothelial growth factor.

Osteoblasts on the surface of the graft can survive transplantation and contribute to osteogenesis. Cancellous bone is thought to be more osteogenic than cortical bone as it has a low density porous structure that allows diffusion of nutrients and growth factors. Subsequently, mesenchymal stem cells in the graft are induced to differentiate and propagate.

Allografts

An allograft is sourced from a different individual to the patient, but of the same species. Allografts are osteoconductive and osteoinductive. Graft processing usually means that any capacity for osteogenesis is eliminated. Many of the drawbacks of autograft harvesting are avoided because the harvesting procedure is separate from grafting. Preparations of allografts that can be produced as 'off the shelf' products include cancellous chips, cortical grafts and demineralized bone matrix (DBM). Disease transmission, immunological stimulation and graft rejection are potential drawbacks, but these problems are substantially reduced by appropriate graft processing and are rarely encountered in dogs and cats. Although the clinical results may be more variable with allografts than autografts, another advantage is that they are not volume limited. The use of allografts is gradually increasing in frequency; they are used in approximately one-third of human bone grafting procedures in the USA, with an estimated 1.5 million human allografts used annually. One additional problem of allografts is graft sourcing; the allograft must come from another individual of the same species, either alive or dead.

Canine and feline allografts are sourced from individuals within a specific weight and age range, a full vaccination history and good health records. Testing for a wide range of infectious agents may be performed to minimize disease transmission. Once harvested, the allograft is processed to reduce the risk of disease transmission; depending on treatment this may degrade biological and mechanical properties. Graft preparation options include fresh, frozen or freeze-dried forms of cortical or cancellous bone. Veterinary allografts are typically frozen, demineralized and/or irradiated, which eliminates live cells; therefore, osteogenesis is not possible. Fresh preparations are rarely used due to the risk of disease transmission and stimulation of the immune system.

Cancellous bone chips

Cancellous bone chips are highly porous, osteoconductive and used as autogenous graft extenders or void fillers. They do not provide structural support and have minimal biological activity. Osteoinductive properties may be present, depending on tissue handling, sterilization and processing post harvesting. Processing usually involves the removal of soft tissues, cellular and marrow elements. Cancellous bone chips are morsellized into small fragments, around 1 to 4 mm in diameter, freeze-dried and irradiation-sterilized (Figure 14.1a). The morsellized cancellous bone can be moulded and applied into any defect. Cancellous bone can also be supplied as blocks or dowels; these products are of fixed shape and size that can be altered by trimming the edges (Figure 14.1b).

Cortical grafts

Cortical grafts are prepared as described above, and the cortical bone is then cut to a specified width and length (Figure 14.1c). The advantage of these grafts is that anatomical shape and some strength are maintained. Although a cortical graft is used as a mechanical spacer and it should eventually osteointegrate, it is initially a non-vascularized graft that could theoretically act as a foreign body and become a sequestrum. Cortical struts, ring grafts, intercalary sections and even whole bones (Figure 14.1d) are commercially available but the indications for application are rare: for example, limb sparing for osteosarcoma patients or significant diaphyseal bone loss following trauma.

Demineralized bone matrix

DBM is an allograft produced from cortical bone that is decalcified using hydrochloric acid and thus chemically sterilized; it may be additionally sterilized by irradiation. DBM contains protein growth factors including naturally occurring bone morphogenic proteins that are liberated by the demineralization process. These proteins are highly osteoinductive. The demineralized bone also retains trabecular type I collagen structure, which is osteoconductive, but structural rigidity and mechanical strength are lost. The level of demineralization should be carefully controlled as it can affect osteoinductive capacity.

A range of DBM products exist for canine and feline applications including powder, granules, gel, putty and strips. Most commonly, DBM is used as a powder that is mixed into a paste, or as a putty (Figure 14.2). DBM can be used alone or in combination with other products such as autografts, cancellous chips, or other bone graft substitutes. Despite the theoretical osteoinductive benefits of DBM and its rapidly growing popularity, few human studies have demonstrated comparable efficacy of DBM to autogenous bone grafts; however, efficacy appears to be comparable in dogs (Hoffer *et al.*, 2008). In human

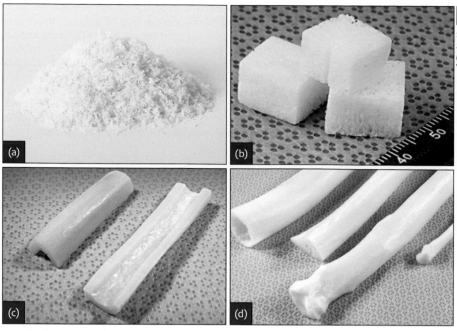

14.1 Allografts. (a) Fine cancellous bone chips. (b) Cancellous blocks. (c) Cortical strut. (d) Cortical sections and whole bone allografts.
(a, Courtesy of Veterinary Tissue Bank; bcd, Courtesy of Veterinary Transplant Services)

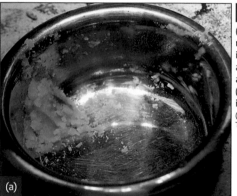

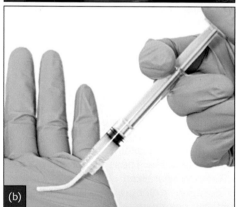

14.2
(a) DBM powder, rehydrated intraoperatively and ready for application.
(b) DBM putty in injectable form.
(Courtesy of Veterinary Tissue Bank)

orthopaedics, DBM may be used alone or in combination with other products, but is usually used as an extender to augment autogenous bone grafts rather than as a replacement. Similarly, in veterinary applications the optimal use of DBM may be in combination with autografts. Despite this, there is an increasing trend to use DBM alone or a mix of DBM and cancellous chips as the sole grafting material in elective surgeries such as arthrodesis, fracture repair, osteotomy and defect filling, with apparently favourable results.

Growth factors

Osteoinductive growth factors can be utilized for bone graft applications following selection and purification.

Bone morphogenic proteins

BMPs are a group of naturally occurring proteins that belong to the TGF-β superfamily of growth factors. At least 20 different subtypes of BMPs have been identified. The *in vivo* function of BMPs is to signal and regulate bone and cartilage formation. They are potent inducers of angiogenesis, progenitor and stem cell migration, stem cell proliferation, differentiation and maturation. The net effect is strong osteoinduction and osteopromotion. Recombinant human (rh) BMP-2 and BMP-7 have been developed and licensed for clinical use in humans with favourable results. The structure of BMPs is highly conserved across species; therefore products developed for humans can be suitable for use in dogs and cats, and have been used with good effect (Kirker-Head *et al.*, 2007; Bernard *et al.*, 2008). However, concerns regarding overstimulation of cells and unwanted side effects including ectopic bone formation, soft tissue swelling and tumour formation have been identified.

The *in vivo* half-life of rhBMP is very short; therefore, the proteins quickly disappear following application. A more sustained effect is desirable for osteoinduction, so slow-release formulations have been developed by impregnating the rhBMP into carrier matrices such as absorbable collagen sponge. Which BMP is best, the optimal quantity and the optimal concentration are all unknown, although some formulations are known to work better than others. Biologically inappropriate doses of BMPs probably account for some of the unwanted side effects including ectopic new bone formation and soft tissue swelling.

Historically, BMP products have been prohibitively expensive for most veterinary applications. Recently a preparation containing rhBMP-2 on a bovine type I collagen sponge carrier matrix was licensed for diaphyseal fracture repair in dogs (TruScient®) (Figure 14.3). The data sheet contained warnings regarding over-exuberant bone formation that could be detrimental in periarticular or perispinal fractures. At the time of print this product is no longer commercially available.

Other growth factors

Platelet-rich plasma (PRP) contains a mixture of growth factors that are involved in the initial orchestration of haemostasis at the fracture site, including platelet-derived growth factor, TGF-β, vascular endothelial growth factor, fibroblast growth factor beta, and insulin-like growth factor. These are all osteopromotive and platelet concentrates promote osteoblast proliferation and differentiation, but their role in promoting bone healing is controversial and clinical evidence validating the use of PRP to enhance fracture healing is lacking; it is rarely used as a grafting product.

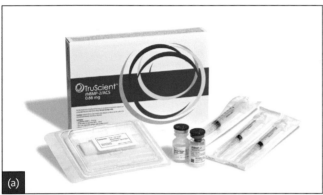

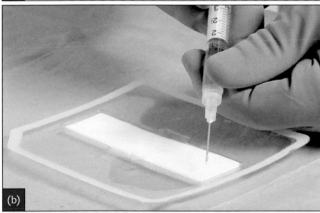

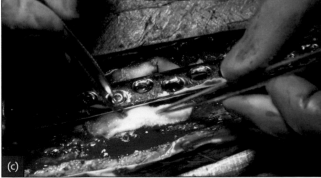

14.3 Recombinant human BMP-2 (rhBMP-2) product. (a) Packaging, vials of active product and sterile water for reconstitution, syringes for mixing and application, and bovine collagen carrier matrix. (b) Application of reconstituted rhBMP-2 on to the collagen sponge. (c) Application of rhBMP-2-soaked collagen sponge into an *in vivo* fracture site.
(Courtesy of Zoetis UK Ltd, UK)

Mesenchymal stem cells and tissue engineering

Mesenchymal stem cells are pluripotent cells that can differentiate into cell lineages important in fracture healing, including osteoblasts and osteoclasts. These stem cells can be harvested from the bone marrow, blood, muscle or adipose tissue of the patient. The stem cells are then cultured in the laboratory and induced to differentiate and multiply. Finally, the differentiated cells are implanted into the patient. This technique has the advantage of being non-immunogenic and should not transmit disease. Disadvantages include expense, the need for two separate patient procedures with a lengthy delay (weeks) between them, and the potential for *in vitro* bacterial contamination. Currently, the timescale, quality control and challenge of achieving sufficient cell populations and lineages to reliably influence bone healing are so problematic that this technique is not used as a bone graft alternative.

In the context of bone grafting, tissue engineering refers to the combination of different grafting technologies to create the 'ultimate' bone graft. For example, a product could be created that combines live cells for osteogenesis with growth factors for osteoinduction, which is seeded on to a perfect scaffold to maximize osteoconduction and osteopromotion. Bone tissue engineering is very much in its infancy; in human medicine other tissue engineering successes have included cartilage, bladder and heart valves.

Alloplastic grafts

Alloplastic grafts are synthetic bone graft products. A wide variety are available but few are used in veterinary medicine. The ideal alloplastic graft would be osteoconductive and osteoinductive, and should be manufactured from material with similar material properties to bone. Most alloplastic grafts are manufactured from hydroxyapatite, which is the naturally occurring mineral component of bone. However, common problems with alloplastic grafts include low and unpredictable resorption rates, poor handling properties such as excessive brittleness, poor clinical results and inflammatory foreign body reactions. For these reasons, although a number of products are available, they are rarely used in small animal veterinary applications.

Ceramics are osteoconductive calcium phosphate synthetic scaffolds, usually tricalcium phosphate (TCP) or hydroxyapatite. These are neither osteogenic nor osteoinductive when used alone, and provide no immediate structural support. However, osteoid (bone) is produced directly on to the ceramic surface, which facilitates osteointegration. Highly biocompatible porous TCP ceramic is gradually replaced by bone ingrowth whereas hydroxyapatite is resorbed much more slowly. Because hydroxyapatite is brittle and undergoes slow resorption, it acts as a stress concentrator, which is undesirable, therefore it is often used in combination with other materials.

Injectable calcium phosphate (Norian® SRS®) is a ceramic composite that has osteoconductive properties. It contains liquid α-TCP that is injected into the fracture site or bone defect; this then hardens *in situ* without an exothermic reaction, avoiding potential thermal necrosis of surrounding tissue including bone. The compressive strength of Norian® SRS® is similar to cancellous bone. Over time, the TCP undergoes remodelling and is gradually replaced by bone.

Bioactive glass is a hard and brittle composite of calcium, phosphate and silicon dioxide that is osteoconductive and osteointegrates. Bone bonds to bioactive glass very well. However, bioactive glass is very strong and resists drilling and shaping; therefore, it is difficult to work with and to affix to adjacent host bone.

Glass ionomer cements are composites of calcium, aluminium and silicate glass mixed with polyacrylic acid to produce a porous cement paste. This sets within 10 minutes, is biocompatible, has good compressive strength and a modulus of elasticity comparable to cortical bone. It is also osteoinductive and osteointegrates. Its disadvantage is that it is brittle. These products are used with human dental implants.

Non-biological osteoconductive substrates are polymers, composites or fabricated metals such as porous tantalum. These are non-immunogenic, have excellent biocompatibility and are used for their osteoconductive properties. Such products are infrequently used but porous tantalum vertebral spacers can be used for cervical spinal fusion surgery, and a tantalum metal endoprosthesis has been used following resection of a distal radial osteosarcoma in a dog (MacDonald and Schiller, 2010). The reasons for using porous tantalum are that the metal is strong and has a relatively low modulus similar to bone, it is highly fatigue resistant, and the porous structure theoretically allows bone ingrowth and osteointegration.

Type I collagen is abundant in extracellular bone matrix and is involved with many important stages of osteogenesis including mineral deposition, vascular ingrowth and growth factor binding. The primary use of collagen in bone grafting is as a carrier matrix for osteoinductive factors such as BMPs. Collagen can also be used as a composite with other bone graft products such as hydroxyapatite, TCP or bone marrow.

Composite alloplastic grafts combine the mechanical structural properties of alloplastic graft materials with osteoinductive or osteogenic properties of other grafting products.

Ideal bone graft properties

The ideal bone graft should be osteoinductive, osteoconductive and osteogenic; it should rapidly osteointegrate, and should be easily, readily and inexpensively available. In addition, it should carry no risk to the recipient patient including disease transmission, should be non-immunogenic, and not be associated with harvesting problems such as donor site morbidity. Unfortunately, no such 'perfect' product exists. Autograft is widely accepted as the gold standard for bone grafting applications in human and veterinary orthopaedics, but harvesting involves an additional surgical procedure with potential risk of donor site morbidity. Recent developments in bone graft substitutes have been significant. Allografts have become more widely used, especially cortico-cancellous allografts used as osteoconductive graft volume expanders, and DBM for osteoinduction. The combination of allograft with autograft, and indeed DBM allograft alone, appears to achieve good outcomes for bone healing with few associated problems. In the future, tissue engineering such as the use of mesenchymal stem cells combined with alloplastic grafts and BMP-type products could more closely approximate the perfect bone graft. However, it is unlikely that simple cancellous autograft will be completely replaced or superseded in the foreseeable future.

References and further reading

Bacher JD and Schmidt RE (2008) Effects of autogenous cancellous bone on healing of homogenous cortical bone grafts. *Journal of Small Animal Practice* **21**, 235–245

Bernard F, Furneaux R, Adrega Da Silva C and Bardet JF (2008) Treatment with rhBMP-2 of extreme radial bone atrophy secondary to fracture management in an Italian Greyhound. *Veterinary and Comparative Orthopaedics and Traumatology* **21**, 64–68

Boudrieau RJ, Tidwell AS, Ullman SL and Gores BR (1994) Correction of mandibular nonunion and malocclusion by plate fixation and autogenous cortical bone grafts in two dogs. *Journal of the American Veterinary Medical Association* **204**, 744–750

Faria MLE, Lu Y, Heaney K *et al.* (2007) Recombinant human bone morphogenetic protein-2 in absorbable collagen sponge enhances bone healing of tibial osteotomies in dogs. *Veterinary Surgery* **36**, 122–131

Hoffer MJ, Griffon DJ, Schaeffer DJ, Johnson AL and Thomas MW (2008) Clinical applications of demineralized bone matrix: a retrospective and case-matched study of seventy-five dogs. *Veterinary Surgery* **37**, 639–647

Innes JF and Myint P (2010) Demineralized bone matrix in veterinary orthopaedics: a review. *Veterinary and Comparative Orthopaedics and Traumatology* **23**, 393–399

Kirker-Head CA, Boudrieau RJ and Kraus KH (2007) Use of bone morphogenetic proteins for augmentation of bone regeneration. *Journal of the American Veterinary Medical Association* **231**, 1039–1055

MacDonald TL and Schiller TD (2010) Limb-sparing surgery using tantalum metal endoprosthesis in a dog with osteosarcoma of the distal radius. *Canadian Veterinary Journal* **51**, 497–500

Ragetly GR and Griffon DJ (2011) The rationale behind novel bone grafting techniques in small animals. *Veterinary and Comparative Orthopaedics and Traumatology* **24**, 1–8

Schena CJ (1983) The procurement of cancellous bone for grafting in small animal orthopedic surgery; a review of instrumentation, technique, and pathophysiology. *Journal of the American Animal Hospital Association* **19**, 695–704

Séguin B, Walsh PJ, Mason DR *et al.* (2003) Use of an ipsilateral vascularized ulnar transposition autograft for limb-sparing surgery of the distal radius in dogs: an anatomic and clinical study. *Veterinary Surgery* **32**, 69–79

Tshamala M and VanBree H (2006) Osteoinductive properties of the bone marrow; myth or reality. *Veterinary and Comparative Orthopaedics and Traumatology* **19**, 133–134

Vertenten G, Gasthuys F, Cornelissen M, Schacht E and Vlaminck L (2010) Enhancing bone healing and regeneration: present and future perspectives in veterinary orthopaedics. *Veterinary and Comparative Orthopaedics and Traumatology* **23**, 153–162

OPERATIVE TECHNIQUE 14.1

Harvesting of an autogenous cancellous bone graft

PREOPERATIVE CONSIDERATIONS

Harvest sites are chosen for ease of surgical access, minimizing patient trauma and for a good supply of cancellous bone. Common harvest sites include:

- Proximal lateral humerus at the base of the greater tubercle
- Ilial wing, dorsal or lateral
- Proximal lateral femur at the base of the greater trochanter
- Medial or lateral distal femoral condyle
- Medial proximal tibial metaphysis.

POSITIONING

Dependent on harvest site.

EQUIPMENT EXTRAS

Gelpi retractors; bone-holding forceps; drill/osteotome; Volkmann curette; syringe/galley pot.

SURGICAL TECHNIQUES

The anatomical landmarks and access point are identified and a limited surgical approach (usually 2–3 cm long) is made to a superficial part of the bone.

Access is maintained using Gelpi retractors oriented at 90 degrees to each other and/or bone-holding forceps (Figure 14.4a).

An access hole is made in the bone using a drill for long bones, or an osteotome for the ilial wing. The hole should be as small as possible to minimize the risk of bone fracture, but large enough to allow a harvesting instrument to be passed.

The harvesting instrument, for example a Volkmann curette, is inserted into the access hole and used to scoop out cancellous bone from the medullary cavity (Figure 14.4b). Care is taken not to damage the cortical bone, in particular by levering the instrument forcefully against the edge of the access hole.

Immediately following collection, the bone graft is temporarily stored, either in a blood-soaked swab or an appropriate container such as the plunger of a syringe or a galley pot until use (Figure 14.4c).

Wound closure

Routine.

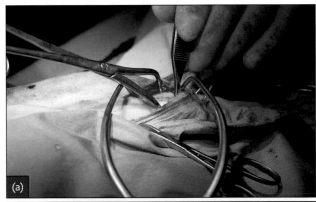

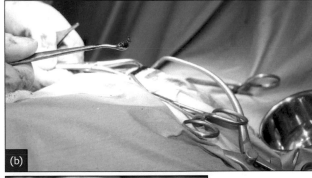

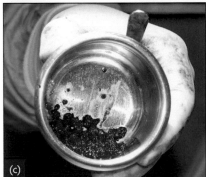

14.4 Collection of a cancellous bone autograft from the proximal humerus of a dog. (a) Use of Gelpi retractors and bone-holding forceps to expose the surgical site and immobilize the bone, prior to drilling a monocortical access hole. (b) Collection of cancellous bone autograft using a Volkmann curette. (c) Temporary storage of collected cancellous bone in a galley pot.

Chapter 15

Minimally invasive osteosynthesis

Antonio Pozzi and Stan Kim

Minimally invasive osteosynthesis (MIO) involves the application of implants for fracture stabilization without making an extensive surgical approach to expose the fracture site. The bone segments are reduced using indirect reduction techniques (without direct manipulation of the bone at the fracture site). In the case of plate fixation of long bone fractures, small insertion incisions are made in the skin at each end of the fractured bone and an epiperiosteal tunnel is made to connect the incisions using blunt dissection. The implant, typically applied in a bridging fashion, is inserted through one of the insertion incisions and tunnelled under the soft tissues, spanning the fracture site (Figure 15.1). When managing articular, physeal or metaphyseal fractures with MIO, other implants such as screws or Kirschner (K) wires may be used percutaneously though small stab incisions (Figure 15.2).

MIO is not a new concept. In human orthopaedic trauma, minimally invasive external skeletal fixation (ESF) and intramedullary nailing have been performed since the beginning of the 20th century. In the veterinary field, percutaneous external fixation and intramedullary pinning were first described more than 20 years ago, although open approaches were still employed more commonly. However, more recently, the introduction of new and improved implants and indirect reduction techniques have led to increased interest in MIO (Hudson *et al.*, 2009). The basic principles of **biological osteosynthesis**, developed to improve biology in the treatment of fractures (see Chapter 8) are directly applicable to MIO. In **open but do not touch (OBDNT)** techniques (Aron *et al.*, 1995), bone

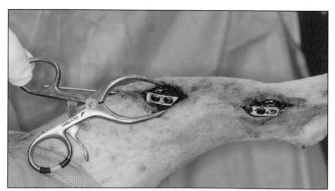

A tibial fracture in a dog has been reduced with an intramedullary pin and a plate placed through the insertion skin incisions. Note that the insertion skin incisions are small and expose only two or three plate holes. Additional screws can be placed through stab incisions.

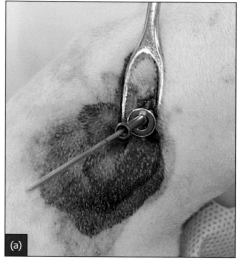

(a)

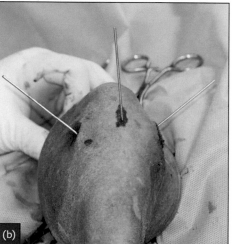

(b)

15.2 (a) A cannulated screw is inserted percutaneously to stabilize a condylar fracture following reduction with vulsellum forceps. (b) Percutaneous K-wires have been used to manage a proximal tibial physeal fracture with MIO.

alignment is achieved without direct manipulation of the fragments through an open approach (Johnson, 2003). Exposure of the full length of the fractured bone and its landmarks allows direct evaluation of alignment. In MIO, similar indirect reduction techniques are used to restore length and alignment, but intraoperative fluoroscopy is used to evaluate fracture apposition and to guide implant placement, rather than direct visualization.

In biological terms, MIO techniques confer an advantage over open fracture fixation techniques by minimizing the iatrogenic soft tissue trauma incurred during surgery. Traditionally, anatomical reduction often required extensive exposure and manipulation of the fractured bone to facilitate accurate reconstruction of the fracture fragments. In contrast, one of the benefits of MIO is preservation of local blood supply and fracture haematoma. Recent studies have demonstrated that minimally invasive plate osteosynthesis (MIPO) causes less disruption of periosteal blood supply (Garofolo and Pozzi, 2013) (Figure 15.3) and earlier vascularization of the fracture callus compared to open plating (Pozzi *et al.*, 2012b). The process of bone healing is dependent on numerous interactions between biological and mechanical factors. Two principal concerns are whether there is adequate blood supply and whether there is effective stability to allow a fracture to achieve bony union. Previous studies comparing the pattern of bone healing between fractures treated by open plating or by MIPO showed that dogs treated with MIPO healed in 4 weeks. In the fractures stabilized using open plating, callus was only apparent 8 weeks following surgery (Pozzi *et al.*, 2012b). These findings would suggest that the difference in the pattern of fracture healing between MIPO and open plating may be dependent on both mechanical and biological factors (Perren, 1975). 'Relative stability', a condition where an acceptable amount of interfragmentary displacement is present, provides a mechanical environment that promotes indirect or secondary bone healing (Baumgaertel *et al.*, 1998; Goodship *et al.*, 1998). Techniques that achieve relative stability, such as ESF, bridging plating or interlocking nailing, are generally indicated for MIO of comminuted long bone fractures, whilst absolute stability techniques may be employed for open compression plating of simple fractures and for articular fractures.

Case selection and preoperative considerations

Despite the perceived benefits associated with MIO, several criteria must be considered when determining whether a case should be managed in a minimally invasive manner or whether an open approach should be used (Figure 15.4). Most focus on the ability to successfully perform closed reduction of the fracture and maintain reduction whilst the implants are placed; extensive previous experience with traditional fracture management techniques is required to consistently achieve a successful outcome, and specialized instrumentation is useful in some cases.

In most cases, closed reduction is more challenging than open reduction, as the soft tissue envelope around the fracture site is left predominantly intact and direct manipulation of the fracture margins is prohibited. Thus, reduction techniques such as toggling and levering cannot be performed; moreover, it is not usually feasible to maintain reduction with direct application of bone reduction forceps. Fracture segments must be adequately mobile and manoeuvrable using techniques in which the bone can be manipulated in regions that are remote from the fracture site, such as temporary external fixation (Figure 15.5) (see Operative Technique 15.1). Important case-related factors that must be assessed include the chronicity of the fracture, the age of the animal, the location of the fracture, size of the bone segments and the degree of displacement. Orthogonal radiographs of the affected limb as well as careful palpation of the fracture site should be performed. Generally, the interval between trauma and surgery should be less than 3 days because muscle contraction, formation of soft tissue callus and local adhesions can greatly hinder the relative mobility of the fracture fragments. This is especially apparent in skeletally immature animals. In addition, skeletally immature animals have a tremendous capacity to achieve rapid union, and thus the benefits of MIO techniques may not be as apparent when compared to older subjects. Bone segments that have extensive soft tissue coverage such as the femur or humerus are more difficult to manipulate than bones that are located more superficially. Extremely small fracture fragments, particularly those seen in cats or toy-breed dogs, are also challenging to reduce accurately. Finally, it is more challenging to perform MIO in animals with highly displaced fractures; the ideal candidates have minimal displacement of the major fragments.

Another important consideration is whether the fracture site itself should be opened to obtain perfect apposition of the fracture margins. For simple fractures, it is useful to reconstruct anatomically and provide interfragmentary compression, in order to achieve optimal construct stability. Fixation can rarely be applied in anything other than a

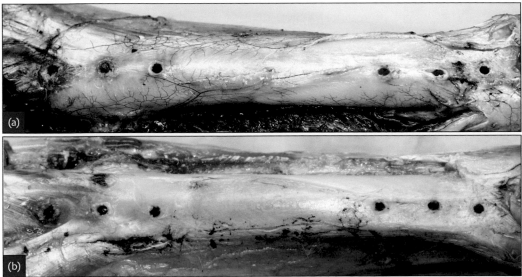

15.3 Photographs of cadaveric radii injected with blue latex and India ink to evaluate extraosseous blood supply in specimens that underwent (a) minimally invasive plate osteosynthesis (MIPO) and (b) open reduction and internal fixation (ORIF). There is markedly improved preservation of periosteal vasculature and less extravasation with MIPO when compared to ORIF.
(Reproduced from Garofolo and Pozzi (2013) with permission from *Veterinary Surgery*)

Technique	Indications	Limitations
MIO	• Comminuted fractures • Long bone fractures • Acute fractures • Minimally displaced fractures • Well aligned delayed union	• Intraoperative radiography or fluoroscopy may be necessary • Not possible to compress fracture • Learning curve • Need for indirect reduction • Less suitable for simple fractures (especially oblique)
ORIF	• Simple fractures • Both long bone and articular fractures • Long-standing fractures • Non-union or delayed union requiring ostectomy	• Need for direct reduction • Extensive surgical exposure leads to increased risk of delayed union and/or infection

15.4 Indications for and limitations of minimally invasive osteosynthesis (MIO), and open reduction and internal fixation (ORIF).

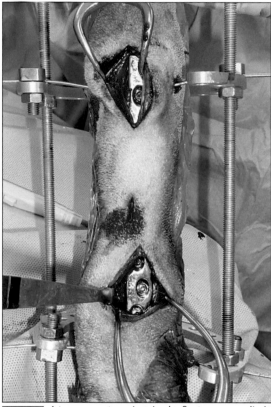

15.5 A temporary two-ring circular fixator was applied to a radius for reducing a mid-diaphyseal fracture. A broad 3.5 mm limited contact dynamic compression plate was used in MIPO fashion for definitive fracture fixation.

bridging fashion when minimally invasive techniques are adopted, which leads to substantially more stress being placed on the implant. Conversely, MIO may be particularly advantageous with comminuted diaphyseal fractures, where preservation of the fracture haematoma and minimal iatrogenic disruption to the fracture is desirable. Articular fractures can be very challenging because perfect reduction and interfragmentary compression is almost always indicated. In the authors' experience, indirect anatomical reduction of articular fractures is most achievable when the surgery is performed within 24 hours of the fracture occurring. These 'fresh' fractures can often be reduced without extensive manipulation; however, if appropriate reduction is not achieved with the first

few attempts prompt conversion to an open approach is recommended, as optimal anatomical reconstruction of articular fractures should not be sacrificed for the sake of a minimally invasive treatment.

Whether an open fracture warrants a minimally invasive procedure also varies according to the individual case characteristics. For open fractures, there are no definitive, evidence-based guidelines that incorporate minimally invasive options. In general, Gustilo and Anderson grade I open fractures may be surgically managed as though they were closed; grade II and III fractures are likely to require thorough wound exploration and decontamination, and have much of the fracture already exposed (see Chapter 12). Nevertheless, adopting the main principle of MIO by performing only necessary and careful soft tissue dissection adjacent to the fracture site is likely to be beneficial.

Whilst MIO can be executed without additional equipment beyond what is necessary for traditional repair, there are several tools that will greatly facilitate the procedure. Foremost, intraoperative radiography or fluoroscopy is highly recommended (Figure 15.6). This allows for accurate evaluation of reduction, as well as precise positioning of implants. It is also valuable to have more than one method of performing closed reduction available at the time of surgery, such as temporary ESF or a reduction table. For MIPO, locking plate systems may be advantageous in certain scenarios compared to traditional dynamic compression plating (Miller and Goswami, 2007). Locking plates do not require precise contouring and may confer some mechanical advantages. Conversely, purely locking systems do not allow the implant to be used to assist reduction, and it can be difficult to angle screws away from adjacent joints. If available, implants that allow use of either locking or conventional screws are preferred (see Chapter 10).

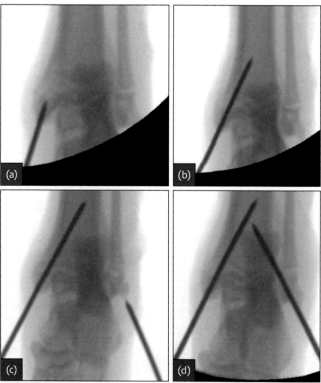

15.6 (a–d) Serial fluoroscopic images of cross pin placement for a distal tibial physeal fracture in a cat. Use of fluoroscopy greatly facilitates accurate insertion point, insertion length and pin trajectory.

Principles of specific fixation methods using minimally invasive osteosynthesis

External skeletal fixation

ESF can be an excellent technique for surgical fracture management that minimizes disruption to fracture biology. A more complete discussion on the components, types, mechanics, indications and application of external fixators is provided in Chapter 10.

There are many advantages to choosing ESF when deciding to treat a fracture using a minimally invasive technique:

- Control and manipulation of bone segments in a closed manner using ESF components is vastly superior to indirect manual traction or application of traditional bone-holding forceps alone. In particular, circular components are able to provide excellent biaxial control when applied circumferentially around the affected limb (Farese et al., 2002)
- Fractures can be gradually distracted intraoperatively in a controlled manner by sequentially loosening, applying traction and tightening multiple connecting elements to acutely manage overridden segments
- Although application of ESF has been associated with a relatively high degree of postoperative morbidity, it is possible to place percutaneous fixation pins with minimal exposure of bone. The limited surgical approach required for pin insertion and the ability to remove the implants after fracture healing makes ESF a reasonable choice for many open fractures
- Unlike with internal fixation, small adjustments to the constructs can be performed postoperatively to improve fracture reduction and limb alignment. These corrections may be particularly useful when performing MIO, because of the risk of malalignment associated with this technique.

There are several major disadvantages of ESF:

- Pin tract discharge and infection is extremely common, particularly where there is a thick soft tissue envelope in a high-motion area such as the proximal limb
- Femoral and humeral fracture stabilization with ESF is also challenging because the proximity of the body wall limits the surgeon's ability to provide biaxial support
- Whilst additional fixation elements can be placed to make a frame stronger, the position of the connecting rods away from the neutral axis of the bone is mechanically inferior when compared to bone plating or intramedullary fixation
- Daily maintenance of the frame is required from the owner, and these cases must be re-evaluated frequently.

Minimally invasive plate osteosynthesis

MIPO involves making small insertion incisions remote to the fracture and developing an epiperiosteal tunnel between these incisions. The plate is inserted through the soft tissue tunnel and fixed to the bone with screws, which are placed through the insertion incisions or through additional stab incisions (Hudson et al., 2009) (see Operative Techniques 15.2–15.5).

Preoperative preparation is essential to the execution of MIPO. As the fracture site is not exposed, each step of the surgical procedure, including reduction and implant application, needs to be planned ahead to avoid long surgical times and unnecessary exposure to ionizing radiation.

Patient evaluation

As in standard fracture treatment, appropriate assessment of the patient is important for correct decision making. A detailed history, physical examination and appropriate preoperative imaging studies should be performed. Timing of the surgery relative to the trauma is an important factor because indirect reduction may be challenging for long-standing fractures. Other factors, such as haemodynamic stability, are also important because longer anaesthesia time may be required when performing MIPO, especially whilst gaining experience with the technique.

Fracture evaluation

Orthogonal radiographs of the fractured bone, including proximal and distal joints, are necessary. In selected cases, it may be helpful to acquire computed tomography scans and evaluate three-dimensional reconstructions of the fractured bone for detailed planning. Radiographs of the intact contralateral bone are often very helpful; accurate contouring of the implant based on images of the contralateral intact bone may shorten surgical time and allow use of the plate for indirect reduction. Fracture configuration is also considered. MIPO is most applicable to comminuted diaphyseal or metaphyseal fractures, which may not be amenable to anatomical reduction (Figure 15.7); however, MIPO can also be utilized for some simple transverse fractures if anatomical reduction can be achieved (Figure 15.8). Long plates are typically applied in a bridging fashion to stabilize comminuted fractures, dissipating strain over the comminuted segment. In a retrospective study comparing antebrachial fractures treated with MIPO or open plating, simple fractures were more likely to have translational malalignment than comminuted fractures (Pozzi et al., 2012a). In our experience, MIPO techniques may be attempted for simple fractures, but if good reduction cannot be accomplished easily the procedure should be revised to an open plating technique.

Choice of implant

The evolution of MIPO in human orthopaedics was accelerated by the development of locking plates. Locking plates have both mechanical and biological advantages:

- The periosteal blood supply beneath the plate is not compromised because compression between plate and bone does not occur; this may improve healing and decrease the risk of cortical bone necrosis and infection (Baumgaertel et al., 1998)
- The plate does not need to be perfectly contoured, because the bone is not pulled towards the plate whilst tightening the screw; for this reason, locking plates are often used for MIPO
- Locking plate constructs may be mechanically advantageous compared to non-locking constructs, especially in soft bone.

Disadvantages of locking plates include:

- An inability to use the plate to assist reduction as can be achieved using a pre-contoured non-locking plate
- An increased risk of inserting screws into adjacent joints when the plate is applied to metaphyseal fractures
- Unique mechanisms of mechanical failure such as screw shearing and screw 'slicing' through bone.

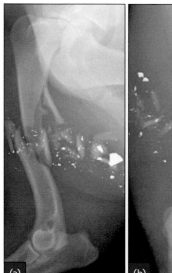
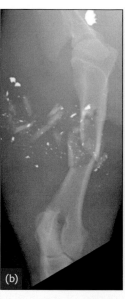
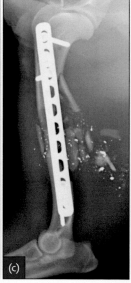
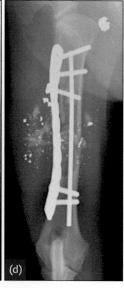

15.7 Preoperative (a) mediolateral and (b) craniocaudal radiographs of a highly comminuted mid-diaphyseal humeral fracture due to a gunshot injury in a dog. Postoperative (c) mediolateral and (d) craniocaudal radiographs. A pin–plate construct was used in MIPO fashion to stabilize the fracture.

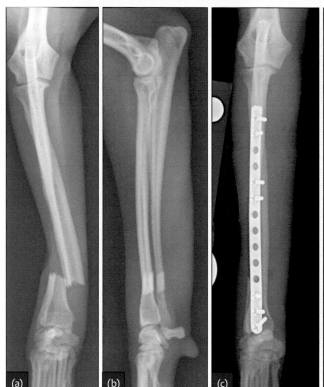

15.8 Preoperative (a) craniocaudal and (b) mediolateral radiographs of a short oblique distal diaphyseal antebrachial fracture in a dog. Postoperative (c) craniocaudal and (d) mediolateral radiographs. A plate was applied to the radius in MIPO fashion to stabilize the fracture. Note that MIPO techniques can still be adopted in non-comminuted injuries, provided accurate reduction can be achieved.

Several different locking plate systems are available (see Chapter 10). Systems with combination holes that allow placement of a locking screw or a conventional non-locking screw are preferred in most cases since, if applied correctly, they can confer advantages of locking and non-locking systems.

The selection of an appropriate length plate is a very important step in the preoperative planning. Appropriate plate length is dependent on the location and configuration of the fracture, as well as the intended functional application of the plate. In bridge plating, longer implants lower the pull-out force acting on screws and allow better distribution of the bending forces along the plate (see Chapter 4). Sanders *et al.* (2002) compared 6-, 8- and 10-hole 3.5 mm dynamic compression plates fixed on canine cadaveric ulnae that were then tested by four-point bending to failure. This study revealed that ten-hole plates with four screws widely spread on the fracture fragment failed at higher peak loads than six-hole plates with six screws, supporting the recommendation to use longer plates with fewer screws as these provide superior bending strength than shorter plates with a greater number of screws.

Percutaneous pinning and percutaneous screw fixation

When Steinmann pins or K-wires (hereafter collectively referred to as pins) are used alone to stabilize fractures in a minimally invasive fashion (see Figure 15.2), the procedure is known as percutaneous pinning. Some fractures amenable to lag screw fixation as the primary method of stabilization may also be approached in a minimally invasive manner. Placement of pins or screws through small stab incisions may confer significant advantages compared to traditional open pinning, including decreased postoperative pain, accelerated healing and decreased iatrogenic trauma to important structures such as the physes and periarticular tissues. Although percutaneous pinning can be utilized with a high success rate, appropriate case selection, fluoroscopic guidance and surgeon experience are required if it is to be attempted.

All traditional principles of intramedullary pinning, cross-pinning and lag screw fixation apply when considering the use of percutaneous fixation (see Chapters 10 and 11). Salter–Harris type I and II physeal fractures (see Chapter 2) are the most amenable to percutaneous pinning as they usually have some inherent stability following reduction, and thus sufficient stabilization can be achieved solely by use of pins. In addition, these fractures can often be reduced with minimal manipulation (Figure 15.9). Percutaneous lag screw fixation may be most suited to Salter–Harris type III and IV fractures as well as certain sacroiliac luxations.

Reduction can be difficult as the epiphyseal segments are typically small. The precise technique of closed reduction depends on the location of the fracture and the direction and degree of displacement of the epiphysis; generally, the manoeuvre involves indirect manual manipulation of the fragments with traction and gentle leverage (Skaggs, 2006). Maintenance of reduction can be aided in some cases by placement of a small temporary K-wire or percutaneous application of pointed reduction forceps; this is especially applicable to Salter–Harris type IV fractures of the humeral condyle (see Figure 15.2). Following reduction, small (10 mm) approaches are made down to the periosteum over the proposed implant insertion sites, to allow placement of the definitive fixation. The approaches should be large enough to be able to countersink the pins sufficiently or tighten the screws, and to check that the implants are seated adequately. Whilst immature bone may be soft enough to place pins by hand, power drills are preferred for optimal accuracy. An oscillating drill function is useful to prevent soft tissues from entangling around the pin during insertion.

Intraoperative fluoroscopy should be used before, during and after application of the implants to ensure optimal positioning. Without fluoroscopy, it is often extremely difficult to place implants accurately due to the limited exposure. Pins must be seated into the trans cortex, carefully measured, backed out, and then cut to length accurately such that they can be countersunk to beneath the surface of the bone without protruding into soft tissue. Accurate screw sizing is less problematic, so long as the depth gauge is appropriately seated against bone and does not entrap soft tissue during its use.

References and further reading

Aron DN, Palmer RH and Johnson AL (1995) Biologic strategies and a balanced concept for repair of highly comminuted long bone fractures. *Compendium on Continuing Education for the Practicing Veterinarian* **17**, 35–47

Baumgaertel F, Buhl M and Rahn BA (1998) Fracture healing in biological plate osteosynthesis. *Injury* **29** (Suppl 3), 3–6

Farese JP, Lewis DD, Cross AR *et al.* (2002) Use of IMEX SK-circular external fixator hybrid constructs for fracture stabilization in dogs and cats. *Journal of the American Animal Hospital Association* **38**, 279–289

Field JR and Tornkvist H (2001) Biological fracture fixation: a perspective. *Veterinary and Comparative Orthopaedics and Traumatology* **14**, 169–178

Field JR, Tornkvist H, Hearn TC, Sumner-Smith G and Woodside TD (1999) The influence of screw omission on construction stiffness and bone surface strain in the application of bone plates to cadaveric bone. *Injury* **30**, 591–598

Garofolo S and Pozzi A (2013) Effect of plating technique on periosteal blood supply of the radius in dogs: a cadaveric study. *Veterinary Surgery* **42**, 255–261

Gautier E and Sommer C (2003) Guidelines for the clinical application of the LCP. *Injury* **34**, 63–76

Goodship AE, Cunningham JL and Kenwright J (1998) Strain rate and timing of stimulation in mechanical modulation of fracture healing. *Clinical Orthopaedics and Related Research* **355**, Suppl S105–115

Hudson C, Pozzi A and Lewis DD (2009) Introduction to minimally invasive plating osteosynthesis in dogs. *Veterinary and Comparative Orthopaedics and Traumatology* **22**, 175–182

Johnson AL (2003) Current concepts in fracture reduction. *Veterinary and Comparative Orthopaedics and Traumatology* **16**, 59–66

Miller DL and Goswami T (2007) A review of locking compression plate biomechanics and their advantages as internal fixators in fracture healing. *Clinical Biomechanics* **22**, 1049–1062

Perren SM (1975) Physical and biological aspects of fracture healing with special reference to internal fixation. *Clinical Orthopaedics and Related Research* **138**, 175–194

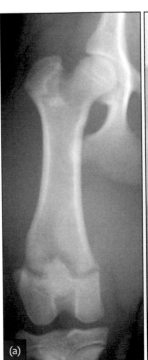
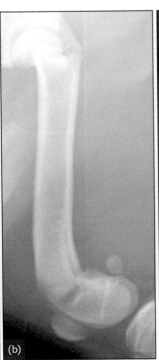
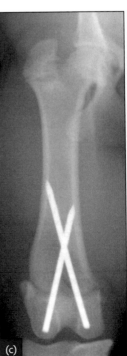
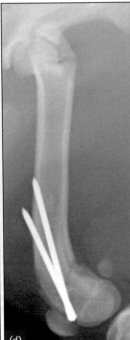

15.9

Preoperative (a) craniocaudal and (b) mediolateral radiographs of a distal femoral Salter–Harris type II fracture in a dog. Postoperative (c) craniocaudal and (d) mediolateral radiographs. Percutaneously placed cross pins were used to stabilize the fracture.

→ **OPERATIVE TECHNIQUE 15.1 CONTINUED**

USE OF A PRE-CONTOURED PLATE

A pre-contoured plate used with cortical screws can aid in indirect reduction because the shape of the plate will determine the alignment of the fracture fragments after tightening the screws (Figure 15.14). The plate is contoured to a radiograph of the contralateral intact bone and then inserted through the skin incisions. After assessing the position of the plate and the anticipated reduction with orthogonal fluoroscopic views, cortical screws are placed in each fragment to pull the fragments to the plate. Then further screws can be placed to complete the fixation. Implants that allow use of either locking or cortical screws are preferred because they may allow a combination of screws to be placed.

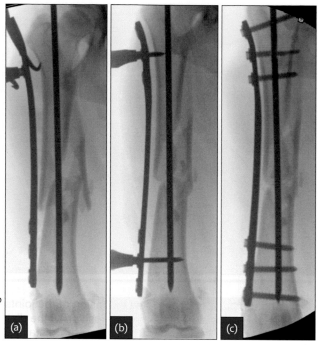

15.14 Sequential fluoroscopic images showing indirect reduction of a femoral fracture using a pre-contoured plate. (a) The plate is slid into the epiperiosteal tunnel. (b) Pin stoppers, instruments similar to push-pull devices, are used to pull the bone fragments towards the plate. (c) Screws are applied to complete the fixation.

OPERATIVE TECHNIQUE 15.2

Minimally invasive application of a plate to the humerus

POSITIONING

The dog is positioned in dorsal recumbency with a foam pad placed under the shoulder to allow intraoperative fluoroscopy (limb held vertically to allow the fluoroscope to rotate 360 degrees around it). Elevation of the shoulder relative to the chest allows imaging of the proximal humerus without interference from the sternum, an important consideration in deep-chested dogs. It is easier to rotate the dog into lateral recumbency for the surgical dissection and plate insertion. If a radiolucent surgical table is available the entire procedure can be performed with the dog in lateral recumbency.

ASSISTANT

Useful in the initial phase of the procedure when performing indirect reduction.

SURGICAL TECHNIQUES

Reduction

Indirect reduction is performed using an IM pin inserted in normograde (see Operative Technique 20.10), proximodistal fashion under fluoroscopic guidance. The pin is directed away from the radial nerve, in a caudomedial direction. Bone reduction forceps can be inserted through the insertion incisions and used to manipulate the fragments whilst directing the IM pin in the medullary canal.

→ **OPERATIVE TECHNIQUE 15.2 CONTINUED**

Approach

A craniolateral approach is usually performed; a medial approach is used less commonly. For a craniolateral approach a 3 cm long skin incision is made over the greater tubercle and then through the deep fascia along the lateral border of the brachiocephalicus muscle (Figure 15.15). After retraction of the brachiocephalicus muscle and the fascia, the distal insertion of the acromial part of the deltoideus muscle is incised and elevated. The distal window is obtained by making a limited approach to the distal humeral metaphysis and lateral epicondyle. A submuscular tunnel is created by passing either Metzenbaum scissors or a large periosteal elevator from the distal to the proximal incision, deep to the brachialis muscle. The tunnelling instrument must be passed along the cranial aspect of the humerus and kept in contact with the humeral cortex to avoid injury to the radial nerve lateral to the distal humerus.

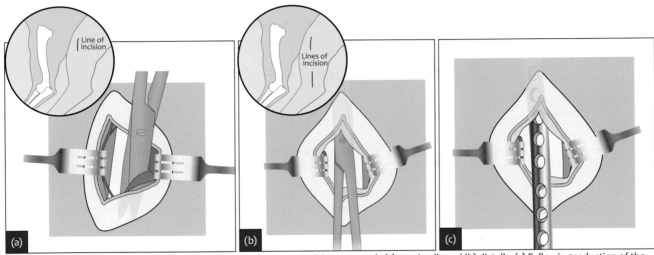

15.15 Minimally invasive application of a plate to the humerus. Incisions are made (a) proximally and (b) distally. (c) Following reduction of the fracture and creation of an epiperiosteol tunnel a pre-contoured plate is applied.

Application of plate

A combination of an IM pin and a plate is frequently used. The IM pin facilitates indirect reduction, maintains alignment during plate application and improves mechanical stability. Following pin placement, the pre-contoured plate is inserted through the epiperiosteal tunnel, taking care to avoid iatrogenic injury to the radial nerve. The plate is generally applied to the cranial or craniolateral aspect of the bone. In comminuted fractures the plate can be used as an indirect reduction tool (Figure 15.16).

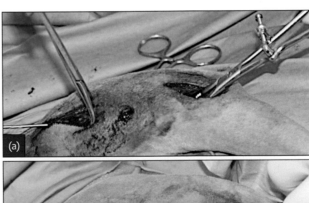

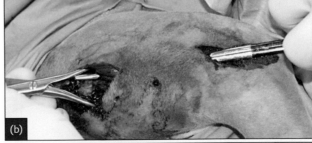

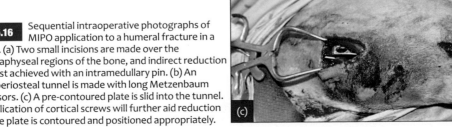

15.16 Sequential intraoperative photographs of MIPO application to a humeral fracture in a dog. (a) Two small incisions are made over the metaphyseal regions of the bone, and indirect reduction is first achieved with an intramedullary pin. (b) An epiperiosteal tunnel is made with long Metzenbaum scissors. (c) A pre-contoured plate is slid into the tunnel. Application of cortical screws will further aid reduction if the plate is contoured and positioned appropriately.

OPERATIVE TECHNIQUE 15.3

Minimally invasive application of a plate to the radius

POSITIONING

The patient is positioned in dorsal recumbency with foam pads placed under both shoulders. Depending on the reduction technique, the limb is typically extended caudally for the approach and placement of implants.

ASSISTANT

Useful in the initial phase of the surgery when performing indirect reduction.

SURGICAL TECHNIQUES

Reduction

The authors' preferred method of reduction is by use of a temporary circular external fixator. The initial fixation wire is placed in the mediolateral plane through the distal fracture segment, adjacent and parallel to the distal articular surface of the radius. In dogs with distal metaphyseal fractures, the wire is placed to allow placement of a plate screw both proximal and distal to the wire. The wire is attached to the distal ring of the pre-assembled fixator using wire fixation bolts and nuts. A second fixation wire is then placed through the proximal radial metaphysis in the mediolateral plane and attached to the proximal ring in a similar fashion to the first wire. The fracture is distracted to length by turning the nuts on the threaded connector bars. Rotational alignment is evaluated by observing the plane of flexion and extension of the carpus relative to that of the elbow. Rotational malalignment can be corrected by shifting the position of the distal wire about the circumference on the distal ring. Translational malalignment can be improved by sliding the distal fracture segment along the distal wire.

Approach

After the fracture segments have been aligned, proximal and distal insertion incisions are created. The radiocarpal joint is identified by palpation and a craniolateral skin incision is made, centred over the distal radial metaphysis. The deep antebrachial fascia is then incised between the tendon of the extensor carpi radialis muscle and the tendon of the common digital extensor muscle. The oblique abductor pollicus longs muscle should be avoided if possible. A periosteal elevator or Metzenbaum scissors are used to develop the epiperiosteal tunnel from distal to proximal. A proximal craniolateral or craniomedial incision is made after measuring and marking the proximal extent of the plate on the skin. For a craniomedial approach, the antebrachial fascia is incised between the extensor carpi radialis and the pronator teres muscles. For a craniolateral approach, the extensor muscle bellies are separated to expose the bone (Figure 15.17).

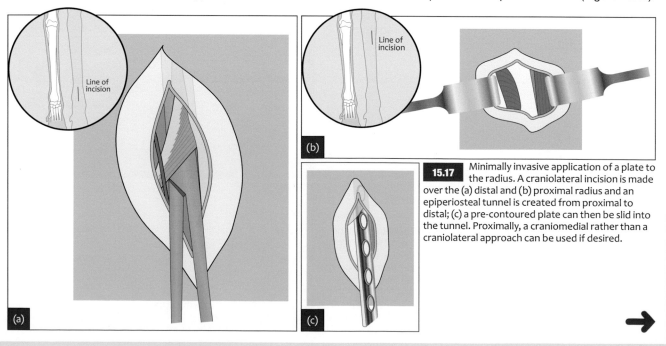

15.17 Minimally invasive application of a plate to the radius. A craniolateral incision is made over the (a) distal and (b) proximal radius and an epiperiosteal tunnel is created from proximal to distal; (c) a pre-contoured plate can then be slid into the tunnel. Proximally, a craniomedial rather than a craniolateral approach can be used if desired.

→ **OPERATIVE TECHNIQUE 15.3 CONTINUED**

Application of plate

The plate is inserted from the proximal incision if the distal fracture segment is caudally displaced and from the distal incision if the distal fracture segment is cranially displaced. After plate insertion, orthogonal fluoroscopic images of the antebrachium are acquired to evaluate the position of the plate. The plate is appropriately positioned over the distal radial segment first and a screw is inserted in the distal screw hole in the plate. The position of the plate over the proximal radial segment is then confirmed and a screw is placed in the proximal end of the plate. One to three screws are then placed in both the proximal and distal radial fracture segments (Figure 15.18).

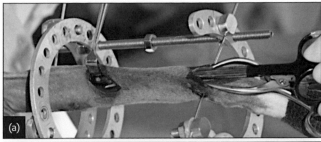
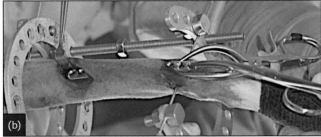
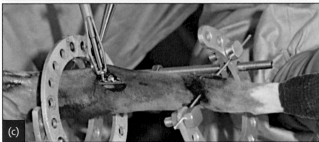

15.18 Sequential intraoperative photographs of MIPO application to an antebrachial fracture in a dog. (a) Two small incisions are made over the metaphyseal regions of the bone, and indirect reduction is first achieved with a temporary circular fixator. (b) A pre-contoured plate is slid into the epiperiosteal tunnel. (c) Application of cortical screws will further aid in reduction if the plate is contoured and positioned appropriately.

OPERATIVE TECHNIQUE 15.4

Minimally invasive application of a plate to the femur

POSITIONING

The patient is positioned in lateral recumbency, as caudally as possible on the table, with the fractured limb uppermost. Use of a radiolucent operating table is highly recommended in order to facilitate lateromedial radiographic views during surgery. Alternatively, a dense sheet of plexiglass (or other strong radiolucent material) can be placed on a traditional table, which is used to support the caudal aspect of the patient. The contralateral femur should be positioned cranially with the hip flexed, to ensure there is no superimposition with the affected side during imaging. Prior to sterile preparation and draping, it is useful to confirm that orthogonal radiographs of the affected bone can be performed.

ASSISTANT

Useful in the initial phase of the surgery when performing indirect reduction.

→ **OPERATIVE TECHNIQUE 15.4 CONTINUED**

Reduction

Indirect reduction of the fracture is best performed using an IM pin inserted in normograde fashion (see Operative Technique 23.4) under fluoroscopic guidance. The pin is 'walked' off the greater trochanter until it falls into the intertrochanteric fossa; caution is needed to avoid iatrogenic injury of the sciatic nerve. Bone reduction forceps are inserted through the insertion incisions and used to manipulate the proximal fragment whilst directing the IM pin in the medullary canal. Manipulation of bone segments with temporary transcortical half pins can also be helpful.

Approach

Lateral approaches to the proximal (Figure 15.9a) and distal (Figure 15.9b) femur are made. Proximally, an incision is made from the greater trochanter extending a short distance distally. The superficial and deep leaves of the fascia lata are incised at the cranial border of the biceps femoris muscle. The vastus lateralis muscle is partially elevated off the proximal metaphysis. Hohmann or self-retaining retractors are used cranially and caudally to provide optimal exposure. For the distal approach, a longitudinal incision is made laterally at the level of the patella extending proximally. The fascia lata is incised at the cranial border of the biceps femoris muscle. The vastus lateralis muscle is retracted cranially and the biceps femoris muscle is retracted caudally with Hohmann or self-retaining retractors; this is facilitated by ligation and transection of branches from the distal caudal femoral artery and vein. A submuscular tunnel is created by passing either Metzenbaum scissors or a large periosteal elevator from the distal to the proximal incision (Figure 15.9c).

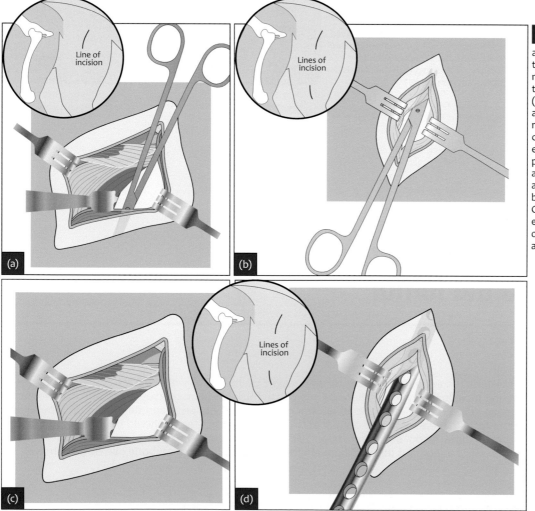

15.19 Minimally invasive application of a plate to the femur. Incisions are made (a) proximally over the greater trochanter and (b) distally over the lateral aspect of the femoral metaphysis. (c) Following creation of an epiperiosteal tunnel, (d) a pre-contoured plate is applied to the bone. Linear alignment of the bone is best achieved using an IM. Great care is needed to ensure torsional alignment of the bone as the plate is applied.

→ **OPERATIVE TECHNIQUE 15.4 CONTINUED**

Application of plate

A combination of an IM pin and a plate is frequently used. With the pin in place, an appropriately sized bone plate is pre-contoured to the lateral surface of the bone based on radiographs of the contralateral femur. Mild torsional contouring of the plate is required, as the greater trochanter is oriented slightly caudally. Initial use of cortical screws in each segment allows the plate to be used to assist reduction. Distally, the plate and screws should be carefully positioned such that there is no interference with the patellofemoral or femorotibial joints. One to three further cortical or locking screws are then placed proximally and distally to further stabilize the construct (Figure 15.20). At least one screw in the proximal segment should engage the calcar region.

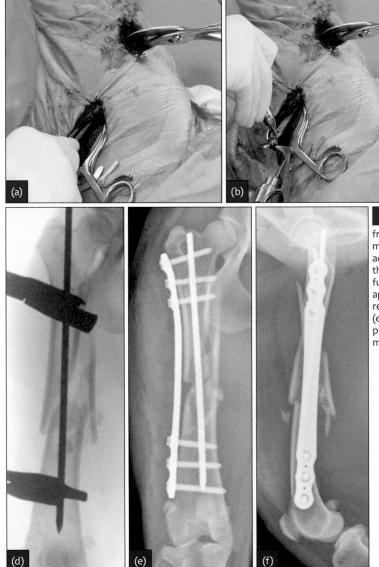

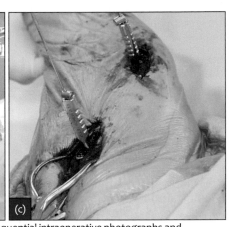

15.20 Sequential intraoperative photographs and fluoroscopic images of MIPO application to a femoral fracture in a dog. (a) Two small incisions are made over the metaphyseal regions of the bone, and indirect reduction is first achieved with an IM pin. (b) A pre-contoured plate is slid into the epiperiosteal tunnel. (c) Application of pin stoppers will further aid in reduction if the plate is contoured and positioned appropriately. (d) Intraoperative radiograph of indirect reduction achieved with an IM pin. Postoperative (e) craniocaudal and (f) mediolateral radiographs of the pin–plate construct. Ideally, the IM pin could have been seated more distally.

OPERATIVE TECHNIQUE 15.5

Minimally invasive application of a plate to the tibia

POSITIONING

The patient is positioned in dorsal recumbency at the end of the surgical table. A Mayo stand can be used to support the limb during plate application. As the limb is off the table, a fluoroscope can easily be used to image the tibia in both sagittal and coronal planes.

ASSISTANT

Useful in the initial phase of the surgery when performing indirect reduction.

SURGICAL TECHNIQUES

Reduction

Various techniques of indirect reduction can be used for tibial fractures. The IM pin technique is a simple way to achieve distraction, reduction and alignment of the fracture fragments. A temporary two-ring circular fixator can also be applied to the tibia and used to distract the fracture segments and to facilitate and maintain reduction during plate application. The proximal and distal fixation wires are placed in the medial-to-lateral plane in locations that will not impair implant insertion and fixation. The distal wire can be placed through the talus if desired, to allow full exposure of the distal fracture segment.

Approach

A longitudinal incision is made over the medial aspect of the proximal tibia. The tendons of insertion of the sartorius, gracilis and semitendinosus muscles are incised and elevated. Caudal retraction of these muscles allows exposure of the medial aspect of the proximal tibia. A skin incision is then made over the medial aspect of the distal tibia (Figure 15.21). A submuscular tunnel is developed under the skin, carefully sparing the medial saphenous artery and vein. Blunt dissection with Metzenbaum scissors allows the tunnel to be extended from distal to proximal.

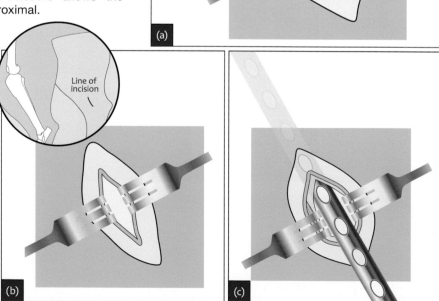

15.21 Minimally invasive application of a plate to the medial aspect of the tibia. An incision is made (a) proximally and (b) distally. (c) Following creation of an epiperiosteal tunnel, a pre-contoured plate is slid into it and applied to the bone.

→ **OPERATIVE TECHNIQUE 15.5 CONTINUED**

Application of plate

The plate is pre-contoured based on radiographs of the contralateral limb and inserted from either the proximal or distal incision. Temporary fixation with a push-pull device allows evaluation of limb alignment and implant positioning using fluoroscopy (Figure 15.22). Adjustments to plate contouring and plate position can be made before fixing the plate with screws. The most proximal and distal screws are placed first; use of cortical screws allows the plate to be used to aid fracture reduction. After reassessing limb alignment, further cortical or locking screws are placed through the insertion incisions. Additional screws can be added through stab incisions if necessary.

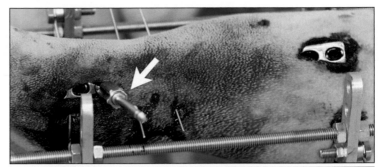

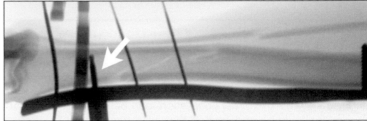

15.22 A push-pull device (arrowed) placed in the distal aspect of the plate allows the plate to be secured and its position checked with fluoroscopy. In addition, the push-pull device aids reduction of the fracture if a pre-contoured plate is used.

Chapter 16

Non-surgical management of fractures

Jon Dyce

The management of long bone fractures using casts and splints pre-dates other means of repair. With appropriate case selection, the results achieved by rigid bandaging, otherwise known as external coaptation, can be excellent. However, it should be appreciated that, with the advent of more sophisticated fixation techniques, optimal fracture management is now less likely to involve primary coaptation. The aim of this chapter is to review the principles of non-surgical fracture management. It does not give a comprehensive list of fractures suitable for non-surgical management, and the reader is directed to the chapters on specific fractures for guidance in individual cases (see Chapters 17–27).

Cast biomechanics

Coaptation of fractures does not result in rigid immobility but should impart sufficient stability for fracture healing to occur. As rigid bone fixation is not achieved, healing will proceed by secondary bone union, with radiographically obvious callus formation. Therefore, aspects of the local fracture environment that favour callus formation will significantly influence selection for cast or splint management.

The ability of a cast to immobilize a fracture depends on the stiffness of the cast, the intimacy of the cast layer to the bone and the location of the fracture within the cast (Tobias, 1995). The stiffness (or resistance to bending) is determined by the choice of cast material and the application technique. Of the forces acting at the fracture site, bending is neutralized well by a cylinder cast, but compressive, torsional, shearing and distractive forces are counteracted relatively poorly. Consequently, inherently unstable fractures (including avulsion fractures) are not suitable for coaptation. Casting materials are stronger in tension than compression, so cast failure is likely to occur on the concave aspect of any angulation. A spine moulded from cast material may be applied to reinforce this vulnerable surface.

Cast management of fractures proximal to the elbow and stifle is precluded by the proximity of the body wall and by the presence of large muscle masses around the humerus and femur, which result in poor mechanical coupling between the cast and bone. Application of excessive cast padding to more distal fractures will produce a similar effect.

The fracture should be located centrally within the cast, as cast purchase on the proximal and distal limb is necessary for stabilization. The axiom that the joint proximal and distal to the fracture should be immobilized is a useful guide, but fractures with considerable intrinsic stability (e.g. minimally displaced, isolated distal radial or ulnar fractures) may not require extension of the cast beyond the proximal joint.

Indications for casting

The following criteria should be considered when assessing the suitability of a fracture for cast management.

Fracture configuration

Relatively stable fractures, for example those with greenstick (incomplete) and interdigitating transverse configurations, are the most suitable for casting. If a fracture is minimally displaced, particularly in the immature animal, the periosteum is more likely to be intact and will contribute to fracture stability.

Casting may be appropriate for those cases where one member of paired bones is fractured and the intact bone contributes significant support; for example, fracture of the radius with an intact ulna, or fewer than three metapodial fractures. Simple oblique or spiral fractures are generally not good candidates for coaptation, because of the intrinsic instability of the fracture plane. Similarly, comminuted fractures are rarely suitable for casting as collapse of the fracture site is likely to occur.

Fracture location

The biomechanics of cast application and the difficulty of manipulative reduction preclude satisfactory coaptation of proximal limb fractures.

Intra-articular fractures proximal to the carpus and tarsus almost invariably dictate open reduction and internal fixation, and coaptation is not recommended. However, selected fractures of the carpus and tarsus can have a good clinical outcome without internal fixation, and coaptation may therefore be appropriate (see Chapter 25). A successful outcome is unlikely if significant avulsion forces act on the fracture fragment, for example, an oblique fracture of the base of metacarpal V or an avulsion fracture of the plantar distal calcaneus. These fractures are frequently associated with traumatic carpal hyperextension and proximal intertarsal subluxation with plantar instability,

BSAVA Manual of Canine and Feline Fracture Repair and Management, 2nd edition. Edited by Toby Gemmill and Dylan Clements. ©BSAVA 2016

respectively. Coaptation would offer a poor prognosis for resolution of postural collapse in such cases.

Growth plate fractures occur in young dogs with good osteogenic potential, but the advantage of an early return to weight bearing offered by internal fixation, and the likelihood of complications of cast management of such juxta-articular fractures make cast management a poor option. Salter–Harris type I fractures of the distal radius are a special case and may be managed by casting alone or by cross-pin fixation and adjunctive coaptation. The latter technique, where an intrinsically weak repair is protected by a secondary fixation, is referred to as **adaptation osteosynthesis**.

Fracture reduction

Reduction should be performed without an open surgical approach, to conserve the soft tissue envelope and limit vascular compromise to the fracture site. The fracture is reduced with care, using a combination of linear traction and toggling of the bone ends. Following manipulation of transverse fractures, the fracture should appear more than 50% reduced on both orthogonal radiographic projections. Although anatomical reduction is the ideal, it is rarely achieved and is certainly not a prerequisite for success.

Muscle masses in the proximal limb and soft tissue swelling may preclude fracture palpation and therefore adequate manipulative reduction.

If there is a delay to fracture management, muscle contracture and callus formation will progressively impede reduction. If adequate reduction is not possible then open reduction and alternative fixation must be considered.

Signalment

In general, limbs can be maintained comfortably in casts for 4 to 6 weeks. Candidates for coaptation should therefore produce adequate bridging callus within this period. Younger animals form callus more readily and on this criterion are better subjects for casting, but the rapidly growing juvenile is more likely to encounter complications associated with restricted limb growth within the cast. The use of splinted bandages is therefore favoured in immature dogs and has the advantage of ease of splint exchange.

The specific physiology of distal radial and ulnar fractures in toy breed dogs (Welch et al., 1997) results in an unacceptably high incidence of failure following cast management. Operative fixation using plate and screws is the recommended standard of care (see Chapter 21).

> **WARNING**
>
> Distal radial/ulnar fractures in toy breeds should not be casted

Chondrodystrophic and obese dogs are difficult to cast effectively, because of limb conformation, and therefore alternative methods of fracture management are generally indicated.

Intended role of the patient

Whilst casting of, for example, radial/ulnar or tibial fractures is frequently possible, it is unlikely to be the optimal management for athletic and working animals. Expectations of function should be discussed with owners prior to fracture coaptation.

Cost

Economy is frequently cited as an indication for cast management of fractures. However, the cost of materials used in cast application is likely to exceed that of disposable materials used in simple operative stabilization such as external skeletal fixation. The incidence of complications leading to additional expense (e.g. pressure sores, cast breakage, malunion) should also be considered (Meeson et al., 2011). The time commitment to fracture convalescence is similar for both treatment regimens.

Cast construction

A cast typically comprises several layers: a contact layer (generally stockinette), a padding layer, a compression layer and the circumferential cast material.

Casting materials

For many decades, plaster of Paris was the only available casting material (Hohn, 1975). Plaster of Paris products are still produced, but are messy to apply, take many hours to reach weight-bearing strength, deteriorate when wet and are relatively heavy and brittle. Excellent conformability, radiolucency and economy are its redeeming qualities, but a number of alternative casting materials are now available that are superior in many key respects. Predictably, none is ideal (see below). For reviews of casting materials see Houlton and Brearley (1985) and Langley-Hobbs et al. (1996). Currently, the author uses a standard resin-impregnated fibreglass (such as Vetcast™, 3M™) for all small animal cast applications, and finds this a versatile splinting material. This consistently allows construction of well tolerated, light, strong and durable casts. Any increase in material cost is justified by the likelihood of the initial cast delivering bone union without complications.

Properties of the ideal casting material include:

- High strength/weight ratio
- Easy to apply
- Short time to reach maximum strength after application
- Conformable
- Durable
- Radiolucent
- Water resistant but 'breathable'
- Easy and safe to remove
- Reusable
- Economical.

Cast application

If there is significant soft tissue swelling associated with the fracture at the time of initial examination, casting should be delayed and a splinted bandage or non-rigid compressive (Robert Jones) bandage should be applied to the limb following fracture reduction, until this swelling has subsided. Typically, this will take 2 to 3 days.

Any skin wounds should be debrided and, if appropriate, closed primarily. Full cylinder casting of exudative wounds should be avoided, and appropriate standards of wound care followed (see *BSAVA Manual of Canine and Feline Wound Management and Reconstruction*). The hair coat is clipped if it would interfere with cast application. The limb should be clean and dry. Following appropriate preparation, adhesive tape stirrups (e.g. zinc oxide or micropore tape) can be applied to the limb to prevent distal migration of the cast (Figure 16.1a). Tapes may be placed on the dorsal and palmar/plantar, or medial and lateral aspects of the foot. Tape adhesion to the large metapodial footpad is discouraged as epidermal sloughing can result. The free ends of the tapes are temporarily secured to a tongue depressor. Stockinette is rolled up the limb to incorporate any wound dressing, and is tensioned to eliminate creases (Figure 16.1b). Cast padding is wound on to the limb with a 50% overlap on each turn. Two to three layers generally suffice. Particular care is taken to ensure even padding over pressure points. Excessive padding about pressure points should be avoided and consideration should be given to increasing the padding in adjacent depressed regions with, for example, doughnuts of orthopaedic foam, cast padding or stockinette placed around the prominence.

Next, a compressive layer is applied in a similar manner to compact the padding. Application of correct tension is necessary but difficult to quantify. Too tight and it will act as a tourniquet; too loose and it will allow chafing and fail to stabilize the fracture.

The cast material is applied with appropriate tension, again with a 50% overlap on each turn (Figure 16.1c). Care is taken to maintain this overlap over the convex aspect of joints. If the material requires wetting to activate the hardening process, then the temporary application of cling film around the limb can keep the cast padding dry, and prevent adhesion of the resin to the underlying compressive layer. A 1–2 cm margin of cast padding is left exposed proximal and distal to the cast (Figure 16.1d). Two or three layers of cast material are generally applied. Manufacturers' recommendations regarding wetting and handling should be followed. Tension is increased as the cast is applied proximal to the elbow or stifle to give a snug fit about the muscle masses and to prevent loosening.

It is important that an appropriate limb posture is maintained during casting and that indentations are not produced in the cast by the fingers. Once the cast has hardened, the stockinette and padding are rolled down and secured to the cast with adhesive tape (Figure 16.1e). The stirrups are peeled apart, twisted through 180 degrees and bound to the distal cast with adhesive tape (Figures 16.1fg). The pads and nails of the axial digits should remain exposed (Figure 16.1h).

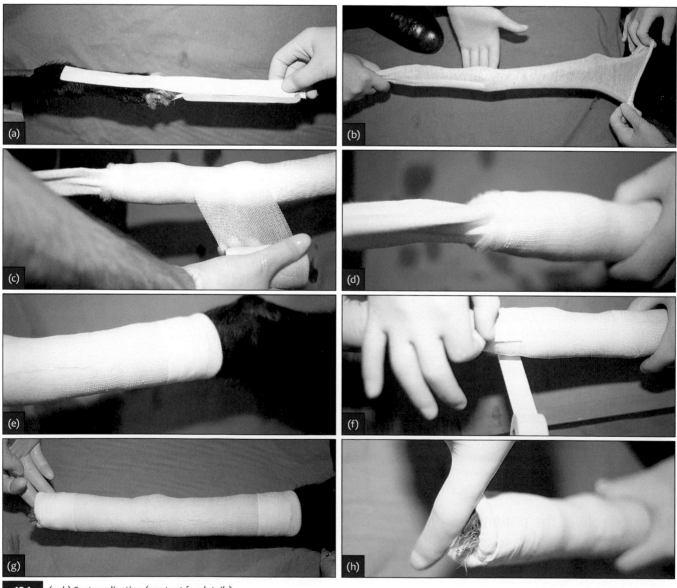

16.1 (a–h) Cast application (see text for details).

To facilitate removal, the cast may be bivalved by cutting along its medial and lateral aspects and then bandaged with strong adhesive tape. However, this will diminish some of the material properties of the cast. Cutting along the cranial and caudal, rather than medial and lateral, aspects may have less impact on the material properties, although this is rarely performed.

With the resin-embedded fibreglass materials, weight-bearing strength will have been reached by the time of recovery from anaesthesia.

Medication with non-steroidal anti-inflammatory drugs is useful to limit soft tissue swelling and to provide analgesia. The requirement for ongoing treatment should be reassessed after 3 to 5 days.

Cast maintenance

> **WARNING**
>
> Amputation may be the price paid for poor cast management

The majority of patients managed in a cast will be discharged to the care of their owners until cast removal. It is therefore essential that owners are educated in daily cast monitoring and that the development of complications is reported at the earliest opportunity. It is a sobering fact that a significant amount of litigation arises from poorly managed casts. Written instructions should always be given out at discharge and owners must understand their responsibility in cast maintenance.

Points to monitor are swelling of the toes or proximal limb, toe discolouration and coolness, skin abrasion about the toes or proximal cast, cast loosening, angular deformity, damage, breakage, discharge or foul odour. Chewing at the cast may be a response to discomfort and should be investigated. In addition, deteriorating weight-bearing function of the cast limb and signs of general ill health (e.g. inappetence, dullness) may suggest the development of complications within the cast. It is sensible to schedule routine weekly appointments for cast assessment for the duration of casting. Rapidly growing dogs and other high-risk patients may require more frequent assessment.

Excessive activity will compromise cast survival and predispose to complications; therefore cage rest is recommended, with minimal leash walking exercise for toileting purposes only. The cast must be kept clean and dry. Whilst outside, a polythene foot bag or protective bandage boot is applied. This must be removed when the patient is inside to avoid the cast becoming saturated with moisture.

> **WARNING**
>
> Bandage covers should be removed at all other times to prevent moisture build-up within the cast

Bedding materials such as straw can migrate between cast and skin, and should be avoided. Kennelled dogs can be successfully managed in casts provided that monitoring is diligent and hygiene good.

Cast removal

The time course for development of clinical union will be around 3 to 6 weeks, depending on individual patient and fracture factors. Radiography should be performed (see Chapter 6) to confirm adequate progression towards fracture healing, prior to cast removal. Note that in 3- to 4-month-old puppies, in which long bone fractures are commonly coapted, fracture healing is often permissive of return to unsupported weight bearing within 2 weeks. Although plaster shears can be used to remove most casting materials, an oscillating circular saw is most suitable. Bilateral incisions are made in the cast (Figure 16.2a), taking care not to damage underlying tissue. The two halves are then prised apart using cast spreaders (Figure 16.2b) and the underlying bandage materials are removed (Figure 16.2c).

After cast removal the gross physical stability of the fracture should be confirmed by manipulation. It is important that a regimen of progressively increasing controlled exercise is enforced. The goal is stimulation of callus remodelling without jeopardizing fracture repair.

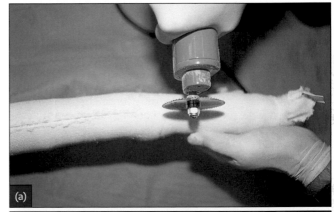

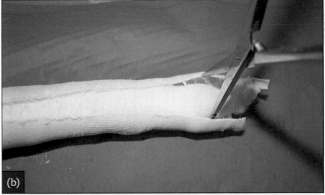

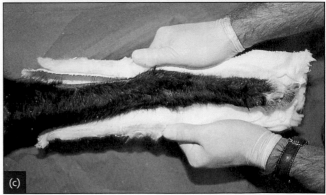

16.2 (a–c) Cast removal (see text for details).

Complications

Joint stiffness

Limb immobilization will cause progressive joint stiffness; this is an inevitable consequence of cast management (Tomlinson, 1991). It is most marked in those patients with periarticular soft tissue damage, which exacerbates periarticular fibrosis and adhesion. It is common to cast joints in extension and, therefore, compromised joint flexion is to be expected following cast removal. The degree of compromise may be overcome (e.g. in the carpus) by immobilizing the joint in a mild degree of flexion. Degrees of fracture disease, a syndrome of stiffness, periarticular fibrosis, cartilage degeneration, muscle atrophy and osteoporosis, can occur (see Chapter 28). This is seen particularly following cast application to the proximal hindlimb in young dogs with unstable distal femoral fracture, where quadriceps contracture and the resultant genu recurvatum are devastating complications.

> **WARNING**
>
> Avoid stifle immobilization in skeletally immature animals

Joint laxity

Laxity is a particular complication in rapidly growing young dogs, especially of large breeds. Carpal hyperextension associated with palmar carpal ligament laxity and carpal and digital flexor insufficiency is most commonly seen after coaptation for radial/ulnar fractures (Figure 16.3). Further coaptation is not appropriate if the healed fracture is stable. Posture in the majority of such cases will resolve spontaneously with return to unsupported weight-bearing.

Limb swelling

Excessive tension during cast application will cause attenuation of lymphatic and venous drainage and consequently distal limb oedema. This is likely to be seen within hours of cast application. It may therefore be sensible to hospitalize the patient overnight to observe any early complications of casting. Ongoing soft tissue swelling within a properly pressurized cast will also cause distal limb oedema, but this will manifest later after application. Limb swelling is a potentially serious complication and requires diligent monitoring and appropriately rapid intervention.

Pressure sores

Bony prominences such as the olecranon, accessory carpal bone, calcaneus and the distal metacarpals and metatarsals are particularly vulnerable to skin trauma (Figure 16.4). Two mechanisms are responsible: pressure necrosis and abrasion. Good application technique and appropriate cast monitoring will significantly reduce the incidence and severity of such complications. Direct skin trauma and a moist environment within the cast predispose to bacterial dermatitis. Staphylococcal organisms are generally responsible. The development of full thickness skin wounds can permit extension of infection to underlying tissues and necrotizing cellulitis can become established. There may be few systemic clinical signs of deterioration and a purulent discharge staining the cast may be the first obvious sign. Decubitus sores can require intensive and prolonged management (Anderson and White, 2000) and prevention of this complication by good bandaging technique is a point of emphasis.

Abrasion of the toes caused by a cast that is too short or tight should be managed by cast replacement rather than piecemeal reconstruction or local trimming.

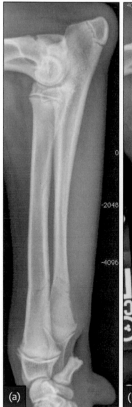
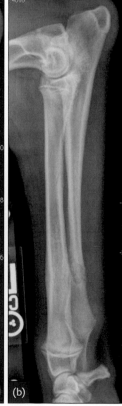
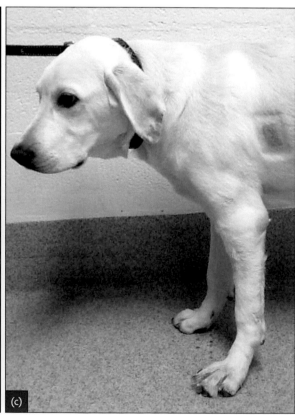

16.3 (a) Greenstick fracture of the left distal radial diaphysis and minimally displaced complete oblique fracture of the distal ulnar diaphysis in a 6-month-old Labrador Retriever. (b) After 3 weeks of coaptation in a splinted bandage there is bridging periosteal callus formation about the radial fracture plane. (c) Immediately after splint removal there is carpal and digital hyperextension affecting the left forelimb associated with disuse atrophy. Restoration of normal posture should be expected within 2 to 3 weeks.

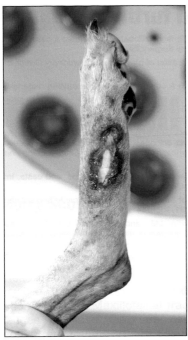

16.4 Pressure sore over the medial aspect of the distal metatarsus in a 4-year-old Border Collie. Bone is exposed in the wound. A cast had been applied to manage an isolated, mid-diaphyseal fracture of the fifth metatarsal bone. The wound eventually healed, but required several weeks of ongoing management with dressings.

Cast loosening

As the acute soft tissue swelling about the fracture subsides, the snug fit of the cast is lost. This will predispose to fracture instability and abrasion within and about the cast. Long-term casting will inevitably be associated with muscle atrophy and similar loosening.

Delayed union, malunion and non-union

Correct case selection and good casting technique should prevent fracture repair failure. Torsional misalignment is easily introduced when bandaging unstable fractures and diligence in application is required to preserve alignment. Compromised fracture healing is more likely to be seen in association with any of the above complications. The frequent removal and reapplication of a cast may contribute to movement at the fracture plane and failure of repair; therefore, cast changes should be minimized or should be performed with the patient under heavy sedation or even general anaesthesia. Delayed union, malunion and non-union are discussed in detail in Chapter 31.

Re-fracture

Re-fracture rarely occurs following cast removal if there is radiographic evidence of bridging callus formation.

Splinted bandages

Splinted bandages can be used in the place of cylinder casts and require less exacting technical application. Splints tend to be less durable, requiring more frequent replacement, and there is some relative loss of mechanical strength, but they can be effective in providing adequate stability for long bone fractures distal to the elbow and stifle, particularly in the immature dog.

Splints are useful in the management of fractures distal to the metacarpus/metatarsus as all toes can be supported and not subjected to weight-bearing. Selected phalangeal fractures are commonly managed in foot splints (see Chapter 26). Ready-made plastic and metal 'metasplints' are available. Customized splints are readily made from casting materials and have the advantage of better conformability. Metacarpal fractures managed with non-mouldable splints are more likely to develop palmar bowing during fracture healing. The components of the splinted bandage are essentially the same as the cast, but without a rigid circumferential external layer. Padding is placed between the toes before bandaging to prevent interdigital sores. The splint is enclosed in the compressive layer and this is then covered with a flexible cohesive bandage. In general, for fractures distal to the carpus/tarsus the foot is enclosed in the splinted bandage, whereas the toes remain exposed for more proximal fractures.

Fractures of the tarsus may be immobilized by cranial or lateral splints made from casting materials or thermally sensitive plastic; these customized splints are preferred to 'off the shelf' pre-contoured lateral splints.

Other bandages

Support bandages such as the Spica splint and Schroeder–Thomas extension splint have historically been used for primary fracture management, but in contemporary small animal orthopaedics they are not the first choice as they are associated with very high complication rates. Similarly, non-weight-bearing slings such as the Velpeau, carpal and Ehmer slings are usually considered only as adjunctive means to protect relatively fragile internal fixation or reduced luxation.

In cases such as scapular and pelvic fractures that are not candidates for surgical intervention, it is rare that such bandage support will improve the prognosis or time of convalescence compared with more conservative management. The likely incidence of complications of bandaging should also be considered.

External coaptation in fractures of the skull and spine

Specific issues relating to the management of skull and spinal fractures are covered in Chapters 17 and 18, respectively.

Non-surgical management without external support

A number of fractures – for example, fractures of the pubis and ischium that do not involve the load-bearing sacral-ilial-acetabular axis, or fractures of vertebral transverse processes that do not involve the spinal canal – are adequately supported by the local soft tissues and best managed without any additional support.

Management involves attention to ongoing analgesia, rest in an appropriately sized pen with flooring that offers a sure footing, and provision of comfortable bedding. In all cases in which ambulation is difficult, good quality nursing should be practised, with supervision of defecation and urination. The use of hand-held supportive slings should be considered to assist dogs when they are taken out.

alveolus serves as a stress riser. Extraction of teeth in the fracture line should only be performed if there is severe periodontitis, or if the tooth roots are fractured or loose and cannot be stabilized. Teeth with fractures of the crown involving the root can often be salvaged, but may require root canal therapy or future extraction. Disruption of the blood supply to the teeth along the fracture line may cause inflammation of the pulpal tissues, leading to periapical abscessation; such teeth should be monitored closely during the postoperative period and if this complication occurs the tooth should be treated as appropriate

- **Restore correct dental occlusion.** Restoration of normal/preoperative dental occlusion and jaw function are paramount. Small malalignments that are well tolerated in diaphyseal fractures of the appendicular skeleton are often unacceptable in the mandible or maxilla. In dogs with normal dental morphology, correct occlusion is achieved when the mandibular canine tooth is positioned in the middle of the space between the maxillary lateral incisor and canine tooth (Figure 17.1) and the cusp of the mandibular fourth premolar is positioned between the maxillary third and fourth premolars. Malocclusion results in complications such as delayed fracture healing, impaired mastication, abnormal tooth wear, accumulation of plaque and tartar, periodontal disease and degenerative disease of the TMJ.

The dominant muscle pull on the mandible is from the temporalis, masseter and the medial and lateral pterygoid muscles, whose combined effect is to close the jaw. In the dog, these muscles are very strong and are capable of generating large forces. The only muscle whose action is to open the jaw is the relatively weak digastricus muscle, which attaches to the ventral aspect of the mandibular body. The primary force acting on the mandible during mastication is bending which induces maximum tensile stress at the oral or alveolar aspect of the mandible. The rostral fragment of a fractured mandible will therefore displace in a caudoventral direction (Figure 17.2). Shear, rotational and compressive forces are much less significant,

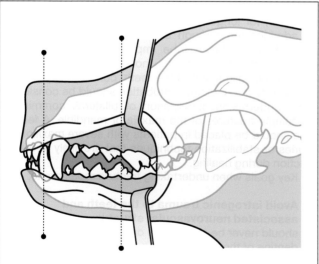

17.1 Schematic view of the canine skull showing normal dental occlusion. The mandibular canine tooth is positioned in the middle of the space between the maxillary lateral incisor and canine tooth (rostral dotted line) and the cusp of the mandibular fourth premolar is positioned between the maxillary third and fourth premolars (caudal dotted line).

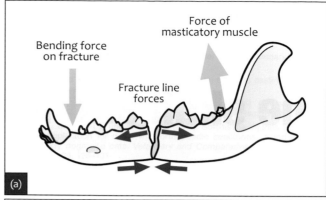

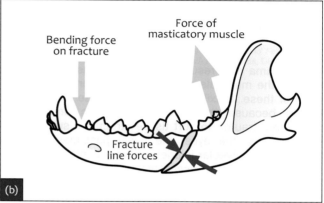

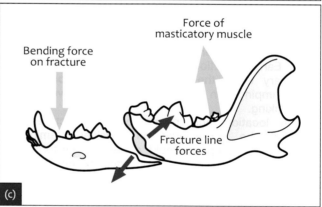

17.2 Biomechanics of mandibular fractures. (a) A fracture perpendicular to the long axis of the body of the mandible will tend to open at the dorsal end of the fracture line. (b–c) For oblique fractures, stability will depend on the angle and direction of the obliquity. (b) A fracture line that runs from dorsocaudal to ventrorostral is favourable because muscle forces compress the fracture line and it will be inherently stable. (c) A fracture line that is oriented from dorsorostral to ventrocaudal is unfavourable because muscle forces lead to distraction of the rostral fragment.

particularly when fractures are unilateral due to the splinting effect of the intact hemimandible. To take advantage of the tension-band principle, implants should ideally be placed on the alveolar border unless this is likely to jeopardize the tooth roots and the neurovascular structures in the mandibular canal. For simple mandibular fractures, the direction of the fracture line will influence the inherent stability of the fracture and should be considered when choosing the method of fixation (Figure 17.2). A fracture line that runs from dorsocaudal to rostroventral is favourable biomechanically because muscle forces compress the fracture surfaces and it will be inherently more stable than other fracture configurations. The distribution of forces on the maxilla differs from the mandible and it is generally accepted that the maxilla is subjected to less strain. The maxilla is attached to the remainder of the head with areas of thickened bone (or buttresses) that support the dental arches and act to transmit the occlusal forces to the base of the skull. The three primary buttresses are the medial (or rostral) nasomaxillary, the lateral zygomatico-maxillary and the caudal pterygomaxillary (Figure 17.3). Following fracture, reconstruction of the lateral and medial buttresses alone will be sufficient to restore stability and alignment. The lateral buttress is repaired first. Fractures not involving the buttresses may occasionally still benefit from fixation, for example if they adversely affect cosmetic appearance or compromise support for the incisor teeth.

Almost all fractures of the mandible are open, owing to the tight attachment of the gingiva to the underlying bone. The use of perioperative broad-spectrum antibiotics has been associated with a reduced incidence of complications in open mandibular fractures in dogs. Continued post-operative administration of antibiotics in humans has been questioned (Lovato and Wagner, 2009), but the significance of this in small animals is uncertain, and antibiotics are usually continued in the postoperative period. Cefalexin or amoxicillin/clavulanate (co-amoxiclav) are good empirical choices; animals with concurrent severe periodontal dis-ease may benefit from the addition of clindamycin or metronidazole because they are effective against the types of anaerobic bacteria associated with this condition.

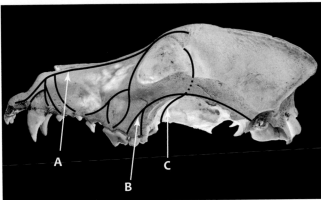

17.3 Lateral view of the skull showing the three primary lines of buttress support. The lines of the buttress support follow the thicker sections of bone (as identified by transillumination). A = the medial (or rostral) nasomaxillary buttress; B = the lateral zygomaticomaxillary buttress; C = the caudal pterygomaxillary buttress.

Techniques for managing maxillofacial fractures

The three broad categories of technique used for maxillo-facial fracture management are closed or minimally inva-sive, open/surgical and salvage procedures.

Closed or minimally invasive management of maxillofacial fractures

With the exception of interdental wiring/interdental acrylic splinting, all of these techniques are forms of biological osteosynthesis that rely on keeping the mouth closed or partially closed. Fracture reduction and stabilization is achieved through occlusal alignment by interdigitation of the teeth of the upper and lower dental arcades. If possible a gap (5–20 mm depending on the size of the patient) should be left between the upper and lower incisors to allow for the animal to lap a semi-liquid diet. In some patients proper occlusion can only be maintained by closing the jaws so that no gap is left and the animal is fed through a feeding tube. The disadvantages of all mouth closure methods are as follows:

- Interference with normal masticatory function
- Less stability than an appropriate open reduction
- Delay in return to normal eating and drinking
- Risk of heat stroke due to interference with panting
- Risk of aspiration pneumonia if the animal regurgitates or vomits
- Less suitable for cats and contraindicated in brachycephalic dogs because of interference with breathing
- A period of immobilization may lead to soft tissue contracture and reduced range of TMJ motion.

External coaptation of the muzzle

Indications for external coaptation muzzle include:

- Stable fractures of the mandible and maxilla with minimal displacement
- Fractures in young animals (<6 months), provided occlusion is satisfactory
- Unilateral or bilateral fissure or incomplete (greenstick) fractures
- Minimally displaced fractures of the ramus of the mandible including the condyloid process
- Fractures secondary to periodontitis where there is insufficient bone stock to accept implants
- As a temporary means of stabilization before definitive repair
- As an adjunct to other methods of stabilization.

External support using a muzzle fashioned from adhe-sive tape (Figure 17.4), or a commercially available nylon muzzle, is a practical, cheap and non-invasive method of managing selected jaw fractures. It is essential to establish that an animal can breathe normally through its nose before application of a muzzle. Despite its common usage, there are drawbacks, some of which are similar to those for external coaptation of limb fractures:

- Reliance is placed on the owner for daily maintenance of the muzzle
- Dermatitis may develop under the muzzle
- Some patients may not tolerate application of a muzzle.

Interarcade wiring

Depending on the location of the fracture, dental occlusion is maintained by the placement of interarcade wires either around the incisor teeth, through drill holes in the alveolar ridge just caudal to the canine teeth, or between the tooth roots of the maxillary fourth premolar and the mandibular first molar bilaterally. The technique has been largely super-seded by other methods of maintaining mouth closure and is not commonly employed.

Maxillomandibular external skeletal fixation

A variable number of fixation pins or Kirschner wires are placed laterally across the maxilla and mandible and connected using either elastic bands or epoxy putty connecting bars (Figure 17.5). The technique may be most useful for cats with caudal mandibular fractures. Complications include trauma to tooth roots during pin application and pin tract infection.

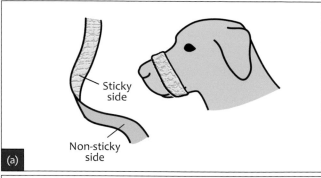

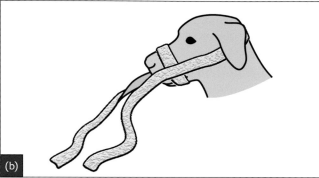

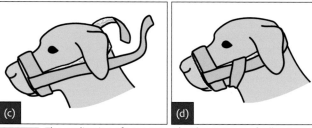

17.4 The application of a tape muzzle. Three pieces of adhesive tape are used for the basic muzzle. (a) The first piece encircles the muzzle (sticky side out). (b) A second strip of tape is then placed around the back of the head with each end running alongside the muzzle (sticky side out). The ends should be of sufficient length to fold back behind the ears again after a third piece of tape has been applied. (c) A third strip of tape is placed around the muzzle (sticky side down) to bind in the second piece. The ends of the second piece are now folded back on themselves and anchored behind the head. (d) A fourth strip acting as a chin strap may be added.

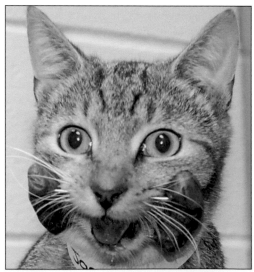

17.5 Maxillomandibular ESF in a 3-year-old cat. Wires are driven laterally across the maxilla and mandible, avoiding the tooth roots. Following reduction of the fracture the jaw is opened slightly and acrylic applied to link the ends of the pins.
(Courtesy of T Gemmill)

Intercanine acrylic bonding

Intercanine acrylic bonding (see Operative Technique 17.1) is a method of interarcade fixation (Figure 17.6) that has been used for all types of canine and feline mandibular fractures except symphyseal or very rostral fractures. The technique is best restricted to cats and very small dogs with caudal mandibular fractures and four intact canine teeth in which other more invasive methods of fixation are not applicable. Unlike maxillomandibular external skeletal fixation (ESF), there is no risk of iatrogenic damage to the teeth and periodontal structures; however, the fixation may be less robust.

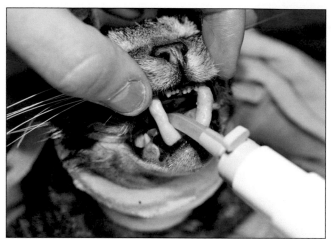

17.6 Intercanine acrylic bonding. Note that the mouth has been left partially open to allow the intake of liquidized food.

Bi-gnathic encircling and retaining device

This technique is a simple method to restrict maxillomandibular movement through the application of a nylon suture, which encircles both the mandible and maxilla (see Operative Technique 17.1). The technique is cheaper and simpler to apply than canine acrylic bonding and has the advantage of easy removal of the appliance by the owner using a pair of scissors if there is an emergency (Figure 17.7) (Nicholson *et al.* 2010). However, the bi-gnathic encircling and retaining device (BEARD) does not provide rigid fixation unless the mandible is closed. The technique is most successful when used for caudal mandibular fractures in puppies, small-breed dogs and cats.

Labial reverse suture through buttons

This technique is similar in its application to the BEARD except that the mattress sutures are placed in the midline of the lower lip and passed subcutaneously into the oral cavity, on either side of the mandible. The sutures cross the oral cavity rostral to the canine teeth, and then pass subcutaneously to exit the skin either side of the maxilla (Figure 17.8). The sutures are placed through buttons to distribute the pressure. This method can be indicated in cases where there is caudoversion of the mandibular canine teeth, sometimes seen in cats that have fallen from a height. However, rigid stabilization of the fracture is not achieved and secondary tissue complications can be seen.

Interdental wiring and interdental acrylic splinting

Interdental wiring is commonly used for the management of human jaw fractures and has been adapted for use in dogs, either as the sole method of repair for maxillary fractures and simple transverse mandibular body fractures

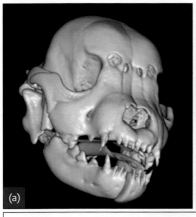
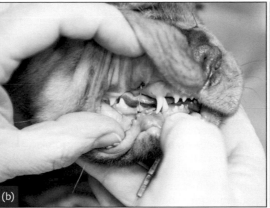
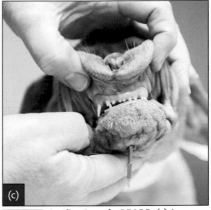

17.7 Application of a BEARD. (a) A three-dimensional reconstructed CT image of a 9-week-old puppy with a fracture of the ramus of the mandible and separation of the mandibular symphysis. (b–c) A cerclage wire was placed to stabilize the symphysis and a BEARD. Note that an oesophagostomy tube has also been placed (b = lateral view; c = rostral view). (d) The position of the suture is shown in a cat.

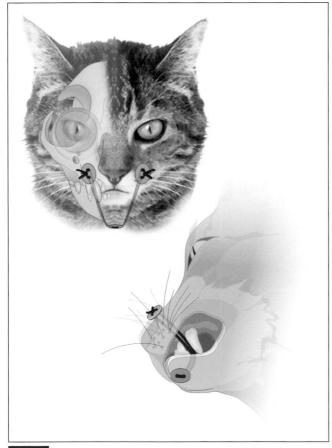

17.8 Application of a labial reverse suture through buttons.

(see Operative Technique 17.1), or as an adjunct to other techniques for the repair of more complex fractures. Advantages include the low cost of materials and relative ease of application in dogs. Unfortunately, the dental anatomy of the dog and cat does not lend itself to this technique because of the large interdental spaces and the tendency of the wire to slip off the teeth. The technique is most applicable to dogs with stable mandibular mid-body fractures that have intact and healthy dentition. It can be used as an alternative to muzzle coaptation as it is more likely to restore occlusion whilst avoiding the potential complications associated with the use of a muzzle.

An alternative method of interdental fixation is the use of acrylic or dental composite to construct an interdental splint that is bonded directly to the teeth (Operative Technique 17.1). Reinforcement of the acrylic with interdental wiring is advisable as this significantly increases the strength of the repair compared with wire or acrylic alone. The combination of interdental wiring and acrylic splinting is a versatile technique that is quick and simple to perform, and avoids the risk of iatrogenic damage to the tooth roots and neurovascular structures of the mandibular canal. An inherent disadvantage of any intraoral appliance is the development of stomatitis and gingivitis secondary to entrapment of food particles between the appliance and the gingiva for the time it is *in situ*.

Open/surgical management of maxillofacial fractures

Surgical techniques for the management of maxillofacial fractures include interfragmentary or interosseous wiring, ESF and bone plating. These techniques are indicated particularly when fractures are bilateral and/or comminuted, where there are fracture gaps, in patients that lack teeth, in large-breed dogs and in the revision of other repair techniques.

Interfragmentary wire fixation

Interfragmentary or interosseous wiring, which involves the placement of wire directly across a fracture line, is a versatile and economical technique when properly performed. However, it is an invasive procedure, requires very careful case selection and is unforgiving of technical errors and it is therefore rarely used as the sole method of repair. The exception is cerclage wiring of the mandibular symphysis. Interfragmentary wiring in general is not suitable for repair of fractures with comminution that cannot be reconstructed.

External skeletal fixation

The use of ESF with an acrylic connecting bar permits the placement of numerous pins of differing sizes and at variable angles, and the splint can be curved around the jaw rostrally to incorporate bilateral pins (Figure 17.9) (see Operative Technique 17.3). For the maxilla, pins can be placed immediately dorsal to the hard palate in a laterolateral direction. Indications include fractures where there is comminution and those where there are deficits due to loss of bone or teeth or gross soft tissue injury. The use of circular ESF for repair of bilateral fractures of the caudal aspect of the mandible has also been described (Marshall *et al.*, 2010).

Pin breakage is much less of a problem following repair of jaw fractures than with fractures of the weight-bearing bones of the appendicular skeleton, because the forces on the jaw are of lower magnitude and can be more easily controlled by appropriate postoperative care. ESF is applicable to a wide variety of fracture configurations; it can be applied in a minimally invasive fashion and implants are placed away from the fracture site. Complications include pin tract infection and injury to the tooth roots or neurovascular structures if the pins are not placed carefully. There is increased morbidity with pins placed caudally because they penetrate the large masseter muscle.

Bone plating

Bone plating provides an opportunity for rigid fixation, rapid return to pain-free normal function and primary bone healing (Operative Technique 17.4). However, application can involve considerable disruption of soft tissues, which may compromise healing. Furthermore, there is a risk of damage to the tooth roots and neurovascular structures during screw placement, which may lead to endodontic disease. Application of the plate on the tension side of the bone near the alveolar border is biomechanically advantageous but is not recommended because of the likelihood of interference with the tooth roots and the risk of complications due to gingival erosion over the implants. The plate should therefore be placed on the ventral third of the lateral surface of the mandible; if necessary, a second plate can be placed on the ventral surface (Figure 17.10).

Plating is often the preferred treatment for medium or large-breed dogs with unstable unilateral or bilateral mandibular mid or caudal body fractures. Locking plates are preferred, particularly those that enable the surgeon to angle the screws away from the tooth roots. Locking plates have been shown to be biomechanically superior to conventional plates when applied to the thin cortical bone of the mandibular ramus (Miller *et al.*, 2011). Smaller implants can be used than for equivalent long bone fractures because the bones are non-weight bearing and, if there is a danger of impinging a tooth root, screws may be inserted in monocortical fashion.

Maxillofacial mini-plates specifically designed for the treatment of humans with maxillofacial trauma have also been used for repair of mandibular and maxillary fractures in dogs and cats (Boudrieau, 2012); these are particularly useful for maxillary fractures and for mandibular fractures in smaller patients.

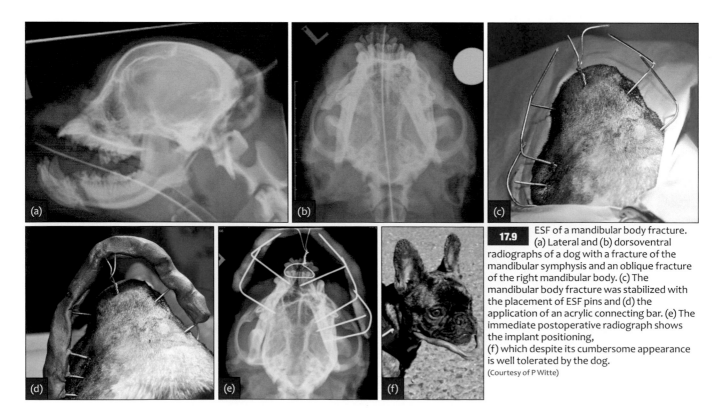

17.9 ESF of a mandibular body fracture. (a) Lateral and (b) dorsoventral radiographs of a dog with a fracture of the mandibular symphysis and an oblique fracture of the right mandibular body. (c) The mandibular body fracture was stabilized with the placement of ESF pins and (d) the application of an acrylic connecting bar. (e) The immediate postoperative radiograph shows the implant positioning, (f) which despite its cumbersome appearance is well tolerated by the dog.
(Courtesy of P Witte)

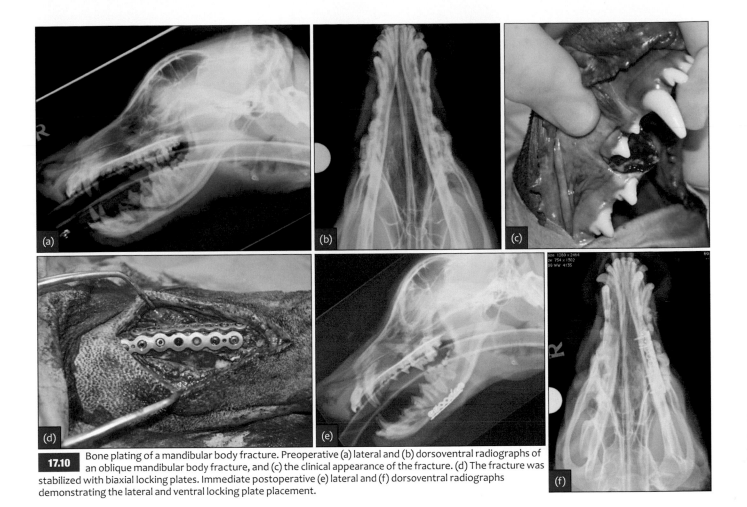

17.10 Bone plating of a mandibular body fracture. Preoperative (a) lateral and (b) dorsoventral radiographs of an oblique mandibular body fracture, and (c) the clinical appearance of the fracture. (d) The fracture was stabilized with biaxial locking plates. Immediate postoperative (e) lateral and (f) dorsoventral radiographs demonstrating the lateral and ventral locking plate placement.

Salvage procedures

Salvage procedures should generally be limited to those cases where primary repair has failed and resulted in loss of function or cases where primary repair is likely to fail because extensive trauma or infection precludes adequate reduction and stabilization.

Partial mandibulectomy/maxillectomy

Partial mandibulectomy/maxillectomy are salvage procedures that are indicated for patients with fractures which cannot be repaired using other techniques. Indications include non-union fractures, severely comminuted fractures and pathological fractures in animals with advanced periodontitis. These techniques are widely used for the management of oral neoplasia and are well tolerated in dogs and cats (see the *BSAVA Manual of Canine and Feline Head, Neck and Thoracic Surgery*). Hemimandibular instability and TMJ degeneration are inevitable sequelae of mandibulectomy (Umphlet *et al.*, 1988), though often are of limited or no clinical significance.

Mandibular condylectomy and meniscectomy

This is a salvage procedure that is indicated for patients with painful non-union fractures, temporomandibular osteoarthritis or ankylosis attributable to periarticular fibrosis. The technique is well tolerated in normal dogs (Tomlinson and Presnell, 1983).

Management of specific fractures

Fractures of the mandible

Fractures of the mandible are relatively common, accounting for between 11% and 23% of all fractures in cats and 1.5% and 2.5% in dogs. In previous studies (Umphlet and Johnson, 1988; Umphlet and Johnson, 1990) road traffic accidents were the most frequent cause, followed by fights, falls and iatrogenic, associated with dental extractions. In two recent canine studies, dog fights were the commonest cause of mandibular (Kitshoff *et al.*, 2013), and mandibular and maxillary fracture (Lopes *et al.*, 2005), and young dogs were most frequently affected.

Decision making in mandibular fracture repair

Developing an appropriate treatment plan involves selecting the technique that will be associated with the least morbidity and achieve a successful outcome in the shortest period of time. The choice of technique will be influenced by the size, age and use of the animal, the location of the fracture, concurrent injuries and financial considerations. Treatment options in cats are limited by the small size of the fracture fragments, the irregular shape of the bones and the thin cortical bone.

Traditionally, orthopaedic surgeons have tended to view the jaw as a modified long bone and have therefore favoured the use of metal implants such as ESF and plates. On the other hand, veterinary dentists, with more of a tendency to focus on the dentition and associated neurovascular structures, have favoured the use of less invasive techniques such as intraoral acrylic splints. There is merit in both approaches, but ultimately the choice of technique will be based on the preferences and expertise of the surgeon and the equipment available.

A lack of available expertise or equipment for optimum repair should prompt consideration of referral.

Fractures of the mandibular symphysis

The symphysis of the mandible is a fibrocartilaginous joint or synchondrosis uniting the right and left mandibular bodies. The joint is flexible and permits a small amount of independent movement of the two hemimandibles. The simplest method of repair is the use of a cerclage wire (Figure 17.11) (see Operative Technique 17.2). Healing of the symphyseal joint is assessed by clinical examination, rather than radiography prior to wire removal.

Fractures of the body of the mandible

The body of the mandible is the tooth-bearing portion of the bone. The premolar and molar regions are the most common sites of jaw fractures in the dog (Umphlet and Johnson, 1990; Lopes *et al.*, 2005; Kitshoff *et al.*, 2013). If the fracture is inherently stable almost all repair techniques are applicable and the simplest method that will provide adequate stability with the least potential for complications should be chosen. Muzzle fixation is often

adequate for fractures where there is innate stability, especially for immature dogs where healing is expected to be rapid, provided the canine teeth are able to occlude normally when the mouth is gently closed. The stability of the fracture will depend on the location and direction of the fracture line (see Figure 17.2). Umphlet and Johnson (1990) found that clinical union for canine mandibular fractures in the premolar region occurred in an average time of 9 weeks (range 4–16 weeks). Overall, it was found that the more caudally located the fracture, the longer the time required for healing.

The ventral surgical approach is preferred for access to most mandibular fractures (Johnson, 2014) (see Operative Technique 17.4). Bilateral fractures immediately caudal to the canine teeth or in the rostral premolar region can be managed using either ESF or interdental wire and acrylic splinting. The latter technique avoids the risk of further damage to the blood supply and tooth roots when implants are placed in the rostral fragment. Rostral mandibulectomy can also be considered where there is extensive trauma or severe periodontitis.

For comminuted fractures in small dogs and cats where the canine teeth are intact and stable, the canine teeth can be bonded together or a BEARD can be used to maintain normal occlusion during the healing process. Where there are multiple small fragments of bone and broken teeth, an alternative approach for comminuted fractures, or for animals with severe periodontitis, is partial mandibulectomy.

Interdental wiring can be considered for reasonably stable fractures without comminution or bone loss. Locking bone plates or interdental wiring combined with

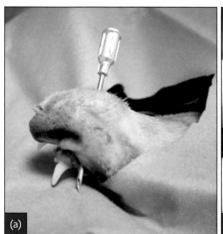
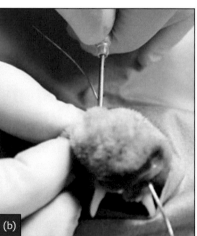
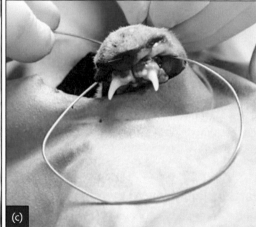

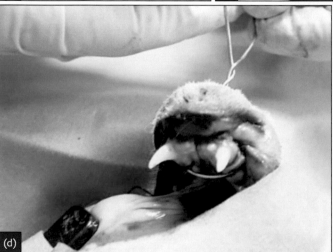

17.11 Circumferential wiring of a mandibular symphyseal fracture in a cat. (a) A small midline incision is made on the chin ventral to the canine teeth and a large bore (16 G) hypodermic needle is inserted through the incision to emerge intraorally through the mucosa just lateral and caudal to the canine tooth. (b) A 0.8 mm wire is passed through the needle to emerge orally. The procedure is then repeated on the opposite side, with the wire passed through the oral end of the needle to emerge ventrally. (c) The hypodermic needle is withdrawn and the loop of wire is pulled tight. (d) The fracture is reduced and the two ends of the wire are twisted together to stabilize the fracture. The wire is cut and the twisted ends are bent over to lie under the skin surface.

acrylic splinting can be used for unstable mandibular body fractures provided, in the case of the latter technique, there are two intact teeth on either side of the fracture line. ESF can also be considered if there is adequate bone stock in the caudal fragment for fixation pins. Interdental wiring is not applicable to cats since there are only three cheek teeth in each hemimandible.

Where fractures are bilateral or there is comminution or loss of bone stock, bone plating using a locking plate or ESF is a more appropriate method of repair. Plating is not generally a good choice for cats, for young dogs with growing teeth, or in cases where there is gross soft tissue trauma.

Fractures of the vertical ramus of the mandible

The vertical ramus is the caudal non-tooth-bearing part of the bone. It has three processes: the coronoid process, the condyloid or articular process and the angular process. The mandibular notch is located between the coronoid and the condyloid processes; the angle of the mandible is its caudoventral portion. Due to its protected location, fractures of the ramus are less common than fractures of the body of the mandible. The ramus differs from the rest of the mandible in that the bone is thinner and weaker (in its central portion <1.0 mm thick in the cat and only a few mm in large dogs) and, because of its shape, it is more difficult to hold in alignment using internal fixation. However, the bone is surrounded by broad muscular insertions over its entire surface, the coronoid process in particular being well protected by the overlying zygomatic arch and masseter muscle. Fractures in this region are usually closed, stable and minimally displaced. If significant malocclusion is present, concomitant TMJ luxation or fracture/luxation should be suspected.

Muzzle fixation or the application of a BEARD is the preferred technique for most fractures of the ramus in dogs. In cats, if fixation is required, interarcade canine acrylic bonding or application of a BEARD is generally preferable to the use of a muzzle. Maxillomandibular ESF can be used as an alternative, but is more invasive than the other techniques. The preferred option for grossly displaced or unstable fractures, especially in larger dogs, is plating (locking plates or mini-plates) (see Operative Technique 17.4). Dental malocclusion as a complication of fracture repair is less common in this region of the mandible (Umphlet and Johnson, 1990).

Fractures of the condyloid process

Condylar fractures are reported to be uncommon and are often associated with fractures of the rostral mandibular body or mandibular symphysis. However, condylar fracture is easily overlooked even when radiographic examination is performed; the more recent widespread use of CT imaging for animals with maxillofacial trauma has shown that these fractures are much more common than previously reported (Figure 17.12). As with other articular fractures, rigid internal fixation and an early return to function have been recommended. However, most fractures are minimally displaced and internal fixation is difficult because of the small size of the fragments and the inaccessibility of the joint. In most cases good results can be obtained with non-surgical management, and postoperative periarticular fibrosis is avoided. A partial mouth closure technique is applied for 2 to 4 weeks and the animal is fed a semi-liquid diet. Clinical union takes an average of 11 weeks (range

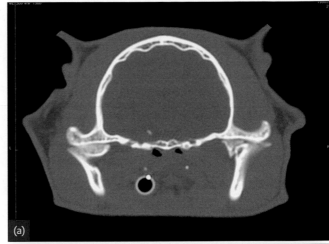

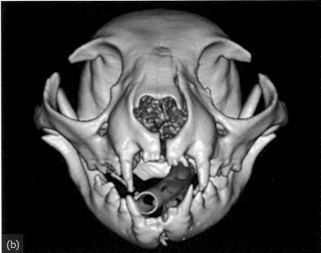

17.12 (a) Transverse CT image of a cat at the level of the TMJs showing a fracture of the medial aspect of the right condyloid process. This is a common injury in cats and is often not appreciated on radiographs. (b) Three-dimensional reconstruction of the images of the same cat showing a concurrent median fracture of the hard palate and mandibular symphysis.

10–13 weeks) (Umphlet and Johnson, 1990). In some cases a fibrous union may develop because of motion at the fracture site, but good mandibular function may still result. Displaced fractures of the condyle are usually best treated by condylectomy (see Operative Technique 17.5).

Fractures of the maxilla

Fractures of this region account for approximately 1–2% of all fractures in the dog and cat (Figure 17.13). In addition to the maxilla itself, which bears all of the cheek teeth, the term maxilla is used here to refer to the incisive (formerly premaxilla), palatine, nasal, zygomatic, lacrimal and frontal bones. There is often epistaxis due to concurrent trauma to the nasal turbinates, but haemorrhage tends to be self-limiting and is rarely of great clinical concern, provided reduction of the fractured bones is achieved.

The majority of fractures are stable and minimally displaced and can be treated conservatively or using external coaptation. As the muscular forces on the maxilla are less than those on the mandible, less rigid fixation is required and a fibrous union may produce a satisfactory functional result, provided dental occlusion has not been compromised. Fractures that communicate with the nasal cavity or the sinuses are likely to be contaminated and the patient should be treated with antibiotics, as in any other open

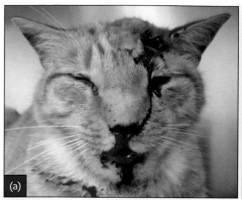
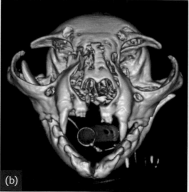
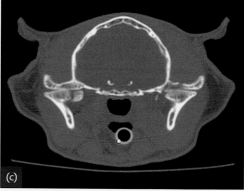

17.13 (a) Cat with multiple fractures of the mandible and maxilla including a median fracture of the hard palate and a fracture of the mandibular symphysis. (b) Three-dimensional reconstructed CT image of the same cat. (c) Transverse CT image at the level of the TMJs showing fractures of the condyloid processes and the mandibular fossa region of the temporal bone on the right.

fracture. Frontal bone fractures may develop subcutaneous emphysema if fracture fragments penetrate the frontal sinus. These rarely require surgical intervention unless they impinge on the orbit, in which case consideration should be given to removal of small fragments and stabilization of larger fragments. Non-surgical treatment may require aspiration of the emphysema, if extensive, followed by application of a compressive dressing to prevent recurrence. Fractures of the zygomatic arch are relatively common and may require surgery if they interfere with mastication or compress ocular structures. An occasional complication of the healing of fractures of the zygomatic arch or the ramus of the mandible is the production of excessive bony callus that interferes with normal jaw movement. This condition is treated by resection of a portion of the zygomatic arch and fibrous tissue adhesions as necessary. The surgical approach is made through the skin and platysma muscle directly over the bone. For complex fractures of the maxilla and mandible, the mandible is usually repaired first, starting caudally and working rostrally, with symphyseal separations repaired last. The mandible then serves as a template for the maxilla, which is repaired next starting with the side that is least severely injured. Temporary fixation of the maxilla to the mandible may facilitate repair and ensure correct dental occlusion.

Most of the standard fixation techniques are applicable for comminuted or displaced fractures of the maxilla, particularly interfragmentary wiring, and interdental wire and acrylic splinting. ESF can be used for bilateral or severely comminuted maxillary fracture repair. There must be sufficient bone stock caudal to the fracture line to allow placement of the fixation pins, which are usually inserted parallel to the hard palate, with the teeth held in the correct alignment using at least two half pins for each major fragment. Once inserted, the pins may be used to manipulate the bone fragments to achieve dental occlusion before they are embedded in acrylic. Plating, in combination with interfragmentary wiring if necessary, is the preferred approach for fractures that compromise the maxillary buttresses in medium- and large-breed dogs. The surgical approach should be made directly over the site of the fracture, although, for multiple fractures (especially along the nose), a dorsal midline approach with retraction of soft tissues laterally may be best to avoid neurovascular structures. Care should be taken to avoid the infraorbital artery and nerve exiting through the large infraorbital foramen of the maxilla, which lies dorsal to the septum between the third and fourth maxillary premolars. The osseous lacrimal canal should be avoided when drilling holes for orthopaedic wire in the small lacrimal bone in the rostral margin of the orbit.

Intraoral approaches are used for fractures of the hard palate or along the dental arcade. Median fracture of the hard palate or nasal bones is common in the cat and may be seen as one component of the specific triad of injuries (thoracic injury, facial trauma and extremity fractures) that occurs when an animal jumps or falls from a height and lands on its forelimbs and chin.

Traumatic clefts of the hard palate can often be repaired using soft tissue debridement, apposition of the bony structures by digital pressure and primary closure of soft tissue with simple interrupted sutures. If more support is required, wire is placed perpendicular to the fracture line and anchored between the teeth on either side of the buccal cavity (usually the fourth premolars or carnassial teeth in the cat, and additionally the canine teeth in the dog). It is preferable to bury the wire by passing it between the bone and the mucoperiosteum rather than leaving it exposed. Conservative treatment of this injury risks the development of an oronasal fistula, which is far more difficult to manage.

Postoperative management of jaw fractures

Postoperative care for all animals with jaw fractures includes the feeding of a soft food diet until the fracture has healed. In cases where long-term nutritional support or where difficulty in eating a liquid or soft diet are anticipated, an oesophagostomy or gastrostomy tube should be placed at the time of fracture repair. In animals with oral wounds or where an intraoral appliance has been used for fracture repair, the mouth should be rinsed daily with warm water or dilute chlorhexidine mouthwash. Intraoral appliances may cause trauma to soft tissues and will inevitably cause a degree of stomatitis and gingivitis secondary to food entrapment between the appliance and the gingiva. This problem generally resolves spontaneously within 7 days of removal of the appliance.

Problems encountered in managing jaw fractures

There are two situations where an increase in the frequency of complications of fracture repair can be predicted:

- **Fractures where there is severe comminution or bone loss.** External skeletal fixators and bone plates are the best techniques for bridging deficits. A cancellous bone graft should be used for all fractures where a problem is anticipated if an open approach is performed. Substantial defects may be managed as partial mandibulectomies requiring no further treatment;

alternatively, plate fixation and application of a bone graft or graft substitute may be performed

- **Fractures where there is advanced periodontal disease.** More than 80% of dogs older than 6 years and 95% of dogs aged 12–14 years have periodontitis, which can lead to destruction of bone and soft tissue (Lommer, 2012). If an animal has clinically significant periodontal disease, a complete dental prophylaxis should be performed, with dental extractions as appropriate, at the same time as fracture fixation. Pathological fracture may occur in animals with severe periodontitis as a result of minimal trauma through an alveolus already weakened by osteolysis. These animals are also at risk of iatrogenic fracture as a result of attempted extraction of teeth where there has been extensive bone loss but the teeth are still securely maintained in their sockets. Management of iatrogenic fractures is frequently complicated by bone loss and the presence of poor quality osteopenic bone with limited osteogenic potential, and infection secondary to the periodontitis. Typically, these patients are geriatric small-breed dogs with incomplete dentition caused by previous extractions or shedding of teeth. Internal fixation is generally a poor option because of the poor bone quality. Judicious extraction of diseased teeth is indicated where there is periapical abscess formation, though this may result in further weakening of the bone. Options for fracture management are limited to long-term mouth closure techniques or partial mandibulectomy, depending on the type of fracture. A functional result is to be expected for fractures that are unilateral and stable, even in cases where the bone fails to heal. For unstable fractures, especially when bilateral, it may be preferable to perform a primary mandibulectomy rather than risk a prolonged and potentially unsuccessful attempt at fracture repair (Manfra Maretta, 2012).

Complications

Complications of jaw fractures and jaw fracture management are essentially the same as those described for fractures of the appendicular skeleton, but with the addition of problems relating to the dentition. Complications include osteomyelitis, delayed union, non-union, malunion and malocclusion, bone sequestration, facial deformity, oronasal fistula, temporomandibular degenerative joint disease and temporomandibular ankylosis. Complications were reported in 34% of mandibular fractures in 105 dogs (Umphlet and Johnson, 1990) and 24.5% of mandibular fractures in 62 cats (Umphlet and Johnson, 1988) – figures which are higher than those for long bone fractures. The most frequent complication in dogs and cats was dental malocclusion which, besides adversely affecting function, increases the risk of delayed union and non-union by increasing the forces of leverage against the fixation device. Treatment for this complication is determined by the severity of the associated clinical signs. Options include immediate removal of the fixation device followed by correct reduction and fixation, and extraction or orthodontic movement of the maloccluded teeth. Malocclusion secondary to segmental defects may be corrected by bone grafting and plate fixation. In cats correction of malocclusion secondary to stable impaction fractures of the maxilla can be performed by realignment of the mandibular symphysis. Temporomandibular ankylosis is not an uncommon sequela in any cat with TMJ trauma and clients should be forewarned of this possibility. Pseudo-ankylosis, where fibrous bands form between the zygomatic arch and the mandible, is also occasionally encountered.

Fractures of the calvaria

Fractures of the calvaria are uncommon; this may be due in part to the fact that most animals are either killed outright or die soon after injury as a result of severe brain trauma. These fractures are frequently associated with injury to the underlying neurological structures.

Animals with severe head trauma are often compromised in terms of their neurological, respiratory and cardiovascular status, and constitute a medical emergency. In a small proportion of cases rapid surgical intervention may also be indicated. Details of medical therapy for head injury are described in standard neurology texts (see *BSAVA Manual of Canine and Feline Neurology*). Imaging of the injured area (including advanced imaging if indicated) and thoracic radiography should be performed, preferably under general anaesthesia once the patient is in a stable condition.

Many skull fractures (Figure 17.14) can be managed conservatively. Fractures of the base of the skull are rarely treated because of the severity of the injury and their inaccessibility for surgical intervention. The benefits of surgical intervention must be weighed against the complications of administering a general anaesthetic to a neurologically compromised patient. In the absence of neurological deterioration, surgery may be delayed for 24–48 hours if time is needed for patient stabilization. Surgical intervention may be indicated in the following circumstances:

- Open fractures
- Fractures where there are depressed fragments
- Retrieval of contaminated or necrotic bone fragments or foreign material
- Persistent leakage of cerebrospinal fluid
- Evacuation of haematomas and control of haemorrhage
- For decompression, where there is a deteriorating neurological status despite medical therapy.

The surgical approach to the calvaria is made with the patient positioned in ventral recumbency with the head elevated above the level of the heart. Compression of the jugular veins must be avoided as this increases intracranial pressure and the likelihood of intraoperative haemorrhage.

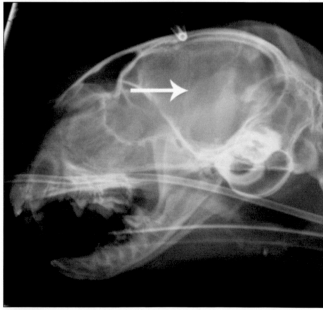

17.14 Lateral radiograph of a cat with a fracture of the calvaria (arrowed).

A midline skin incision is made extending from the external occipital protuberance to the level of the eyes (Johnson, 2014) (Figure 17.15). Alternatively, a lateral curved incision may be made, depending on the location of the fracture. The superficial temporal fascia is incised and the temporalis muscle elevated subperiosteally and retracted laterally to expose the area of the fracture. Multiple holes are drilled in the calvaria around the periphery of the fracture, enabling the insertion of small instruments to elevate the fragments. Unstable fragments can be removed even if large since the temporalis muscle provides adequate protection of the underlying brain parenchyma.

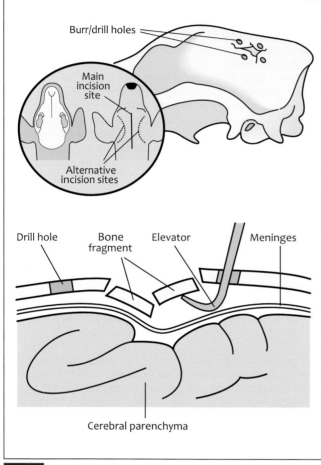

17.15 Exposure and reduction of fractures of the calvaria.

References and further reading

Bar-Am Y, Pollard RE, Kass PH and Verstraete FJ (2008) The diagnostic yield of conventional radiographs and computed tomography in dogs and cats with maxillofacial trauma. *Veterinary Surgery* **37**, 294–299

Boudrieau RJ (2012) Maxillofacial fracture repair using miniplates and screws. In: *Oral and Maxillofacial Surgery in Dogs and Cats*, ed. FJM Verstraete and MJ Lommer, pp. 293–308. Saunders Elsevier, Philadelphia

Brockman D and Holt D (2005) *BSAVA Manual of Canine and Feline Head, Neck and Thoracic Surgery*. BSAVA Publications, Gloucester

Glyde M and Lidbetter D (2003) Management of fractures of the mandible in small animals. *In Practice* **25**, 570–585

Johnson KA (2014) *Piermattei's Atlas of Surgical Approaches to the Bones and Joints of the Dog and Cat, 5th edn*. Elsevier Saunders, St. Louis

Kitshoff AM, de Rooster H, Ferreira SM and Steenkamp G (2013) A retrospective study of 109 dogs with mandibular fractures. *Veterinary and Comparative Orthopaedics and Traumatology* **26**, 1–5

Lommer MJ (2012) Principles of exodontics. In: *Oral and Maxillofacial Surgery in Dogs and Cats*, ed. FJM Verstraete and MJ Lommer, pp. 97–114. Saunders Elsevier, Philadelphia

Lopes FM, Gioso MA, Ferro DG *et al.* (2005) Oral fractures in dogs in Brazil – a retrospective study. *Journal of Veterinary Dentistry* **22**, 86–90

Lovato C and Wagner JD (2009) Infection rates following perioperative prophylactic antibiotics *versus* postoperative extended regimen prophylactic antibiotics in surgical management of mandibular fractures. *Journal of Oral and Maxillofacial Surgery* **67**, 827–832

Manfra Maretta S (2012) Maxillofacial fracture complications. In: *Oral and Maxillofacial Surgery in Dogs and Cats*, ed. FJM Verstraete and MJ Lommer, pp. 333–341. Saunders Elsevier, Philadelphia

Marshall WG, Farrell M, Chase D and Carmichael S (2010) Maxillomandibular circular external skeletal fixation for repair of bilateral fractures of the caudal aspect of the mandible in a dog. *Veterinary Surgery* **39**, 765–770

Miller EI, Acquaviva AE, Eisenmann DJ, Stone RT and Kraus KH (2011) Perpendicular pull-out force of locking *versus* non-locking plates in thin cortical bone using a canine mandibular ramus model. *Veterinary Surgery* **40**, 870–874

Nicholson I, Wyatt J, Radke H and Langley-Hobbs SJ (2010) Treatment of caudal mandibular fracture and temporomandibular joint fracture-luxation using a bi-gnathic encircling and retaining device. *Veterinary and Comparative Orthopaedics and Traumatology* **23**, 102–108

Platt S and Obly N (2013) *BSAVA Manual of Canine and Feline Neurology, 4th edn*. BSAVA Publications, Gloucester

Schwarz T, Weller R, Dickie AM, Konar M and Sullivan M (2002) Imaging of the canine and feline temporomandibular joint: a review. *Veterinary Radiology and Ultrasound* **43**, 85–97

Soukup JW, Mulherin BL and Snyder CJ (2013) Prevalence and nature of dentoalveolar injuries among patients with maxillofacial fractures. *Journal of Small Animal Practice* **54**, 9

Tomlinson J and Presnell KR (1983) Mandibular condylectomy effects in normal dogs. *Veterinary Surgery* **12**, 148–154

Umphlet RC and Johnson AL (1988a) Mandibular fractures in the cat. A retrospective study. *Veterinary Surgery* **17**, 333–337

Umphlet RC and Johnson AL (1990) Mandibular fractures in the dog. A retrospective study of 157 cases. *Veterinary Surgery* **19**, 272–275

Umphlet RC, Johnson AL, Eurell JC and Losonsky J (1988b) The effect of partial rostral hemimandibulectomy on mandibular mobility and temporomandibular joint morphology in the dog. *Veterinary Surgery* **17**, 186–193

Verstraete FJM and Lommer MJ (2012) *Oral and Maxillofacial Surgery in Dogs and Cats*. Saunders Elsevier, Philadelphia

OPERATIVE TECHNIQUE 17.1

Intraoral techniques

PREOPERATIVE CONSIDERATIONS

When using these techniques, pharyngostomy or tracheostomy intubation is recommended in order to provide unobstructed access for application and to assess occlusion. The teeth should be cleaned and their surfaces should be slightly roughened using a coarse dental pumice mix. Patients treated with a device that restricts opening of the oral cavity (e.g. intercanine acrylic or a BEARD) may require the placement of an oesophagostomy tube to facilitate tube feeding postoperatively.

POSITIONING

For mandibular fracture repair the patient should be placed in sternal recumbency; for maxillary fracture repair, the patient should be placed in dorsal recumbency.

ASSISTANT

No.

EQUIPMENT EXTRAS

Orthopaedic wire (0.5–0.6 mm); 18–20 G hypodermic needle; wire twisters; wire cutters; leader line (BEARD); dental composite.

SURGICAL TECHNIQUES

Interdental wiring

Fractures often involve at least one of the roots of the adjacent teeth; therefore, the wire should normally incorporate a minimum of two teeth on either side of the fracture line. The modified Stout multiple loop wiring technique is commonly utilized for dogs. In this technique, repetitive loops of wire are placed around a minimum of two teeth on either side of the fracture. The loops should be situated on the lingual side of the interdental spaces of the mandibular teeth and the labial side of the interdental spaces of the maxillary teeth. Once a sufficient number of teeth have been incorporated in the loops, the free end of the wire is threaded through all the loops (Figure 17.16a). The loops are then twisted tight and bent to lie flat interdentally (Figure 17.16b). The size of wire used in dogs is usually 0.5–0.6 mm. Wire slippage from the teeth can be prevented by using an 18–20 G hypodermic needle positioned subgingivally between the teeth as a wire passer. Overtightening of the wire must be avoided because this causes opening of the ventral side of the fracture line.

Interdental acrylic or composite

A combination of acrylic or composite with wire is recommended (Figure 17.16c). The wire is placed first as described above. Self-curing composite (also termed 'cold-cure') is preferable to methyl-methacrylate as it is non-exothermic, easier to apply and does not produce any toxic fumes. Depending on the type of material used, the teeth may need to be etched using phosphoric acid gel according to the manufacturer's instructions, to improve adhesion to the enamel. A thin layer of petroleum jelly can be applied to protect the soft tissues. Composite is applied directly from an applicator gun (a syringe with a mixing tip; Figure 17.16d) to conform to the shape of the crowns and interdigitate with the wire twists. Mandibular splints are created on the labial and lingual

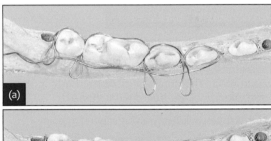
(a)

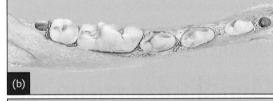
(b)

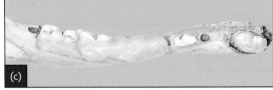
(c)

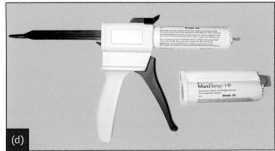
(d)

17.16 (a) Interdental wire placement on the mandible of a large-breed dog using 0.6 mm diameter orthopaedic wire in a Stout loop pattern. The loops should be placed on the lingual aspect. (b) The loops are then twisted tight and bent to lie flat interdentally. (c) 'Cold-cure' dental acrylic is applied over the interdental wiring. The acrylic is applied bilaterally on the premolars and on the lingual aspect only caudal to the first molar tooth. (d) 'Cold-cure' temporary crown and bridge material in a re-usable applicator gun. ➡

→ **OPERATIVE TECHNIQUE 17.1 CONTINUED**

surfaces of the first to third premolar teeth, but only on the lingual surface of the fourth premolar and molars, to allow for the scissor bite of the carnassial teeth. Maxillary splints are created primarily on the labial surfaces of the maxillary teeth. Care must be exercised to prevent entry of the composite into the fracture site, as this can compromise bone healing. Once the material has cured any sharp edges are removed using an acrylic burr and occlusion is checked.

Intercanine acrylic bonding

The upper and lower canine teeth are bonded together using acrylic or composite, to provide the same functional effect as a muzzle. Dental composite is easier to apply than acrylic, is non-exothermic and does not produce any toxic fumes. The mouth is left partially open (approximately 5–10 mm between the upper and lower incisors for a cat) to allow the intake of liquidized food (see Figure 17.6). Depending on the type of material used, the canine teeth may need to be etched using phosphoric acid gel, according to the manufacturer's instructions, to improve adhesion to the enamel. Dental composite can be applied directly from an applicator gun (syringe with mixing tip). A modification of this method involves the use of thin-walled cylinders (e.g. portions of a large-diameter drinking straw) as moulds to create columns of acrylic connecting ipsilateral canine teeth – the 'Corinthian method' (Glyde and Lidbetter, 2003). The teeth are inserted into the pre-filled straws and the jaw is held in alignment whilst the material hardens. The bonding often breaks within 4–6 weeks; otherwise, it is removed once the fractures have healed.

Bi-gnathic encircling and retaining device

A subcutaneous loop of nylon (leader line) (18 G for cats, 27–36 G for dogs) is placed using a large-bore hypodermic needle as a suture passer around the maxilla, incisive and nasal bones, and the mandible just caudal to the canine teeth (see Figure 17.7). The nylon emerges from the skin ventral to the mandible where it is secured with a crimp. Following placement of the suture, occlusion is checked to ensure that it is still correct.

POSTOPERATIVE MANAGEMENT

Postoperative antibiotic therapy is indicated if the fracture is open. Patients treated with any device which restricts opening of the oral cavity (e.g. intercanine acrylic or a BEARD) should be monitored carefully during recovery from anaesthesia and the early postoperative period, as breathing may be compromised if the patient's nasal cavity is obstructed. The surgeon must be ready to remove the device rapidly if required. Soft food should be fed or a feeding tube used until the fracture has healed.

OPERATIVE TECHNIQUE 17.2

Mandibular symphyseal wiring

POSITIONING

Dorsal recumbency with the neck extended.

ASSISTANT

No.

EQUIPMENT EXTRAS

Orthopaedic wire (0.8–1.2 mm for dogs, 0.6–0.8 mm for cats); a large-bore hypodermic needle (a 16 G hypodermic needle for 0.8 mm wire); wire twisters; wire cutters.

SURGICAL TECHNIQUES

Orthopaedic wire is placed using a large-bore hypodermic needle as a wire passer. The needle is inserted through a small incision in the skin of the chin (see Figure 17.11a) and passed along the lateral aspect of the mandible. The needle should exit the gingiva just caudal to the canine tooth at the junction of the attached gingival and alveolar mucosa (see Figure 17.11b). The wire is then passed through the needle, which is withdrawn and the procedure is repeated on the opposite side (this time passing the oral wire end through the needle so that both ends exit through the skin incision (see Figure 17.11c). The wire is tightened by twisting the ends together until stability is achieved (see Figure 17.11d), being careful to maintain perfect reduction of the symphysis by observing the alignment of the lower →

incisor arcade. The wire is cut leaving two or three twists and then bent over to lie under the skin surface. The skin incision is closed with a single suture. The wire can be removed after 6–12 weeks under general anaesthesia or can be left *in situ* if it does not cause any problems.

An alternative intraoral approach, which avoids having to make a skin incision at the time of wire removal, is preferred by some surgeons. The lip is retracted and the needle is inserted at the junction of gingival and alveolar mucosa to exit the skin in the ventral midline. The wire is passed through the needle and the needle is withdrawn. The needle is then inserted in an identical fashion on the opposite side of the mouth. The end of the wire is located and passed through the needle before the needle is withdrawn. The wire is twisted caudolateral to one of the canine teeth. The wire is cut leaving two or three twists and bent over to lie along the gingival mucosa so that it will not traumatize the tongue or lower lip. To remove the wire it is cut on the side opposite the twist at the gingival margin. The twist is then grasped and the wire is removed, thus avoiding contamination of tissue by the intraoral portion of the wire.

OPERATIVE TECHNIQUE 17.3

Application of external skeletal fixation to the mandible or maxilla

POSITIONING

Dorsal recumbency with the neck extended for application to mandibular fractures; sternal recumbency for application to maxillary fractures.

ASSISTANT

Optional.

EQUIPMENT EXTRAS

Threaded fixation pins (0.9–2.4 mm diameter depending on patient size); electric low-speed drill; pin cutters; acrylic or epoxy putty; plastic tubing (if required to make an acrylic connecting bar).

SURGICAL TECHNIQUES

Approach

Fixation pins are placed ventrally on the mandible through small stab incisions avoiding the tooth roots. For maxillary fractures, pins are placed transversely immediately dorsal to the hard palate from the cutaneous surface of the upper lip, without penetration of the mucosal surface.

Reduction and fixation

When using ESF to repair a mandibular or maxillary fracture it is essential to perform pharyngostomy or tracheostomy intubation to allow assessment of dental occlusion. At least two, and preferably three, pins of the correct diameter are placed in each main fragment to provide rigid fixation. Pre-drilling with a drill bit either the same diameter or slightly smaller than the diameter of the pin shaft is recommended for all but the 0.9 mm pins. If standard fixation pins are used they should be notched or bent over to lie parallel to the skin to increase the strength of the pin–acrylic interface. The acrylic can be injected in the liquid phase into flexible plastic tubing or a Penrose drain that has been placed over the pins. Alternatively, acrylic allowed to set to its dough phase, or an epoxy putty, can be moulded over the fixation pins by hand. A final check of occlusion is made, and the jaw is prevented from moving whilst the acrylic is curing. In some instances, standard ESF clamps and connector bars can be used instead of the acrylic, but this is less common.

POSTOPERATIVE MANAGEMENT

Postoperative antibiotic therapy is indicated as most fractures are open. The pin sites should be cleansed daily with sterile saline or a dilute chlorhexidine solution and an antibacterial ointment can be applied until granulation tissue has formed at the pin sites. The patient should be re-examined twice weekly for the first 2 weeks then weekly until fixator removal. Soft food should be fed until the fracture has healed.

OPERATIVE TECHNIQUE 17.4

Ventral approach and plate application to the mandibular body

POSITIONING

Dorsal recumbency with the neck extended following pharyngostomy or tracheostomy intubation. If access to the oral cavity is required to assess occlusion, repeated irrigation is performed with a dilute povidone–iodine solution.

ASSISTANT

Optional.

EQUIPMENT EXTRAS

Gelpi retractors; bone-holding forceps; periosteal elevator; bone plates, cortical screws and corresponding equipment for application (titanium variable angle locking plate systems are preferred by the author).

SURGICAL TECHNIQUES

Approach

Exposure of the mandible is achieved by incising the thin sheet-like platysma muscle, which is then retracted laterally with the fascia and skin (Figure 17.17). If necessary, exposure of the medial aspect of the bone can be increased by separating the mylohyoideus muscle from the medial edge of the mandible and retracting it medially. For access to caudal body fractures, an incision is made in the intermuscular septum between the masseter and the digastricus muscles. Elevation and reflection of the periosteal attachment of the digastricus muscle is performed to expose the shaft of the mandible. It is important to identify and protect the large facial vein and accompanying nerve trunks.

Reduction and fixation

For simple fractures, anatomical reduction of the fracture using bone-holding forceps followed by routine plate application will restore dental occlusion. Comminuted fractures or fractures with gaps must be reconstructed using occlusion to determine the accuracy of the reduction. The plate is applied to the ventral third of the lateral surface of the mandible ensuring that the screws avoid the tooth roots. With standard non-locking plates, precise contouring of the plate is required if malocclusion is to be avoided when the screws are tightened.

POSTOPERATIVE MANAGEMENT

Postoperative antibiotic therapy is recommended as most fractures are open. Radiographs are generally obtained every 4 to 6 weeks to assess fracture healing. Soft food should be fed until the fracture has healed. Plates are normally left *in situ*.

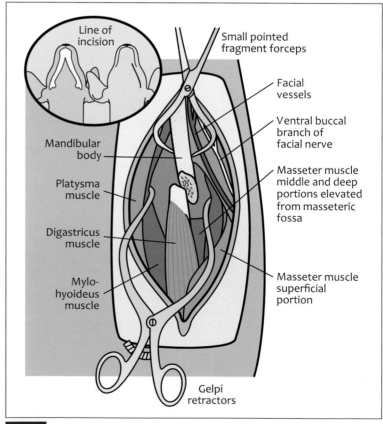

17.17 Ventral exposure of a mandibular body fracture (see text for details).

OPERATIVE TECHNIQUE 17.5

Surgical approach to the temporomandibular joint and condylectomy

POSITIONING

Lateral recumbency with the head supported.

ASSISTANT

Optional.

EQUIPMENT EXTRAS

Gelpi retractors; high speed burr; rongeurs.

SURGICAL TECHNIQUES

Approach

The skin incision is made along the ventral border of the zygomatic arch and crosses the TMJ caudally (Figure 17.18). The platysma muscle and fascia are incised and retracted with the skin. The attachment of the origin of the masseter muscle on the zygomatic arch is incised and subperiosteal elevation is performed. The parotid duct and branches of the facial nerve are avoided. Reflection of the tissue ventrally exposes the lateral surface of the TMJ. The condyle and interior of the joint are exposed by wide excision of the joint capsule.

Reduction and fixation

Displaced fractures involving the condyloid process are not usually reconstructable and condylectomy is performed. All bone fragments of the condyloid process are excised and condylectomy is performed at the base of the neck of the condyloid process at the level of the mandibular notch (Figure 17.19) using a bone burr or rongeurs. The meniscus is left *in situ* if it is undamaged; this may be important in the formation of a functional pseudoarthrosis.

POSTOPERATIVE MANAGEMENT

Soft food should be fed for 4 to 6 weeks. If it is necessary to immobilize the TMJ after stabilization of any other fractures, it should not be for longer than 2 weeks to avoid periarticular fibrosis and reduced range of mouth opening.

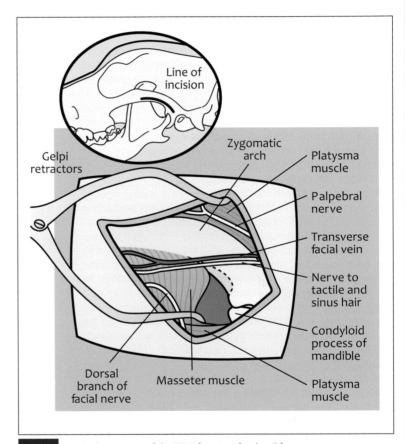

17.18 Surgical exposure of the TMJ (see text for details).

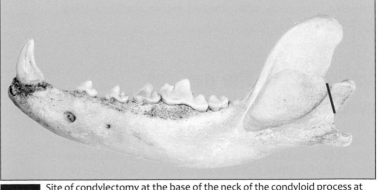

17.19 Site of condylectomy at the base of the neck of the condyloid process at the level of the mandibular notch (red line).

Chapter 18

The spine

Malcolm McKee

Traumatic injuries involving the vertebral column and spinal cord are relatively common in small animal practice. The principal injuries are vertebral fractures, vertebral luxations and disc extrusions. They most commonly result from road traffic accidents. Other forms of trauma include collision with stationary objects, falls from heights and bite injuries. Less frequent non-traumatic causes of pathological vertebral fracture include neoplasia, infection and osteoporosis. Of key importance is the potential for concomitant injury to the spinal cord or cauda equina as varying degrees of neurological dysfunction may result from compression, contusion or laceration of neural tissue.

Dogs and cats with acute spinal cord injury should be considered as emergencies. In addition, care should be taken to avoid additional injury in cases with vertebral instability. Patients should be thoroughly evaluated in view of the potential for concomitant life-threatening injuries to other body systems. Open reduction and internal fixation of vertebral fractures and luxations is often indicated in order to decompress the spinal cord, reduce pain and aid nursing care and rehabilitation; however, surgery can be challenging and thus referral to a specialist should be considered. Selected fractures and luxations with inherent vertebral stability and minimal neurological deficits may be managed non-surgically with cage confinement or external splinting. Traumatic disc extrusions in the absence of vertebral instability involve rupture of the previously healthy annulus fibrosus and rapid extrusion of nucleus pulposus into the vertebral canal. Due to their high water content, these 'explosive' discs tend to be minimally or non-compressive and thus surgery is rarely indicated. The prognosis in patients with traumatic vertebral fractures and luxations that retain pain perception is generally favourable, especially when treated within a short period of time following injury.

Evaluation of the patient

Physical examination

Dogs and cats with traumatic vertebral injuries should be handled with care as they are often distressed and in significant pain. The use of a muzzle is advisable. Avoidance of further spinal cord injury is of paramount importance. A temporary splint may be applied or, especially when being transported, the animal may be strapped to a rigid board or stretcher.

A thorough clinical examination is essential since trauma that is sufficient to cause a vertebral fracture or luxation may result in significant concomitant injuries. Particular reference should be made to the cardiopulmonary system and the patient should be monitored for evidence of pneumothorax, cardiac dysrhythmia and shock. Animals with neck trauma should be carefully checked for evidence of hypoventilation because cervical spinal cord injury may affect intercostal and diaphragmatic muscle innervation. Concurrent pelvic trauma may be difficult to detect in non-ambulatory patients. Rectal examination and careful assessment of pelvic symmetry may be helpful. Failure to detect pelvic fractures and sacroiliac separations may result in an overestimation of the severity of spinal cord injury.

Neurological examination

A detailed neurological examination (see the *BSAVA Manual of Canine and Feline Neurology*) should enable the level of vertebral column injury to be identified and the severity of spinal cord damage to be graded (Figure 18.1). Malalignment of the spine may be palpable, or indeed visible or audible, and there may be external evidence of trauma such as bruising. Certain postural reaction tests (e.g. hemiwalking and wheelbarrowing) should be avoided due to the possibility of vertebral instability and further spinal cord trauma. The severity of cord injury is primarily determined based on the presence or absence of motor function (purposeful limb movement) and conscious

Grade	Neurological dysfunction
1	Spinal pain (no neurological deficits)
2a	Mild, ambulatory paraparesis/tetraparesis
2b	Moderate, ambulatory paraparesis/tetraparesis
2c	Severe, ambulatory paraparesis/tetraparesis
3	Non-ambulatory paraparesis/tetraparesis
4	Paraplegia/tetraplegia
5a	Paraplegia/tetraplegia; urinary incontinence; loss of superficial (digital pressure) pain perception
5b	Paraplegia/tetraplegia; urinary incontinence; loss of deep pain perception
5c	Grade 5b and evidence of ascending-descending myelomalacia

18.1 Grading system for spinal cord injury. The combination of tetraplegia and loss of deep pain perception is rare; cervical spinal cord injuries of this severity tend to be fatal.

pain perception caudal to the lesion. Wherever possible, narcotic analgesics should only be given after the neurological examination as they can alter these findings. Evidence of conscious pain perception may be as obvious as vocalization or attempting to bite; however, it may be as subtle as an alteration in breathing pattern or heart rate. The presence or absence of deep pain perception (as assessed with painful stimulation, such as the application of pliers to periosteum, e.g. metatarsals, tibia, tail) is an extremely important prognostic factor.

Three key points should be considered when attempting to neurolocalize the lesion in patients with traumatic spinal cord injuries.

- There may be injury at more than one area of the vertebral column. It is particularly important to be aware that lower motor neuron (LMN) lesion deficits may mask the effect of concomitant upper motor neuron lesion (UMN) deficits. The possibility of concurrent peripheral nerve damage, for example brachial plexus avulsion, should also be considered.
- Traumatic spinal injuries may cause 'spinal shock' – a phenomenon where segmental spinal reflexes are temporarily reduced or absent caudal to the area of spinal cord injury (Smith and Jeffery, 2005). Recognition of this condition is important since it may explain discrepancies between neurolocalization on examination and imaging findings.
- Dogs with severe cord injury and loss of deep pain perception may develop progressive myelomalacia that ascends and descends the spinal cord (Olby et al., 2003). This distressing condition may be recognized on neurological examination due to evidence of multi-segment injury, for example, hyporeflexic patellar and pelvic limb withdrawal reflexes and absence of the cutaneous trunci reflex caudal to the thoracolumbar junction. Once recognized these animals should be euthanased to avoid death by respiratory paralysis.

WARNINGS

- Interpretation of the neurological examination can be challenging in the presence of cardiovascular shock and/or other injuries; if there is doubt, it is best to repeat the examination after the patient has been stabilized
- It is essential to remember that the withdrawal of a limb is not evidence of pain perception; it may be a reflex. The patient must show a behavioural response, such as vocalization, attempting to bite, or turning the head
- Serial neurological examinations are important to detect changes in neurological status
- Instability of the vertebral column can have devastating consequences. Sudden displacement may result in spinal cord laceration or compression. Even minor instability may produce deterioration in neurological status due to repeated contusion of the spinal cord. Therefore, great care must be exercised when handling the patient

---

Differential diagnosis

Diagnosis is generally straightforward from the history and neurological findings; however, on occasions the owner may be unaware of trauma. In these cases other causes of acute onset neurological dysfunction must be considered,

and femoral pulses assessed to rule out the possibility of thromboembolism.

Common causes of acute onset neurological dysfunction include:

- Degenerative or traumatic intervertebral disc extrusion
- Ischaemic myelopathy (e.g. fibrocartilaginous embolism)
- Developmental atlantoaxial subluxation.

Uncommon causes of acute onset neurological dysfunction include:

- Pathological vertebral fracture:
  - Neoplasia (e.g. osteosarcoma)
  - Oseopenia (e.g. nutritional secondary hyperparathyroidism, Cushing's disease)
  - Infection (e.g. osteomyelitis, discospondylitis)
- Spontaneous spinal haemorrhage (e.g. coagulopathy, *Angiostrongylus*)
- Non-osseous neoplasia (possible with associated haemorrhage)
- Acute inflammatory central nervous system disorders.

Imaging the vertebral trauma patient

Conventional radiography is the most common technique used to investigate vertebral trauma patients and is generally sufficient to diagnose the majority of fractures and luxations. It is, however, insensitive at detecting the presence of fracture fragments within the vertebral canal, or spinal cord compression or swelling. Myelography may play a role but is seldom indicated and can carry significant risk to the patient. Computed tomography (CT) and magnetic resonance imaging (MRI) provide superior bone and soft tissue detail respectively and are becoming increasingly widely available. Each have advantages and disadvantages, and both greatly aid surgical planning. If, however, a vertebral fracture or luxation is detected in the region of neurolocalization and neurological deficits and pain are mild, advanced imaging may not be necessary as the prognosis with appropriate management is generally good.

It is important to remember that images do not necessarily represent the position of the vertebrae at the time of trauma. This is one explanation for the poor correlation that often exists between the degree of vertebral displacement and the severity of the neurological dysfunction. Conversely, many dogs with significant displacement of vertebral fractures and luxations, especially in the cervical and caudal lumbar spine, retain pain perception and variable motor function. This is primarily due to the large ratio of vertebral canal to spinal cord or cauda equina diameter.

WARNING

Since images do not necessarily represent the position of vertebrae at the time of trauma, the prognosis must be assessed on the basis of the neurological examination rather than the imaging findings

---

Survey radiography

Radiography (or CT) of the chest is mandatory in all spinal trauma cases to detect potentially life-threatening problems, such as pulmonary contusion and pneumothorax.

Rupture of the diaphragm and rib fractures are less common. Radiography (or CT) of the pelvis should be performed if there is any doubt regarding possible injury.

General anaesthesia is generally mandatory when imaging the spine in order to obtain diagnostic images. Caution should be exercised when intubating animals with cervical fractures or luxations. Likewise, great care is necessary when moving and positioning all spinal trauma patients because of the possibility of vertebral instability that may be exacerbated in anaesthetized patients due to abolishment of the protective role of the paraspinal and abdominal musculature.

Lateral radiographs should primarily focus on the region of neurolocalization; however, the entire vertebral column should be imaged in animals where there is a clinical suspicion of more than one lesion (Figure 18.2). Since LMN lesion deficits can mask UMN lesion deficits, the C1–C5 region should be imaged when there are C6–T2 deficits and the T3–L3 region when there are L4–S3 deficits. Ventrodorsal radiographs may be obtained using a horizontal X-ray beam technique. If this is not possible the value of such views should be questioned and extreme caution should be employed if the patient is moved to dorsal recumbency in view of the possibility of exacerbating vertebral instability and spinal cord injury.

Stressed view radiographs are seldom necessary; however, on occasion they can provide valuable information regarding vertebral stability. For example, vertebral subluxations with minimal displacement and traumatic disc extrusions may be difficult to differentiate on survey radiographs, especially in the thoracic spine where there is superimposition of rib heads. Stressed views may aid differentiation and this information can be critical for management (Figure 18.3). The risk of further spinal cord injury is significant and thus flexion or extension of the spine should be incremental and performed with great care; fluoroscopy should be used where possible.

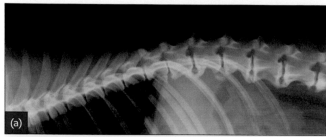

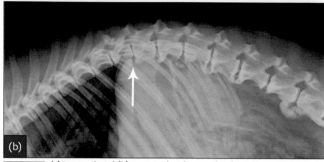

18.3 (a) Neutral and (b) stressed radiographs demonstrating vertebral instability at T11–T12 with ventral displacement of the caudal vertebrae evident on the mildly flexed projection (arrowed). Narrowing of the T11–T12 intervertebral disc was noted on the neutral radiograph; however, the subluxation was not apparent.

Myelography

Myelography may reveal spinal cord swelling or compression due to bone fragments, haemorrhage or disc material, and this information may influence surgical planning, for example the need for a decompressive procedure. Marked spinal cord swelling may, however, attenuate the subarachnoid space so that contrast agent fails to define areas of compression. The technique has largely fallen out of favour because of the need to manipulate the spine during injection of contrast agent, and the potential for side effects including increased pressure within the vertebral canal and seizures. Advanced imaging techniques that are less invasive such as CT or MRI are preferable to myelography. Myelography may, however, be considered in the following situations when more advanced imaging is not available:

- Survey films are normal or inconclusive (e.g. cases with spinal haemorrhage, spinal cord concussion or subtle invertebral disc extrusion
- Survey radiographic findings are inconsistent with neurological findings (e.g. thoracolumbar luxation in a patient with absent patellar reflexes).

Myelography enables space-occupying lesions to be localized:

- Extradural (e.g. fracture, luxation, disc material, bone fragments, haemorrhage)
- Intradural–extramedullary (e.g. haematoma)
- Intramedullary (e.g. haematoma, spinal cord oedema).

The vast majority of spinal trauma lesions are extradural.

18.2 Radiograph of a cat that sustained multiple vertebral and pelvic injuries including luxation of L4–L5 and L7–S1. Note the concomitant bilateral ilial wing fractures and left ischial fracture. A left sacral fracture is also present.

Computed tomography

CT provides excellent detail of fracture fragments and can identify fractures that are not visible on plain radiographs (Kinns *et al.*, 2006; Draffan *et al.*, 2009) (Figure 18.4). It is particularly useful when planning surgery since two-dimensional cross-sectional or three-dimensional volume rendered images enable accurate assessment of implantation angles, implant size and orientation of affected vertebrae (Figure 18.5). It is also valuable postoperatively for assessing implant positioning and the possibility of violation of the vertebral canal or other important structures. Key limitations of CT include relatively poor assessment of spinal cord parenchyma and limited detection of compressive disc material or haematoma within the canal.

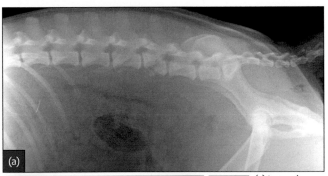

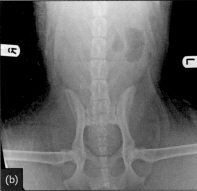

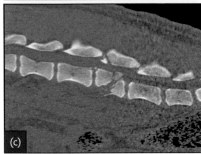

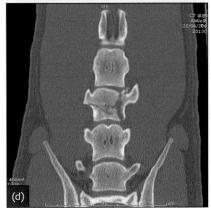

18.4 (a) Lateral and (b) ventrodorsal radiographs and (c) lateral and (d) ventrodorsal reconstructed CT images of a dog with an L5 fracture. These images demonstrate the superiority of CT multiplanar reformatted images compared to conventional radiography. Identification of the comminuted nature of the L5 vertebral fracture with CT aided surgical planning.

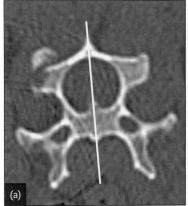

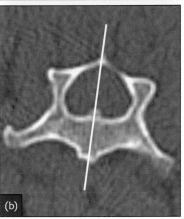

18.5 Transverse CT images showing (a) C6 and (b) C7 in a dog with a C6–C7 vertebral luxation. Note the rotational malalignment of the two vertebrae with each rotated in opposite directions. The white line indicates the sagittal plane of the vertebra; in a normal dog these should be parallel to each other. Failure to recognize this feature could result in malpositioning of implants and life-threatening spinal cord injury.

Magnetic resonance imaging

MRI is excellent at imaging the spinal cord parenchyma and also the paraspinal muscles, intervertebral discs and ligamentous structures, all of which contribute to vertebral stability (Johnson *et al.*, 2012). It is useful for detecting sequelae of spinal cord trauma including myelomalacia and syrinx formation, and is the imaging technique of choice when investigating traumatic disc extrusions. However, MR images of bone are relatively poor and thus it can be difficult to identify fracture lines in vertebrae, which is important when planning implant placement. Additionally, MRI acquisition times are longer than for other imaging modalities.

Management of the spinal trauma patient

The appropriate management of traumatic spinal injuries necessitates an understanding of:

* Pathophysiology of acute spinal cord injury
* Spinal biomechanics
* Types of spinal injury.

Pathophysiology of acute spinal cord injury

Acute spinal cord injury following vertebral trauma may be considered as primary or secondary. Primary injury is due to varying degrees of cord contusion, laceration and compression (by bone, disc material, other soft tissue or blood), each of which may be exacerbated by ongoing vertebral instability. Spinal cord contusion results in axonal disruption, vascular damage, grey matter haemorrhage and cord oedema. Spinal cord compression causes nerve conduction blockage, interruption of neuronal axoplasmic flow, demyelination, axonal degeneration, reduced vascular perfusion, and neuronal and supporting tissue necrosis.

Vertebral trauma can also initiate secondary injury to the spinal cord via metabolic processes that are self-perpetuating (Olby, 2010). Severely injured spinal cord tissues release chemicals, including oxygen free radicals, cytokines, inflammatory mediators and catecholamines that are associated with ionic disturbances and complex metabolic processes such as lipid peroxidation. The result is reduced spinal cord blood flow (hypotension), ischaemia (hypoxia), haemorrhage, inflammation, oedema and further destruction of neuronal tissue. In severe cases these vicious metabolic cycles may transverse, ascend and descend the spinal cord until they result in death by respiratory paralysis, a process known as progressive myelomalacia.

In milder spinal trauma cases injured neuronal tissue is gradually replaced with a glial scar, and a syrinx (cavity) may develop within the spinal cord as a late feature in some patients.

Spinal biomechanics

Traumatic vertebral column injuries may be caused by bending, rotational, axial (compressive) or shear forces; naturally occurring injuries tend to result from a combination of these forces. The same forces need to be resisted when managing vertebral fractures and luxations. The ideal stabilization technique (surgical or external splinting) should be based on the disruptive forces and identification of the structures that have been damaged. Structures that provide strength in the normal vertebral column may be divided into dorsal and ventral compartments (Figure 18.6).

Dorsal compartment structures:

* Articular facets/joint capsules
* Vertebral lamina/pedicles
* Supraspinous ligament
* Interspinous ligament.

Ventral compartment structures:

* Vertebral body
* Intervertebral disc
* Dorsal longitudinal ligament
* Ventral longitudinal ligament
* Intertransverse ligament.

The three most important contributors to vertebral stability are the vertebral bodies, the intervertebral discs and the articular facets. Vertebral bodies and (to a lesser extent) articular facets resist bending and axial forces, whereas ligamentous structures and facet joint capsules provide tensile strength (Smith and Walter, 1988; Patterson and Smith, 1992). Lateral bending and rotational stability are derived from the intervertebral discs and articular facets (Shires et al., 1991; Schulz et al., 1996). It should be considered that vertebral column injuries with failure of more than one of these three key components is associated with vertebral instability, regardless of the degree of displacement seen on imaging; clinically, this is the most common scenario.

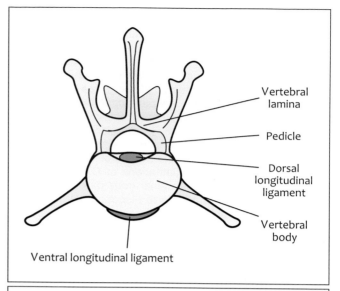

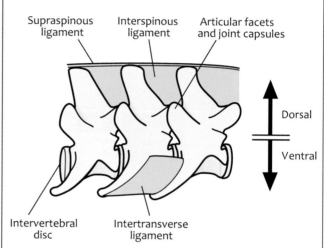

18.6 Dorsal and ventral compartment structures of the vertebral column.

Types of vertebral injury

Traumatic vertebral injuries occur most commonly between stable and more mobile parts of the vertebral column, such as the thoracolumbar junction, although any vertebra(e) may be affected. Injuries may be divided into three groups on the basis of which structures are affected:

* Dorsal compartment injury (e.g. articular facet fracture)
* Ventral compartment injury (e.g. intervertebral disc extrusion)
* Combined compartment injury (e.g. vertebral body fracture and articular facet luxation).

Combined compartment injuries are the most common. Dorsal compartment injury in combination with vertebral body fracture is the most serious, allowing bending, rotational and shear displacement, as well as axial vertebral collapse (Figure 18.7). In contrast, injury to the dorsal compartment structures in combination with vertebral subluxation is less serious since a ventral buttress remains (Figure 18.8). Disc extrusions are inherently stable, because of an intact ventral buttress and articular facets. Isolated dorsal compartment injuries are uncommon and are often of limited clinical significance.

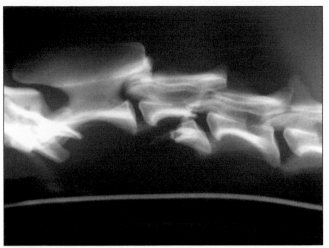

18.7 A C3 fracture with concomitant luxation of the C3–C4 facets in a Lurcher. This is a combined dorsal and ventral compartment injury that has resulted in gross vertebral instability.

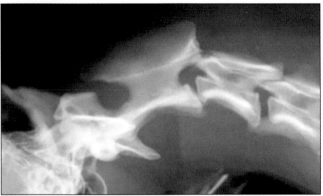

18.8 A C2–C3 luxation in a Weimaraner. The intact vertebral bodies are providing a ventral buttress and contributing to vertebral stability (compare with Figure 18.7).

General principles of management

It is essential that vertebral fractures and luxations with concomitant neurological dysfunction are treated promptly. The key objectives are to manage:

- Spinal pain
- Secondary spinal cord injury
- Spinal cord compression
- Vertebral instability.

The need for surgery should be considered according to individual status. Decompression of the spinal cord and/or stabilization of the vertebral column are frequently indicated. These techniques are often technically demanding and thus referral of the patient to a surgical specialist should be considered. A temporary splint should be applied, or alternatively the patient may be strapped to a rigid board, in order to reduce the possibility of further spinal cord injury during transport.

Management of spinal pain

Vertebral fractures and luxations often cause severe pain. Therefore it is important that patients are regularly monitored and where appropriate assigned a pain score. Analgesics should be administered as soon as possible to avoid sensitization or 'wind-up', and they should be given preoperatively to reduce the requirement postoperatively. A multimodal approach to pain management is most effective. The two key groups of drugs are narcotic analgesics (e.g. fentanyl and methadone) and non-steroidal anti-inflammatory drugs (NSAIDs). Opioids cause respiratory depression and thus should be used with caution in patients with intracranial, cervical and chest injuries. NSAIDs should also be used with care as spinal surgery patients in general have a tendency for gastrointestinal ulceration. They are contraindicated in animals that have recently been administered corticosteroids. Drugs active against neuropathic pain, such as gabapentin, are often helpful and methocarbamol, a centrally acting skeletal muscle relaxant, and diazepam may reduce the pain associated with muscle spasm.

> **WARNING**
>
> Failure to surgically reduce and stabilize vertebral fractures and luxations may prevent effective medical pain management

Management of secondary spinal cord injury

There has been a vast amount of research on the pathogenesis and management of secondary spinal cord injury. Unfortunately, as with the primary injuries associated with contusion and laceration, there are many secondary events that remain untreatable. The key current medical methods of managing acute spinal cord injury in vertebral trauma patients are to reduce or prevent hypotension, hypoxia and lipid peroxidation (and other metabolic processes) (Olby, 2010).

The judicious use of intravenous fluids is indicated to aid maintenance of spinal cord blood flow, especially when the patient is anaesthetized, as the injured spinal cord is unable to regulate its own perfusion. Monitoring of mean systemic arterial pressure is advisable in order to avoid hypertension, which may increase cord haemorrhage and oedema. Maintaining arterial oxygenation is also of prime importance.

The use of corticosteroids remains controversial, despite their antioxidant properties that can theoretically mitigate against the effect of oxygen free radicals by inhibiting lipid peroxidation in cell membranes. In controlled multicentre clinical trials in humans, methylprednisolone sodium succinate has been demonstrated to have dubious efficacy and there is currently no evidence that it is beneficial in naturally occurring spinal cord injury in animals. Furthermore, administration has been associated with a high incidence of diarrhoea and melaena. Other corticosteroids, such as dexamethasone, should never be administered, as no beneficial effects have been demonstrated and they may result in potentially serious and even lethal gastrointestinal complications, especially when used in combination with NSAIDs.

> **WARNING**
>
> The evidence to support the use of corticosteroids for acute spinal cord injury is extremely limited, and the use of corticosteroids can be associated with severe side effects

Management of spinal cord compression and vertebral instability

The presence and extent of spinal cord compression and vertebral instability are key factors in determining whether surgical or conservative management is most appropriate when managing vertebral fractures and luxations. Decompression is primarily achieved by realigning fractured or luxated vertebrae; removal of material from the vertebral canal via laminectomy or hemilaminectomy is rarely necessary. Internal (or external) fixation is the most effective method of stabilizing unstable vertebrae compared to external splinting or cage rest.

The following factors aid decision making when managing spinal trauma patients.

Neurological factors:

- Nature of spinal lesion
- Grade of spinal cord injury
- Degree of spinal cord compression
- Evidence of vertebral instability
- Severity of spinal pain
- Anatomical location of injury
- Interval between injury and presentation.

Other factors:

- Size of the patient
- Concurrent orthopaedic injuries
- Concurrent non-orthopaedic injuries
- Disposition and function of the patient
- Available equipment and expertise
- Financial restrictions and owner compliance.

Surgery is generally indicated in non-ambulatory patients and those that are deteriorating, have unstable spines, or have significant pain. Reduction and fixation of vertebral fractures and luxations allows early pain-free ambulation and unimpeded physiotherapy, including hydrotherapy, compared with conservative management. This is particularly important in large dogs, where the required level of nursing care should not be underestimated. In addition, surgery generally reduces the hospitalization and recovery times and thus the incidence of decubital ulcers and other complications of prolonged recumbency. Conservative management may be considered with select cervical and caudal lumbar fractures and luxations in particular, since the vertebral canal to spinal cord ratio is relatively large compared to the thoracolumbar spine, and thus the risk of a devastating deterioration in neurological function is lower. It is essential, however, that these patients are carefully monitored for evidence of deterioration.

Non-surgical management

External splinting and/or cage rest are advocated in the majority of non-surgical patients with vertebral fractures and luxations.

External splinting

External splints are most applicable to thoracolumbar fractures and luxations in animals with an intact ventral buttress or intact facets. They are not recommended for combined compartment injuries since their ability to counteract major disruptive forces is limited. Back splints

may be used as the sole means of providing stability or as an adjunct to internal fixation techniques. The following advantages and disadvantages are worthy of consideration.

Advantages of back splints:

- Inexpensive
- Unlikely to cause harm during application
- Can move patient safely when applied
- Less expertise/equipment required.

Disadvantages of back splints:

- Require intact ventral or dorsal buttress
- Significant risk of decubital ulcers
- Hindrance of manual bladder expression
- Inability to manage concurrent traumatic chest and abdominal wounds
- Necessity to monitor/adjust splint on a weekly basis
- Often not well tolerated, particularly by cats.

> **WARNING**
>
> Significant complications may result from pressure sores and urine scalding if a high level of nursing care is not practised with back splints

Back splints may be constructed from aluminium sheeting or thermoplastic materials. Mason metasplints are an alternative in small dogs and cats (Figure 18.9). They are secured to the patient with Velcro® straps or sticking plasters. The former may allow the splint to be changed, or adjusted, more readily. The reader is referred to Patterson and Smith (1992) for further details.

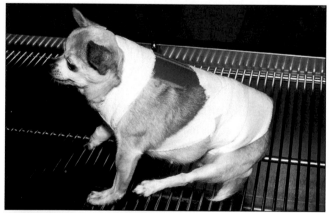

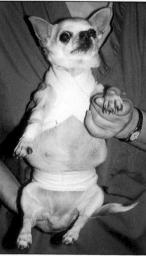

18.9 A Mason metasplint provided temporary vertebral stabilization in this Chihuahua with a mid-thoracic fracture–luxation.

Cage confinement

Some animals with cervical, caudal lumbar and lumbosacral fractures and luxations may respond favourably to strict cage confinement (Figure 18.10). Closed reduction of these injuries is extremely difficult and provision of adequate stability with external splints is practically impossible. The two key disadvantages of cage confinement are the possibility of prolonged pain and the risk of vertebral instability increasing spinal cord compression and neurological dysfunction.

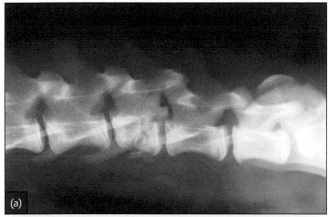

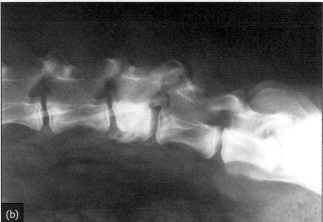

18.10 (a) Lumbar fracture–luxation in an immature Labrador Retriever with mild paraparesis which was managed by cage confinement. (b) By 10 weeks post-trauma the fracture had healed and the neurological deficits had resolved.

Surgical management

Surgery is the most reliable method to accurately reduce (realign) fractures and luxations, decompress the spinal cord, and stabilize affected vertebrae. It is important to recognize that incomplete reduction is preferable to accurate realignment if the latter results in additional neural tissue injury. A thorough knowledge of vertebral anatomy is essential in view of the potential for inadvertent placement of implants and iatrogenic injury of important structures including the spinal cord. Preoperative cross-sectional CT or MR images can be useful for determining insertion angles and the size of implants. Having access to a cadaver spine can also be helpful. Ideally the surgical technique employed should be sufficiently rigid to encourage fracture or luxation healing and strong enough to withstand the intrinsic and extrinsic forces exerted on the vertebral column during this period.

Biomechanics of spinal fixation techniques

The potential postoperative bending (especially flexion), rotational, axial and shear forces that may disrupt vertebral fracture or luxation fixation techniques must be carefully considered. The possibility of inadvertent injury when nursing paretic and ataxic patients is significant. It has been estimated that the bending moment at the thoracolumbar junction in a 45 kg dog, supported by the chest with the pelvic limbs hanging free, is greater than three times the strength provided by vertebral body plating (Walter *et al.*, 1986).

The following biomechanical properties of fixation techniques should be considered when planning surgery and postoperative management:

- When subjected to bending, vertebral body plating is the most strong and most rigid single technique; however, for unilaterally applied plates the strength at failure is only one-third the strength of the normal intact spine (Walter *et al.*, 1986)
- When subjected to rotational deformation, vertebral body pins and bone cement provided the greatest stability and strength compared with other techniques (Waldron *et al.*, 1991).

Choice of fixation technique

Many vertebral fixation techniques have been described, including vertebral body screws/pins and bone cement, vertebral body plates, external skeletal fixation, modified segmental fixation, tension-band fixation, spinous process plating/wiring and facet screwing/wiring. The choice of technique depends on characteristics of the vertebral injury and biomechanical factors.

Fracture/luxation characteristics:

- Location of the injury
- Potential for accurate reduction
- Necessity of laminectomy/hemilaminectomy.

Biomechanical factors:

- Inherent fracture/luxation stability
- Ability of technique to counteract disruptive forces
- Size and activity of the patient
- Concurrent orthopaedic injuries.

Techniques that utilize the vertebral bodies (ventral compartment) are generally preferred since the dorsal compartment structures are inherently weak and implant failure is not unusual; vertebral body screws/pins and cement and vertebral body plates are the two most common procedures.

Screws (or pins) and bone cement is the most versatile technique because the placement of implants in vertebral bodies is not dictated by holes in a plate. It is thus possible to place implants in a bicortical manner with avoidance of fracture lines and important anatomical structures; bicortical fixation confers significantly more strength than unicortical fixation. As a result, the technique is appropriate for the majority of vertebral fractures and luxations. Locking screws with cement are preferable to cortical screws with an equivalent thread diameter as their strength is greatly increased by the larger core diameter. If pins are used rather than screws, pre-drilling minimizes thermal necrosis of bone and microfractures, which reduce pin stability. In addition, the depth of the vertebral body can be measured accurately prior to pin insertion. To prevent the drill bit 'walking' on the surface of the vertebral bone a small hole can be made using a burr or Kirschner (K) wire. Threaded pins are preferable to smooth pins. Following insertion, screws and pins can be bent to improve the implant–cement interface. Polymethylmethacrylate bone cement with a short liquid phase and long dough phase is advantageous to other preparations when moulding around spinal implants.

A variety of bone plates may be applied to the vertebral column. Locking plates with fixed angle screws may be advantageous compared to conventional plates in the thoracolumbar spine because they 'stand off' the vertebrae and interfere less with regional spinal nerves. However, in the cervical spine fixed angle screws have a tendency to loosen by slicing through the bone since they are generally placed in a unicortical manner to minimize the possibility of entering the vertebral canal or transverse foramina. In contrast to conventional plates, the string-of-pearls (SOP) plate can be contoured with 6 degrees of freedom, which is important when applying a plate to multiple vertebrae in the thoracolumbar spine with natural kyphosis (McKee and Downes, 2008). Great care must be exercised when applying locking plates since the angle of screw insertion is generally determined by the plate, and it is possible to place screws into fracture lines or damage vital structures during screw insertion.

Screw/pin implantation in vertebrae

Extreme caution is necessary when placing screws or pins in vertebrae due to the proximity of important neural and vascular structures, such as the spinal cord and aorta. Cross-sectional imaging, such as CT, has enabled the determination of 'safe implantation corridors' (Figure 18.11), although given the spectrum of variation of these corridors in normal dogs it is preferable to rely on those defined using the CT scan of the individual patient, rather than the published values.

In the cervical spine, the width of the implantation corridor is small if violation of the vertebral canal and transverse foraminae (containing the vertebral artery) is to be avoided. In general, as the implant insertion angle increases, the risk of transverse foramen penetration increases and the risk of vertebral canal penetration decreases. The implications for vertebral artery damage in dogs and cats appear to be less severe than in humans; however, haemorrhage from this vessel can be substantial. In the thoracolumbar spine there are several important structures that lie in close proximity to the ventral aspect of the vertebrae, including the aorta, the azygous vein, the pleurae and the lungs. There is thus a risk of life-threatening haemorrhage or pneumothorax when placing screws or pins that engage the ventral cortex of these vertebrae. Although not without risk, bicortical placement of implants in the lumbar spine has a wider margin of safety than in the thoracolumbar spine.

The value of decompressive surgery

Spinal cord decompression is not usually necessary when vertebral alignment and stability have been restored. Decompression is thus only indicated if there is evidence on preoperative imaging of compression due to a large haematoma, bone fragments or disc material. As little bone as possible should be removed due to the potential for restrictive laminectomy membrane formation, and

	Mean	Range
C2	50	45–60
C3–C6	36	30–45
C7	48	45–55
T10	22	20–25
T11	28	25–35
T12	30	25–35
T13	44	40–45
L1–L6	60	55–65
L7	0	0
S1	5	0–15

18.11 (a) Implantation angles in canine vertebrae: (b) C4 and (c) L3. The angle (star) is defined as that between the sagittal plane of the vertebra and the implantation corridor. Note that cervical vertebrae are approached ventrally, and thoracolumbar vertebrae dorsolaterally.
(Modified from Watine et al., 2006)

procedures that preserve articular facets are favoured because facet removal is very destabilizing (Shires et al., 1991; Schulz et al., 1996). The technique of choice is primarily governed by the method of vertebral fixation, since this dictates the surgical approach to the affected area.

General comments on postoperative management

Postoperative management is an extremely important aspect when caring for neurosurgical patients. The priorities are analgesia, emptying the bladder, physiotherapy and reducing the risk of complications of recumbency. Antimicrobial agents, if considered necessary, should be used perioperatively (see Chapter 8). Faeces should be monitored for evidence of melaena or fresh blood, because gastrointestinal ulceration is not uncommon in spinal injury patients treated with anti-prostaglandin drugs.

Patients must be kept clean and dry on non-retentive, well padded bedding and checked regularly for the development of urine or faecal scald or decubital ulcers over pressure points. A high standard of nursing care is essential in order to prevent bladder distension and urinary tract infections in incontinent animals. The bladder must be emptied at least three times daily and urine samples regularly analysed. Pharmacological therapy, such as bethanechol and phenoxybenzamine, may occasionally be beneficial. Recumbent animals should be turned regularly to reduce the risk of decubital ulcers and pneumonia.

Regular physiotherapy and hydrotherapy to promote limb use and reduce muscle atrophy are invaluable; where necessary professional assistance should be sought. Large and giant dogs that are unable to ambulate can be challenging to nurse and may require assistance with a belly band, chest harness or mobility cart.

Prognosis

The prognosis depends on a number of factors, the most important of which are the severity of the neurological dysfunction and the duration of the injury. In general, cases that retain pain perception and some degree of voluntary motor function have a good prognosis provided they are managed appropriately and promptly. Serial neurological examinations are an important factor in assessing the prognosis more accurately since a functional recovery is less likely if there is no improvement within 4 weeks of the initial injury. It is also important to note that surgical experience can critically affect the outcome and surgical procedures should not be attempted without appropriate training.

Cervical fractures and luxations are associated with a guarded prognosis if the patient is tetraplegic or hypoventilating; delayed treatment worsens the prognosis (Hawthorne *et al.*, 1999). Less severe cervical injuries have a good prognosis when managed appropriately by experienced surgeons. Thoracolumbar fractures and luxations generally have a good prognosis provided deep pain perception remains intact. Patients with no voluntary motor function and with urinary incontinence have a guarded prognosis and cases with loss of pain perception rarely recover (McKee, 1990; Selcer *et al.*, 1991; Kuntz *et al.*, 1995; Olby *et al.*, 2003; Bruce *et al.*, 2008). Recent research suggests the latter cases may benefit from transplantation of autologous olfactory mucosal ensheathing cells (Granger *et al.*, 2012). Although this procedure can lead to improved motor function in some cases it is not currently readily available. Lumbosacral fractures and luxations in patients that retain pain perception generally have a good prognosis since injured spinal nerves tolerate concussion and compression better than spinal cord parenchyma. Cats with sacrocaudal injuries usually recover urinary continence if they retain good anal tone, and perineal and tail base pain perception on initial examination (Tatton *et al.*, 2009). Cats that do not become continent within 1 month generally fail to regain urinary function (Moise and Flanders, 1983; Smeak and Olmstead, 1985).

References and further reading

Aikawa T, Shibata M and Fujita H (2013) Modified ventral stabilization using positively threaded profile pins and polymethylmethacrylate for atlantoaxial instability in 49 dogs. *Veterinary Surgery* **42**, 683–692

Anderson A and Coughlan AR (1997) Sacral fractures in dogs and cats: a classification scheme and review of 51 cases. *Journal of Small Animal Practice* **38**, 404–409

Beaver DP, MacPherson GC, Muir P *et al.* (1996) Methylmethacrylate and bone screw repair of seventh lumbar vertebral fracture-luxations in dogs. *Journal of Small Animal Practice* **37**, 381–386

Bruce CW, Brisson BA and Gyselinck K (2008) Spinal fracture and luxation in dogs and cats: a retrospective evaluation of 95 cases. *Veterinary and Comparative Orthopaedics and Traumatology* **21**, 280–284

Carberry CA, Flanders JA, Dietze AE *et al.* (1989) Nonsurgical management of thoracic and lumbar spinal fractures and fracture/luxations in the dog and cat: a review of 17 cases. *Journal of the American Animal Hospital Association* **25**, 43–54

Draffan D, Clements D, Farrell M *et al.* (2009) The role of computed tomography in the classification and management of pelvic fractures. *Veterinary and Comparative Orthopaedics and Traumatology* **22**, 190–197

Garcia J, Milthorpe BK, Russell D *et al.* (1994) Biomechanical study of canine spinal fracture fixation using pins or bone screws with polymethylmethacrylate. *Veterinary Surgery* **23**, 322–329

Granger N, Blamires H, Franklin RJ *et al.* (2012) Autologous olfactory mucosal cell transplants in clinical spinal cord injury: a randomized double-blinded trial in a canine translational model. *Brain* **135**, 3227–3237

Griffiths IR (1978) Spinal cord injuries: a pathological study of naturally occurring lesions in the dog and cat. *Journal of Comparative Pathology* **88**, 303–315

Hawthorne JC, Blevins WE, Wallace LJ *et al.* (1999) Cervical vertebral fractures in 56 dogs: a retrospective study. *Journal of the American Animal Hospital Association* **35**, 135–146

Johnson P, Beltran E, Dennis R *et al.* (2012) Magnetic resonance imaging characteristics of suspected vertebral instability associated with fracture or subluxation in eleven dogs. *Veterinary Radiology and Ultrasound* **53**, 552–559

Kinns J, Mai W, Seiler G *et al.* (2006) Radiographic sensitivity and negative predictive value for acute canine spinal trauma. *Veterinary Radiology and Ultrasound* **47**, 563–570

Kuntz CA, Waldron D, Martin RA *et al.* (1995) Sacral fractures in dogs: a review of 32 cases. *Journal of the American Animal Hospital Association* **31**, 142–150

McAnulty JF, Lenehan TM and Maletz LM (1986) Modified segmental spinal instrumentation in repair of spinal fractures and luxations in dogs. *Veterinary Surgery* **15**, 143–149

McKee WM (1990) Spinal trauma in dogs and cats: a review of 51 cases. *Veterinary Record* **126**, 285–289

McKee WM and Downes CJ (2008) Vertebral stabilisation and selective decompression for the management of triple thoracolumbar disc protrusions. *Journal of Small Animal Practice* **49**, 536–539

Moise NS and Flanders JA (1983) Micturition disorders in cats with sacrocaudal vertebral lesions. In: *Current Veterinary Therapy VIII*, ed. RW Kirk, pp. 722–726. WB Saunders Company, Philadelphia

Olby N (2010) The pathogenesis and treatment of acute spinal cord injuries in dogs. *Veterinary Clinics of North America: Small Animal Practice* **40**, 791–807

Olby N, Levine J, Harris T *et al.* (2003) Long-term functional outcome of dogs with severe injuries of the thoracolumbar spinal cord: 87 cases (1996–2001). *Journal of the American Veterinary Medical Association* **222**, 762–769

Pare B, Gendreau CL and Robbins MA (2001) Open reduction of sacral fractures using transarticular implants at the articular facets of L7-S1: 8 consecutive canine patients (1995–1999). *Veterinary Surgery* **30**, 476–481

Patterson RH and Smith GK (1992) Backsplinting for treatment of thoracic and lumbar fracture/luxation in the dog: principles of application and case series. *Veterinary and Comparative Orthopaedics and Traumatology* **5**, 179–187

Platt S and Olby N (2013) *BSAVA Manual of Canine and Feline Neurology, 4th edn.* BSAVA Publications, Gloucester

Schulz KS, Waldron DR, Grant JW *et al.* (1996) Biomechanics of the thoracolumbar vertebral column of dogs during lateral bending. *American Journal of Veterinary Research* **57**, 1228–1232

Selcer RR, Bubb WJ and Walker TL (1991) Management of vertebral column fractures in dogs and cats; 211 cases (1977–1985). *Journal of the American Veterinary Medical Association* **198**, 1965–1968

Shires PK, Waldron DR, Hedlund CS *et al.* (1991) A biomechanical study of rotational instability in unaltered and surgically altered canine thoracolumbar vertebral motion units. *Progress in Veterinary Neurology* **2**, 6–14

Smeak DD and Olmstead ML (1985) Fracture/luxations of the sacrococcygeal area in the cat. A retrospective study of 51 cases. *Veterinary Surgery* **14**, 319–324

Smith GK and Walter MC (1988) Spinal decompressive procedures and dorsal compartment injuries: comparative biomechanical study in canine cadavers. *American Journal of Veterinary Research* **49**, 266–273

Smith PM and Jeffery ND (2005) Spinal shock – comparative aspects and clinical relevance. *Journal of Veterinary Internal Medicine* **19**, 788–793

Tatton B, Jeffery N and Holmes M (2009) Predicting recovery of urination control in cats after sacrocaudal injury: a prospective study. *Journal of Small Animal Practice* **50**, 593–596

Waldron DR, Shires PK, McCain W *et al.* (1991) The rotational stabilising effect of spinal fixation techniques in an unstable vertebral model. *Progress in Veterinary Neurology* **2**, 105–110

Walter MC, Smith GK and Newton CD (1986) Canine lumbar spinal internal fixation techniques: a comparative biomechanical study. *Veterinary Surgery* **15**, 191–198

Watine S, Cabassu JP, Catheland S *et al.* (2006) Computed tomography study of implantation corridors in canine vertebrae. *Journal of Small Animal Practice* **47**, 651–657

Weh JM and Kraus KH (2007) Use of a four pin and methylmethacrylate fixation in L7 and the iliac body to stabilize lumbosacral fracture-luxations: a clinical and anatomic study. *Veterinary Surgery* **36**, 775–782

OPERATIVE TECHNIQUE 18.1

Atlantoaxial subluxation (C1–C2)

BACKGROUND

Atlantoaxial subluxation is most commonly a developmental disorder in small dogs; however, trauma may occasionally disrupt a previously normal articulation. The author's fixation technique of choice is to place screws in the ventral aspects of C1 and C2 and encase them in bone cement (Aikawa *et al.*, 2013). Careful consideration of implant corridors is necessary. Additional screws may be placed across the articular facets in large dogs, although it can be difficult to achieve the desired angle.

WARNINGS

- Dorsal approaches that rely on passing a suture ventral to the dorsal arch of the axis carry a significant risk of life-threatening iatrogenic injury to the medulla oblongata, either directly through contact, or indirectly because of flexion at the atlantoaxial articulation that is necessary to pass the suture
- Great care is necessary to avoid additional spinal cord injury associated with increased flexion of the cranial cervical spine, especially at induction of anaesthesia, during imaging, when the patient is being prepared for surgery and when positioning on the operating table

POSITIONING

Dorsal recumbency with the cranial cervical spine extended over a sandbag (which effectively reduces the subluxation). The thoracic limbs are pulled caudally in a symmetrical manner and secured to the table. Gentle traction is applied by means of tapes that are passed around the maxillary canine teeth and secured to the surgery table cranially (Figure 18.12a).

PRACTICAL TIP

Symmetrical positioning of the patient is critical

ASSISTANT

Useful.

EQUIPMENT EXTRAS

Gelpi retractors; periosteal elevator; small curette or pneumatic burr; drill; locking or cortical screws; threaded pins and corresponding instrumentation for insertion; drill bit (or gouge and mallet) for making hole for collection of bone graft; dental tartar scraper; bone cement; demineralized bone matrix.

SURGICAL TECHNIQUES

Approach

A midline incision is made from cranial to the larynx to the manubrium. The sternohyoideus muscles are separated and the right sternothyroideus muscle is sectioned near the thyroid cartilage (Figure 18.12b). The trachea, oesophagus and left common carotid sheath are retracted to the left.

PRACTICAL TIP

An oesophageal stethoscope aids identification of the oesophagus

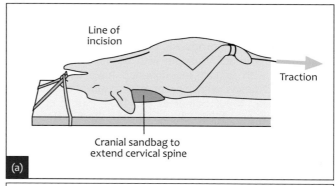

(a)

Line of incision

Traction

Cranial sandbag to extend cervical spine

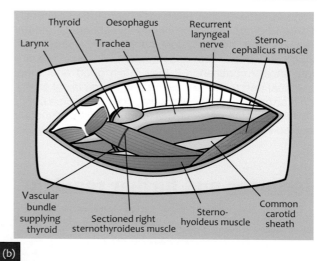

Thyroid   Oesophagus   Recurrent laryngeal nerve

Larynx   Trachea   Sterno-cephalicus muscle

Vascular bundle supplying thyroid

Sectioned right sternothyroideus muscle

Sterno-hyoideus muscle

Common carotid sheath

(b)

18.12   Ventral surgical approach to C1–C2.

→ OPERATIVE TECHNIQUE 18.1 CONTINUED

The prominent ventral process of the atlas is palpated and the tendons of the longus colli muscles are dissected from this structure and retracted laterally. The atlantoaxial synovial joints are opened (viscous synovial fluid is generally visible) and the articular cartilage is removed with a small burr or curette.

Reduction and fixation

The aforementioned traction is released, whilst extension of the spine is maintained. Screws are placed in the pedicles of C1 and the caudal vertebral body of C2 (entry point is midline); the thin central body of the axis provides little purchase for implants. When using facet screws they are positioned at an angle of 30 degrees away from the midline and 20 degrees dorsally. The facet screws are placed in a positional manner, and all screws used are 5–8 mm longer than the length measured with the depth gauge. The screws are placed leaving the extra threaded length exposed ventral to the bone. Cancellous bone is obtained from the proximal aspect of a humerus and packed in and around the joint spaces to promote fusion. Alternatively, demineralized bone matrix may be used. Polymethylmethacrylate bone cement is placed around the screws and lavaged with saline, preferably cooled, to dissipate heat during hardening (Figure 18.13).

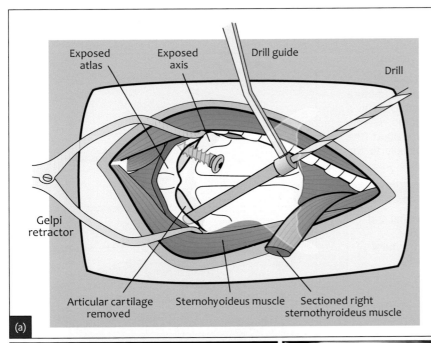
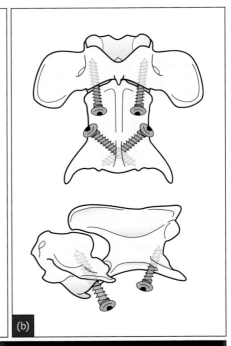
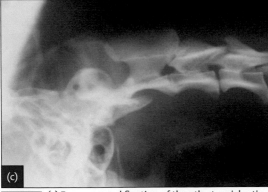
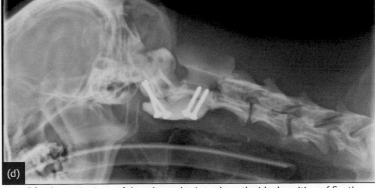

18.13 (a) Exposure and fixation of the atlantoaxial articulation. (b) Schematic views of the atlas and axis to show the ideal position of fixation screws in the pedicles of C1 and the caudal aspect of the C2 vertebral body. (c) Preoperative and (d) postoperative lateral radiographs showing repair of a traumatic atlantoaxial subluxation in a Dachshund using screws and cement. Note the C2–C3 block vertebra.

Wound closure

Routine, including repair of the right sternothyroideus muscle.

POSTOPERATIVE MANAGEMENT

Strict rest for 6 weeks. Harness preferable to collar.

WARNINGS

- Excessive cement is to be avoided in order to reduce the possibility of tracheal or oesophageal injury
- Monitor closely for potential bradycardia and hypoventilation

OPERATIVE TECHNIQUE 18.2

Cervical fractures and luxations (C2–T1)

BACKGROUND

The axis is the most frequently fractured cervical vertebra due to the concentration of force in this area, which is a transition point between the atlanto-occipital unit and the caudal cervical spine. The body of the axis is invariably displaced dorsally relative to the dens and the atlas.

Fractures and luxations of the cervical spine are most appropriately stabilized with vertebral body screws or pins and bone cement. It may be necessary for the construct to span more than two vertebrae; for cranial C2 fractures implants may be placed across the articular facets or into the pedicles of C1. Dorsal facet fixation may be considered in cervical luxation cases as an alternative to vertebral body screws/pins and cement, since the intact vertebral bodies provide a ventral buttress that significantly contributes to vertebral stability. Facet screwing or wiring is particularly appropriate in cases where one or both cranial processes of the caudal vertebra displace dorsal to the articular processes of the cranial vertebra, since a dorsal approach is generally necessary in order to reduce the luxated facet joint(s).

POSITIONING

Dorsal recumbency with the affected region of the spine extended over a sandbag (to aid reduction of the fracture or luxation). The thoracic limbs are pulled caudally in a symmetrical manner and secured to the table. Gentle traction is applied by means of tapes around the maxillary canine teeth that are secured cranially to the surgery table (Figure 18.14a).

PRACTICAL TIP

Symmetrical positioning of the patient is critical and this is aided by gentle cervical traction (Figure 18.14a). Traction also aids reduction of the fracture/luxation. Hyperextension should be avoided

ASSISTANT

Useful.

EQUIPMENT EXTRAS

Hohmann and Gelpi retractors; periosteal elevator; locking or cortical screws; threaded pins and corresponding instrumentation for insertion; drill; drill bits; bone cement.

SURGICAL TECHNIQUES

Approach

A midline incision is made from the larynx to the manubrium. The sternocephalicus and sternohyoideus muscles are separated (Figure 18.14b) and branches of the caudal thyroid vein are cauterized. The trachea, oesophagus and left common carotid sheath are retracted to the left. The prominent ventrally directed transverse processes of C6 are a useful landmark. The longus colli muscles are elevated from the affected vertebrae and retracted laterally (Figure 18.14c).

PRACTICAL TIP

An oesophageal stethoscope aids identification of the oesophagus

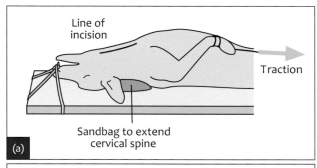

(a)

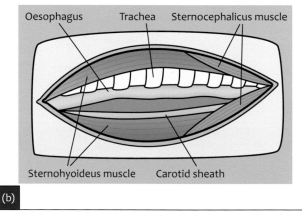

(b)

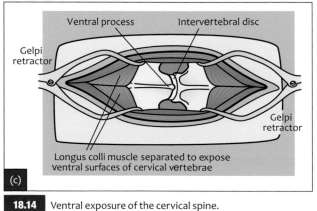

(c)

18.14 Ventral exposure of the cervical spine.

→ OPERATIVE TECHNIQUE 18.2 CONTINUED

Reduction and fixation

The caudal segment is generally displaced dorsally. Reduction is achieved by careful leverage with a Hohmann retractor and gentle traction/countertraction. K-wires or small bone screws may be used to temporarily stabilize bone fragments or unstable intervertebral spaces whilst definitive fixation is applied.

A minimum of two screws or pins should be placed in pre-drilled holes both cranial and caudal to the fracture or luxation; the entry point is in the ventral midline. Implants are directed between the vertebral canal and transverse foramina and ideally the trans (far) cortex should be penetrated. Polymethylmethacrylate bone cement is placed around the screws or pins and lavaged with saline, preferably cooled, to dissipate heat during hardening (Figures 18.15 and 18.16).

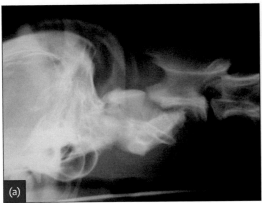
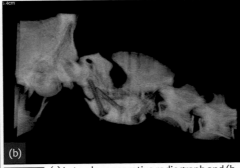
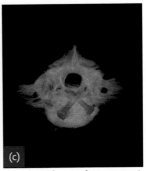

18.15 (a) Lateral preoperative radiograph and (b–c) postoperative semitransparent volume rendered hardware reconstructed CT images of a C2 fracture in a Labrador Retriever that was stabilized with screws and cement.

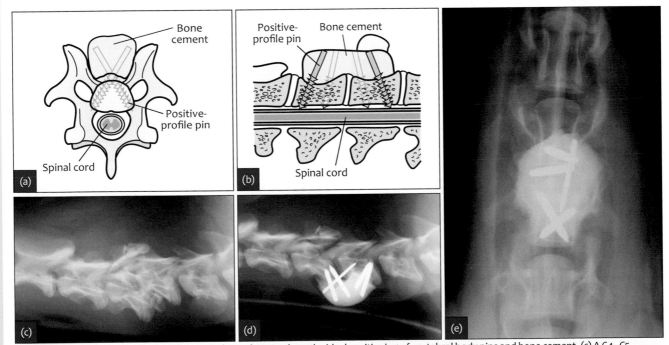

18.16 (a–b) Schematic views of the cervical vertebrae to show the ideal positioning of vertebral body pins and bone cement. (c) A C4–C5 luxation in a 6-month-old Dobermann. (d) Lateral and (e) ventrodorsal postoperative radiographs of the case shown in (c). Fixation was achieved using vertebral body positive-profile threaded pins and bone cement.

Wound closure

Routine, including apposition of the longus colli muscles where possible.

POSTOPERATIVE MANAGEMENT

Strict rest for 6 weeks. Harness preferable to collar. Dressing generally not helpful.

WARNINGS

- Severe intraoperative haemorrhage can occur with C2 fractures and reduction can be challenging
- Excessive cement is to be avoided in order to reduce the possibility of tracheal or oesophageal injury
- Monitor closely for potential bradycardia and hypoventilation

OPERATIVE TECHNIQUE 18.3

Thoracic fractures and luxations (T1–T8)

BACKGROUND

Injuries in this area of the spine are, fortunately, uncommon. Luxations are inherently stable because of an intact ventral buttress, the ribs and the epaxial musculature. Utilization of the vertebral bodies is extremely difficult because of their triangular cross-section, the relative lack of bone stock in the centre of the vertebrae and the presence of the heads of the ribs. Dorsal spinous process plating or wiring is an applicable technique, especially for the management of luxations in this region of the spine. Alternatively, affected vertebrae may be exposed and stabilized with screws/pins/cement or plates and screws via a transthoracic approach.

POSITIONING

Ventral recumbency (symmetrical).

ASSISTANT

Yes.

EQUIPMENT EXTRAS

Gelpi and Hohmann retractors; periosteal elevator; plastic or metal spinal plates; bolts and nuts; spanners; drill and drill bit for metal plates; orthopaedic wire and twisters.

SURGICAL TECHNIQUES

Approach

Dorsal midline with elevation and retraction of the epaxial muscles from the dorsal spinous processes and dorsal laminae (Figure 18.17).

Reduction and fixation

Towel clamps or artery forceps attached to the dorsal spinous processes cranial and caudal to the fracture or luxation may be distracted with a Gelpi retractor. Alternatively, an assistant may apply traction and counter-traction. The tip of a small Hohmann retractor can be placed under the lamina of the ventrally displaced vertebra and levered on the lamina of the dorsal vertebra to aid final reduction. Reduction is maintained using traction and countertraction by an assistant. In addition, non-fractured facet joints may be stabilized with K-wires.

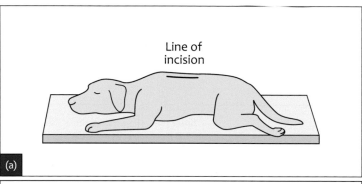

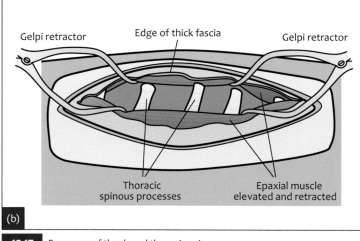

18.17 Exposure of the dorsal thoracic spine.

Fixation is achieved using paired metal or plastic plates secured to the dorsal spinous processes by bolts placed either through (metal) or between (plastic) the processes. Alternatively, wire may be placed around the dorsal spinous processes (Figure 18.18).

PRACTICAL TIP

Position plates or wire as ventrally as possible on the processes

WARNING

The spinous processes are inherently weak and failure due to implant slippage, fracture or avascular necrosis is not uncommon

→ **OPERATIVE TECHNIQUE 18.3 CONTINUED**

Wound closure

Routine, including the midline tendinous raphe.

POSTOPERATIVE MANAGEMENT

Strict confinement for 6 weeks. Consider use of external splint in large dogs with mid to caudal thoracic injuries since the fixation technique is inherently weak. Belly band support.

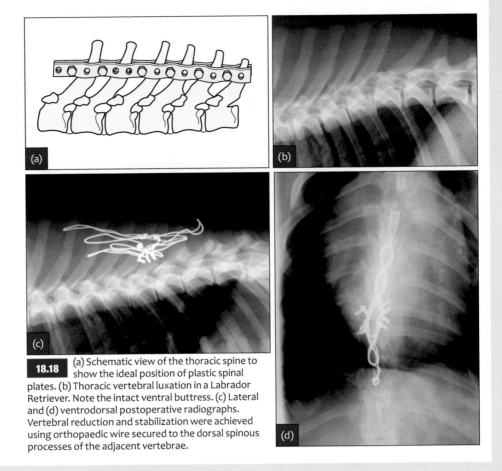

18.18 (a) Schematic view of the thoracic spine to show the ideal position of plastic spinal plates. (b) Thoracic vertebral luxation in a Labrador Retriever. Note the intact ventral buttress. (c) Lateral and (d) ventrodorsal postoperative radiographs. Vertebral reduction and stabilization were achieved using orthopaedic wire secured to the dorsal spinous processes of the adjacent vertebrae.

OPERATIVE TECHNIQUE 18.4

Thoracolumbar fractures and luxations (T12–L3)

BACKGROUND

Vertebral body plates can be readily applied in this region of the spine and bilateral plating may be performed in large dogs. Alternatively, vertebral body screws or pins and bone cement can be applied (see Operative Technique 18.5).

POSITIONING

Ventral recumbency.

ASSISTANT

Useful.

EQUIPMENT EXTRAS

Gelpi and Hohmann retractors; periosteal elevator; drill and drill bits; bone plates; locking and cortical screws and corresponding instrumentation for insertion.

→ **OPERATIVE TECHNIQUE 18.4 CONTINUED**

SURGICAL TECHNIQUES

Approach

Dorsal approach with elevation and retraction of the epaxial muscles. In the thoracic region, resection (or disarticulation) of rib heads and removal of the short transverse processes are required.

Reduction and fixation

Reduction is achieved by traction/countertraction and leverage with a Hohmann retractor.

PRACTICAL TIP

Intact articular facet processes may be used to assess accuracy of reduction

Articular facets may be luxated and require careful reduction. There is inherent stability if facet processes are intact (they may be secured with a transarticular K-wire). The bone plate is positioned on transverse process ostectomy sites in the thoracic region and at the junction of the transverse processes and vertebral bodies in the lumbar region. Locking plate/screw systems may provide additional security compared to non-locking systems. Screws should engage a minimum of four cortices cranial and caudal to the fracture or luxation taking care to observe the optimal implantation angles. It is essential that they are directed ventral to the vertebral canal (Figure 18.19).

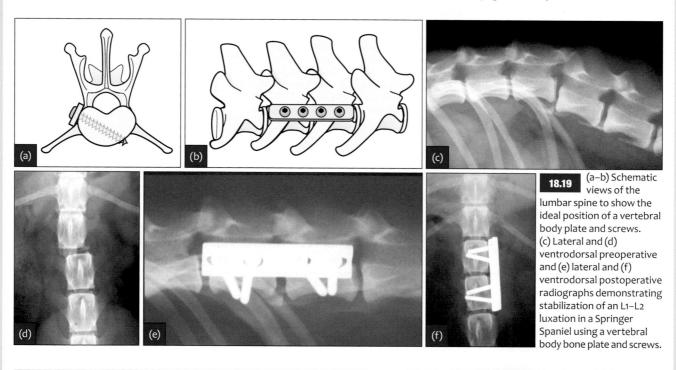

18.19 (a–b) Schematic views of the lumbar spine to show the ideal position of a vertebral body plate and screws. (c) Lateral and (d) ventrodorsal preoperative and (e) lateral and (f) ventrodorsal postoperative radiographs demonstrating stabilization of an L1–L2 luxation in a Springer Spaniel using a vertebral body bone plate and screws.

PRACTICAL TIP

Ascertain appropriate plate size from preoperative radiographs. In order to avoid inappropriate screw placement, identify intervertebral disc spaces with a hypodermic needle

WARNING

Inappropriate plate positioning or angle of drilling may result in catastrophic iatrogenic spinal cord injury, or implant loosening

Wound closure

Routine, including repair of the lumbodorsal fascia.

POSTOPERATIVE MANAGEMENT

Strict rest for 6 weeks. Belly band support.

OPERATIVE TECHNIQUE 18.5

Caudal thoracic fractures and luxations (T8–T12); lumbar fractures and luxations (L3–L7)

BACKGROUND

Vertebral body screws, or pins, and bone cement are less likely to interfere with important pelvic limb spinal nerves compared with plates in the L3–L7 region of the spine. In addition, screw placement is not determined by plate holes, giving more versatility in screw placement.

POSITIONING

Ventral recumbency with pelvic limbs positioned alongside the abdomen (Figure 18.20a).

ASSISTANT

Yes.

EQUIPMENT EXTRAS

Gelpi and Hohmann retractors; periosteal elevator; locking and cortical screws; threaded pins and corresponding instrumentation for insertion; drill and drill bits; bone cement; pin cutters.

SURGICAL TECHNIQUES

Approach

The affected vertebrae are exposed via a dorsal midline approach with elevation and retraction of the epaxial musculature (Figure 18.20b).

Reduction and fixation

Towel clamps or artery forceps attached to the dorsal spinous processes cranial and caudal to the fracture or luxation may be distracted with a Gelpi retractor. Alternatively, an assistant may apply traction and countertraction. The tip of a small Hohmann retractor can be placed under the lamina of the ventrally displaced (usually caudal) vertebra and levered on the lamina of the dorsal (usually cranial) vertebra to aid final reduction. Reduction may often be maintained with screws or K-wires placed across intact articular processes. Manual reduction by the assistant surgeon is occasionally necessary. Screws or threaded pins (pre-drilled) are placed bilaterally in the vertebral bodies where the transverse processes originate. A minimum of two screws or pins, and preferably three, should be placed both cranial and caudal to the fracture or luxation, taking care to observe the optimal implantation angles. Bone cement is placed around the implants and lavaged with saline to dissipate heat during hardening (Figure 18.21).

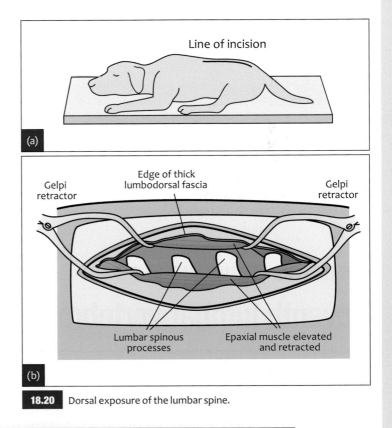

(a) Line of incision

(b) Gelpi retractor — Edge of thick lumbodorsal fascia — Gelpi retractor — Lumbar spinous processes — Epaxial muscle elevated and retracted

18.20 Dorsal exposure of the lumbar spine.

WARNING

Protect vital pelvic limb spinal nerves. Excessive cement may make wound closure difficult. Ensure implants do not unduly penetrate the abdominal (or thoracic) cavity, since they may result in vascular injury (immediate or delayed): measure the required length in the bone prior to placement

→ **OPERATIVE TECHNIQUE 18.5 CONTINUED**

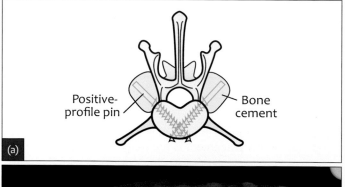

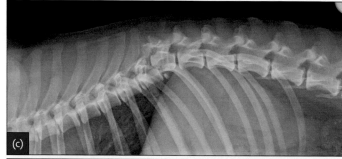

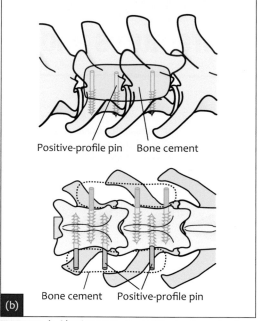

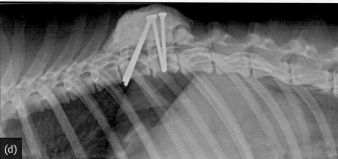

18.21 (a–b) Schematic views of the lumbar spine to show the ideal position of vertebral body pins and bone cement. Lateral (c) preoperative and (d) postoperative radiographs demonstrating stabilization of a T10–T11 fracture–luxation in an Irish Setter using screws and cement. This dog had retained deep pain perception caudal to the lesion despite the severity of vertebral displacement in this region of the spine.

Wound closure

Routine, including, where possible, repair of the lumbodorsal fascia.

POSTOPERATIVE MANAGEMENT

Strict rest for 6 weeks. Belly band support.

OPERATIVE TECHNIQUE 18.6

Seventh lumbar vertebra fractures (L7)

BACKGROUND

Injury to L7 typically involves an oblique fracture of the vertebral body and luxation of the articular facets with cranioventral displacement of the caudal segment. L7 fracture–luxations may be markedly displaced yet result in only mild neurological deficits because the vertebral canal is relatively spacious, containing the cauda equina rather than the spinal cord. Many dogs have difficulty ambulating due to severe pain rather than neurological dysfunction. Rigid fixation with screws or pins and bone cement enables predictable bone healing. Transilial pinning techniques have been described; however, they do not provide rigid fixation or reliably maintain fracture reduction.

→ **OPERATIVE TECHNIQUE 18.6 CONTINUED**

POSITIONING

Ventral recumbency with pelvic limbs positioned alongside the abdomen (Figure 18.22a).

ASSISTANT

Useful.

EQUIPMENT EXTRAS

Gelpi and Hohmann retractors; periosteal elevator; drill and drill bits; locking and cortical screws; threaded pins and corresponding instrumentation for insertion; spiked washers; pin cutters; bone cement.

SURGICAL TECHNIQUES

Approach

The lumbosacral spine is exposed via a dorsal midline approach with elevation and retraction of the epaxial musculature. Articular facets L7–S1 are identified (Figure 18.22b).

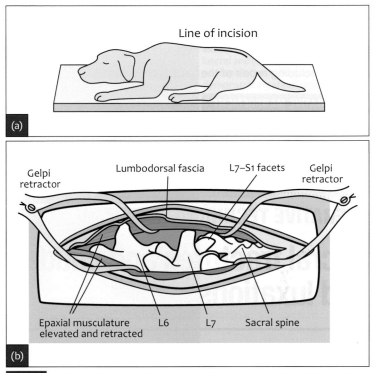

(a)

(b)

18.22 Dorsal exposure of the lumbosacral spine.

Reduction and fixation

Towel clamps attached to the dorsal spinous processes of L7 and the sacrum may be distracted with a Gelpi retractor. Alternatively, an assistant may apply traction and countertraction. The tip of a small Hohmann retractor can be placed under the lamina of the L7 vertebra and levered on the dorsal lamina of L6 to aid final reduction. Reduction may be maintained with screws placed across luxated articular facet processes. Screws (or threaded pins) are placed in the vertebral bodies of L7 (or L6) and the ilial bodies, or alternatively pedicle implants may be placed in L7 and the sacrum (entry point is the base of the cranial articular processes). These screws may be driven into the ilium if necessary (Figure 18.23).

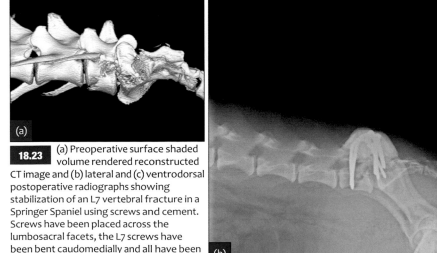

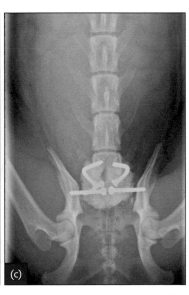

(a)

18.23 (a) Preoperative surface shaded volume rendered reconstructed CT image and (b) lateral and (c) ventrodorsal postoperative radiographs showing stabilization of an L7 vertebral fracture in a Springer Spaniel using screws and cement. Screws have been placed across the lumbosacral facets, the L7 screws have been bent caudomedially and all have been incorporated into the bone cement.

(b)

(c)

→ **OPERATIVE TECHNIQUE 19.1 CONTINUED**

These fractures are preferably managed with locking plates rather than with traditional screw and plating systems. Fragment displacement can occur with traditional systems if contouring is inaccurate.

Scapular fractures are well vascularized and generally heal rapidly. The muscular attachments between the scapula and the body wall will also tend to dissipate the forces of weight-bearing. These factors permit the use of weaker plates than those considered appropriate for lower limb fractures. In general, locking systems up to 2.7 mm are adequate for scapular body fractures in most patients. In larger dogs two plates can be placed, one either side of the scapular spine; the plates should be staggered slightly to avoid screw impingement.

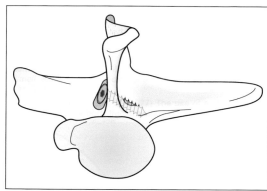

19.15 Transverse view of the scapula showing ideal screw and plate positioning.

WARNING

Care must be taken to avoid iatrogenic damage to structures medial to the scapula including the brachial plexus, axillary artery and the thorax. It is also important to be aware of the suprascapular nerve which passes under the acromial process (see Figure 19.16c). This should be identified and protected when positioning the plate on the distal fragment

POSTOPERATIVE MANAGEMENT

Depending on the stability achieved surgically, a modified Velpeau or a scapular support bandage may be applied for 2–3 weeks. The patient should be restricted to short lead exercise for 4–6 weeks.

Implant removal is usually only undertaken if there are problems associated with its continued presence, such as screw loosening or infection.

OPERATIVE TECHNIQUE 19.2

Fractures of the scapular neck

POSITIONING

Lateral recumbency with affected limb uppermost.

ASSISTANT

Ideally.

EQUIPMENT EXTRAS

Gelpi self-retaining retractors; pointed reduction forceps; osteotome and mallet and/or bone cutting forceps for osteotomy; drill; Kirschner (K) wire and cerclage wire set; pin/wire cutters; appropriately sized screw and plate system (locking system may be preferable to conventional plating system).

SURGICAL TECHNIQUES

Approach

A lateral incision is made, commencing at the mid-point of the scapular spine curving caudally over the proximal third of the humerus (Figure 19.16a). The deep fascia over the spine is incised and retracted cranially and caudally (Figure 19.16b). The acromial process is osteotomized and retracted with the acromial head of the deltoideus muscle distally (Figure 19.16c). The osteotomy should leave sufficient bone attached to the deltoideus muscle to permit later reattachment.

→

→ **OPERATIVE TECHNIQUE 19.2 CONTINUED**

The supraspinatus and infraspinatus muscles are either retracted or freed from their humeral attachment in order to permit greater visualization of the fracture site. Exposure of the lateral and caudal aspects of the scapular neck is gained by tenotomy of the infraspinatus or teres minor muscle. Proximal retraction of the supraspinatus muscle requires osteotomy of the greater tubercle of the humerus.

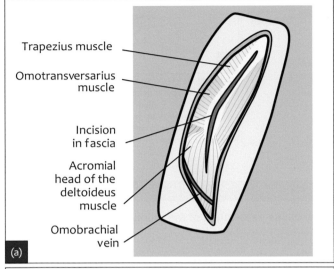

(a)

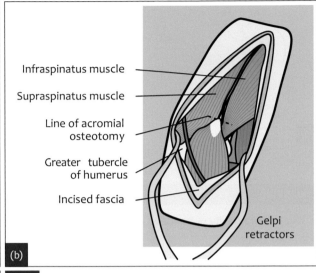

(b)

19.16 Surgical approach to the scapular neck and glenoid.

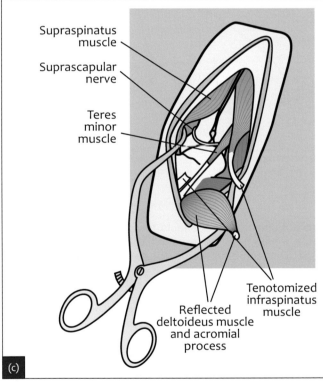

(c)

WARNING

The suprascapular nerve should be identified and avoided

Articular component

Articular components of the fracture, where present, should be addressed first (Figure 19.17). Accurate reduction of the articular surface is important and can be achieved by a combination of gentle leverage and the application of fragment-holding forceps. A small incision in the lateral joint capsule will allow inspection of the articular surface to assess the accuracy of reduction. The articular components are then stabilized with a lag screw placed craniocaudally or caudo-cranially. This screw should be positioned such that it does not interfere with any plate screws that may subsequently be placed (see Figure 19.18). The fracture may now be treated as a simple scapular neck fracture.

→

→ **OPERATIVE TECHNIQUE 19.2 CONTINUED**

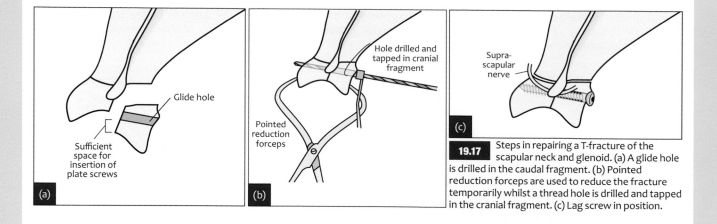

19.17 Steps in repairing a T-fracture of the scapular neck and glenoid. (a) A glide hole is drilled in the caudal fragment. (b) Pointed reduction forceps are used to reduce the fracture temporarily whilst a thread hole is drilled and tapped in the cranial fragment. (c) Lag screw in position.

WARNING

The glenoid cavity is concave and distal screw placement may cause penetration of the articular surface

Scapular neck component

The scapular neck fracture is reduced by a combination of linear traction and gentle leverage. Great care should be taken to avoid damaging any articular repair that has been performed. T-plates are often used for fracture stabilization since they optimize bone purchase in the small distal fragment (Figures 19.18 and 19.19).

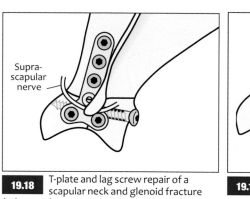

19.18 T-plate and lag screw repair of a scapular neck and glenoid fracture (T-fracture).

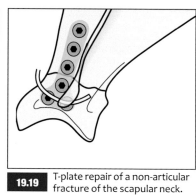

19.19 T-plate repair of a non-articular fracture of the scapular neck.

Wound closure

The surgical site should be closed in layers. The greater tubercle, if osteotomized, should be reattached with pins and tension-band wire. The infraspinatus and teres minor muscle tenotomies are repaired with a Bunnell–Mayer or horizontal mattress suture pattern using polydioxanone (PDS) or a non-absorbable suture material. The acromial osteotomy is repaired using wire sutures or pins and a tension-band wire (Figure 19.20).

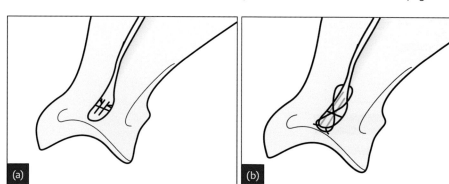

19.20 Acromial process osteotomy repair. (a) Wire suture. (b) Pin and tension-band wire.

POSTOPERATIVE MANAGEMENT

Depending on the stability achieved surgically, a modified Velpeau or a scapular support bandage may be applied for 2–3 weeks. The patient should be restricted to short lead exercise for 4–6 weeks.

OPERATIVE TECHNIQUE 19.3

Fractures of the supraglenoid tuberosity

POSITIONING

Lateral recumbency with affected limb uppermost.

ASSISTANT

Ideally.

EQUIPMENT EXTRAS

Gelpi self-retaining retractors; osteotome and mallet and/or bone-cutting forceps and/or sagittal saw for osteotomy; pointed reduction forceps; drill; K-wire and cerclage wire set (for pin and tension-band repair); pin/wire cutters; appropriately sized screw set (for lag screw fixation).

SURGICAL TECHNIQUES

Approach

See Operative Technique 19.2. It may be necessary to osteotomize the greater tubercle of the humerus and to reflect the brachiocephalicus muscle cranially to facilitate adequate exposure.

Reduction and fixation

Two small K-wires are inserted in a caudoproximal direction. A tension-band wire is placed around the K-wires and anchored proximally through a bone tunnel (Figure 19.21a). Care should be taken to protect the suprascapular nerve when applying the tension-band wire.

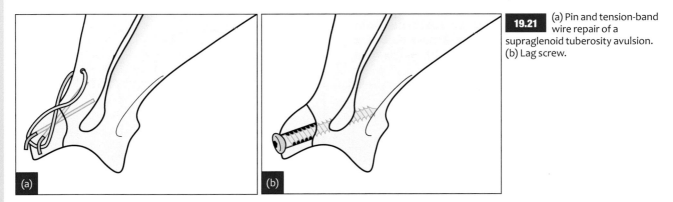

19.21 (a) Pin and tension-band wire repair of a supraglenoid tuberosity avulsion. (b) Lag screw.

Alternatively, a single screw is placed in lag fashion, inserted in a caudoproximal direction. This procedure is facilitated by pre-drilling and tapping the screw hole in the scapular body prior to reduction of the fracture. The glide hole is then drilled in the avulsed fragment and the screw inserted (Figure 19.21b). The additional use of a spiked washer will engage the biceps tendon and prevent the screw head from being driven into the soft cancellous bone of the tuberosity as it is tightened.

Excision of the avulsed fragment may be appropriate for chronic injuries or where small fragment size makes anatomical reduction and fixation impractical. Concurrent tenodesis to the proximal humerus can be considered in these cases.

Wound closure

The surgical site should be closed in layers. The greater tubercle, if osteotomized, should be reattached with pins and tension-band wire.

POSTOPERATIVE MANAGEMENT

A Velpeau or off-weight-bearing sling is indicated for 2 weeks postoperatively, with exercise severely restricted for 4 weeks.

Chapter 20

The humerus

Steve Clarke

The humerus lies within the brachium, articulating proximally with the scapular glenoid to form the shoulder joint and distally with the radius and ulna to form the elbow joint. The canine and feline humeri are largely similar; however, some important species-specific anatomical variations exist. Overall, the complex bony anatomy, muscular coverage and neurovascular structures, particularly in the distal third of the humerus, present a challenge for the fracture surgeon with regards to both surgical exposure and implant placement.

In a survey by Phillips (1979), humeral fractures accounted for 7.7% of canine fractures and 4.4% of feline fractures. In the cat the distal humeral diaphyseal and supracondylar regions are fractured most commonly, which is in contrast to the dog where the humeral condyle is more frequently affected (Phillips, 1979; Vannini *et al.*, 1988). Humeral fractures can often be associated with major trauma and as such the patient should receive a thorough clinical assessment on initial presentation to assess for significant non-orthopaedic injuries.

Fractures of the proximal humerus

Proximal humeral fractures are rare, most often being the result of direct trauma. In skeletally immature animals, Salter–Harris Type I (Figure 20.1a) and II fractures are most likely, and require open reduction and internal fixation using Kirschner (K) wires or small intramedullary (IM) pins (see Operative Technique 20.1). In most cases surgical repair offers a good prognosis. A Salter–Harris Type III fracture (Figure 20.1b), where the epiphysis is fractured through the articular surface separating the greater tubercle and humeral head, is very rare. Articular surface disruption requires accurate anatomical reconstruction, with the cranial and caudal fragments being stabilized with K-wires (see Operative Technique 20.2). Less commonly, this fracture configuration can be seen in skeletally mature patients, which necessitates more mechanically robust fixation. The greater tubercle fragment is stabilized using a pin and tension-band wire and the humeral head using a lag screw and anti-rotation K-wire. More complex comminuted fractures of the articular surface of the humeral head are extremely rare. Non-surgical management can be considered for non-reconstructable humeral head fractures, with immobilization of the thoracic limb achieved by use of a Velpeau sling. If significant unremitting discomfort is present or if longer-term limb function is unsatisfactory then shoulder arthrodesis can be considered.

Proximal metaphyseal fractures are also uncommon. When present, close scrutiny of the signalment, history and fracture configuration is required as pathological fractures are not uncommon in this region. Proximal diaphyseal fractures mostly occur in the proximity of the deltoid tuberosity. Contraction of the deltoideus and latissimus dorsi muscles results in caudal displacement of the proximal fragment. Multiple fixation choices can be considered dependent on the precise fracture configuration; these may include IM devices, external skeletal fixation (ESF) or plates and bone screws.

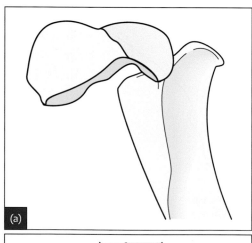

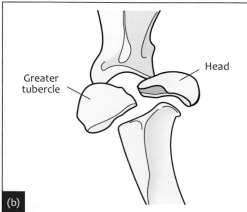

20.1 (a) Salter–Harris type I and (b) Salter–Harris type III separation of the proximal humeral epiphysis.

Humeral diaphyseal fractures

Whilst internal fixation using plates and screws remains commonplace, the shift in emphasis from anatomical reconstruction to a more biological approach (see Chapter 8) means that only two- or three-piece fractures are likely to be anatomically reconstructed, with more comminuted fractures being managed using bridging osteosynthesis techniques.

Despite its complex shape, the humeral diaphysis is amenable to plate application on its cranial, lateral or medial surfaces. The aspect to which the bone plate is applied is largely based on fracture location. Despite a more complex approach to the medial aspect of the humerus (see Operative Techniques 20.3 and 20.4), the medial surface of the humerus provides a relatively flat surface where minimal plate contouring is required (Figure 20.2). Distally, particularly in the dog, the greater width and flatter profile of the medial supracondylar ridge in comparison to its lateral counterpart makes for less technically challenging plate application, as well as allowing a bone plate to span the entire length of the humerus; this is useful when fractures of the distal diaphyseal region are present. In the cat, a supracondylar foramen is present at the distal extent of the medial supracondylar ridge, through which the median nerve and brachial artery pass. Consideration must be given to mobilization and retraction of these structures when applying a bone plate in this region (see Operative Technique 20.4).

The lateral approach to the humerus (see Operative Techniques 20.5 and 20.6) is less complex; however, great care must be taken to identify and protect the radial nerve on the lateral aspect of the distal humeral diaphysis.

> **WARNING**
>
> Failure to identify and protect the radial nerve can result in neuropraxia and thoracic limb paresis or complete radial nerve paralysis

Lateral plate application to the distal humerus can be complicated by a disparity in size between the diaphysis and the lateral supracondylar ridge, which may necessitate application of a smaller plate than is desirable (Figure 20.3). It can be further complicated due to the greater degree of plate contouring which is often required, given the complex profile of the lateral supracondylar ridge. The suitability of cranial plate application is dependent on fracture location. If the fracture is located more distally in the diaphysis, the amount of available bone stock in the distal fracture fragment is limited by the presence of the supratrochlear foramen (Figure 20.3) in the dog and the incomplete supratrochlear foramen in the cat, which

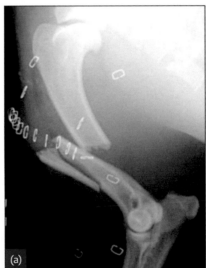
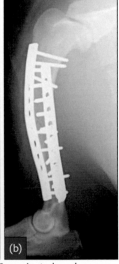

(a)   (b)

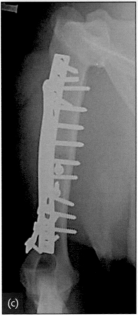

(c)

20.3 (a) Comminuted grade 2 open humeral fracture in an 11-year old Staffordshire Bull Terrier. (b) Mediolateral and (c) craniocaudal radiographs showing that the large cranial fragment has been anatomically reduced and stabilized using two 2.7 mm lag screws. The humeral diaphysis was then anatomically reduced and stabilized using orthogonal bone plates – a lateral 2.7 mm locking compression plate (LCP) and a cranial 2.7 mm dynamic compression plate (DCP). The proximal humerus would have readily accommodated a 3.5 mm bone plate and screws, however the narrower lateral supracondylar ridge would not, hence the 2.7 mm plates were used. Although the fracture had been anatomically reconstructed the lateral LCP in isolation was not considered mechanically robust enough given both the poor biology and high mechanical challenge that this fracture presented. Note how the supratrochlear foramen limits the distal extent of cranial plate application.

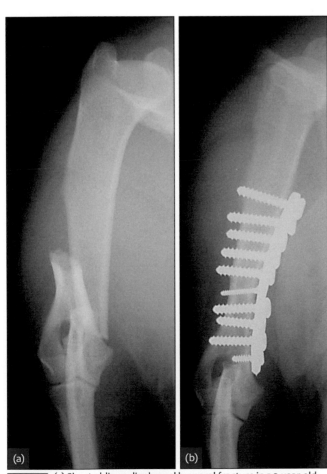

(a)   (b)

20.2 (a) Short oblique diaphyseal humeral fracture in a 3-year-old Cavalier King Charles Spaniel. (b) The humeral diaphysis has been anatomically reconstructed using a 1.5 mm lag screw. A veterinary cuttable plate has been applied to the medial aspect of the humerus. Minimal contouring of the bone plate was required.

may prevent a plate of appropriate size and length from being applied. As such, proximal to mid-diaphyseal fractures are most amenable to either cranial or lateral plate application. Proximally the cranial aspect of the humerus is the tension surface.

Bridging osteosynthesis techniques (Figures 20.4 and 20.5) are most likely to include pin–plate (Reems *et al.*, 2003), ESF (Langley-Hobbs *et al.*, 1997) and, less commonly, interlocking nails (Moses *et al.*, 2002). Bridging osteosynthesis provides an opportunity for the surgeon to utilize a biologically sparing surgical technique such as 'open but do not touch' or 'minimally invasive plate osteosynthesis' (MIPO). When ESF is used in the humerus (see

Operative Technique 20.12), type 1a configurations are most often used in combination with an IM pin (Langley-Hobbs *et al.*, 1997) to optimize construct mechanics. Alternatively, hybrid configurations using a full pin or a ring distally connected to a type 1 frame proximally can be considered. Close attention should be paid to using appropriate safe zones (Marti and Miller, 1994; Langley-Hobbs and Straw, 2005) for ESF pin placement.

The distal diaphysis lies immediately proximal to the supracondylar region of the humerus and, as a consequence, fractures in both regions are managed in similar ways. Distally, the caudal aspect of the humerus is the tension surface.

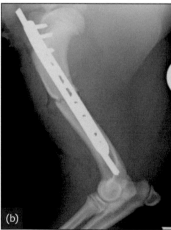

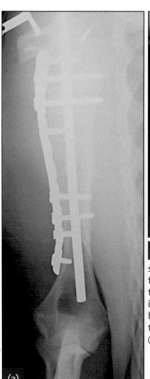

20.4 (a) Comminuted humeral diaphyseal fracture in a 4-year-old Springer Spaniel. (b) This fracture is non-reconstructable and has been managed using a bridging osteosynthesis technique comprising a type 1a ESF construct and an IM pin. Allogenic cancellous bone chips were placed at the fracture site.

20.5 (a) Craniocaudal and (b) mediolateral radiographs showing a mid-diaphyseal humeral fracture stabilized using a pin–plate technique. The IM pin has been seated into the medial aspect of the distal humerus and the bone plate placed on the lateral aspect of the humerus.
(Courtesy of J Pink)

Fractures of the distal humerus

The humeral condyle is composed of lateral and medial portions, the capitulum and the trochlea respectively, which create an uneven articular surface (Figure 20.6). The capitulum articulates with the radial head, whilst the trochlea articulates with both the radius and the ulna. The lateral and medial epicondyles are prominent bony landmarks, which provide the origin for the collateral ligaments and the carpal and digital extensor/flexor muscles respectively; they provide useful reference points during surgery. The humeral condyle is attached to the humeral diaphysis by the lateral and medial supracondylar ridges, which in the dog are separated by the supratrochlear foramen. In the dog the lateral supracondylar ridge is smaller than its medial counterpart, and is also offset laterally from the humeral diaphysis. In comparison, the distal humerus in the cat has an incomplete supratrochlear foramen, a supracondylar foramen (Figure 20.7), and both the medial and lateral supracondylar ridges are wider and thicker, which may in part explain why fractures through the humeral condyle occur less commonly in the cat than the dog (Vannini *et al.*, 1988).

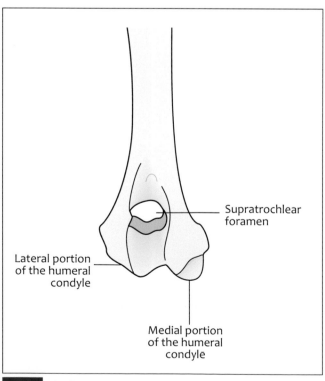

20.6 The distal humerus in the dog.

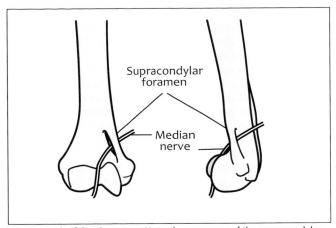

20.7 The feline humerus. Note the presence of the supracondylar foramen at the distal extent of the medal supracondylar ridge, through which the median nerve and brachial artery pass.

Distal humeral diaphyseal and supracondylar fractures

These fractures are most often caused by significant trauma. Supracondylar fractures communicate with the supratrochlear foramen, whereas distal diaphyseal fractures do not. Fractures in either location can be simple or comminuted. Although fracture fixation is complicated by the close proximity to the elbow joint and the limited bone stock in the distal humerus for implant placement, either internal fixation or ESF can be used. In patients where rapid healing is expected, pin fixation in isolation may be sufficient (e.g. IM pin and K-wire; see Operative Technique 20.13); however, in most cases pins are used in combination with a type 1a ESF construct with the IM pin being 'tied in' (Figure 20.8). In the skeletally mature patient, more robust fixation is required and internal fixation with bone plate application, to either the medial or both the lateral and medial aspects of the distal humerus, is generally performed (see Operative Techniques 20.9 and 20.13). If applying only a medial bone plate, a K-wire can be placed across the lateral supracondylar fracture; this technique is useful in smaller patients. Bone plate fixation can also be used in the skeletally immature patient if desired (Figure 20.9). ESF application with a 'tied-in' IM pin can also be useful, particularly when comminution of either region is present and bridging osteosynthesis is desired. When distal bone stock is limited hybrid ESF configurations can be useful, such as a modified type 1 ESF construct; a full pin across the humeral condyle is attached to a lateral connecting bar by second acrylic connecting bar (Guerin *et al.*, 1998). A linear/circular system can also be used with the distal circular component attached to either a full transcondylar pin or transcondylar olive wires. The ring is then connected to a type 1 frame proximally (Silva *et al.*, 2012).

Incomplete ossification of the humeral condyle

Aetiopathogenesis

Incomplete ossification of the humeral condyle (IOHC) is an enigmatic cause of forelimb lameness, for which the aetiopathogenesis remains poorly understood. Although reported sporadically in a variety of breeds, in the UK it is seen most commonly in English Springer Spaniels, with the prevalence in this breed estimated at approximately

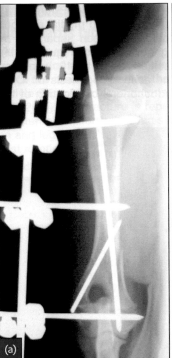
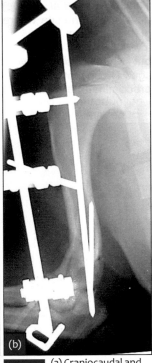
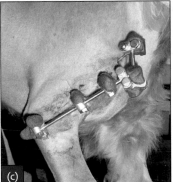

20.8 (a) Craniocaudal and (b) mediolateral radiographs of a supracondylar fracture in a 4-month-old Cocker Spaniel, which has been stabilized using an IM pin and a type 1a external skeletal fixator. Note the distal position of the IM pin and the use of the humeral condyle for the most distal external fixator pin. (c) The IM pin has been 'tied in' to the external skeletal fixator.

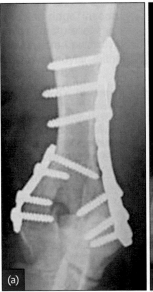
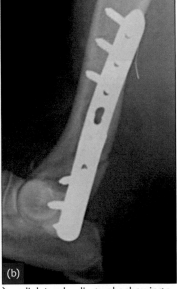

20.9 (a) Craniocaudal and (b) mediolateral radiographs showing a supracondylar humeral fracture in a 6-month-old Springer Spaniel which has been stabilized using bilateral bone plate application. A 2.7 mm locking compression plate (LCP) has been placed medially and a 2.0/2.7 mm veterinary cuttable plate laterally. In this case the use of non-locking screws with the medial LCP allows for more variation in direction of screw orientation, which can be helpful when placing plate screws in the distal humerus.

OPERATIVE TECHNIQUE 20.2

Salter–Harris type III fractures of the proximal humerus

POSITIONING

Lateral recumbency with the affected limb uppermost.

ASSISTANT

Yes.

EQUIPMENT EXTRAS

Appropriately sized K-wires or IM pins; orthopaedic wire; chuck; drill; pliers/wire twisters; pin/wire cutters; Gelpi and Hohmann retractors; pointed reduction forceps; Kern or Burns bone-holding forceps.

SURGICAL TECHNIQUES

Approach

An approach to the lateral aspect of the shoulder, proximal humerus and scapula is performed (see Operative Technique 19.2). Tenotomy of the tendon of insertion of the infraspinatus muscle is necessary to give good exposure of the shoulder and also to allow the humeral shaft to be pulled distally using Kern forceps (positioned as in Figure 20.21) during exposure of the fracture surfaces. The joint capsule (or its remains) are reflected to allow inspection of the articular surfaces. The fractured humeral head usually loses all soft tissue attachments and is found impacted in the soft tissues caudal to the shoulder.

Reduction and fixation

At this stage the proximal humeral shaft is rotated out of the incision; the humeral head is located and placed in its correct position on the metaphysis. It can be held in place by one of two methods. In the first, K-wires are driven down from the articular surface through the head into the metaphysis. The wires are cut flush with the joint surface and then countersunk. Alternatively, two or three K-wires can be driven in normograde fashion from the cranial, craniolateral and craniomedial aspect of the metaphysis up into the humeral head (Figure 20.23a). To allow maximum purchase in the head, each K-wire is advanced until its point just penetrates the articular surface. The wire is then retracted until the tip lies just below the surface. The distal ends of the wires are cut close to the surface of the metaphysis.

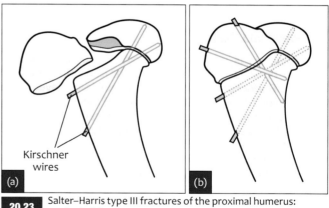

Kirschner wires

20.23 Salter–Harris type III fractures of the proximal humerus: method of fixation.

If there is a fracture of the lesser tuberosity and the fragment is unstable, K-wire fixation can be carried out at this stage. The humeral head is placed back into the glenoid. The avulsed greater tuberosity of the humerus is grasped with pointed reduction forceps and reattached to the metaphysis with two or three diverging K-wires driven from the craniolateral surface of the tubercle into the caudal aspect of the metaphysis (Figure 20.23b).

Wound closure

Remnants of the joint capsule are sutured. The infraspinatus muscle tenotomy is repaired with an appropriate suture pattern. Routine layered closure is performed to appose the superficial layers.

POSTOPERATIVE MANAGEMENT

Exercise is restricted for 4 to 6 weeks. In growing animals implants should ideally be removed once fracture union is complete (4 to 8 weeks), but in practice they are generally left *in situ* unless loosening causes soft tissue problems.

OPERATIVE TECHNIQUE 20.3

Medial approach to the humeral diaphysis for bone plate application

POSITIONING

Lateral recumbency with the affected limb dependent and pulled cranially. The contralateral limb is pulled caudally to lie over the thoracic wall and secured in place. A restraining band placed under the axilla of the contralateral limb and secured to the table can help with traction.

ASSISTANT

Not essential but helpful.

EQUIPMENT EXTRAS

Self-retaining retractors; Hohmann retractors; appropriate plating kit and screws; IM pins (if required for pin–plate fixation); hand chuck; drill; reduction forceps.

SURGICAL TECHNIQUES

Approach

A skin incision is made from the proximal aspect of the humerus to the epicondylar region distally. An incision in the deep fascia is made along the caudal border of the brachiocephalicus muscle and along the distal border of the superficial pectoral muscle. The brachiocephalicus muscle is retracted cranially, exposing the insertion of the superficial pectoral muscle on the humeral shaft. The insertion is incised proximally to the level of the cephalic vein and elevated from the bone. To allow more proximal exposure, the superficial pectoral muscle is divided and the deep pectoral insertion is incised along the humeral shaft, which exposes the biceps brachii muscle. Retraction of the biceps muscle caudally results in the best exposure of the proximal and mid shaft of the humerus. The biceps muscle should be retracted carefully as the underlying neurovascular structures – the median and musculocutaneous nerves and the brachial artery and vein – will be retracted with it. Exposure of the distal shaft of the humerus is achieved by cranial retraction of the biceps brachii muscle, although first the neurovascular structures need to be separated from the caudal border of the muscle.

Wound closure

The superficial pectoral muscle insertion and deep fascia are reattached. The remainder of the wound is closed routinely.

OPERATIVE TECHNIQUE 20.4

Medial approach to the distal humerus for bone plate application

POSITIONING

Lateral recumbency with the affected limb dependent and pulled cranially. The contralateral limb is pulled caudally to lie over the thoracic wall and secured in place. A restraining band placed under the axilla of the contralateral limb and secured to the table can help with traction.

→

OPERATIVE TECHNIQUE 20.6

Lateral approach to the distal humerus for bone plate application

POSITIONING

Lateral recumbency with the affected limb uppermost. A restraining band placed under the axilla of the dependant limb and secured to the table can help with traction.

ASSISTANT

Not essential but helpful.

EQUIPMENT EXTRAS

Self-retaining retractors; Hohmann retractors; appropriate plating kit and screws; IM pins (if required for pin–plate fixation); hand chuck; drill; reduction forceps.

SURGICAL TECHNIQUES

Approach

Exposure of the distal aspect of the lateral humerus (e.g. for supracondylar or condylar fractures) can be achieved by this approach. A skin incision is made passing slightly caudal to the lateral epicondyle. It extends distally in the region of the proximal ulna. Proximally, the incision can extend to the mid shaft of the humerus if required, being dictated by the fracture location. The lateral head of the triceps muscle is exposed and the deep fascia is incised along the cranial aspect of the triceps muscle, extending distally over the extensor muscles (Figure 20.27a). Retraction of the fascia cranially and the triceps muscle caudally reveals the condylar region of the humerus (Figure 20.27b). The radial nerve emerges from between the lateral head of the triceps and courses distally in association with the brachialis muscles. To expose the humeral condyle for a uni- or dicondylar fracture, elevation of the extensor carpi radialis muscle from the supracondylar ridge exposes both the bone and the underlying joint capsule. The joint capsule can be incised to expose the humeral condyle. To facilitate bone plate application in this region the approach can be extended proximally as detailed in Operative Technique 20.5. Retraction of the brachialis muscle and radial nerve cranially and the triceps muscle caudally exposes the lateral aspect of the humeral shaft.

Wound closure

The joint capsule is closed routinely. If possible the extensor carpi radialis muscle is reattached to the distal humerus or the fascia overlying the anconeus muscle. Following closure of the fascia the remaining wound closure is routine.

PRACTICAL TIP

The extent to which the radial nerve is exposed and indeed visualized will be dictated by the fracture location. For a unicondylar fracture the nerve is often not visualized, although if more proximal access is required, for example for concomitant plate application, care needs to be taken to identify and protect the nerve, both during dissection and retraction

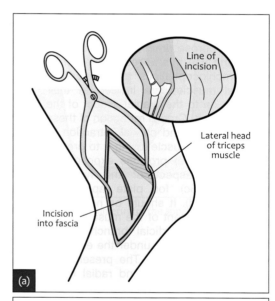

(a)

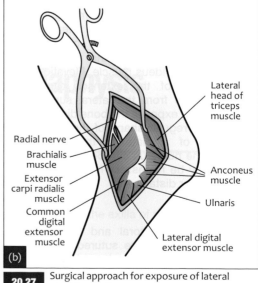

(b)

20.27 Surgical approach for exposure of lateral condylar fractures.

OPERATIVE TECHNIQUE 20.7

Lateral condylar fractures

POSITIONING

As for Operative Technique 20.6.

ASSISTANT

Not necessary.

EQUIPMENT EXTRAS

K-wires and associated wire instrumentation; drill; Gelpi self-retaining retractors; pointed reduction forceps; vulsellum forceps; appropriately sized bone screw and plating kits.

SURGICAL TECHNIQUES

Approach

As for Operative Technique 20.6. It is important to elevate the muscle (both the extensor carpi radialis and the anconeus muscles) from the lateral supracondylar ridge fracture as accurate identification of this fracture is imperative. Once the lateral humeral condyle is exposed, it is hinged on its collateral ligament running distally to expose the fracture site (Figure 20.28a), allowing evacuation of any haematoma. With the lateral condyle in this position the exposed articular surfaces of the radius and ulna can be inspected. On occasions a concomitant small fracture of the medial coronoid process may be present; if so it can be removed at this point.

Reduction and fixation

Irrespective of the method of transcondylar lag screw placement, it is important to ensure that the fracture can be accurately reduced in the first instance. Reduction is achieved by applying digital pressure to the lateral condyle directing it into the appropriate position.

Ideally condylar reduction is maintained by the application of pointed reduction forceps across the humeral condyle (see Figure 20.28b). In skeletally immature dogs where the bone is soft, vulsellum forceps can be a useful alternative to single point reduction forceps. Alternatively, reduction can be maintained using a K-wire, across either the supracondylar region or the humeral condyle (Figure 20.28cd). A transcondylar lag screw is then placed. There are two methods of preparing the drill hole for the transcondylar lag screw: outside-in and inside-out.

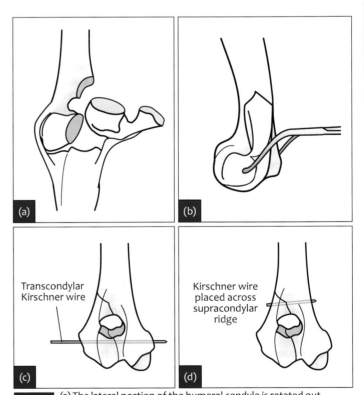

20.28 (a) The lateral portion of the humeral condyle is rotated out laterally on its collateral ligament to allow inspection of the fracture site and removal of the fracture haematoma. (b–d) Methods of maintaining reduction of lateral condylar fractures during transcondylar screw placement.

PRACTICAL TIP

Following reduction, the humeral articular surface cannot be easily observed. Its proximocaudal aspect can be inspected if the elbow joint is flexed and the anconeus muscle retracted, allowing assessment of the condylar reduction. In most cases satisfactory reduction of the humeral articular surface is more likely if the lateral supracondylar ridge fracture is also accurately reduced

→ **OPERATIVE TECHNIQUE 20.9 CONTINUED**

Reduction and reattachment of either the medial or lateral humeral condyle on to the humeral shaft followed by repair of the resultant unicondylar fracture

This technique is perhaps best suited to fracture configurations where a large supracondylar component is present. Whether the medial or lateral aspect is reconstructed is dictated by the fracture configuration and preference of individual surgeon; however, most often the medial aspect is stabilized first. **The disadvantage of this method is that if the supracondylar region is not perfectly anatomically reconstructed, it will then not be possible to anatomically reconstruct the resultant unicondylar fracture, which will result in articular surface malalignment.** Via a medial approach to the distal humerus, the medial aspect of the distal humerus is reduced and stabilized appropriately, most commonly using a bone plate and screws (Figure 20.33ab). Depending on the fracture configuration it may be possible to use lag screws, K-wires or cerclage wire to stabilize the fragment before the bone plate is applied. Subsequently, the patient is rolled over to allow a lateral approach to the distal humerus. The lateral condylar fracture is repaired appropriately as described in Operative Technique 20.7 (Figure 20.33c). In most situations the lateral supracondylar ridge fracture is stabilized using an appropriate bone plate and screws.

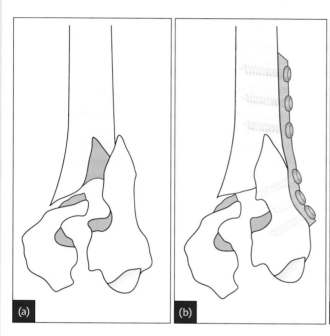

(a)   (b)   (c)

20.33 Reduction and fixation of a dicondylar fracture by reduction and reattachment of either the medial or lateral humeral condyle on to the humeral shaft followed by repair of the resultant unicondylar fracture. (a–b) The medial humeral condyle is anatomically reduced and stabilized using a bone plate. (c) Subsequently the lateral condylar fracture is repaired using a transcondylar lag screw and bone plate (see text for details).

Wound closure

As for Operative Techniques 20.4 and 20.6.

PRACTICAL TIPS

- The range of motion of the elbow in both flexion and extension should be repeatedly checked throughout surgery
- The use of non-locking screws/fixation allows flexibility in plate screw orientation, which is desirable in these fractures

---

POSTOPERATIVE MANAGEMENT

At the discretion of the surgeon, a bandage can be placed for 2 to 5 days following surgery to limit postoperative swelling. Extension of the elbow and abduction of the limb allow the bandage to be extended to the proximal humeral region. Strict rest (other than regular lead walks for toileting purposes) is recommended for the initial 4 weeks after surgery, followed by a gradual increase in controlled lead activity until re-examination of the patient at approximately 6 weeks postoperatively. Ideally, follow-up radiographs should be obtained at the time of re-examination before activity is increased further. Although the patient is strictly rested, early controlled mobilization of the limb is imperative.

OPERATIVE TECHNIQUE 20.10

Intramedullary pinning

BACKGROUND

IM pinning of the humerus is commonly used in both humeral diaphyseal and distal third humeral fractures. **The inability of an IM pin to resist rotational forces means it should not be used as the sole method of fixation and as such additional fixation is required.** In rare situations it can be combined with cerclage wire (Figure 20.34), but more commonly it is used in combination with an ESF construct (see Figure 20.8), or a bone plate and screws (see Figure 20.5). Pin placement can be either **retrograde** from the fracture site into the proximal or distal fragment or **normograde** from either the proximal or distal humerus.

PREOPERATIVE PLANNING

Radiographs of both the contralateral and fractured humerus aid surgical planning. The diameter and length of the IM pin required will be dictated by the size of the humerus, location of the fracture and fixation method being used. Historically, when an IM pin was placed as the sole device or when used in combination with cerclage wire for the repair of diaphyseal fractures, the largest diameter IM pin which filled the medullary cavity as tightly as possible was used. If an external skeletal fixator is to be used, or a pin–plate construct is to be created, the size of the IM pin must be reduced to around 35–50% of the diameter of the medullary cavity. Downsizing of the IM pin is also required when dealing with more distal humeral fractures, as it must pass through the medullary cavity of the medial supracondylar ridge and be seated in the medial humeral epicondyle (see Figures 20.8 and 20.35a). In this situation, the IM pin used should still fill the majority of the medullary cavity of the medial supracondylar ridge; an IM pin approximately 35% of the craniocaudal diameter of the distal humeral medullary cavity will fill the entire medullary cavity of the medial supracondylar ridge (Milgram *et al.*, 2012). In the cat, the absence of a supratrochlear foramen and the frequent absence of a medullary canal in the distal humerus may hinder or prevent placement of an IM pin into the medial humeral epicondyle; when a pin can be placed, only pins up to 1.6 mm in diameter can be placed safely through the medial supracondylar ridge (Langley-Hobbs and Straw, 2005). In comparison, with a more proximal fracture location in either species a larger diameter IM pin can be used, which is seated distally immediately proximal to the supratrochlear foramen (see Figures 20.34 and 20.35b). In this situation in the cat, the size of pin should be no greater than 2.4 mm (Langley-Hobbs and Straw, 2005).

POSITIONING

Lateral recumbency with the affected limb either up or down depending on whether a medial or lateral approach is being made.

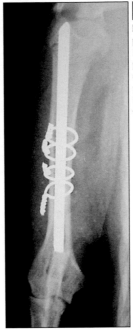

20.34 An oblique humeral fracture in a 4-month-old kitten has been stabilized using an IM pin and cerclage wire. Note how the IM pin occupies all of the narrowest part of the medullary canal. When using a pin this size it has to be seated proximal to the supratrochlear fossa in the cat and the supratrochlear foramen in the dog.

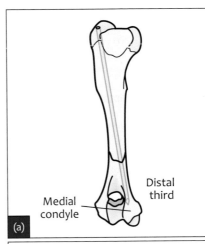

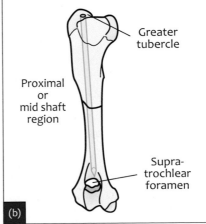

20.35 IM pin placement for humeral fractures.
(a) For more distal fractures, a smaller pin is used which is placed into the medial epicondyle.
(b) For more proximal fractures, a larger pin is used which is seated distally immediately proximal to the supratrochlear foramen.

Distal third

Medial condyle

(a)

Greater tubercle

Proximal or mid shaft region

Supra-trochlear foramen

(b)

→ **OPERATIVE TECHNIQUE 20.10 CONTINUED**

ASSISTANT

Not essential but may be helpful depending on the procedure being performed.

EQUIPMENT EXTRAS

Appropriate IM pins; pin cutters; hand chuck; drill; cerclage wire and appropriate wire instrumentation; Gelpi self-retaining retractors; reduction forceps; appropriately sized bone screw and plating kits; ESF equipment.

SURGICAL TECHNIQUES

Approach

Will depend on the specific procedure and the additional fixation system being used.

Retrograde pin placement

The IM pin is secured in an appropriate hand chuck and driven from the fracture site into the proximal fragment. The shoulder is kept flexed and the pin directed proximally towards the lateral aspect of the greater tubercle. Bone-holding forceps applied to the fragments make driving the pin easier. After the tip of the pin has penetrated and exited the proximal humerus, the Jacobs chuck is removed distally and attached to the proximal aspect of the pin, which is then withdrawn further proximally until the fracture can be reduced. The pin is then driven into the distal fracture fragment. If the pin is to be seated below the supratrochlear foramen, slight medial bowing of the fracture fragments can help direct the pin medially through the supracondylar ridge into the medial epicondyle. In distal diaphyseal or supracondylar humeral fractures, retrograde pinning of the *distal* fragment has been advocated to improve accuracy of pin placement within the medial epicondyle. However, *ex vivo* studies have shown that retrograde pinning of the distal humeral fragment can lead to penetration of the humeral condylar articular surface or peri-articular structures such as the ulnar nerve (Cohen *et al.*, 2012; Milgram *et al.*, 2012).

Normograde pin placement

The IM pin can be driven into the humerus from either its proximal or distal aspect, although the former is most common. The proximal entry point is just lateral to the greater tubercle. Once the fracture is exposed, bone-holding forceps applied to the proximal fragment make driving the pin easier. Placement and seating within the distal humeral fragment are as described for retrograde pin placement. Normograde pin insertion from the distal aspect of the medial epicondyle in the dog and cat removes the possibility of humeral condylar articular surface violation that can be associated with retrograde pinning of the distal humeral fragment.

- **Distal canine entry point** – distal aspect of the caudal part of the medial epicondyle (Milgram *et al.*, 2012) (Figure 20.36a).
- **Distal feline entry point** – immediately medial to the humeral trochlea and cranial to the caudal cortex of the medial epicondyle (Cohen *et al.*, 2012) (Figure 20.36b). In the cat accuracy is ensured by a limited open approach. Pre-drilling to create a pilot hole for the IM pin is advised, with the drill hole being directed into the centre of the medullary cavity of the distal humeral diaphysis and advanced until the medullary cavity is entered. A 1.5 mm diameter IM pin with the end bevelled and inserted using a hand chuck is recommended. Inserting the pin with the bevelled end directed against the lateral cortex prevents penetration of the distal lateral humeral cortex.

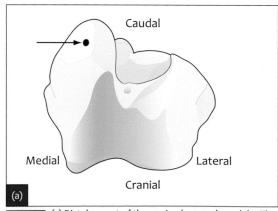
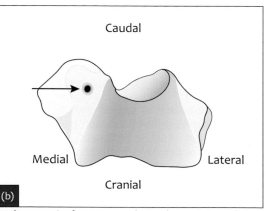

20.36 (a) Distal aspect of the canine humeral condyle. The distal entry point for normograde pin placement is on the distal aspect of the caudal part of the medial epicondyle (arrowed) (Milgram *et al.*, 2012). (b) Distal aspect of the feline humeral condyle. The distal entry hole is pre-drilled, starting immediately medial to the humeral trochlea and cranial to the caudal cortex of the medial epicondyle (arrowed) (Cohen *et al.*, 2012).

→ **OPERATIVE TECHNIQUE 20.10 CONTINUED**

> **PRACTICAL TIP**
>
> When placing an IM pin, and in particular with a comminuted fracture, great care should be employed to minimize disturbance of the fracture site to reduce any compromise of the fracture biology

When used in combination with an external skeletal fixator, the IM pin usually exits the proximal humerus and is 'tied in' to the external skeletal fixator (see Figure 20.8). In comparison, when used with cerclage wire or with a bone plate, the pin should be cut as close to the humerus as possible (see Figure 20.34). Although this can be done using pin cutters or a hacksaw, the length of IM pin required can be measured preoperatively from a radiograph of the contralateral humerus. The IM pin is cut part way through at the predetermined point using a hacksaw. Once inserted to the appropriate length the pin can be easily broken flush with the humerus. This technique is only suitable with normograde pin placement. The cut region is protected within the chuck during pin insertion until final seating is required, to prevent the pin breaking prematurely.

Wound closure

As for Operative Techniques 20.3–20.6.

POSTOPERATIVE MANAGEMENT

Will depend on the final technique which is performed.

OPERATIVE TECHNIQUE 20.11

Pin–plate application

POSITIONING

Lateral recumbency with the affected limb up if applying a lateral or cranial plate.

ASSISTANT

Not essential but may be helpful depending on the procedure being performed.

EQUIPMENT EXTRAS

Appropriate IM pins; pin cutters; hand chuck; drill; Gelpi self-retaining retractors; reduction forceps; appropriately sized bone screw and plating kits.

SURGICAL TECHNIQUES

Approach

As for Operative Technique 20.5.

> **PRACTICAL TIP**
>
> Preoperative radiographs of the contralateral humerus allow for assessment of the required IM pin diameter and length. They also allow for assessment of an appropriate size and length of bone plate, which can be pre-contoured

Reduction and fixation

Ideally, when pin–plate fixation is used the pin should extend further distally than the plate. The pin will have a better frictional interface with the cancellous bone at the proximal and distal aspect of the bone; the greater the frictional interlock between the pin and the bone, the more effective the construct. Although dependent on the fracture configuration, to achieve this in the humerus will usually require the IM pin to be directed distally through the medial supracondylar ridge into the medial epicondylar region. The bone plate is then placed on the lateral or cranial aspect of the humerus.

→

→ **OPERATIVE TECHNIQUE 20.11 CONTINUED**

An appropriately sized IM pin is placed in either a normograde or retrograde manner as described in Operative Technique 20.10. Excessive manipulation of the fracture site should be avoided. The IM pin will help axially align the main fragments and re-establish appropriate bone length.

> **PRACTICAL TIP**
>
> It may be helpful to cut the tip off the IM pin as it appears at the fracture site. The now blunt end can be used to 'push' the distal (or proximal) humeral fragment, re-establishing bone length whilst minimizing the risk of cortical bone penetration

The bone plate is then applied to the lateral or cranial aspect of the humerus (see Figure 20.5). Although the minimum number of bone screws that should be used in a plate–rod construct is unclear, it has been recommended that at least five cortices should be engaged in the proximal and distal fragments; a mix of mono- and bicortical screws can be used. Distally it is important to be sure that any screws placed in the supracondylar ridge do not interfere with the anconeal process when they exit the trans cortex and enter the supratrochlear foramen. Following plate application the IM pin is cut as close to the humerus as possible or broken off if its length was predetermined and the IM pin partially cut prior to surgery.

Wound closure

As for Operative Technique 20.5.

POSTOPERATIVE MANAGEMENT

Strict rest (other than regular lead walks for toileting purposes) for the initial 6 weeks after surgery is recommended. Follow-up examination and radiography at around 6 weeks postoperatively should be undertaken before activity is increased further. Although the patient is strictly rested, early mobilization of the limb is imperative. The implants are left in place unless they cause specific problems.

OPERATIVE TECHNIQUE 20.12

Linear external skeletal fixation of the humerus

PREOPERATIVE CONSIDERATIONS

External skeletal fixator application in the humerus is challenging. There are no safe corridors for ESF pin insertion in the humerus, although hazardous corridors (relatively safe areas) are present in both the cat (Langley-Hobbs and Straw, 2005) and the dog (Marti and Miller, 1994) in the proximal craniolateral and distal lateral epicondylar/condylar regions (Figure 20.37). As such, attention to ESF pin placement is paramount to avoid transfixation of muscle bellies and neurovascular structures. Distally in the supracondylar/epicondylar region, the ESF pins should be placed through an open approach (either the main surgical incision or via stab incisions) to ensure their placement between muscle groups and to avoid the radial nerve. The proximal location of the humerus does not allow for complex frame configurations, so the ESF construct is almost always combined with an IM pin to optimize the frame stiffness. The severity of the fracture will ultimately dictate the number of ESF pins that are placed in each of the main fracture fragments. In general, three pins can be safely placed in the proximal zone and two or three pins in the distal zone.

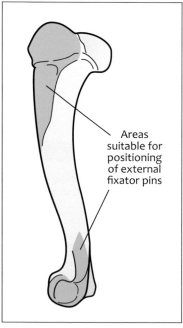

20.37 Areas suitable for ESF pin placement in the canine humerus (Marti and Miller, 1994). Similar areas are present in the feline humerus (Langley-Hobbs and Straw, 2005).

Areas suitable for positioning of external fixator pins

→ **OPERATIVE TECHNIQUE 20.12 CONTINUED**

PRACTICAL TIP

With distal diaphyseal or supracondylar fractures, where distal bone stock is limited, hybrid ESF configurations can be useful. Using linear ESF, a full pin is placed across the humeral condyle and then attached to a lateral connecting bar by a second curved connecting bar fashioned from metal or acrylic. A linear/circular system can also be used with the circular component attached to either a full transcondylar pin or transcondylar olive wires (see Figure 20.20)

POSITIONING

Lateral recumbency with the affected limb uppermost.

ASSISTANT

Not essential but may be helpful.

EQUIPMENT EXTRAS

Appropriate IM pins; pin cutters; hand chuck; drill; drill bits; Gelpi self-retaining retractors; reduction forceps; ESF equipment.

SURGICAL TECHNIQUES

Approach

As for Operative Technique 20.5.

PRACTICAL TIP

Preoperative radiographs of the contralateral humerus allow for assessment of the required IM pin diameter and length, and the size of ESF pins which will be required

Reduction and fixation

An appropriately sized IM pin is placed in either a normograde or retrograde manner as described in Operative Technique 20.10. The distal placement of the pin will be dictated by the fracture location. Excessive manipulation of the fracture site should be avoided. The IM pin will help axially align the main fragments and re-establish appropriate bone length (Figure 20.38a). Subsequently the ESF construct is applied. The most proximal and distal pins are placed first (Figure 20.38b). All pins should be pre-drilled. In distal diaphyseal humeral fractures, the most distal pin will need to be placed through the humeral condyle; this can be done through a stab incision. When a more proximal fracture is present and the distal fragment is long, the most distal pin can be placed just proximal to the supratrochlear foramen. Clamps are placed on a connecting bar and loosely attached to the ESF pins. Once fracture alignment is deemed satisfactory, the clamps are tightened. The remaining ESF pins are placed (Figure 20.38c). The transcondylar pin and the lateral epicondylar/supracondylar pins are the most challenging to place. In the cat a transcondylar pin between 1.5 and 2.2 mm should be used (Langley-Hobbs and Straw, 2005), being angled from just cranial and distal to the lateral epicondyle to exit craniodistal to the medial epicondyle. The more proximal pin(s) in the distal fragment should be placed through an open approach to ensure the radial nerve is avoided on the lateral aspect of the humerus. In the cat this pin should be angled in a distolateral to proximomedial direction, so it penetrates the bone at least 20 mm proximal to the medial epicondyle in order to avoid the supracondylar foramen and its neurovascular contents on the medial aspect of the humerus. Following placement of the ESF construct, the IM pin is generally 'tied in' to the ESF frame (Figure 20.38c).

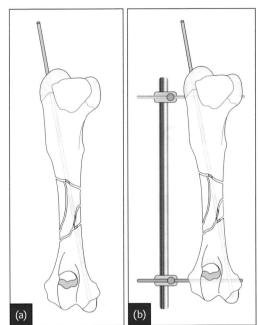

(a)　(b)

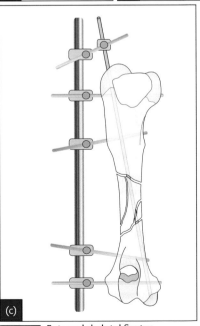

(c)

20.38 External skeletal fixator placement in combination with an IM pin (see text for details).

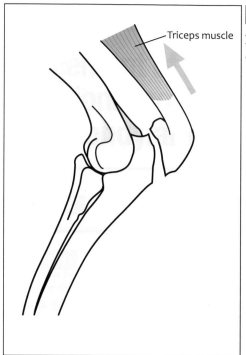

21.1 Avulsion fracture of the olecranon.

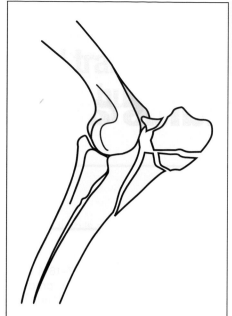

21.3 Comminuted fracture of the proximal ulna.

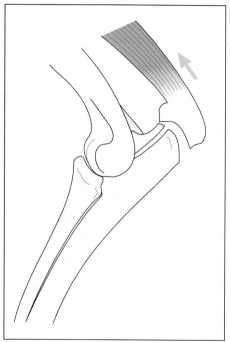

21.4 Avulsion fracture of the olecranon and fractured anconeal process.

proximal to the midpoint of the trochlear notch (Figure 21.2) can be managed with tension-band wire application, ideally with pins placed perpendicular to the fracture line and the tension-band wire applied caudally to counteract the pull of the triceps muscle (see Operative Technique 21.1). If the proximal fragment is large enough, more robust bone plate fixation can also be considered.

Comminuted ulnar fractures (Figure 21.3) and/or fractures distal to the midpoint of the trochlear notch with or without fracture to the anconeal process (Figure 21.4) are ideally reconstructed with Kirschner (K) wires and lag screws, and then stabilized with a neutralization plate (see Operative Technique 21.3). The plate can be applied caudally or laterally. An interlocking nail was successfully

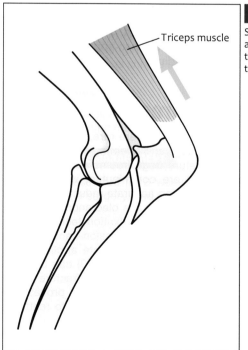

21.2 Simple, intra-articular fracture through the trochlear notch.

utilized in one reported case for stabilization of a comminuted radial and ulnar fracture where accurate reduction of fragments was not possible (Gatineau and Plante, 2010). In most cases, such an application would be challenging due to the size and shape of the bone and hence its use is restricted to larger dogs; application of a plate is preferred in most cases.

Fractures of the proximal diaphysis of the ulna with concurrent displacement of the radial head were first described in humans by Monteggia in 1814. These have been classified according to the direction of radial displacement into four types (Schwarz and Schrader, 1984):

- Type I – cranial dislocation of the radial head with concurrent fracture of the ulna (the most frequently observed configuration) (Figures 21.5 and 21.6)
- Type II – caudal dislocation of the radial head with concurrent fracture of the ulna

- Type III – lateral or craniolateral dislocation of the radial head with concurrent fracture of the ulnar diaphysis
- Type IV – cranial dislocation of the radial head with ulnar and radial diaphyseal fractures. In the immature patient it is possible to have concurrent proximal radial physeal fracture.

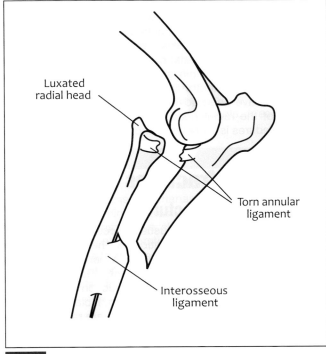

21.5 Type I Monteggia fracture.

Wadsworth (1993) suggested these fractures are caused by a direct blow to the caudal aspect of the ulna when the antebrachium is extended, usually in road traffic trauma, a fall or a bite. Displacement of the radial head occurs with stretching or tearing of the annular ligament and concurrent contraction of the biceps brachii and brachialis muscles. Separation of the radial and ulnar diaphyses may occur with interosseous ligament rupture.

Radial head chip fractures (Schwarz and Schrader, 1984) or medial coronoid process fractures may be observed in association with Monteggia fractures. The medial coronoid process appears to displace ventromedially (Figure 21.6d); this is rarely considered clinically significant. Non-reducible small radial head fragments can be excised, although their significance is unclear.

The goal of treatment is restoration of the humeroradial joint and annular ligament with reduction and stabilization of ulnar and/or radial diaphyseal fractures. Collateral ligaments should also be assessed for injury (Figure 21.7). In acute injuries where the interosseous ligament remains intact, closed reduction and normograde insertion of a pin into the ulna may be attempted. However, open reduction with internal fixation is preferred in most cases (Figure 21.6cd) (see Operative Technique 21.4).

Radial head fractures

Fortunately, fractures of the proximal metaphysis and the proximal radial growth plate are rare. Fractures to the radial head, especially those involving the articular surface, require accurate reduction and stabilization. However, the surrounding musculature can make exposure for fracture reduction challenging.

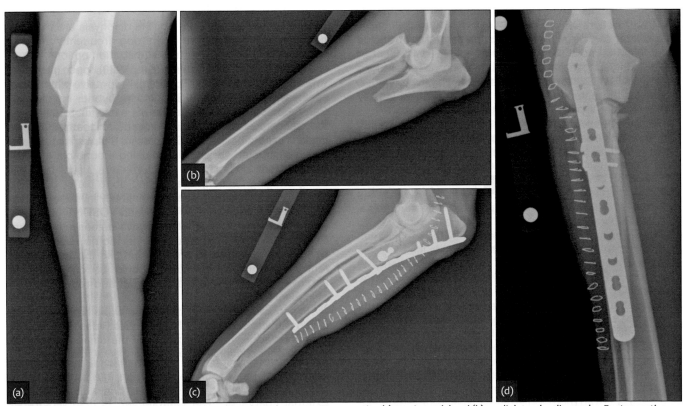

21.6 Type I Monteggia fracture in a 4-year-old, 45 kg Dobermann. Preoperative (a) craniocaudal and (b) mediolateral radiographs. Postoperative (c) mediolateral and (d) craniocaudal radiographs. The radial head was reduced in a closed fashion and the ulnar fracture stabilized with lag screws and a 3.5 mm locking compression plate. Note the fracture of the medial coronoid process ventromedial to the humeroulnar joint on the postoperative craniocaudal view.

mentioned earlier, ulnar plating is also recommended to support comminuted radial fractures that have been stabilized with plating (Figure 21.9). Concurrent stabilization of the ulna, using an IM pin or plate, is also advised in cats.

Locking plates act as 'internal fixators' (see Chapter 10). They do not rely on bone friction for stabilization and therefore act to preserve periosteal vascularization. Some pre-contouring is required to reflect the natural procurvatum of the radius, but accuracy of pre-contouring is not essential.

Long plates that span the length of the radius provide mechanical advantages over shorter plates (Figure 21.10). Long plates lower the pull-out force acting on screws because of an improvement of the working leverage for the screws and better distribution of the bending forces along the plates (Gautier and Sommer, 2003) and, when used in a minimally invasive technique (see Chapter 15), allow plate insertion sites to be away from the fracture site.

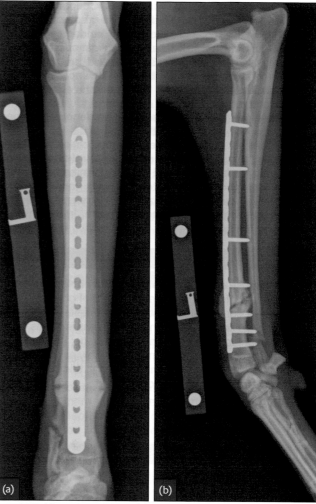

(a)　(b)

21.10 (a) Craniocaudal and (b) mediolateral radiographs taken 6 weeks postoperatively of an antebrachial fracture in a 1-year-old Lurcher, stabilized with a 16-hole 2.7 mm locking compression plate placed using the minimally invasive osteosynthesis technique.

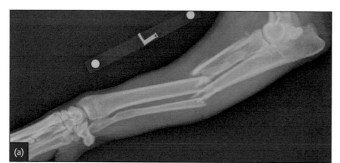

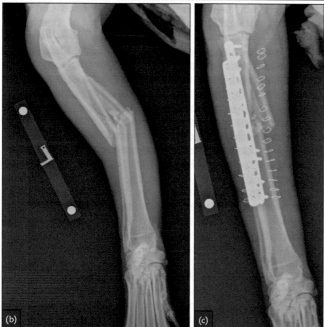

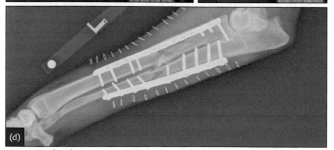

21.9 (a–b) Comminuted fracture of the radius and mid-diaphyseal fracture of the ulna in a 2-year-old German Shepherd Dog. (c–d) The fractures were stabilized with a 14-hole 2.7 mm locking compression plate applied to the cranial radius and a 10-hole 2.7/3.5 mm hybrid dynamic compression plate applied to the caudal ulna.

Diaphyseal fractures in small-breed dogs

Small-breed dogs commonly suffer short oblique or transverse fractures following low trauma. Dogs less than 12 months old are most commonly affected. These fractures have been associated with a complication rate as high as 54% (Larsen et al., 1999) and delayed or non-union has been common historically (Hunt et al., 1980). However, recent studies report better results with lower complication rates (Hamilton and Langley-Hobbs, 2005; Saikku-Backstrom et al., 2005; Haaland et al., 2009; Voss et al., 2009a).

Poor fracture healing is attributed to biomechanical and vascular factors. The small bone diameter and fracture orientation mean that there is minimal bone surface contact at reduction; furthermore, anatomical realignment is hindered by caudolateral displacement of the distal segment created by tension of the carpal and digital flexor muscles (Welch et al., 1997).

Small-breed dogs have decreased vascular density and arborization of vessels at the distal diaphyseal–metaphyseal junction compared to large-breed dogs; they may be more reliant on the nutrient artery as the dominant source for revascularization and subsequent healing (Welch et al., 1997). This is an important consideration when planning fracture management, as increased stability at the fracture site promotes recovery of medullary circulation. In addition, there is limited soft tissue cover and tissue damage during open reduction and compression of the plate against the bone can further affect blood supply to the bone, thereby leading to cortical necrosis and possible osteopenia. Therefore, any surgical intervention is aimed at providing sufficient fracture stabilization whilst limiting vascular interference. Stress protection resulting from excessive implant rigidity can further contribute to osteopenia (Field, 1997; Saikku-Backstrom et al., 2005). It has been recommended that plate removal is performed in small-breed dogs following fracture healing. However, in most cases, osteopenia appears to have minimal clinical significance compared to the risks, such as re-fracture, associated with plate removal (Bernard et al., 2008) (Figure 21.11). Therefore, although use of excessively large plates should be avoided, plate removal is rarely performed.

Multiple fracture stabilization options are reported including non-locking (Larsen et al., 1999), locking (Haaland et al., 2009), absorbable polylactide (SR-PLA 70/30) (Saikku-Backstrom et al., 2005) or T-plates (Hamilton and Langley-Hobbs, 2005), traditional ESF (Laverty et al., 2002), modified ESF using polymethylmethacrylate (PMMA)/acrylic (Bernard et al., 2008), CESF (Piras et al., 2011), tubular ESF and external coaption (DeAngelis et al., 1973; Lappin et al., 1983).

Both casting and stabilization of the radius with an IM pin are unacceptable; casting was associated with an 83% incidence of malunion and non-union, and non-union affected 100% of small-breed dogs treated with IM pins (Lappin et al., 1983). Radial and ulnar atrophy have been demonstrated in small breeds managed with external coaptation for longer than 4 weeks (DeAngelis et al., 1973).

ESF has been shown to be effective for the management of these fractures; however, pin tract problems make the complication rate somewhat variable, ranging from 4 to 50% (Muir, 1997; Hass et al., 2003). Protracted healing time

and subsequent pin loosening can be seen with both conventional and PMMA connecting bars; in addition, with PMMA bars, alterations cannot be made after application. An increased frequency of healing complications is evident in small-breed dogs managed with ESF when compared to larger breeds (Laverty et al., 2002), where 50% of patients less than 5 kg, compared to 10% greater than 5 kg, experienced complications. CESF does not appear to be associated with major complications, osteopenia or loss of carpal range of motion when applied by experienced surgeons proficient with the technique (Piras et al., 2011), although application of CESF in these smaller patients can be technically challenging.

Fractures to the radius in small-breed dogs are generally simple and rarely open, and therefore lend themselves well to internal stabilization with plates; hence this is preferred in most cases.

For very small dogs, 1 mm and 1.5 mm implants are available, which address the limited bone stock available for implant purchase. Although successful outcomes can be readily achieved using dynamic compression plates or cuttable plates, the negative effect of bone–plate contact area on periosteal vascularity can be minimized using limited-contact dynamic compression plates or locking plates. Implants of a composition with a lower modulus of elasticity (e.g. titanium alloy) limit the potential for implant-induced osteoporosis and the need for implant removal. In addition, remodelling of bone after fracture repair is more active with titanium (Field, 1997). However, titanium implants are more expensive and hence appropriately sized stainless steel implants are used in most cases.

Healing can be encouraged with cancellous autograft, allograft and osteoinductive substances (see Chapter 14); rhBMP-2 reconstituted and applied to bovine type I absorbable collagen sponge can be an effective treatment for radial bone atrophy secondary to fracture management (Bernard et al., 2008).

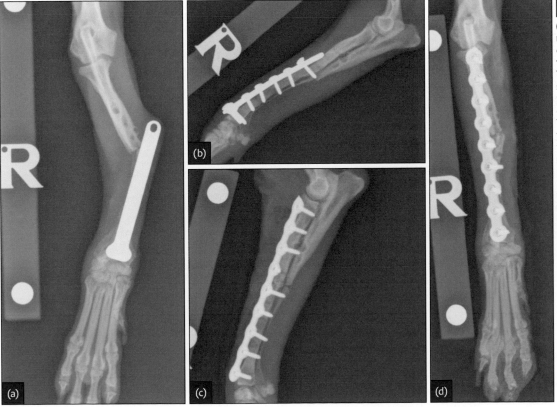

21.11
(a) Craniocaudal and (b) mediolateral radiographs of a mid-antebrachial fracture in a 3-year-old Yorkshire Terrier. Revision surgery had already been performed to replace the original implant with a T-plate; the bone then fractured through one of the original screw holes. (c) Mediolateral and (d) craniocaudal radiographs showing stabilization of the fracture with a 2mm titanium plate applied to the cranial radius.

Reported complications following bone plating in small-breed dogs include radial resorption, re-fracture through screw holes and implant failure (plate breakage or screw pull-out) with subsequent angular deformity (Larsen *et al.*, 1999; Haaland *et al.*, 2009). Minor complications can include skin erosion, stress protection osteopenia, thermal conduction, synostosis, ulnar resorption and loss of carpal flexion.

Plate breakage results from failure to reconstruct simple fractures (see Chapter 4) or from inadequate plate choice and underestimation of plate length (Haaland *et al.*, 2009); therefore, care must be taken to select an implant with sufficient length and rigidity to allow fracture healing and limb usage, but not too rigid so as to create stress protection. Complications using the locking compression plate appear to be lower (Haaland *et al.*, 2009) when compared to other osteosynthesis techniques (Hunt, 1980).

Distal radial and ulnar fractures

Distal physeal fractures

Distal physeal fractures of the radius and ulna (Figure 21.12) are relatively common in immature animals and are easily overlooked where there is minimal displacement, or where other, more obvious fractures coexist on the limb, diverting the clinician's attention. Whilst commonly attributed to a significant fall, minor trauma such as a leap from a chair can induce a physeal fracture. Prompt examination may reveal swelling at the site with associated pain on palpation. Physeal fractures may result in premature growth plate closure; owners should be warned of the possibility of subsequent limb length deficits and angular or rotational deformities. If displacement is present, early closed reduction should be attempted and may be managed with external coaptation (for around 3 weeks). Non-reducible fractures or those with persistent instability require open reduction and stabilization, most commonly using small pins (see Operative Technique 21.10).

Styloid fractures

Radial styloid fractures are often intra-articular and result in medial carpal instability, therefore requiring accurate reduction and fixation using lag screws or K-wires with a tension-band wire (Figure 21.13) (see Operative Technique 21.11).

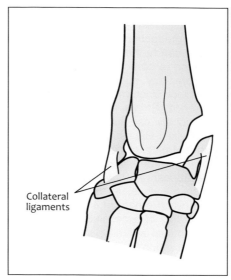

21.13 Avulsion fracture of the radial styloid process with resultant instability of the antebrachiocarpal joint; note that the fracture line is intra-articular.

Collateral ligaments

Ulnar styloid fractures usually result in lateral carpal instability and therefore require open reduction and stabilization using pins and a tension-band wire (see Operative Technique 21.11).

Distal radial metaphyseal fractures in mature dogs

Simple transverse fractures have limited distal bone stock, and access to the fracture is complicated by the presence of the extensor muscles and tendons (see Operative Technique 21.9). Where possible the fracture is reduced and stabilized using a plate applied to the dorsal or medial surface. Hybrid anatomical T-plates have tapered ends with a narrowing plate profile and smaller screw holes in the distal plate to limit extensor tendon interference. If a concurrent ulnar fracture is present it can be stabilized using an IM pin or a plate. Comminuted intra-articular fractures of the distal radius can be stabilized using lag screws with or without K-wires and plates; however, if the comminution is severe it may be necessary to consider immediate pancarpal arthrodesis.

References and further reading

Bernard F, Furneaux R, Adrega Da Silva C and Bardet JF (2008) Treatment with rhBMP-2 of extreme radial bone atrophy secondary to fracture management in an Italian Greyhound. *Veterinary and Comparative Orthopaedics and Traumatology* **21**, 64–68

DeAngelis MP, Olds RB, Stoll SG, Prata RG and Sinibaldi KR (1973) Repair of fractures of the radius and ulna in small dogs. *Journal of the American Animal Hospital Association* **9**, 436–441

Farese JP, Lewis DD, Cross AR *et al.* (2002) Use of IMEX SK-circular external fixator hybrid constructs for fracture stabilization in dogs and cats. *Journal of the American Animal Hospital Association* **38**, 279–289

Field JR (1997) Bone plate fixation: its relationship with implant induced osteoporosis. *Veterinary and Comparative Orthopaedics and Traumatology* **10**, 88–94

Garofolo S and Pozzi A (2013) Effect of plating technique on periosteal vasculature of the radius in dogs: a cadaveric study. *Veterinary Surgery* **42**, 255–261

Gatineau M and Plante J (2010) Ulnar interlocking intramedullary nail stabilization of a proximal radio-ulnar fracture in a dog. *Veterinary Surgery* **39**, 1025–1029

Gautier E and Sommer C (2003) Guidelines for the application of the LCP. *Injury* **34** Suppl 2, 63–76

Haaland PJ, Sjostrom L, Devor M and Haug A (2009) Appendicular fracture repair in dogs using the locking compression plate system: 47 cases. *Veterinary and Comparative Orthopaedics and Traumatology* **22**, 309–315

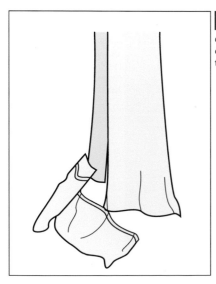

21.12 Salter–Harris type I fracture of the distal radius with concurrent fracture of the distal ulna.

Haas B, Reichler IM and Montavon PM (2003) Use of the tubular external fixator in the treatment of distal radial and ulnar fractures in small dogs and cats. *Veterinary and Comparative Orthopaedics and Traumatology* **3**, 132–137

Hamilton MH and Langley-Hobbs SJ (2005) Use of the AO veterinary mini 'T'-plate for stabilization of distal radius and ulnar fractures in toy breed dogs. *Veterinary and Comparative Orthopaedics and Traumatology* **18**, 18–24

Hunt JM, Aitken ML, Denny HR *et al.* (1980) The complications of diaphyseal fractures in dogs: a review of 100 cases. *Journal of Small Animal Practice* **21**, 103–119

Johnson AL and Schaeffer DJ (2008) Evolution of the treatment of canine radial and tibial fractures with external fixators. *Veterinary and Comparative Orthopaedics and Traumatology* **21**, 256–261

Lappin LJ, Aron DN, Herron HL and Malnati G (1983) Fractures of the radius and ulna in the dog. *Journal of the American Animal Hospital Association* **19**, 643–650

Larsen LJ, Rousch JK and McLaughlin RM (1999) Bone plate fixation of distal radius and ulna fractures in small and miniature breed dogs. *Journal of the American Animal Hospital Association* **35**, 243–250

Laverty PH, Johnson AL and Toombs JP (2002) Simple and multiple fractures of the radius treated with an external skeletal fixator. *Veterinary and Comparative Orthopaedics and Traumatology* **15**, 97–103

Lewis DD, Radasch RM, Beale BS *et al.* (1999) Initial experience with the IMEX circular external skeletal fixation system. Part I: Use in fractures and arthrodeses. *Veterinary and Comparative Orthopaedics and Traumatology* **12**, 108–117

Luc Vallone BS and Schulz K (2011) Repair of Monteggia fractures using an Arthrex Tightrope system and ulnar plating. *Veterinary Surgery* **40**, 734–737

Marti JM and Miller A (1994) Delimitation of safe corridors for the insertion of external skeletal fixator pins in the dog 2: Forelimb. *Journal of Small Animal Practice* **35**, 78–85

McLain DL and Brown SG (1982) Fixation of radius and ulna fractures in the immature dog and cat: a review of popular techniques and a report of eight cases using plate fixation. *Veterinary Surgery* **11**, 140–145

Muir P (1997) Distal antebrachial fractures in toy breeds of dogs. *Veterinary Surgery* **26**, 254–255

Piras L, Cappellari F, Peirone B and Ferretti A (2011) Treatment of fractures of the distal radius and ulna in toy breed dogs with circular external skeletal fixation: a retrospective study. *Veterinary and Comparative Orthopaedics and Traumatology* **24**, 228–235

Pozzi A, Hudson CC, Gauthier C *et al.* (2013) A retrospective comparison of minimally invasive plate osteosynthesis and open reduction and internal fixation for radius-ulna fractures in dogs. *Veterinary Surgery* **16**, 19–27

Robins GM, Eaton Wells R and Johnson K (1993) Customised hook plates for metaphyseal fractures, nonunions and osteotomies in the dog and cat. *Veterinary and Comparative Orthopaedics and Traumatology* **6**, 56–61

Saikku-Backstrom A, Raiha JE, Valimaa T *et al.* (2005) Repair of radial fractures in toy breed dogs with self reinforced biodegradable plates, metal screws, and light weight external coaptation. *Veterinary Surgery* **34**, 11–17

Sardinas JC and Montavon PM (1997) Use of a medial bone plate for repair of radius and ulna fractures in dogs and cats: a report of 22 cases. *Veterinary Surgery* **26**, 108–113

Schwarz PD and Schrader SC (1984) Ulnar fracture and dislocation of the proximal radial epiphysis (Monteggia lesion) in the dog and cat: a review of 28 cases. *Journal of the American Veterinary Medical Association* **185**, 190–194

Voss K, Kull M, Hassig M and Montavon P (2009a) Repair of long bone fractures in cats and small dogs with the Unilock mandible locking plate system. *Veterinary and Comparative Orthopaedics and Traumatology* **22**, 398–405

Voss K, Langley Hobbs SJ and Montavon PM (2009b). Elbow joint. In: *Feline Orthopaedic Surgery and Musculoskeletal Disease, 1st edn*, pp. 359–370. WB Saunders, Philadelphia

Wadsworth PL (1993) Biomechanics of luxation. In: *Disease Mechanisms in Small Animal Surgery, 2nd edn*, ed. MJ Bojrab, pp. 1048–1059. Lea and Febiger, Philadelphia

Wallace AM, De La Puerta B, Trayhorn D *et al.* (2009) Feline combined diaphyseal radial and ulnar fractures. *Veterinary and Comparative Orthopaedics and Traumatology* **22**, 38–46

Wallace MK, Boudrieau RJ, Hyodo K *et al.* (1992) Mechanical evaluation of three methods of plating distal radial osteotomies. *Veterinary Surgery* **21**, 108–113

Welch JA, Boudrieau RJ, Dejardin LM and Spodnick GJ (1997) The intraosseous blood supply of the canine radius: implications for healing of distal fractures in small dogs. *Veterinary Surgery* **26**, 57–61

OPERATIVE TECHNIQUE 21.1

Tension-band application to the proximal ulna

BACKGROUND

Tension-band wiring is suitable for simple fractures of the olecranon proximal to the mid-point of the trochlear notch. In the dog, the ulna is wide proximally and narrows distally with torsion. In the cat, the ulna is thicker than the radius; however, the olecranon is relatively shorter and its caudal surface curves cranially.

POSITIONING

Dorsal recumbency (hanging limb preparation; Figure 21.14). Flex the affected elbow (Figure 21.15) and make a caudolateral approach or extend it cranially and make a caudomedial approach (Figure 21.16). Rolling the patient into lateral recumbency with the affected limb uppermost may be useful when making the caudolateral approach.

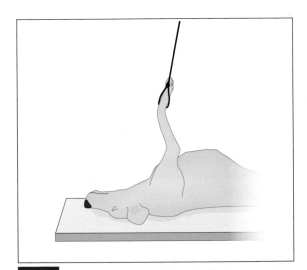

21.14 Dorsal recumbency with hanging limb preparation.

→ **OPERATIVE TECHNIQUE 21.1 CONTINUED**

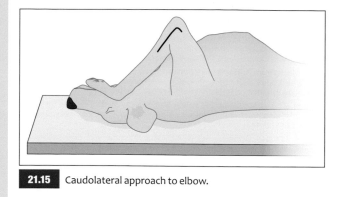

21.15 Caudolateral approach to elbow.

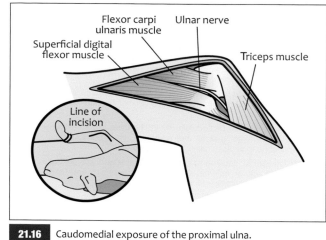

21.16 Caudomedial exposure of the proximal ulna.

ASSISTANT

Ideally.

EQUIPMENT EXTRAS

K-wires (diameter appropriate to size of ulna and the ability to insert two pins in parallel); chuck; drill and drill bits; cerclage wire (0.8 mm diameter for cats and small dogs, 1–1.2 mm for medium to large dogs); wire twisters; pin cutters; bone-holding forceps; periosteal elevator; ± bone plate and screw set; ± parallel drill guide.

SURGICAL TECHNIQUES

Approach

For a caudolateral approach (see Figure 21.15), the skin is incised from the lateral humeral epicondyle along the caudolateral border of the olecranon. Continue the incision through the subcutaneous layer and along the fascial attachment of the ulnaris lateralis muscle laterally to expose the bone surface.

Alternatively, make a caudomedial skin incision (see Figure 21.16) and retract the skin laterally. Continue the incision through the subcutaneous layer and elevate the flexor carpi ulnaris and deep digital flexor muscles.

Reduction and fixation

Parallel K-wires are drilled retrograde from the fracture site, ideally perpendicular to the fracture line. The proximal ulna is held with bone-holding forceps and the first pin is driven from the fracture surface to exit proximolaterally (Figure 21.17a). The pin is backed out until the tip is at the fracture site, and the second pin placed to exit proximomedially (Figure 21.17b). The elbow is extended to facilitate reduction (Figure 21.17c). Once the fracture has been reduced, each pin is driven into the distal ulnar segment to exit the cranial cortex distal to the trochlear notch (Figure 21.17d). A transverse hole is drilled through the caudal ulna distal to the fracture site, at a distance of one to one and a half times the length of the proximal ulnar segment. A double twist, figure-of-eight tension-band wire is applied. One piece of wire is passed under the triceps tendon cranial to the K-wires. These free ends are twisted with a second piece of wire passed through the transverse bone tunnel (Figure 21.17e). The wire should contact the bone under the triceps muscle and the K-wires. The K-wire tips are bent over close to the end of the olecranon, then rotated cranially so that the bent end of the pin lies over the tension-band wire, and close to the bone (ideally medial or lateral to the triceps tendon to avoid irritation by the pin ends).

In smaller dogs and cats, a single pin placed within the IM canal and a wire tension-band may be sufficient. However, if this technique is used, the fracture should be oblique and interlocking to prevent rotational instability, and the pin should extend the length of the proximal third of the ulnar diaphysis.

PRACTICAL TIPS

- When placing larger sized pins, pre-drill a pilot hole with a smaller diameter drill bit as the proximal ulnar bone is very dense
- In smaller breeds it is advantageous to place the pins in the sagittal plane rather than the frontal plane because of their smaller bone diameter. One pin is placed retrograde, the fracture is reduced and a second more caudal pin is placed normograde parallel to the first using a parallel drill guide (Figure 21.18)
- In the cat, the shape of the ulna makes it difficult for fixation pins to be directed into the distocranial ulnar cortex; therefore, they are inserted into the ulnar medullary canal (Voss *et al.*, 2009b)

→ **OPERATIVE TECHNIQUE 21.1 CONTINUED**

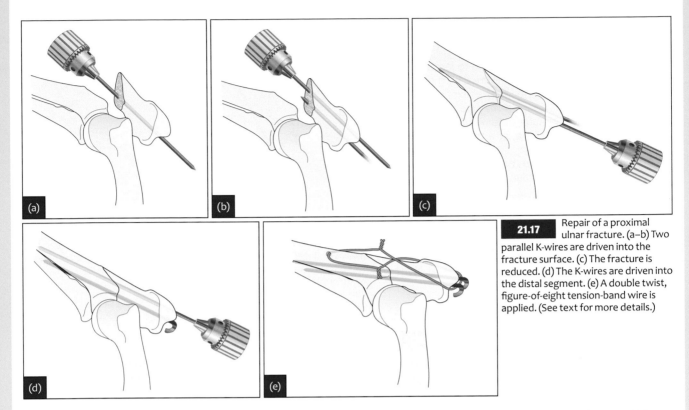

21.17 Repair of a proximal ulnar fracture. (a–b) Two parallel K-wires are driven into the fracture surface. (c) The fracture is reduced. (d) The K-wires are driven into the distal segment. (e) A double twist, figure-of-eight tension-band wire is applied. (See text for more details.)

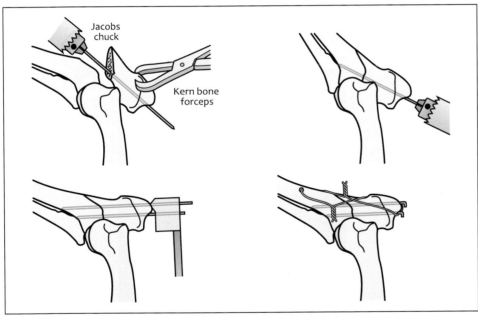

21.18 Repair of a proximal ulnar fracture using pins and a tension-band wire applied with a parallel drill guide. Following reduction of the fracture and placement of the first pin, the second pin is placed using the parallel drill guide.

WARNING

Take care to identify the position of the ulnar nerve and protect it as it runs immediately caudal to the medial humeral epicondyle

Alternative techniques

- The tension-band wire can be placed through a bone tunnel proximally rather than around the pins, to avoid entrapment or irritation of the triceps tendon (Figure 21.19).
- A lagged cortical or cancellous screw can be used in combination with a tension-band wire (Figure 21.20).

→ **OPERATIVE TECHNIQUE 21.1 CONTINUED**

- A neutralization plate applied to the caudal ulna in addition to a K-wire and tension-band wire gives
  additional stabilization in medium to large-breed or over-active dogs (Figure 21.21).
- In active patients or if the internal fixation is tenuous, additional support may be provided with a temporary circular external skeletal fixator applied to the ulna, or a transarticular frame (Figure 21.22).
- A compression plate can be applied to the caudal ulna (see Operative Technique 21.2, Figure 21.23).

Wound closure

Closely appose the external fascia of the flexor carpi ulnaris and ulnaris lateralis muscles. Place a continuous suture into the subcutaneous layer followed by routine closure of the skin.

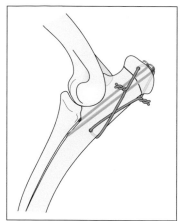
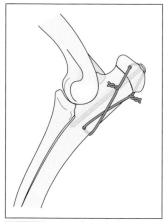

21.19 Olecranon fracture stabilized with K-wire and tension-band wire, with orthopaedic wire placed through bone tunnels in the olecranon and ulnar metaphysis distal to the fracture line.

21.20 Lagged cortical or cancellous screw plus tension-band wire.

POSTOPERATIVE MANAGEMENT AND COMPLICATIONS

Place a Robert Jones dressing immediately postoperatively to limit distal limb swelling. Remove at 48 hours and replace if necessary. Confine to a cage or small room for 6 weeks with controlled lead exercise for 8–12 weeks; include physical therapy to maintain joint range of motion. Repeat radiography at 6–8 weeks to check implant positioning and demonstrate fracture healing. Remove implants as required.

The prognosis is good where appropriate stabilization has been performed. Attention to postoperative rehabilitation is important to assist recovery or elbow range of motion where intra-articular fracture has occurred.

Complications include pin loosening, migration and soft tissue irritation necessitating implant removal.

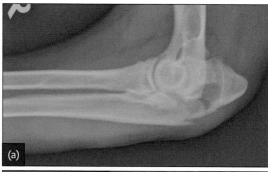
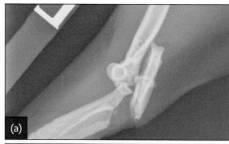
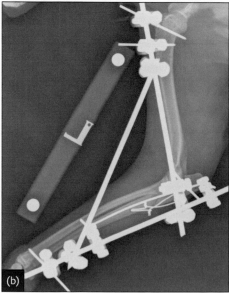

21.22 (a) Type II Monteggia fracture in a 3-year-old cat. (b) Closed radial head reduction was performed and the ulnar fracture stabilized with an IM pin, figure-of-eight tension-band wire and transarticular fixator.

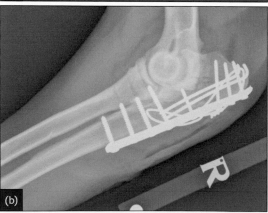

21.21 (a) Intra-articular trochlear notch fracture in a 2-year-old Bernese Mountain Dog. (b) The fracture was stabilized with two parallel K-wires, a figure-of-eight tension-band wire and a caudally applied 3.5 mm dynamic compression plate in neutralization function.

OPERATIVE TECHNIQUE 21.2

Plate application to the caudal ulna for simple fractures

POSITIONING

Dorsal recumbency or lateral recumbency with the affected limb uppermost.

ASSISTANT

Ideally.

EQUIPMENT EXTRAS

Bone-holding forceps; periosteal elevator; Hohmann retractors; bone plate and screw set.

SURGICAL TECHNIQUES

Approach

Caudolateral approach to the proximal ulna (see Operative Technique 21.1). Extend distally along the ulnar diaphysis as necessary.

Reduction and fixation

Following reduction, the plate is accurately contoured and applied to the caudal aspect of the ulna (tension side) to resist the pull of the triceps muscle (Figure 21.23). In some dogs, especially chondrodystrophic breeds, application of a plate to the lateral rather than the caudal aspect of the proximal ulna is more straightforward (see Figure 21.26)

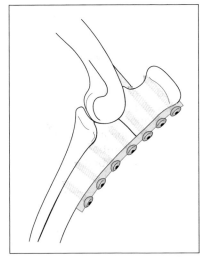

21.23 Trochlear notch intra-articular fracture (single) stabilized with a caudal compression plate.

> **PRACTICAL TIP**
>
> Pre-measure screw depth from radiographs to avoid breaching the ulnar articular surface or caudal radial cortex. Supination and pronation movement will lead to irritation and screw loosening if screws penetrate the radius

> **WARNING**
>
> Do not underestimate the forces exerted by the pull of the triceps muscle. Inadequate plate size will result in implant failure

Wound closure

Closely appose the external fascia of the flexor carpi ulnaris and ulnaris lateralis muscles. Place a continuous suture into the subcutaneous layer followed by routine closure of the skin.

POSTOPERATIVE MANAGEMENT

Place a Robert Jones dressing immediately postoperatively to limit distal limb swelling. Remove at 48 hours and replace if necessary. Confine to a cage or small room for 6 weeks with controlled lead exercise for 8–12 weeks; include physical therapy to maintain joint range of motion. Repeat radiography at 6–8 weeks to check implant positioning and demonstrate fracture healing. Remove implants as required.

The prognosis is good where appropriate stabilization has been performed. Caudally applied plates can cause irritation at their proximal aspect, so it is preferable to use low profile plates. Attention to postoperative rehabilitation is important to assist recovery or elbow range of motion where intra-articular fracture has occurred.

OPERATIVE TECHNIQUE 21.4

Fractures of the ulna with concurrent luxation of the radial head (Monteggia fractures)

POSITIONING

Lateral recumbency with affected limb up.

ASSISTANT

Ideally.

EQUIPMENT EXTRAS

K-wires; chuck; drill and drill bits; wire twisters; pin cutters; bone-holding forceps; periosteal elevator; Gelpi self-retaining retractors; Hohmann retractors; IM pins; bone plate and screw set; plate-bending irons.

SURGICAL TECHNIQUES

Approach

Combined caudolateral approach to the ulna (see Operative Technique 21.1) with lateral approach to the radius (see Operative Technique 21.5) for radial head reduction if required. The integrity of the interosseous ligament limits motion between the radius and ulna and as such can be used to assist fracture stabilization. The feline antebrachium lacks a strong interosseous ligament. The annular ligament encircles the radial head and is attached to the lateral and medial extremities of the radial incisure of the ulna and to the humeral epicondyle on the lateral side (Voss *et al.*, 2009b). The annular ligament together with the joint capsule, lateral and medial collateral ligaments stabilizes the humeroradial joint.

Reduction and fixation

Reduce the radial head by sliding it medially over the humeral condyle with the elbow in a flexed position. Where closed reduction is not possible, perform an open craniolateral approach to the radial head, then perform the same manoeuvre or gently lever a Freer elevator between the radial head and humeral condyle to reduce the radial head. Care must be taken to remove any interposed soft tissues, bone fragments or organized haematoma. Place pointed bone-holding forceps across the radius and ulna for temporary compression and reduction (Figure 21.28). Where possible, repair the annular ligament with sutures. The radius can be transfixed to the ulna with a cortical screw if required; drill holes are made from the caudal ulna into the radial head. Screws can be left slightly long, to facilitate removal in case of screw breakage. Alternatively, transfixation can be achieved with a small pin (for a small dog or cat), or a hemi-cerclage wire or nylon leader line suture placed through bone tunnels in the proximal radius and ulna. If collateral ligament injuries are also present, replacement of these ligaments with prostheses placed through bone tunnels in the

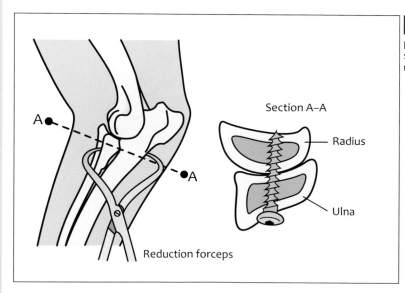

Section A–A

Radius

Ulna

Reduction forceps

21.28 Managing Monteggia fractures. Once reduced, the radial head can be temporarily held in position using pointed reduction forceps. The cross-section shows the position of a transfixing screw to maintain the reduction during healing.

→ **OPERATIVE TECHNIQUE 21.4 CONTINUED**

radius and humerus can be effective, particularly in small dogs or cats (see Figure 21.7). The ulnar fracture can be stabilized with a pin and tension-band wire, (Figure 21.29; also see Figure 21.7) or a plate and screws (see Figure 21.6) with one screw being placed into the radial head if required (Figure 21.30).

- If the ulnar fracture is proximal, the interosseous membrane, annular and interosseous ligaments may be intact. Consequently, if the ulnar fracture can be anatomically reconstructed it may not be necessary to place additional implants into the radius for stabilization, even when the radius appears significantly displaced on the preoperative radiographs (see Figure 21.6).
- If the radial head can be reduced in a closed fashion, the ulnar fracture can be reduced and stabilized with a plate or IM pin.
- Where the ulnar fracture is distal in position, the interosseous and/or annular ligament is likely to be disrupted; therefore, transfixation of the radius to the ulna is required.
- Stability of the annular ligament and collateral ligaments of the elbow joint should be checked after reduction of the radial head and ulnar fracture stabilization.

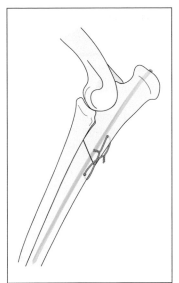

21.29 Monteggia fracture with the proximal ulnar fracture stabilized with an IM pin and figure-of-eight tension-band wire.

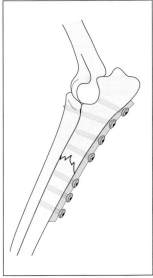

21.30 Monteggia fracture with the proximal ulnar fracture stabilized with a caudally applied plate with one screw placed into the radial head.

WARNING

In immature patients transfixation of the radius and ulna may interfere with independent growth of each bone leading to elbow joint incongruity and antebrachial growth deformities. In addition, pronation–supination movement is likely to break screws placed through the ulna into the radius. Therefore, removal of radioulnar fixation implants at 4 weeks is recommended

PRACTICAL TIP

In cats the radial head can be stabilized with a 1.5 mm positional screw placed from the caudal ulna into the radial head immediately distal to the radioulnar joint surface, so as to avoid the narrow radial isthmus. Alternatively, a suture can be placed through a transverse bone tunnel in the proximal radius to a bone tunnel through the ulna. Simple fractures of the ulna can be stabilized with a figure-of-eight interfragmentary wire applied caudally, an IM pin or a laterally applied plate. Comminuted ulnar fractures are best stabilized with a plate

Alternative technique

The radial head can be maintained in reduction using a toggle and suture system placed between the radius and ulna (Luc Vallone and Schulz, 2011). This is technically less challenging than placement of sutures through transverse bone tunnels, and avoids the potential risk of radioulnar screw breakage.

Wound closure

Close the external fascia of the flexor carpi ulnaris and ulnaris lateralis muscles together. Subcutaneous tissues are closed with a continuous suture pattern followed by routine closure of the skin.

POSTOPERATIVE MANAGEMENT AND COMPLICATIONS

Place a Robert Jones dressing immediately postoperatively to limit distal limb swelling. Remove at 48 hours and replace if necessary. Confine to a cage or small room for 6 weeks with controlled lead exercise for 8 to 12 weeks; include physical therapy to maintain joint range of motion. Where fractures are intra-articular close attention should be paid to elbow function, particularly range of motion. Remove transfixing screws at 3 to 4 weeks postoperatively.

The prognosis is reportedly guarded due to the high incidence of postoperative complications, which include recurrent subluxation of the radial head, fracture non-union, osteomyelitis, traumatic periarticular ossification, osteoarthritis, reduced elbow joint range of motion, nerve damage, synostosis and implant failure (Schwarz and Schrader, 1984).

In the author's experience, the prognosis is better where the interosseous attachments of the radius to the ulna are preserved.

OPERATIVE TECHNIQUE 21.5

Fractures of the proximal radius

POSITIONING

Dorsal recumbency with the affected limb draped to include the shoulder to the carpus, as this enables easier intraoperative assessment of limb alignment (Figure 21.31).

ASSISTANT

Ideally.

EQUIPMENT EXTRAS

K-wires; chuck; drill and drill bits; wire twisters; pin cutters; bone-holding forceps; periosteal elevator; Gelpi self-retaining retractors; Hohmann re-tractors; bone plate and screw set; plate benders; ESF set.

SURGICAL TECHNIQUES

Approach

Craniolateral approach to the proximal radius (Figure 21.32). Make a skin excision from the lateral epicondyle extending distally along the lateral edge of the radius. Continue dissection through the antebrachial fascia and into the intermuscular septum between the extensor carpi radialis and common digital extensor muscles. The extensor carpi radialis muscle is retracted craniomedially and the common and lateral digital extensor muscle groups caudolaterally. The common digital extensor muscle may be incised and retracted and the supinator muscle can be elevated off the radius from the distal insertion site.

> ### WARNING
>
> Note the position of the radial nerve deep to the extensor carpi radialis muscle

If greater exposure is required, make a concurrent medial approach and/or osteotomy of the lateral epicondyle to include the extensor tendons so they can be lifted to expose the fracture site.

Salter–Harris type I fracture

Reduce the fracture with the elbow in flexion. Stabilize with crossed K-wires (Figure 21.33). Drive a K-wire from the proximolateral radial head across the physis and distally into the medial radial cortex. Drive a second K-wire proximally from the lateral aspect of the radial metaphysis across the physis into the medial epiphysis (via the same lateral surgical approach), or from the proximomedial radial head laterodistally into the lateral radial cortex (following a limited proximo-medial approach to the radial head). Bend the tip of each K-wire so the pin is flush with the bone. Cut the tips.

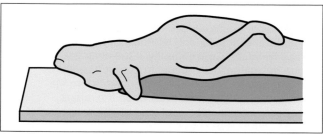

21.31 Repair of proximal radial fractures: the patient is positioned in dorsal recumbency with caudal extension of the affected limb along the body.

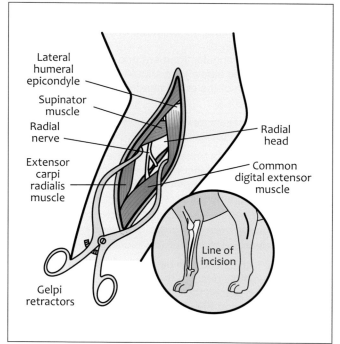

21.32 Repair of proximal radial fractures: lateral exposure of the proximal radius.

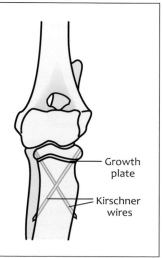

21.33 Repair of a Salter–Harris type I fracture of the proximal radius using crossed K-wires.

→ **OPERATIVE TECHNIQUE 21.5 CONTINUED**

Simple transverse fractures

Simple transverse fractures of the proximal radius can be stabilized with a locking plate or T-plate (1.5, 2, 2.7 mm) applied to the cranial surface. Implant selection depends on available bone stock.

Articular fractures

These require accurate reduction and can be stabilized with lag screws ± K-wires. More complex fractures may require reduction with lag screws or K-wires and the support of a neutralization or buttress plate.

Proximal comminuted fractures of the radius and ulna

These fractures can be challenging where insufficient bone stock is present in the proximal radius. Fixation options include:

- Sole stabilization of the ulna with a plate along the caudal surface of the ulna only
- Type 1 ESF construct attached proximally to the ulna and distally to the radius
- Hybrid ESF construct with stretch ring at the elbow (open aspect of arch cranially), with linear components extending proximally and distally.

Wound closure

Close the external fascia of the extensor carpi radialis muscle to the common digital extensor muscle in a continuous pattern. Subcutaneous tissues are closed with a continuous suture pattern followed by routine closure of the skin.

POSTOPERATIVE MANAGEMENT

Place a Robert Jones dressing immediately postoperatively to limit limb swelling. Remove at 48 hours and replace if necessary. Articular fractures and comminuted fractures, particularly where sole stabilization of the ulna is performed, need external coaptation for 4 to 6 weeks depending on the rigidity required. Confine to a cage or small room for 6 weeks with controlled lead exercise for 8 to 12 weeks; include physical therapy to maintain joint range of motion.

Fractures of the proximal radial epiphysis require exercise restriction for 4 weeks postoperatively. Healing is rapid, so the K-wires can usually be removed 4 weeks postoperatively.

The prognosis depends on the type of fracture and the accuracy of reconstruction. Metaphyseal growth plate fractures carry the best prognosis; however, premature closure and short radius syndrome is possible. Osteoarthritis and reduced elbow range of motion are possible where intra-articular fracture is present. Infection, implant failure, delayed union or non-union are possible complications.

OPERATIVE TECHNIQUE 21.6

Ulnar diaphyseal fractures – intramedullary pinning

POSITIONING

Dorsal recumbency. Flex the affected elbow or extend it cranially. For distal fractures, the patient can be positioned in lateral recumbency.

ASSISTANT

Ideally.

EQUIPMENT EXTRAS

IM pins; chuck; drill and drill bits; cerclage wire; wire twisters; pin cutters; bone-holding forceps; periosteal elevator; Gelpi self-retaining retractors; Hohmann retractors.

→ **OPERATIVE TECHNIQUE 21.6 CONTINUED**

SURGICAL TECHNIQUES

Approach

A small limited caudolateral approach to the ulna is made. Elevate the flexor carpi ulnaris and deep digital flexor muscles medially and the ulnaris lateralis muscle laterally as necessary to expose the fracture site.

Reduction and fixation

The implant is easier to introduce retrograde from the fracture site. It is driven proximally to exit the proximal ulna immediately to one side of the triceps tendon. Reduce the fracture and drive the pin into the distal segment. As the end engages the distal ulna it will distract the fracture ends, which will assist reduction of the radial fracture. If the ulnar pin is maintained for additional fixation, the proximal end is cut and bent to lie flat against the proximal olecranon (Figure 21.34) to avoid tendon irritation for later removal as necessary. Alternatively, the pin can be countersunk. The pin is 50% pre-cut with a hacksaw and then gently driven into the proximal ulna using a hand chuck. The hand chuck is withdrawn along the pin and the pin driven further to ensure the cut is within the proximal olecranon. Gentle bending of the proximal pin encourages breakage at the pre-cut point within the bone or flush with its surface. If protruding it can be seated deeper with a punch and mallet.

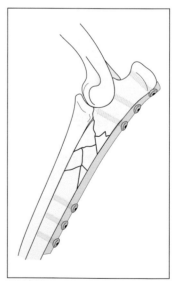

21.34 Simple distal ulnar fracture stabilized with an IM pin.

> **PRACTICAL TIPS**
>
> - The size of pin selected should fit the narrow distal medullary canal
> - When placing large IM pins, pre-drill a pilot hole in the olecranon with a smaller diameter drill bit
> - The pin can be placed retrograde from the fracture site or normograde from the proximocaudal olecranon distal to the point of insertion of the triceps tendon and directed into the distal bone segment; implant size is 1–1.4 mm

Alternative techniques

- The IM pin can be introduced in a closed fashion from the proximal surface of the olecranon and driven normograde to the fracture site. The pin must be maintained parallel to the lateral ulnar cortex to ensure it remains in the medullary canal.
- Plate application to the lateral or caudal ulna is possible (Figure 21.35; also see Figure 21.9). Where plates are used on the radius and ulna in combination, the size of each implant can be reduced.

> **PRACTICAL TIP**
>
> In the cat, plate application to the flat wide aspect of the lateral diaphysis is easier

Wound closure

Routine closure of the fascia between the flexor carpi ulnaris and ulnaris lateralis muscles proximally, and lateral digital extensor muscle distally.

POSTOPERATIVE MANAGEMENT

As for radial diaphyseal fractures (see Operative Techniques 21.7 and 21.8).

21.35 Comminuted proximal ulnar fracture stabilized with caudal plate application in bridging function.

OPERATIVE TECHNIQUE 21.7

Radial diaphyseal fractures – external fixation

POSITIONING

Dorsal recumbency (hanging limb positioning; see Figure 21.14). With the paw attached to a hook in the ceiling, the table can be lowered so that the patient is suspended by the affected limb; therefore, the weight of the patient is used to distract the fracture. The limb can remain in this position for surgery or be dropped for handling by the surgeon.

ASSISTANT

Ideally.

EQUIPMENT EXTRAS

Appropriate ESF sets and transfixation pins; connecting rods; spanners; drill and drill bits; chuck and key; K-wire driver; drill guides; periosteal elevator; reduction forceps; Gelpi self-retaining retractors.

SURGICAL TECHNIQUES

Approach

Limited craniomedial approach to the radial fracture site as required; stab incisions for transfixation pin placement.

Reduction and fixation

As well as the hanging limb positioning, other fracture reduction techniques such as toggling can be used (see Chapter 11). Once applied the ESF frame can be used to distract and align the fracture segments (Figure 21.36).

Consideration of safe corridors (Marti and Miller, 1994) for pin placement is essential. The distal two-thirds of the medial radius is reportedly the only safe corridor for pin placement. The proximal third of the radius is covered by the pronator teres muscle medially and the supinator muscle craniolaterally, which is in turn covered by the extensor muscles laterally. The largest diameter of the radius in the dog lies in a 45-degree oblique craniomedial to caudolateral plane. Conversely, the largest diameter of the feline radius lies in the mediolateral plane. Techniques for pin placement and frame construction are described in Chapter 11.

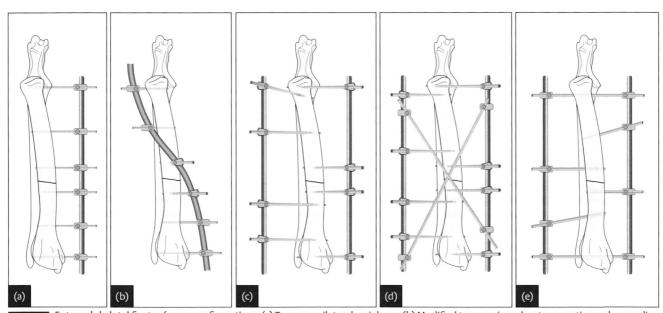

21.36 External skeletal fixator frame configurations. (a) Type 1a; unilateral, uniplanar. (b) Modified type 1 using a bent connecting rod or acrylic tubing. (c) Modified type 1b; unilateral, biplanar. (d) The addition of connecting rods joining the two type 1 elements increases the strength of the type 1b configuration. (e) Modified type 2b with full pins proximally and distally, and half pins distributed along the length of the bone.

→ **OPERATIVE TECHNIQUE 21.8 CONTINUED**

SURGICAL TECHNIQUES

Approach

The radial diaphysis is exposed by a standard skin incision along the craniomedial aspect (Figure 21.37) immediately lateral to the cephalic vein so that this neurovascular bundle can be retracted medially. The antebrachial fascia beneath the skin protects the cephalic vein, two branches of the cranial superficial antebrachial artery and two branches of the superficial radial nerve.

Proximally, extend the incision to reflect the extensor tendons laterally and reveal the pronator teres muscle. This muscle can be elevated from the proximal radius if necessary. Take care as the radial nerve is deep to the supinator muscle.

Distally, continue the incision lateral to the cephalic vein and reflect the neurovascular bundle medially, then reflect the extensor tendons laterally.

For fractures of the proximal radius, a craniolateral approach between the extensor carpi radialis muscle and the common digital extensor muscle is preferred (Figure 21.38). This approach allows concurrent exposure of the ulna. Caution should be exercised as the radial nerve may be encountered crossing the proximolateral aspect of the radius (see Figure 21.32).

Fracture reduction

Techniques for fracture reduction are described in Chapter 11. In addition, the patient's limb can be suspended from a hook during surgical preparation. Subsequent lowering of the surgical table uses the patient's own bodyweight to distract the fracture and fatigue muscle contraction. Placement of an IM pin into the ulnar fracture, a simple two-ring CESF or a type 1 ESF construct will also assist reduction (see Chapter 15).

Cranial plate application

When applied to the cranial surface of the radius, a non-locking plate can be used to reduce and align the fracture. This is particularly useful where the fracture is distal in position and the contracted extensor muscles interfere with reduction. The plate is first secured distally and can then be used to lever the distal segment into position. This requires careful central positioning of the most distal screw, which is not fully tightened until reduction is complete. If reduction remains difficult a second screw can be applied adjacent to the fracture site, the screws tightened to secure the plate to the bone, and leverage applied.

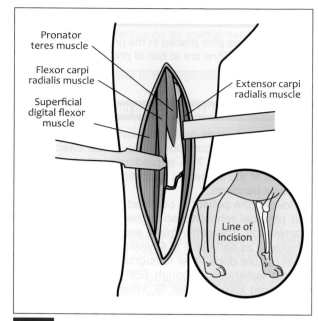

21.37 Craniomedial exposure of the radial diaphysis.

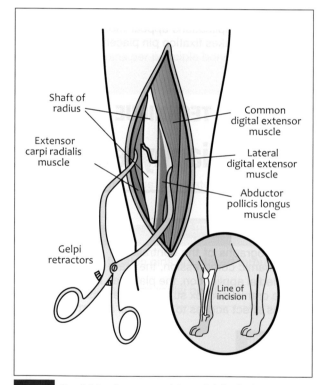

21.38 Craniolateral exposure of the radial diaphysis.

PRACTICAL TIP

In distal or comminuted fractures where the plate is applied dorsally, retraction of the extensor tendons laterally can lead to inadvertent stabilization of the fracture in external rotation or valgus. This can be avoided by positioning the plate under the extensor tendons and making a small incision in the dorsal antebrachial fascia between the common digital extensor tendons and the extensor carpi radialis muscles for screw insertion. Check for alignment throughout the procedure

→ **OPERATIVE TECHNIQUE 21.8 CONTINUED**

Medial plate application

A skin incision is made along the medial aspect of the radius. Take care to maintain the cephalic vein as it crosses distally. Continue the incision through the antebrachial fascia and along the medial fascia of the abductor pollicis longus muscle and elevate as necessary. Mobilization of the extensor tendons is not required. The fracture is reduced and the plate applied in a standard fashion.

PRACTICAL TIP

When plating immature patients, take care to protect the growth plate, avoid excessive stripping of the periosteum (because this results in exuberant callus) and avoid placing screws through the radius into the ulna

---

Implant selection

Fracture planning is essential to avoid stress protection of the bone by the plate (where oversized implants are used) or implant failure (where undersized implants are used). The width of the plate should not exceed the width of the radius. In dogs screw size should not exceed 30% of the bone diameter when placed craniocaudally, or the medullary cavity diameter when placed mediolaterally.

Wound closure

Routine closure of the antebrachial fascia with a simple continuous suture pattern. This is more difficult distally. Routine closure of the skin.

POSTOPERATIVE MANAGEMENT AND COMPLICATIONS

Place a Robert Jones dressing immediately postoperatively to limit distal limb swelling and environmental contamination. Remove at 48 hours and replace if necessary.

The majority of cases repaired with dorsally applied plates return to good function postoperatively. Bone healing is evident at 6 weeks but generally incomplete in mature dogs. Giant breeds are more prone to plate breakage, probably due to their size and the extreme forces placed on the implants; therefore, appropriate implant selection is imperative. Additional stabilization of the ulna, using an IM pin or a plate, can be considered in larger active dogs or when the radial fracture is comminuted (Figure 21.39).

Medial plating is successful in the management of simple transverse fractures, but its use in complex fractures is not documented. Reduced bone–plate contact with medial plate application decreases rotational stability, which may lead to unstable fracture repair where plates are applied in a bridging function for the management of comminuted fractures. This problem can be overcome by applying additional fixation to any ulnar fracture.

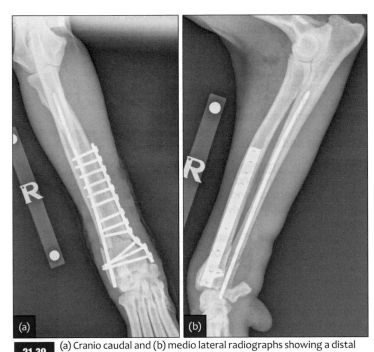

21.39 (a) Cranio caudal and (b) medio lateral radiographs showing a distal third simple transverse antebrachial fracture in 3-year-old Weimaraner stabilized with a 12-hole 2.7 mm dynamic compression plate applied to the medial aspect of the radius and an IM pin in the ulna.

Complications with plates include implant failure, infection, incorrect placement leading to angulation or rotation, thermal conduction, soft tissue irritation and delayed or non-union. Ulnar IM pins may be associated with lameness where soft tissue irritation occurs at the proximal olecranon, which should resolve after pin removal. Implant irritation secondary to screw impingement on the ulna has been reported, and again lameness generally resolves following implant removal.

Implant removal recommendations are based on evidence of bone healing and patient age, and, where present, evidence of broken or loose implants, corrosion, thermal conduction, interference with bone growth, infection, irritation and stress shielding.

→ **OPERATIVE TECHNIQUE 21.11 CONTINUED**

Where bone fragments are too small to reattach, the collateral ligament may be reattached to the bone using a screw and spiked washer or a low-profile suture anchor. The ligament repair can be further supported with non-absorbable suture material or wire placed through bone tunnels or around screws/washers in the styloid process and ulnar/radial carpal bones. Alternatively, a transarticular external skeletal fixator can be applied.

Wound closure

Routine. Check the integrity of the collateral ligaments after any styloid fracture repair.

POSTOPERATIVE MANAGEMENT

Protect any repair with temporary external coaptation. Initially, a Robert Jones bandage is applied to limit swelling. At 2 days postoperatively this can be reduced in size (modified Robert Jones) to include a caudal half splint. This should be changed weekly to limit complications and maintained for 1 to 2 weeks.

Confine to a cage or small room for 2 to 4 weeks with controlled lead exercise for 4 weeks; include physical therapy to maintain joint range of motion.

Chapter 22

The pelvis and sacroiliac joint

Mark Bush

Fractures of the pelvis and sacroiliac (SI) joints are common, accounting for 20–30% of fractures in cats and dogs (Brinker *et al.*, 2006). The aetiology for these injuries is usually high-energy trauma, predominantly road traffic accidents; as such, a pelvic injury should prompt the clinician to thoroughly evaluate the animal for additional injuries. Concurrent injuries should be expected after road traffic accidents; in one study, over 70% of dogs experiencing vehicular trauma were found to have multiple injuries (Streeter *et al.*, 2009).

Initially, emergency care and stabilization of the trauma patient is the primary consideration (see the *BSAVA Manual of Canine and Feline Emergency and Critical Care*). The patient must be thoroughly evaluated in a systematic manner to identify or exclude additional injuries (see Chapter 7). A detailed orthopaedic examination should be performed to check for concurrent fractures of the long bones or disruption of joints. A neurological examination must also be performed; sciatic nerve in-juries are not uncommon in patients with pelvic fractures (see *BSAVA Manual of Canine and Feline Neurology*). Other than cases involving loss of deep pain perception, those with perceived peripheral neurological deficits are still candidates for surgery as there is expectation of a return of neurological function permitting ambulation. However, owners should be advised of the potential for persistent neurological dysfunction, even with successful management of the pelvic fracture. If neurological deficits are identified, it is prudent to reassess the patient following initial cardiovascular stabilization, as the presence of shock can confound interpretation of the neurological examination.

WARNING
Expect additional injuries; examine all systems thoroughly. Look for a second injury, then look for a third

Diagnostic imaging for pelvic fractures requires correctly positioned orthogonal views of the pelvis. Lateral, ventrodorsal hip-extended and ventrodorsal hip-abducted views are performed in most cases; oblique views are also considered on occasions. Computed tomography (CT) can also be very useful for assessing complex fractures of the pelvis, and can allow more detailed surgical planning.

Assessment for surgical or non-surgical management

The anatomy of the pelvis is such that single isolated fractures are uncommon. The box-like configuration means displacement at one site almost invariably requires displacement of at least a second site; the clinician should always evaluate the pelvis with this in mind.

A survey of over 550 cases of small animal pelvic fractures found over 2000 different pelvic fractures in 160 different fracture combinations (Messmer and Montavon, 2004). As such, it is impossible to provide a prescriptive approach to pelvic fracture management. Each case is assessed individually in light of a number of criteria:

- Integrity of the weight-bearing axis
- Pelvic canal diameter
- Fracture duration
- Patient comfort levels
- Concurrent orthopaedic injuries
- Expected outcome/performance
- Financial constraints.

The first consideration in pelvic fracture decision making is the **weight-bearing axis** of the pelvis (Figure 22.1). This comprises the entire acetabulum, the ilial body and the SI joint. Disruption of any part of this axis will compromise locomotor function and consideration should be weighted towards surgical management of the patient. Fractures to bones outside this axis are potentially less significant, and non-surgical management is often appropriate for such injuries.

Secondly, the **pelvic canal diameter** is assessed. Rectal examination can be performed with the patient under general anaesthesia; however, this should be done very cautiously as it is possible to cause iatrogenic rectal perforation. Canal narrowing can be assessed more accurately, and non-invasively, from a ventrodorsal radiographic image or using CT.

The distance between the medial walls of the acetabula is measured, giving an indication of the pelvic canal diameter. This distance should be approximately equal to the width of the sacrum at its cranial border (cats) or caudal border (dogs). Reduction in the pelvic canal diameter by more than 45% is a significant risk factor for the development of megacolon and obstipation in cats (Hamilton *et al.*, 2009); surgical management of the fractures should be strongly considered for these cases. It should be noted

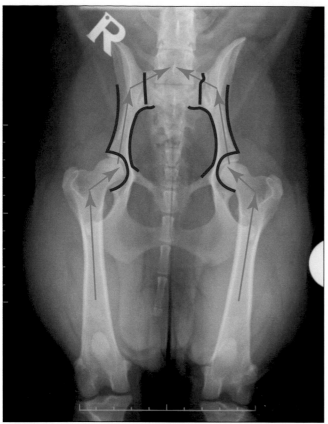

22.1 Ventrodorsal view of the pelvis of a dog showing the weight-bearing axes (green arrows).

that some degree of long-term narrowing of the pelvic canal can be expected following non-surgical management of pelvic fractures, and may be seen despite surgical stabilization of the pelvis if reduction or fixation are suboptimal.

The **duration of the fracture** should be considered. In most cases, pelvic fractures will rapidly develop an effective stabilizing fibrous callus. As a result, fractures of more than 7 to 10 days' duration may prove difficult to reduce surgically. In relatively chronic cases, the clinician should be aware of the potential difficulty in attempting surgery; conservative management may be considered in such cases, particularly where the animal has regained ambulatory function. However, in circumstances where the pelvic canal is significantly narrowed and obstipation is present, surgical management is still advised in most patients. Consideration should be given to pelvic widening alone where obstipation has been present for less than 6 months; if it has been present for longer than 6 months, concurrent sub-total colectomy is also indicated (Colopy-Poulsen et al., 2005).

The overall **comfort level** of the patient must be considered. Surgical correction of pelvic injuries can re-establish the bony anatomy, stabilize fracture fragments and resolve any painful peripheral nerve impingement.

The remaining criteria include: the presence of concurrent orthopaedic injuries, which may indicate surgical management; the expected activity level of the animal postoperatively; and any financial constraints on managing the case. The owner should be allowed to make an informed choice as to how they would like their pet to be managed. Generally, proficient surgical management of pelvic fractures is more likely to consistently result in a more rapid return to comfortable limb use, with a reduced risk of obstipation, compared with non-surgical management.

Non-surgical management of pelvic fractures

The pelvis has substantial soft tissue coverage, which provides a rich extraosseous blood supply and acts as an internal splint for the fragments. This allows certain fractures to be managed non-surgically and accounts for the rapid formation of a stabilizing callus and high rate of bone union following non-surgical management of pelvic fractures.

Non-surgical management usually consists of a 4 to 6 week period of restriction to a suitably sized cage. During this time analgesia should be provided as required and consideration should be given to using faecal softeners or laxatives. Typically a paraffin-based laxative or an osmotic laxative (cat: 0.5–5 ml orally every 8 to 12 hours; dog: 5–25 ml orally every 8 hours) is used with the aim of producing two to three soft stools per day. The patient should be re-evaluated 3 to 4 days after commencing non-surgical management to ensure pain is being adequately managed.

Surgical management of pelvic fractures

Sacroiliac luxation

Luxation of the SI joint is a frequently encountered injury. This may be unilateral, often in conjunction with a contralateral ilial body or acetabular fracture, or it may be bilateral, when the bony integrity of the pelvic architecture may be preserved and the whole pelvis is displaced cranially. Accurate assessment of the SI joint is crucial if luxations are not to be overlooked, or to prevent inadvertent surgery or referral of non-injured cases.

The presence of an SI luxation is best assessed by the contour of the pelvic inlet on a ventrodorsal radiograph of the pelvis. Normally, a smooth transition can be traced between the medial aspect of the ilium and the caudal sacrum as they form the joint (Figure 22.2a). The presence of a step at this point is suggestive of luxation (Figure 22.2b), although the presence of transitional vertebrae in some patients can confuse this appearance. In addition, following unilateral luxations, the ilial wing of the luxated hemipelvis will be displaced cranially with respect to the contralateral ilial wing. A manual assessment of pelvic stability can be made in sedated or anaesthetized cats and slim dogs; the left index finger is placed on the crest of the left ilium and the thumb on the ipsilateral ischiatic tuberosity, the right hemipelvis is similarly held with the right hand and the hemipelves are manipulated to appreciate SI joint instability.

The SI joint comprises two components; the sacroiliac ligamentous component and the crescent-shaped hyaline cartilage-covered synovial component, which forms the articular surface and acts as a landmark for screw placement (Figure 22.3). There is no bony union between the sacrum and ilium.

The SI joint is the site of force transfer from the appendicular to the axial skeleton, so in most cases accurate surgical reduction and stabilization of the joint will facilitate a return to normal, comfortable limb use. Non-surgical management may be appropriate for relatively stable, minimally displaced luxations when animals are already ambulatory and are considered to be comfortable.

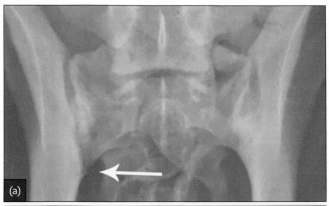

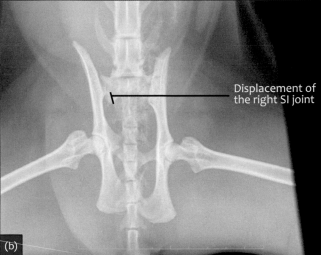

22.2 (a) Ventrodorsal radiograph of canine SI joints. Note the smooth transition between the medial border of the ilial body and the caudal border of the sacrum (arrowed). (b) Ventrodorsal radiograph of a right-sided SI joint luxation in a cat. Note the concurrent ischial and pubic fractures.

A number of techniques have been described for the management of SI luxation, but cortical lag screw fixation is the most reliable method (see Operative Technique 22.1). When performed correctly, a lag screw offers very stable and secure fixation; however, accurate placement of the screw can be challenging and requires a thorough understanding of the anatomy of the sacrum if significant complications are to be avoided. **The location for sacral screw placement is different in the cat and dog.** In both species, the lag screw must engage at least 60% of the sacral width.

When available, fluoroscopic assistance can be useful in ensuring correct screw placement. In cases where accurate identification of the sacral landmarks is not possible or placement of a lag screw is not feasible, the use of a transilial pin or bolt to stabilize the SI joint has been described (Figure 22.4) (see Operative Technique 22.2). However it should be noted that the stability achieved with this technique is inferior to that achieved with lag screw fixation (McCartney *et al.*, 2007). In larger or more active patients, transilial fixation can be applied in addition to a lag screw to provide additional support.

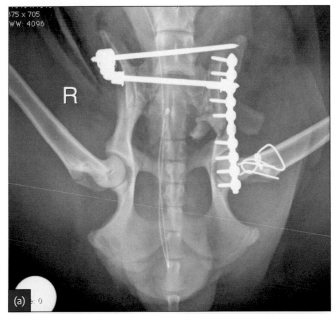

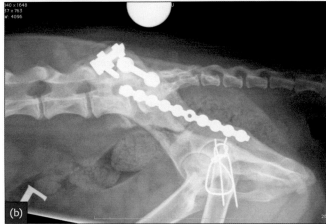

22.4 (a) Ventrodorsal and (b) lateral views of a canine pelvis. A transilial bolt and pin have been used for the management of a sacral fracture. Both implants have been placed dorsal to the sacrum. The animal has had a concurrent contralateral ilial body fracture managed with a string-of-pearls plate and screws placed via a greater trochanteric osteotomy. Transilial implants confer significantly less stability than an SI lag screw and, consequently, should be avoided as the sole means of stabilization of the SI joint if at all possible.

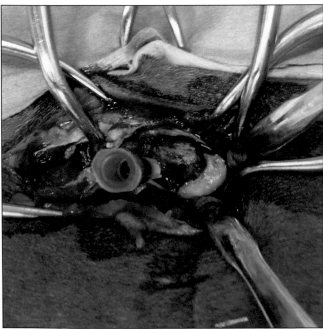

22.3 Intraoperative image of the left sacral articular surface of a cat. The ilial body has been depressed ventrally by a Hohmann retractor. Note the semilunar appearance to the synovial cartilage. The dot indicates the site for pilot hole placement for this case. The needle is positioned just cranial to the point of drill placement.

Bilateral SI luxations can be managed with two screws, one per side, applied separately (Figure 22.5), or with a single trans-sacral screw or bolt applied across both ilia. The trans-sacral screw technique requires perfect screw placement, and should only be attempted under fluoroscopic guidance or using an aiming device.

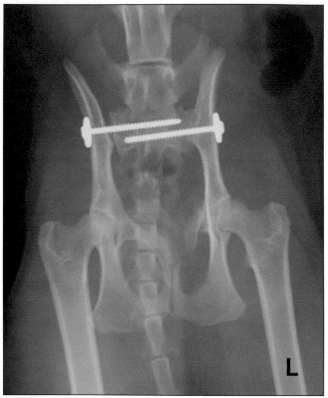

22.5 Ventrodorsal view of a feline pelvis showing bilateral SI joint luxations managed with two 2 mm lag screws and washers. A concurrent fracture of the left pubis is also present.

Fractures of the ilial body

Ilial body fractures are common, occurring in approximately half of feline and canine pelvic fractures. Ilial body fractures lead to disruption of the weight-bearing axis and normally warrant surgical repair.

Ilial body fracture configurations can be simple, short or long oblique or transverse fractures, or can be more complex and comminuted. The preferred management strategy for these fractures is bone plating. Plates are most commonly applied laterally (see Operative Technique 22.3).

Dynamic compression plates (DCPs) are relatively simple to contour to the lateral surface of the ilium. A significant disadvantage of laterally applied DCPs is the quality of bone stock available for screw purchase cranially. Although screws are placed bicortically, the cortices of the cranial ilium are less robust than the cortices of long bones, and the depth of bone available for screw purchase is small, resulting in a short working length of the screw. These factors significantly reduce the pull-out strength of the screws and the resistance of the plate–screw construct to torsional loads. Screw loosening has been shown to occur in over a quarter of small dogs and over 60% of cats with laterally applied bone plates. The consequences of screw loosening include instability of the fragments, patient discomfort and an increased risk of pelvic canal narrowing (Langley-Hobbs et al., 2009). The use of locking

plates can reduce the incidence of screw loosening with laterally applied bone plates, and can mitigate the risk of subsequent pelvic canal narrowing.

Ventral and dorsal plating of the ilial body has been described in dogs and cats respectively (Fitch et al., 2002; Langley-Hobbs et al., 2009). These techniques require the use of screws of a smaller diameter than lateral plating, but allow an increase in the length of screws applied to the fragments. The increased screw length may account for the reduced incidence of screw loosening with dorsally and ventrally applied plates. In addition, the ventral surface of the ilial body is the tension aspect of the bone, which provides a further mechanical advantage over laterally applied plates. However, ventral screw insertion is technically challenging, particularly in well muscled animals where the muscle bulk can limit the surgeon's ability to aim the drill correctly (see Operative Technique 22.4).

In cats, the ilial body is sufficiently straight to allow the application of a dorsal bone plate. The principle advantage offered is that screw loosening is reduced. Dorsal application is less challenging than ventral application as the approach to the dorsal surface can be made more readily and the drill can be aimed without interference from the surrounding musculature. It should be noted that dorsal bone plating is not appropriate for the canine pelvis due to the curvature of the dorsal ilium (see Operative Technique 22.5).

The application of screws across oblique fractures may allow for one or two screws to be lagged through a ventrally or dorsally applied plate. Alternatively, the use of two or three lag screws alone, inserted at the ventral border of the ilium and directed dorsally, has been described in dogs for the management of oblique ilial fractures. The strength and stiffness of lag screw stabilization is greater than that of a laterally applied bone plate (VanGundy et al., 1988); however, as for ventral plate application, orienting the screws correctly can be difficult in well muscled animals.

Ventral fixation can be applied in addition to lateral plate fixation, providing increased strength and stability to fractures of large-breed dogs (Breshears et al., 2004).

Fractures of the cranial part of the ilial wing not involving the weight-bearing axis of the pelvis do not require surgical stabilization and can be managed conservatively.

Fractures of the acetabulum

Acetabular fractures are encountered less commonly than ilial body or SI joint injury and are present in approximately one-fifth of pelvic fractures. In common with other articular fractures, their consequences can be more significant for the long-term outcome of the patient than pelvic fractures in other locations, and their management is less forgiving of minor inaccuracies in repair. It should be borne in mind that surgical management of acetabular fractures can be extremely challenging and, therefore, referral to a specialist centre should be considered.

A misconception has persisted that the caudal third of the acetabulum is non-weight-bearing in cats and dogs, and therefore surgical stabilization is not required. This fallacy may be derived from studies examining loading patterns of the (bipedal) human acetabulum (Dalstra and Huiskes, 1995). However, ex vivo and clinical studies have shown that the caudal aspect of the acetabulum is clearly involved in weight-bearing in (quadrupedal) cats and dogs (Boudrieau and Kleine, 1988; Beck et al., 2005; Moores et al., 2007). A further consideration, which may demonstrate the degree of loading of the caudal third of the acetabulum, is that this is the location of acetabular stress fractures in racing Greyhounds (Wendelburg *et al.*, 1988).

All fractures involving the acetabulum should be considered potential candidates for surgical management, as non-surgical treatment of acetabular fractures in adult animals often leads to disappointing long-term results (Brinker *et al.*, 2006). A study of non-surgically managed caudal acetabular fractures found 80% of cases experienced pain on hip manipulation, half were lame and a third of owners were dissatisfied with the outcome (Boudrieau and Kleine, 1988).

Articular surfaces require perfect reduction and rigid internal fixation to promote primary bone healing without callus production. Where comminution of the dorsal aspect of the acetabulum has occurred, anatomical reduction of the joint can be very challenging and ultimately unrewarding; consideration should be given to immediate femoral head and neck excision. Alternatively, stabilization to allow osseous healing prior to future total hip replacement surgery can be considered.

Fractures involving the medial wall of the acetabulum (Figure 22.6) are managed by repair of the dorsal acetabular rim, as direct stabilization of the medial wall is not possible. Dorsal repair, however, may result in ongoing medial instability of the hip joint, necessitating a salvage procedure.

Bone plates offer the most straightforward method of acetabular fracture repair. The dorsal aspect of the acetabulum is the tension surface of the joint, and provides a suitable surface for plate application (see Operative Technique 22.6). The application of conventional plates (DCPs, reconstruction plates and acetabular plates) to the dorsal acetabulum requires perfect, time-consuming contouring of the plate to the irregularly shaped dorsal acetabulum. Tightening of the screw draws the bone on to

the plate to generate the friction required for stability. This will cause a loss of fracture reduction with imperfectly contoured plates. Several strategies have been developed to counter the need for perfect plate contouring.

Plate luting allows the irregular surface of the dorsal acetabulum to be smoothed by the application of polymethylmethacrylate (PMMA) bone cement between the plate and bone. This has been shown to improve the reduction of repairs, and result in stronger and stiffer fixation than plate repair alone (Anderson *et al.*, 2002).

Locking plates allow the plate to be applied with a small gap between the bone and the plate, as the screw locks into the plate before the bone can be displaced. This gap should be minimal to maximize the strength of the repair (Stoffel *et al.*, 2003). In addition, a plate that is positioned too proudly may impinge on the sciatic nerve. Furthermore, the limited screw insertion angles mandated by some locking plate systems can present difficulties in the application of the plate. A cadaver study found no demonstrable benefit in the application of locking screws compared to conventional screws for the stabilization of acetabular osteotomies (Amato *et al.*, 2008); whether this study was a true reflection of the clinical situation is less certain.

Tension-band techniques can be used to stabilize simple transverse or short oblique fractures. Screws or pins are placed in either fragment and joined by a figure-of-eight tension-band wire (see Operative Technique 22.7). This is only really applicable to immature animals, where rapid healing is expected. Implants should be removed from animals less than 12 weeks of age following healing (Langley-Hobbs *et al.*, 2007). For larger mature animals the technique is modified by the important addition of a Kirschner (K) wire crossing the fracture site and the application of PMMA cement, covering the implants. This composite repair has been shown to provide comparable rigidity to a standard acetabular plate, with greater accuracy of reduction (Lewis *et al.*, 1997; Stubbs *et al.*, 1998). Composite repairs are not suitable for comminuted or long oblique fractures.

Fractures of the ischium and pubis

Fractures of the ischium, ilial wing and pubis are outside the weight-bearing axis of the pelvis and receive substantial splinting from the pelvic musculature. Surgical management of these injuries is rarely indicated and most are managed non-surgically. Plate application to the ischial table or interfragmentary wiring has been described for cases where there is significant instability or marked displacement and pain (Kipfer and Montavon, 2011), but this is not commonly performed.

Postoperative management

Most surgical pelvic fracture repairs offer robust stability; however, activity restriction and appropriate analgesia is still advisable for the first month. Use of an appropriately sized cage or restriction to a small room devoid of furniture is prudent, with periods of short, controlled, on-lead exercise for dogs. Activity can be gradually increased during the first month. Cautious physiotherapy can be considered to help to restore or maintain joint range of motion and muscle mass. More severely affected animals may require the use of a body sling to support the hindquarters in the initial period after surgery. Radiography should be repeated around 6 weeks after surgery to evaluate bone healing and the integrity of the implants.

22.6 A ventrodorsal radiograph of a feline pelvis obtained 12 weeks postoperatively. A fracture of the left acetabulum involved the dorsal and medial aspects. The fracture was stabilized with a 2/2.7 mm veterinary cuttable plate applied to the dorsal acetabular rim via a greater trochanteric osteotomy. The fracture of the medial aspect of the acetabulum has healed. A concurrent fracture of the right femur was stabilized with a plate and screws, and a right SI joint luxation stabilized with a 2.4 mm screw and washer.

References and further reading

Amato NS, Richards A, Knight, TA *et al.* (2008) *Ex vivo* biomechanical comparison of the 2.4 mm UniLOCK reconstruction plate using 2.4 mm locking *versus* standard screws for fixation of acetabular osteotomy in dogs. *Veterinary Surgery* **37**, 741–748

Anderson GM, Cross AR, Lewis DD and Lanz OI (2002) The effect of plate luting on reduction accuracy and biomechanics of acetabular osteotomies stabilized with 2.7 mm reconstruction plates. *Veterinary Surgery* **31**, 3–9

Beck AL, Pead MJ and Draper E (2005) Regional load bearing of the feline acetabulum. *Journal of Biomechanics* **38**, 427–432

Bookbinder PF and Flanders JA (1992) Characteristics of pelvic fractures in the cat. *Veterinary and Comparative Orthopaedics and Traumatology* **5**, 122–127

Boudrieau RJ and Kleine LJ (1988) Non surgically managed caudal acetabular fractures in dogs: 15 cases (1979–1984). *Journal of the American Veterinary Medical Association* **193**, 701–705

Breshears LA, Fitch RB, Wallace LJ, Wells CS and Swiderski JK (2004) The radiographic evaluation of repaired canine ilial fractures (69 cases). *Veterinary and Comparative Orthopaedics and Traumatology* **17**, 64–72

Brinker WO, Piermattei DL and Flo GL (2006) Fractures of the pelvis. In: *Handbook of Small Animal Orthopaedics and Fracture Repair, 4th edn*, p. 433. WB Saunders, Philadelphia

Burger M (2004) Surgical anatomy of the feline sacroiliac joint for lag screw fixation of sacroiliac fracture-luxation. *Veterinary and Comparative Orthopaedics and Traumatology* **17**, 146–151

Colopy-Poulsen SA, Danova NA, Hardie RJ and Muir P (2005) Managing feline obstipation secondary to pelvic fracture. *Compendium of Continuing Education for the Small Animal Practitioner* **42**, 662–669

Dalstra M and Huiskes R (1995) Load transfer across the pelvic bone. *Journal of Biomechanics* **28**, 715–724

DeCamp CE (2012) Fractures of the pelvis. In: *Veterinary Surgery: Small Animal*, p. 801. Elsevier, St Louis

DeCamp CE and Braden TD (1985) The anatomy of the canine sacrum for lag screw fixation of the sacroiliac joint. *Veterinary Surgery* **14**, 131–134

Fitch RB, Hosgood G and Staatz A (2002) Biomechanical evaluation of triple pelvic osteotomy with and without additional ventral plate stabilization. *Veterinary and Comparative Orthopaedics and Traumatology* **15**, 145–149

Hamilton MH, Evans DA and Langley-Hobbs SJ (2009) Feline ilial fractures: assessment of screw loosening and pelvic canal narrowing after lateral plating. *Veterinary Surgery* **38**, 326–333

King L and Boag A (2007) *BSAVA Manual of Canine and Feline Emergency and Critical Care, 2nd edn*. BSAVA Publications, Gloucester

Kipfer NM and Montavon PM (2011) Fixation of pelvic floor fractures in cats. *Veterinary and Comparative Orthopaedics and Traumatology* **24**, 137–141

Langley-Hobbs SJ, Meeson RL, Hamilton MH, Radke H and Lee K (2009) Feline ilial fractures: a prospective study of dorsal plating and comparison with lateral plating. *Veterinary Surgery* **38**, 334–342

Langley-Hobbs SJ, Sissener TR and Shales CJ (2007) Tension band stabilization of acetabular physeal fractures in four kittens. *Journal of Feline Medicine and Surgery* **9**, 177–187

Lanz OI (2002) Lumbosacral and pelvic injuries. *Veterinary Clinics of North America: Small Animal Practice* **32**, 949–962

Lewis DD, Stubbs PW, Neuwirth L *et al.* (1997) Results of screw/wire/polymethylmethacrylate composite fixation for acetabular fracture repair in 14 dogs. *Veterinary Surgery* **26**, 223–234

McCartney WT, Comiskey D and MacDonald B (2007) Use of transilial pinning for the treatment of sacroiliac separation in 25 dogs and finite element analysis of repair methods. *Veterinary and Comparative Orthopaedics and Traumatology* **20**, 38–42

Messmer M and Montavon PM (2004) Pelvic fractures in the dog and cat: a classification system and review of 556 cases. *Veterinary and Comparative Orthopaedics and Traumatology* **17**, 167–183

Moores AL, Moores AP, Brodbelt DC, Owen MR and Draper ERC (2007) Regional load bearing of the canine acetabulum. *Journal of Biomechanics* **40**, 3732–3737

Piermattei DL (2004) The pelvis and hip joint. In: *An Atlas of Surgical Approaches to the Bones of the Dog and Cat, 4th edn*, p. 277. WB Saunders, Philadelphia

Platt S and Olby N (2013) *BSAVA Manual of Canine and Feline Neurology, 4th edn*. BSAVA Publications, Gloucester

Shales CJ and Langley-Hobbs SJ (2005) Canine sacroiliac luxation: anatomic study of dorsoventral articular surface angulation and safe corridor for placement of screws used in lag fixation. *Veterinary Surgery* **34**, 324–331

Shales C, Moores A, Kulendra E *et al.* (2010) Stabilization of sacroiliac luxation in 40 cats using screws inserted in lag fashion. *Veterinary Surgery* **39**, 696–700

Shales CJ, White L and Langley-Hobbs SJ (2009) Sacroiliac luxation in the cat: defining a safe corridor in the dorsoventral plane for screw insertion in lag fashion. *Veterinary Surgery* **38**, 343–348

Stoffel K, Dieter U, Stachowiak G, Gachter A and Kuster MS (2003) Biomechanical testing of the LCP – how can stability in locked internal fixators be controlled. *Injury* **34**, B11–19

Streeter EM, Rozanski EA, Laforcade-Buress A, Freeman LM and Rush JE (2009) Evaluation of vehicular trauma in dogs: 239 cases (January–December 2001). *Journal of the American Veterinary Medical Association* **235**, 405–408

Stubbs PW, Lewis DD, Miller GJ, Quarterman C and Hosgood G (1998) A biomechanical evaluation and assessment of the accuracy of reduction of two methods of acetabular osteotomy fixation in dogs. *Veterinary Surgery* **27**, 429–437

Tomlinson JL (2003) Fractures of the pelvis. In: *Textbook of Small Animal Surgery, 3rd edn*, ed. D Slatter, pp. 1989–2001. WB Saunders, Philadelphia

Vangundy TE, Hulse DA, Nelson JK and Boothe HW (1988) Mechanical evaluation of two canine iliac fracture fixation systems. *Veterinary Surgery* **17**, 321–327

Wendelburg K, Dee J, Kaderly R, Dee L and Eaton-Wells R (1988) Stress fractures of the acetabulum in 26 racing greyhounds. *Veterinary Surgery* **17**, 128–134

OPERATIVE TECHNIQUE 22.1

Sacroiliac luxation – sacroiliac lag screw placement

PREOPERATIVE PLANNING

On a scaled ventrodorsal radiograph of the pelvis, measure the required depth of the sacral pilot hole to a point that is just greater than 60% of the sacral width.

POSITIONING

The animal is placed in lateral recumbency with the affected side uppermost; ventral recumbency with the pelvis and caudal abdomen supported by a small sandbag is preferred by some surgeons.

ASSISTANT

Not essential.

→ **OPERATIVE TECHNIQUE 22.1 CONTINUED**

EQUIPMENT EXTRAS

Gelpi and Hohmann retractors; suitably sized screw and washer; Kern bone-holding forceps.

SURGICAL TECHNIQUES

Approach

A skin incision is made over the dorsal aspect of the ilial spine. The sacrospinalis muscle is incised and elevated at its insertion on the ilial crest (Figure 22.7). Exposure of the dorsal aspect of the sacrum should not be extended medial to the intermediate crests to avoid damage to the sacral nerve outflows. The middle gluteal muscle is elevated ventrally from the lateral aspect of the ilium to a point level with the caudal crest of the ilial spine ('gluteal roll-down').

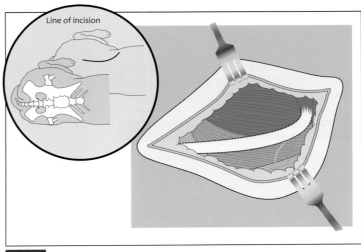

22.7 Dorsal approach to the ilium and SI joint.

Sacral pilot hole

The sacral body is identified by the presence of the C-shaped hyaline cartilage, which is the articular component of the joint. This is occasionally obscured by fibrous tissue. The presence of a vertebral transverse process indicates the approach is too cranial. The ilial wing is depressed ventrally with the use of one or two small, blunt-tipped Hohmann retractors carefully placed with their tips just ventral to the sacral body (see Figure 22.3). Care should be taken to reduce the risk of iatrogenic injury to the lumbosacral plexus. The pilot hole is drilled first.

WARNING

The surgeon should be aware that the site for location of the pilot hole on the wing of the sacrum differs between canine and feline sacra; malpositioning of the pilot hole can have catastrophic results for the patient

The sacral and caudal nerve roots (cauda equina) occupy the spinal canal dorsal to the sacral body, and there are several important structures located ventrally including the lumbosacral nerve plexus and the terminal branches of the aorta. Dorsal or ventral malpositioning of the screw can cause significant damage to these structures (Figure 22.8). Positioning the pilot hole too cranially or caudally in the sacrum will result in poor screw holding and subsequent instability of the repair. The surface area for safe placement of the pilot hole is approximately 1 cm² in large dogs and approximately 0.5 cm² in cats.

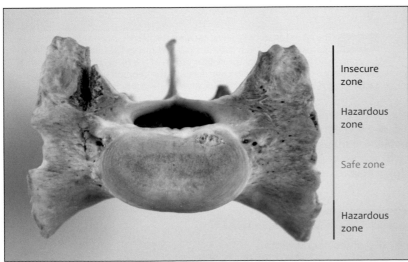

22.8 Transverse view of a canine sacrum highlighting the hazards of screw placement. Note the small proportion of the sacral body that is suitable for screw placement and that both ventral and dorsal malpositioning is hazardous.

Insecure zone

Hazardous zone

Safe zone

Hazardous zone

→ **OPERATIVE TECHNIQUE 22.1 CONTINUED**

The location of the starting point for the pilot hole in canine sacra is a point 60% of the way down the dorsoventral axis and midway between the sacral notch and the cranial aspect of the articular surface (Figure 22.9). The surgeon should be aware of the orientation of the sacrum during surgery by referencing the lateral pelvic radiograph.

For feline sacra, the correct starting point is 1 mm dorsal to the geometric centre of the sacral wing (Figure 22.10).

> **PRACTICAL TIP**
>
> Accurate intraoperative identification of the optimal site for screw placement using these landmarks alone can be unreliable. Although not essential, fluoroscopy is very helpful in ensuring the correct lateral positioning of the patient and accurate placement of the pilot hole

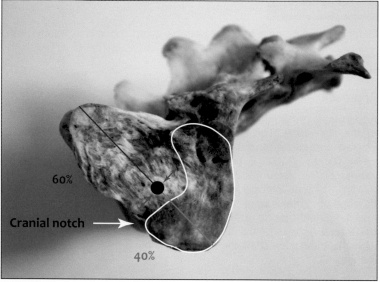

22.9 The lateral aspect of a canine sacrum. The white outline indicates the approximate location of the articular cartilage. The correct site for the placement of the screw is at 60% of the dorsoventral axis and approximately midway between the cranial notch and the cranial aspect of the articular cartilage. A black dot indicates the location of the drill hole for the screw.

It can be helpful to begin the pilot hole with a 1.1 or 1.4 mm K-wire, drilled 2–3 mm into the sacrum. This allows the drill bit to be positioned without slipping from the intended start point during drilling. The pilot hole is then drilled with an appropriate drill bit. If the animal is in perfect lateral recumbency the drill should be vertically oriented; however, it is difficult clinically to ensure the patient is perfectly positioned. Note, due to the orientation of the sacral wing, the drill will not be perpendicular to the craniocaudal orientation of the sacral surface (Figure 22.11a). Placing the screw perpendicular to the sacral surface in this orientation risks penetrating the lumbosacral joint space. Dorsoventral angles have been recommended as 90±4 degrees in the cat (Shales et al., 2009) and 97±4 degrees in the dog (Shales and Langley-Hobbs, 2005). In practice, it is difficult to drill with this degree of accuracy, and the values are predicated on perfect intraoperative positioning of the sacrum and the correct starting location of the drill hole.

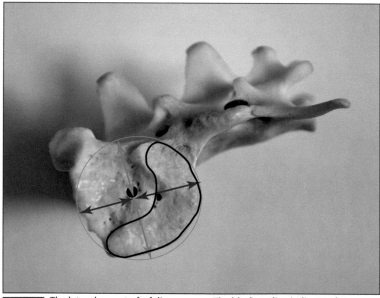

22.10 The lateral aspect of a feline sacrum. The black outline indicates the approximate location of the articular cartilage. The blue circle has been superimposed to demonstrate the circular profile of the feline sacrum. The correct site for placement of the screw is 1 mm dorsal to the geometric centre of the feline sacral wing. A black dot indicates the location of the drill hole for the screw.

A degree of resistance ought to be consistently detected during drilling if the bit is correctly located. The pilot hole should extend to a depth just greater than 60% of the width of the sacrum (this distance should be measured from the preoperative ventrodorsal radiograph). The pilot hole is measured with a depth gauge to confirm the depth is adequate and then tapped if required. Self-tapping cortical screws are preferred. Care should be taken if using a tap to ensure it does not impact on the bone at the end of the pilot hole.

> **WARNING**
>
> Ensure that the SI lag screw engages at least 60% of the sacral width

→ **OPERATIVE TECHNIQUE 22.1 CONTINUED**

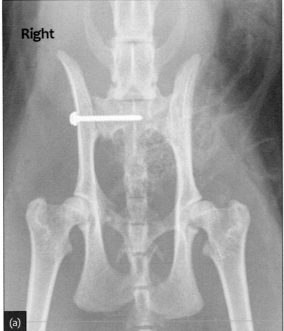

Right

(a)

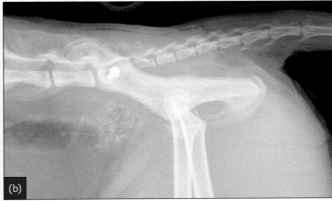

(b)

22.11 Postoperative (a) ventrodorsal and (b) lateral views of the case in Figure 22.2b demonstrating accurate screw placement within the sacral body. The luxation has been stabilized with a 2.4 mm cortical lag screw and a washer. On the ventrodorsal view the screw has been placed across 60% of the sacral width in the true mediolateral plane. Note the sacral surface is angled craniolaterally to caudomedially with respect to the sagittal plane of the patient, therefore the screw is not perpendicular to the sacral surface.

Ilial glide hole

The site for the glide hole in the ilium is identified. The chosen site should be located midway dorsoventrally at a point three-quarters of the way between the cranial and caudal dorsal iliac spines (Figure 22.12). Alternatively, it can be identified by palpating the medial articular surface of the ilium. Pointed reduction forceps are then placed with a point at the desired location on the medial surface, allowing the other point to act as a guide to indicate the position on the lateral aspect of the ilium. The glide hole is drilled with an appropriate drill bit and measured. An attempt should be made to achieve >90% reduction of the SI joint to improve stability.

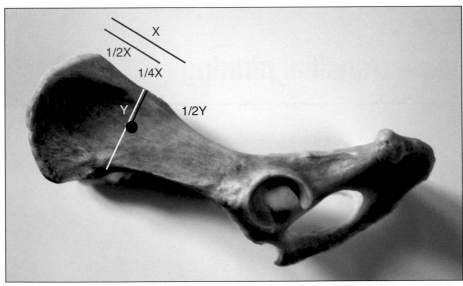

22.12 The lateral aspect of a canine pelvis demonstrating the site for ilial glide hole placement. The chosen site is located midway dorsoventrally at a point three-quarters of the way between the cranial and caudal dorsal iliac spines. X = distance between the cranial and caudal iliac spines; Y = distance between the dorsal and ventral borders of the ilium perpendicular to the iliac crest.

Insertion of lag screw

A screw is chosen that is 2 mm shorter than the combined depth of the pilot and glide holes, to prevent the screw from being driven against the end of the pilot hole and failing to compress the joint. Use of a washer is recommended to reduce the risk of the screw head pulling through the thin ilial bone (see Figure 22.11).

To reduce the luxation, the screw is directed through the glide hole and 3 to 5 mm of the tip is visualized at the medial aspect of the ilium. The pilot hole is identified and the screw tip is directed into the pilot hole. Suction is helpful to clear the sacral surface of blood. Bone-holding forceps are used to manipulate the ilium in order to →

→ **OPERATIVE TECHNIQUE 22.1 CONTINUED**

align the screw tip with the pilot hole. Driving the screw will reduce and compress the SI joint. If the two bones separate during screw driving, the pilot hole has not been engaged.

The optimal screw diameter has not been evaluated, but cortical screw breakage is extremely uncommon. As a rough guide, the author uses 2.4 mm screws for cats and small dogs, 2.7 mm screws for small- to medium-sized dogs, 3.5 mm screws for medium- to large-breed dogs and 4.5 mm screws with or without a second screw for large to giant breeds. Smaller diameter screws are used in the repair of bilateral SI luxations (see Figure 22.5). Cortical screws are used in all cases.

A well placed, single screw of suitable dimensions is adequate for nearly all cases and results in a very low incidence of screw loosening. Other than for giant breeds, placement of a second screw or an additional K-wire is challenging and may well not provide a clinically significant mechanical advantage. Cannulated screws are more expensive and have significantly lower bending resistance than similarly sized regular cortical screws. They offer no advantages for open surgical reduction. Supplementary transilial fixation can be considered in larger or more active patients.

Wound closure

The superficial fascia of the sacrospinalis muscle is sutured to the middle gluteal muscle in a simple continuous pattern using an absorbable monofilament material (e.g. polydioxanone). The periosteum of the dorsal aspect of the ilium is included in the closure. The subdermal tissues are closed according to surgeon preference.

POSTOPERATIVE MANAGEMENT AND COMPLICATIONS

SI lag screws offer robust stability; however, activity restriction and appropriate analgesia are still advisable for the first month. Use of an appropriately sized cage or restriction to a small room devoid of furniture is prudent, with periods of short, controlled, on-lead exercise for dogs. Cautious physiotherapy can be considered to help to restore or maintain joint range of motion and muscle mass. More severely affected animals may require the use of a body sling to support the hindquarters in the initial period after surgery. Radiography should be repeated 6 weeks after surgery to evaluate the repair.

Screw loosening and consequent instability is more likely if the screw has failed to engage the sacrum across 60% of its width. Catastrophic urinary/defecatory dysfunction or fatal haemorrhage could potentially occur if the screw is malpositioned dorsally into the neural canal or ventrally into the iliac vasculature.

OPERATIVE TECHNIQUE 22.2

Sacroiliac luxation – transilial pinning

POSITIONING

The patient is placed in sternal recumbency with sandbags used to raise the ventral aspect of the pelvis and allow the hindlimbs to hang either side.

ASSISTANT

Not essential.

EQUIPMENT EXTRAS

Kern bone-holding forceps; Gelpi retractors; suitably sized bolt with washers and four nuts or an end-threaded pin with an external skeletal fixator clamp.

SURGICAL TECHNIQUES

Approach

Approaches are made over the dorsal aspects of both ilial spines as for Operative Technique 22.1, and bilateral gluteal muscle 'roll-downs' are performed.

→

→ **OPERATIVE TECHNIQUE 22.2 CONTINUED**

Reduction and fixation

The luxation is reduced and held using bone-holding forceps applied to the ilium. A glide hole is drilled in the lateral aspect of the ilial body to exit just dorsal to the dorsal aspect of the SI joint facets. A threaded bolt is driven from laterally to medially, contacting the top of the sacral vertebra, towards the medial aspect of the contralateral ilium. A second glide hole is then drilled from lateral to medial in the contralateral ilium to exit medially at the point of contact with the bolt. The bolt is then advanced though the hole in the contralateral ilium from medial to lateral. A washer and two nuts are applied to each end of the bolt lateral to the ilia, and the long end of the bolt is cut short with a bolt cropper (see Figure 22.4).

It can be difficult to place the glide hole in the contralateral ilium accurately enough to allow the bolt to be advanced through the hole. To circumvent this problem, an end-threaded pin can be used rather than a bolt. The pin is driven across the ilium, dorsal to the vertebra as for the bolt, and the threaded portion of the tip is secured in the contralateral ilial wing. This obviates the need to make a second approach to the contralateral ilium. The smooth end of the pin can then be bent over or an external skeletal fixator clamp can be applied to secure the pin to the ilium. Alternatively an entirely smooth pin can be used, with both ends bent over to engage the ilium; this will require an approach to the contralateral ilium.

WARNING
Transilial repairs alone provide significantly less stability to the SI joint than a single lag screw

Wound closure

See Operative Technique 22.1.

POSTOPERATIVE MANAGEMENT AND COMPLICATIONS

See Operative Technique 22.1. This repair is less stable than lag screw fixation. Greater care should be taken in ensuring adequate postoperative exercise restriction. The bolt or pin may cause irritation of the gluteal muscles.

OPERATIVE TECHNIQUE 22.3

Ilial body bone plating – lateral plate application

PREOPERATIVE PLANNING

Ensure the surgical clip and preparation extends sufficiently caudally to allow an approach to the ischium, if required. Some surgeons like to use the radiographs of the pelvis to pre-contour a bone plate to the lateral surface of the ilium prior to surgery.

POSITIONING

The animal is placed in lateral recumbency with the affected side uppermost.

ASSISTANT

Very helpful.

EQUIPMENT EXTRAS

Large and small pointed reduction forceps; Kern bone-holding forceps; Hohmann and Gelpi retractors; appropriate plate and screw set.

→

→ **OPERATIVE TECHNIQUE 22.3 CONTINUED**

SURGICAL TECHNIQUES

Approach

A skin incision is made over the lateral aspect of the ilium from the ilial crest to the greater trochanter. The middle gluteal muscle is identified and the septum connecting it to the tensor fascia lata muscle is dissected (Figure 22.13a). The middle gluteal muscle is elevated dorsally as required to obtain adequate exposure of the ilium. The origin of the deep gluteal muscle is then elevated from the ilial shaft. The cranial gluteal neurovascular bundle should be preserved (Figure 22.13b). In addition, it can be very helpful to make a caudal approach to the ipsilateral ischium. An incision is made over the ischium and the subdermal fascia is bluntly dissected to expose the bone. Sharp incisions are made into the origins of the muscle dorsal and ventral to the ischium to allow placement of a pair of Kern bone-holding forceps on to the ischial table (Figure 22.14).

Reduction and fixation

The fracture fragments are identified and the fracture is reduced. Fracture reduction is consistently the most difficult aspect of fracture repair. This may be particularly so in larger dogs, or with chronic fractures. Although accurate reduction must be achieved, perfect anatomical reconstruction of the ilial body is not necessary. However, the surgeon should take care to ensure the caudal fragment has been sufficiently lateralized to restore the pelvic canal

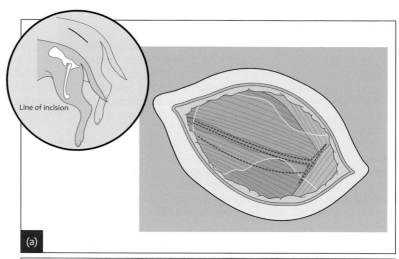

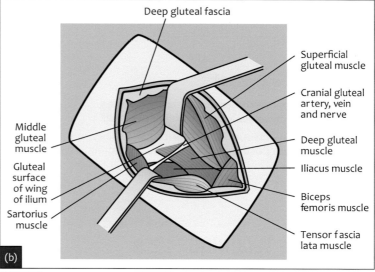

(a)

Line of incision

Deep gluteal fascia

Superficial gluteal muscle

Cranial gluteal artery, vein and nerve

Deep gluteal muscle

Iliacus muscle

Biceps femoris muscle

Tensor fascia lata muscle

Middle gluteal muscle

Gluteal surface of wing of ilium

Sartorius muscle

(b)

22.13 Lateral approach to the ilium.

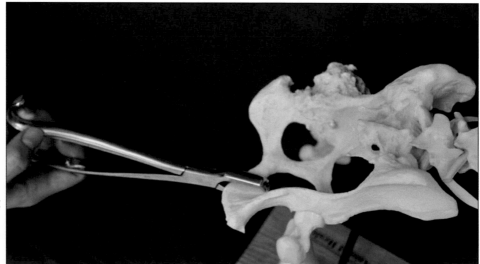

22.14 Model demonstrating the application of Kern bone-holding forceps to the ischial table for the manipulation of pelvic fracture fragments.

→ **OPERATIVE TECHNIQUE 22.3 CONTINUED**

diameter. The caudal fragment can be manipulated using a number of strategies. A Hohmann retractor will help to elevate the medially displaced caudal fragment. In addition, lateral traction applied to the greater trochanter of the femur with pointed reduction forceps may be helpful (Figure 22.15). Where the ipsilateral caudal hemipelvis is intact, an additional caudal approach can be made to the ischial table. A pair of Kern bone-holding forceps is applied to the ischium and used to manipulate the caudal fragment to aid fracture reduction.

Oblique fractures may be reduced and stabilized with reduction forceps applied across the fracture at the dorsal and ventral borders of the ilial body. During reduction of the fracture the forceps are applied and closed; this causes the fragments to slide over each other and into reduction.

Transverse fractures may be more difficult to maintain in reduction. To facilitate this, a temporary K-wire can be driven obliquely across the fracture line. Alternatively, the plate itself can be used to reduce the fracture. A non-locking plate is pre-contoured based on the radiographs. The plate is applied to the bone with the caudal screws placed first. The cranial part of the plate is then pushed against the bone, which draws the caudal fragment into reduction. The cranial screws are then applied; one or two screws should be applied using the 'load' drill guide where possible, to apply compression across the fracture site.

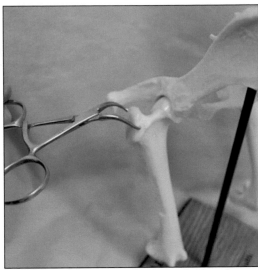

22.15 Model demonstrating the application of pointed reduction forceps to the greater trochanter of the femur for the manipulation of pelvic fracture fragments.

Comminuted fractures can be stabilized by the application of K-wires and lag screws to reduce the fragments where feasible, followed by the application of a neutralization plate. Alternatively, a bridging plate can be applied.

A minimum of three bicortical screws should be applied to the cranial and caudal fragments. Where the caudal fragment has insufficient bone stock to accommodate three screws, a T-plate can be used effectively.

Locking plate technology provides an alternative to conventional screws and plates. The use of locking plates (see Figure 22.4) has been shown to reduce the incidence of screw loosening in laterally applied bone plates and may mitigate the risk of subsequent pelvic canal narrowing. Most locking plates cannot be used to assist with fracture reduction as described above. Plates that allow use of either cortex screws or locking screws are therefore preferred (see Chapter 10).

As a guide, 2 mm DCPs are suitable for cats, 2.4 mm plates for small dogs, 2.7 mm plates for medium-sized dogs and 3.5 mm plates for larger dogs. Giant breeds require double plating.

Wound closure

The middle gluteal muscle is sutured to the sartorius and tensor fascia lata muscles. Subcutaneous tissues and skin are closed in layers according to surgeon preference.

POSTOPERATIVE MANAGEMENT AND COMPLICATIONS

See Operative Technique 22.1. Sciatic nerve injury can result from inadvertent entrapment by retractor tips or bone-holding forceps as the nerve passes close to the dorsomedial border of the ilium.

OPERATIVE TECHNIQUE 22.4

Ilial body bone plating – ventral plate application in canine patients

POSITIONING

The dog is placed in lateral recumbency with the affected side uppermost.

ASSISTANT

Essential.

EQUIPMENT EXTRAS

Large and small pointed reduction forceps; Kern bone-holding forceps; Hohmann and Gelpi retractors; smooth pins of the diameter of the intended screw core; appropriate plate and screw set.

SURGICAL TECHNIQUES

Approach

A standard lateral approach is made to the ilial body (see Operative Technique 22.3) and the iliacus muscle is elevated from the ventral border of the ilium, which is exposed with Hohmann retractors (Figure 22.16). The ilial nutrient artery may be damaged during the approach.

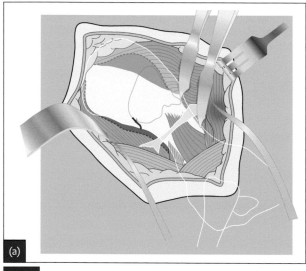
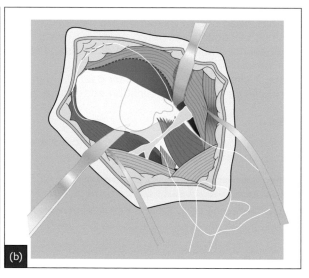

22.16 Approach to the ventral aspect of the ilium.

Reduction and fixation

The fracture is reduced (see Operative Technique 22.3). A DCP is contoured and applied to the ventral aspect of the ilium. The surrounding musculature can make it very difficult to orient the drill bit correctly; a long pin of appropriate diameter can be used instead. Lag screws can be placed through the plate to stabilize oblique fractures. In very large patients biaxial plates (both lateral and ventral) can be applied, which provide very robust fixation.

Wound closure

See Operative Technique 22.3.

POSTOPERATIVE MANAGEMENT AND COMPLICATIONS

See Operative Technique 22.1. Care should be taken not to allow the drill bit to exit the ilial body medially, as this risks encountering the sciatic nerve.

OPERATIVE TECHNIQUE 22.5

Ilial body bone plating – dorsal plate application in feline patients

POSITIONING

The cat is positioned in ventrolateral oblique recumbancy with the affected side uppermost tilted slightly towards the surgeon.

ASSISTANT

Essential.

EQUIPMENT EXTRAS

Large and small pointed reduction forceps; Kern bone-holding forceps; Hohmann and Gelpi retractors; Penrose drain for sciatic nerve retraction.

SURGICAL TECHNIQUES

Approach

The cranial ilium is approached dorsally via a gluteal muscle 'roll-down' (see Figure 22.7). A lateral approach can be made combining craniodorsal and caudodorsal approaches to the hip for more caudal access (Piermattei, 2004).

Reduction and fixation

The fracture is reduced. It can be harder to achieve accurate reduction of the fragments using a dorsal approach than a lateral approach. Care must be taken to protect the sciatic nerve that runs medial to the dorsal ilial body. A 2.0 mm DCP (or 1.5/2.0 mm veterinary cuttable plate, which increases the number of screw holes available with respect to the length of the plate) is contoured to the dorsal aspect of the ilium, with a minimum of two screws in each fragment. A C-shaped drill guide can be used to aim the drill bit correctly; however, the bit should centre itself within the cortices of the ilial body. Oblique fractures can be lag screwed through the plate. Transverse fractures can be compressed using the 'load' drill guide. The range of motion of the hip joint should be evaluated after each caudal screw placement.

Wound closure

See Operative Technique 22.3.

POSTOPERATIVE MANAGEMENT AND COMPLICATIONS

See Operative Technique 22.1. It is possible to inadvertently violate the acetabulum during caudal screw placement.

OPERATIVE TECHNIQUE 22.6

Simple acetabular fractures – bone plate stabilization

PREOPERATIVE PREPARATION

Ensure the surgical clip and preparation extends sufficiently caudally to allow an approach to the ischium.

POSITIONING

The animal is placed in lateral recumbency with the affected side uppermost.

ASSISTANT

Essential.

EQUIPMENT EXTRAS

Kern bone-holding forceps; pointed reduction forceps; Hohmann and Gelpi retractors; Penrose drain for sciatic nerve retraction; osteotome and mallet or sagittal saw for performing a greater trochanteric osteotomy; appropriate plate and screw set, pin and wire set for stabilization of the osteotomy.

SURGICAL TECHNIQUES

Approach

A dorsoventral skin incision is made centred just cranial to the greater trochanter, from the proximal third of the femur ventrally and extending a similar distance dorsally. The fascia lata is incised to expose the superficial gluteal tendon, which is elevated from its insertion at the third trochanter (Figure 22.17a). The middle and deep gluteal tendons are identified, and an osteotome or sagittal saw blade is used to perform a greater trochanteric osteotomy (Figure 22.17b). The osteotomy starts just distal to the insertion of the deep gluteal tendon and is directed medially and proximally at an angle of 45 degrees to the long axis of the femur (Figure 22.17c). Sufficient bone should be osteotomized to allow secure reattachment during closure. The osteotomized bone is reflected dorsally, along with the insertions of the middle and deep gluteal tendons. The sciatic nerve is identified as it crests the ischiatic spine and courses caudolaterally. This is gently dissected free and mobilized with the aid of a small Penrose drain. The external hip rotator muscles and tendons are divided/incised as required to access the dorsal acetabulum (Figures 22.17d and 22.18).

In addition, a caudal approach should be made to the ischium and a pair of Kern bone-holding forceps applied to it to manipulate the caudal fragment, thus aiding fracture reduction (see Operative Technique 22.3 and Figure 22.15).

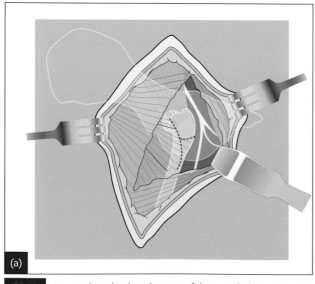
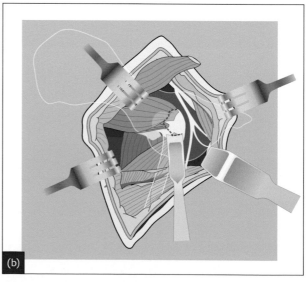

(a) (b)

22.17 Approach to the dorsal aspect of the acetabulum via a greater trochanteric osteotomy. (continues) ▶ →

→ **OPERATIVE TECHNIQUE 22.6 CONTINUED**

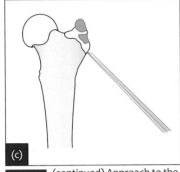

22.17 (continued) Approach to the dorsal aspect of the acetabulum via a greater trochanteric osteotomy.

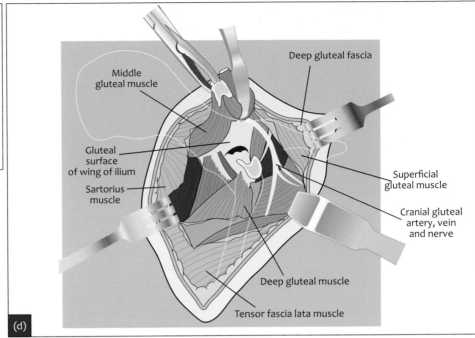

Middle gluteal muscle

Deep gluteal fascia

Gluteal surface of wing of ilium

Superficial gluteal muscle

Sartorius muscle

Cranial gluteal artery, vein and nerve

Deep gluteal muscle

Tensor fascia lata muscle

(d)

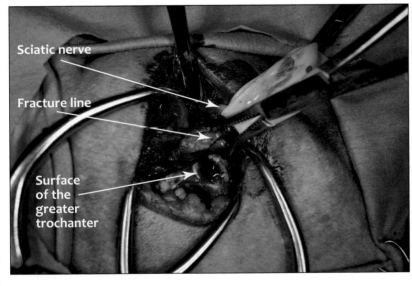

Sciatic nerve

Fracture line

Surface of the greater trochanter

22.18 Intraoperative view of the repair of a feline acetabular fracture. The fracture has been exposed and reduced with a pair of small serrated bone-holding forceps. The surface of the osteotomized greater trochanter is visible. The sciatic nerve has been retracted using a Penrose drain.

Reduction and fixation

Where the joint capsule is intact it is helpful to make a small incision into the dorsal aspect to visualize the reduction of the fragments; distracting the femur distally will open the coxofemoral joint space slightly and improve visualization of the fracture reduction. The fracture is reduced and the fragments are held in temporary reduction with the aid of pointed reduction forceps, avoiding the articular surface. A small K-wire can also be used to temporarily maintain reduction if the fracture configuration is appropriate; normally this will be an oblique fracture.

The plate is contoured to the dorsal aspect of the bone, with a minimum of two screws applied to each fragment (Figure 22.19). Perfect contouring of non-locking plates is mandatory as the plate must be compressed to the bone by the screws to provide stability.

The development of locking screws and plates has reduced the need for perfect contouring of these plates as the screw heads engage the plate and will not pull the fragment out of reduction, thus permitting a small gap between the bone and plate. The construct strength is improved if this distance is minimal. Locking plates can be bulky and most do not allow for alteration in screw direction, which can make screw insertion difficult and potentially risks violating the joint; care should be taken to avoid this. Implant orientation should be considered carefully to account for the shape of the joint (Figure 22.20), and the range of motion of the hip joint should be evaluated after each screw placement.

→ **OPERATIVE TECHNIQUE 22.6 CONTINUED**

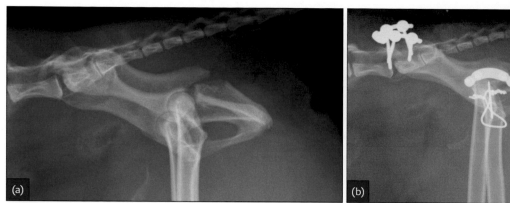

22.19 (a) Lateral radiograph of a feline pelvis showing a caudal acetabular fracture. A sacral fracture was also present. (b) The acetabular fracture has been approached by a greater trochanteric osteotomy, reduced and stabilized with a 4-hole 2 mm acetabular plate. In addition the sacral fracture has been reduced and stabilized with a transilial 2 mm locking plate.

Wound closure

The joint capsule is closed using an appropriately sized monofilament absorbable suture material. The greater trochanteric osteotomy is reduced and stabilized with two appropriately sized K-wires and a figure-of-eight tension-band wire. The superficial gluteal muscle is sutured to the fascia of the lateral vastus muscle. The superficial fascia lata muscle is closed in a continuous pattern of monofilament sutures. The subdermal tissues and skin are closed in layers according to surgeon preference.

POSTOPERATIVE MANAGEMENT AND COMPLICATIONS

See Operative Technique 22.1. Sciatic nerve impairment may be encountered following manipulation of the sciatic nerve. This is normally a temporary problem. Post-traumatic osteoarthritis may develop despite perfect reduction and rigid internal fixation.

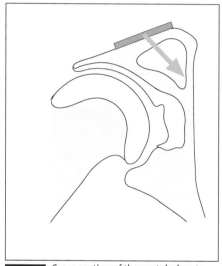

22.20 Cross-section of the acetabulum to indicate the importance of correct screw angulation.

OPERATIVE TECHNIQUE 22.7

Simple acetabular fractures – composite repair using screws, wire and polymethylmethacrylate

WARNING

This technique is only appropriate for simple transverse or short oblique fractures; it should not be used for long oblique or comminuted fracture configurations

POSITIONING

The animal is placed in lateral recumbency with the affected side uppermost.

ASSISTANT

Essential.

EQUIPMENT EXTRAS

Cortical bone screws; K-wires; orthopaedic wire; bone wax; PMMA bone cement.

SURGICAL TECHNIQUES

Approach

A dorsal approach is made to the acetabulum via a greater trochanteric osteotomy (see Operative Technique 22.6).

Reduction and fixation

The fracture is reduced and a K-wire is placed across the fracture line. The use of a K-wire is mandatory to counteract the shear forces experienced by the fragments. A cortical screw is placed into the dorsal aspect of each fragment with the heads remaining sufficiently proud to allow a figure-of-eight tension-band wire to be securely wound around them. The tension-band wire is tightened whilst the surgeon ensures reduction of the fracture is maintained. Bone wax is placed into the heads of the bone screws and PMMA bone cement is then applied in its dough phase to cover the screws and wire (Figure 22.21). Care should be taken to ensure the sciatic nerve is protected from thermal damage as the PMMA polymerizes.

Wound closure

See Operative Technique 22.6. Closure of the joint capsule is not always possible. The greater trochanteric osteotomy is reduced and stabilized with two appropriately sized K-wires and a figure-of-eight tension-band wire.

POSTOPERATIVE MANAGEMENT AND COMPLICATIONS

See Operative Technique 22.1.

Permanent sciatic nerve damage may ensue if the nerve is not sufficiently protected during the exothermic cement polymerization.

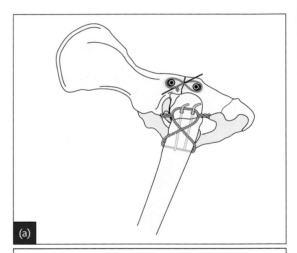

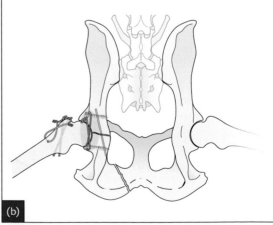

22.21 (a) Lateral and (b) ventrodorsal views of a canine acetabular fracture stabilized with a 1.4 mm K-wire, two 3.5 mm cortical bone screws and a 1.25 mm tension-band wire. The greater trochanteric osteotomy has been stabilized with two K-wires and a tension-band wire.

Chapter 23

The femur

Neil Burton

Femoral fractures occur with high frequency in dogs and cats, representing 45% of all long bone fractures (Unger *et al.*, 1990). Fracture typically occurs following substantial trauma such as a road traffic accident and, as such, individual fracture configuration can vary dramatically. Less commonly, femoral fractures may occur with minimal trauma or spontaneously due to pre-existing bone disease such as neoplasia, for which the distal femur is a predilection site.

Biomechanically, load through the femur is complex and varies as a function of regional anatomy along its length. The femoral diaphysis is eccentrically translated relative to the femoral head and this, combined with a degree of distal procurvatum, renders the lateral and, to a lesser extent, the cranial aspect the tension surfaces of the bone. Femoral fractures have a high incidence of non-union when managed non-surgically; therefore, surgical reduction and internal fixation are indicated in the vast majority of cases.

Fractures of the proximal femur

Proximal femoral fractures are classified as femoral head (epiphyseal), femoral neck (physeal, subcapital and intertrochanteric), trochanteric and subtrochanteric

(Figure 23.1). Of these, physeal fractures are most common in dogs and cats. Fractures are typically seen in animals of less than 1 year of age and are most often a sequel to trauma, although spontaneous physeal fractures have been reported in cats (Craig, 2001) and dogs (Figure 23.2) (Moores *et al.*, 2004); this condition is commonly referred to as slipped femoral capital epiphysis (SFCE). In addition, spontaneous fracture as a sequel to ischaemic necrosis of the femoral head (INFH) may be encountered. Conservative management of fractures typically results in persistent lameness and is not advocated. Therefore, surgical stabilization of simple fractures is indicated, although owners should be counselled regarding the possibility of post-traumatic osteoarthritis or aseptic necrosis occurring due to vascular damage sustained at the time of injury. Comminuted fractures, chronic SFCE or fractures secondary to INFH are usually best managed by femoral head and neck excision or, preferably, total hip replacement.

Femoral head fracture

Stabilization with a screw and anti-rotational Kirschner (K) wire placed via the lateral femoral head/neck junction is indicated (Vernon and Olmstead, 1983) (Operative Technique 23.1).

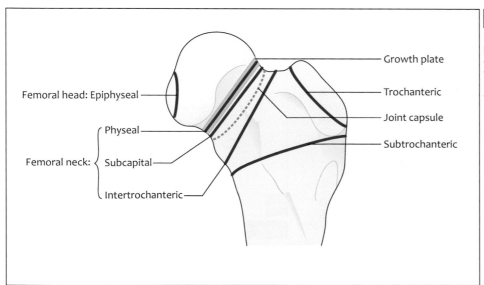

23.1 Fractures of the femoral head, neck and trochanteric region. Physeal fractures occur through the growth plate (blue) and subcapital fractures occur distal to the growth plate but proximal to the insertion of the joint capsule (green). Intertrochanteric fractures occur distal to the joint capsule insertion.

Femoral head: Epiphyseal

Physeal
Femoral neck: Subcapital
Intertrochanteric

Growth plate

Trochanteric

Joint capsule

Subtrochanteric

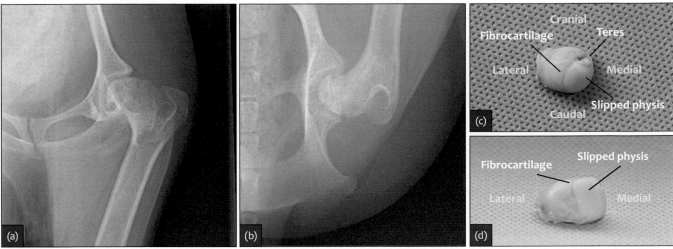

23.2 A slipped capital epiphysis in an 11-month-old Toy Poodle with a 5-week history of left pelvic limb lameness and pain localizing to the left hip joint. (a) Craniocaudal and (b) frog-legged radiographic views showing widening of the coxofemoral joint space and remodelling of the femoral neck and acetabulum. The frog-legged view reveals a step to the epiphysis cranially not evident on the other view, consistent with a slipped capital epiphysis. The slipped physis can be seen on the excised (c) femoral head and (d) neck.

Femoral neck fracture

Techniques for stabilization include lag screw and K-wire, three parallel pins, two parallel pins, and two divergent pins, all placed via a lateral subtrochanteric approach. Lag screw and K-wire and three parallel pin techniques are biomechanically superior based on *ex vivo* studies (Lambrechts *et al.*, 1993) (Figure 23.3) (see Operative Technique 23.2). Stabilization with crossed K-wires placed via a ventral approach has also been described, as have countersunk screws placed from the articular surface, although this technique is not recommended as it is associated with a high incidence of subsequent osteolysis of the femoral neck. Prompt surgical intervention has traditionally been advocated for femoral neck fracture to reduce the risk of femoral head and neck necrosis;

however, development of this complication appears uncommon following internal fixation applied via a lateral subtrochanteric approach (Daly, 1978).

Trochanteric/subtrochanteric fracture

Trochanteric and subtrochanteric fractures are uncommon, the former usually accompanying concurrent epiphyseal separation or coxofemoral dislocation. Trochanteric fracture repair can be performed with paired K-wires and a figure-of-eight tension-band wire (see Operative Technique 23.3). Subtrochanteric fractures may be found in isolation or with femoral neck fracture and are often highly comminuted, necessitating single or double plate, pin-plate or interlocking nail (ILN) fixation.

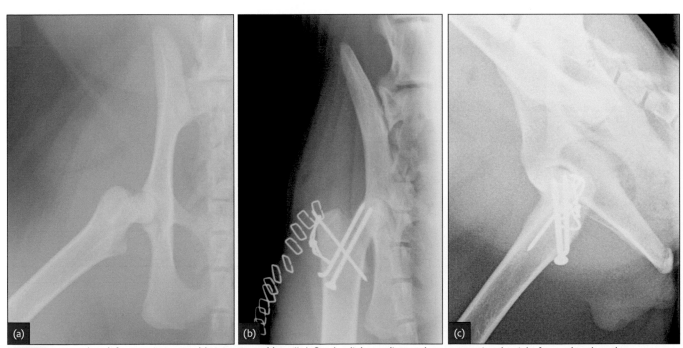

23.3 Femoral neck fracture in 3-year-old Maine Coon. (a) An ill-defined radiolucent line can be seen crossing the right femoral neck on the ventrodorsal radiographic view. Postoperative (b) ventrodorsal and (c) lateromedial radiographic views following stabilization of the fracture with a lag screw and anti-rotational K-wire. A trochanteric osteotomy, performed to aid exposure and reduction of the fracture, was stabilized with a pin and figure-of-eight tension-band wire. Note, the anti-rotational K-wire is not ideally positioned in the femoral head and neck, with limited bone stock on its lateral aspect, and ideally two pins would have been placed to stabilize the trochanteric osteotomy. Fracture healing proceeded uneventfully.

Fractures of the diaphysis

Simple diaphyseal fractures can be treated using rigid anatomical reconstruction. For more comminuted fractures, biological osteosynthesis can be employed with spatial alignment of the proximal and distal fragments without reconstruction, avoiding direct manipulation of intermediate bone fragments. This latter approach can either be performed open via a traditional surgical approach, known as 'open but do not touch' (OBDNT) (see Chapter 8), or closed via limited portals to preserve the soft tissue envelope (see Chapter 15). Fracture configuration is the primary determinant of whether reconstruction is indicated; more comminuted fractures generally lend themselves towards a biological approach. A variety of different implant systems are applicable to stabilization of diaphyseal fractures; the merits of each should be considered during surgical planning.

Intramedullary pin

Biomechanically, the intramedullary (IM) pin affords bending stability but it is poor at resisting concurrent rotation, shear, distraction and compression. As such, an IM pin as the sole means of fracture stabilization cannot be advocated in the vast majority of femoral fractures. Indeed, primary fixation with an IM pin can result in axial collapse of the fracture, proximal pin migration and subsequent sciatic nerve injury (Figure 23.4). The use of an IM pin with the concurrent placement of multiple cerclage wires has been described for the treatment of simple long oblique and spiral fractures, with an IM approximating the diameter of the mid-diaphyseal isthmus being advocated (Beale, 2004) (see Operative Technique 23.4). However, fixation can be tenuous due to the normal procurvatum of the femur, making it challenging to adequately seat an appropriately sized IM pin distally without inducing a recurvatum deformity. Such a deformity will result in incomplete reduction of the fracture, predisposing to fixation failure when cerclage wires have been used. As such, more robust techniques should be considered.

The choice of technique employed for IM pin placement in the femur is paramount as iatrogenic sciatic nerve injury has been associated with IM pinning in 14.3% and 23.1% of dogs and cats, respectively (Fanton *et al.*, 1983). However, sciatic injury is highly unlikely if the pin is placed appropriately. Analysis of normograde and retrograde pinning of simulated proximal, mid-diaphyseal and distal

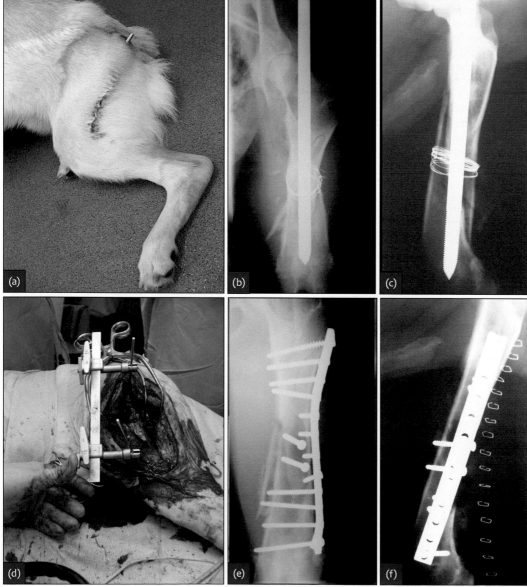

23.4 A comminuted mid-diaphyseal left femoral fracture in a 4-year-old German Shepherd Dog, repaired with an IM pin and cerclage wire 4 weeks previously. (a) Notice marked muscle wastage of the limb and protrusion of the IM pin through the skin. (b) Craniocaudal and (c) mediolateral radiographs at the time of presentation show axial collapse of the fracture and loss of reduction. (d) Intraoperative appearance of the fracture site at the time of revision with distraction of the fracture fragments being performed to restore limb length. (e–f) Postoperative radiographic appearance of the fracture following placement of a lateral 3.5 mm broad dynamic compression plate.

femoral fractures has revealed iatrogenic sciatic damage is significantly less likely to occur if normograde pinning of mid-diaphyseal and distal fractures is adopted; a sciatic nerve injury rate of 53% occurred with retrograde placement for distal femoral fractures (Palmer *et al.*, 1988). In addition, caution should be exercised when considering IM pin placement in immature dogs with open proximal femoral growth plates as proximal femoral deformities such as coxa valga or vara, femoral head and neck malformation, and coxofemoral subluxation may occur as a consequence (Figure 23.5).

Interlocking nail

The femur is well suited to ILN use and the nail can be placed via a minimally invasive direct proximal or distal normograde approach. However, the distal approach necessitates the nail to be recessed subchondrally in the non-weight-bearing distal portion of the trochlear groove of the femur, so direct proximal placement is advocated for most cases. The ILN is a modified IM pin, most commonly employing two to four transverse holes along its length and allowing engagement of a screw or bolt through adjacent bone cortices to lock the nail in place. From a biomechanical perspective, ILN may provide greater resistance to torsional forces than dynamic compression plates (DCPs) and standard IM pins (Dueland *et al.*, 1996). Clinical efficacies of early ILN systems have been reported as favourable in the treatment of femoral fractures in both dogs and cats (Duhautois, 2003). However, 12–14% of animals suffered delayed healing or required adjunctive fixation for successful repair. These complications probably occurred due to limitations in nail design: specifically an inability to adequately resist cyclical torsional and shear forces due to a mismatch between screw/bolt and nail hole dimensions, which precluded rigid interaction. More recently, a novel hourglass-shaped ILN (I-LOC®) has been designed to afford superior mechanical stability by substantially reducing torsional instability (Figure 23.6).

Plate and pin–plate fixation

A plethora of plating systems currently exists for stabilization of long bone fractures including DCPs, limited contact dynamic compression plates (LC-DCPs) and a variety of locking plates (see Chapter 10). Plates can be applied with compression, neutralization or bridging function, via an open approach with anatomical reconstruction of fracture fragments (see Operative Technique 23.5) or via OBDNT or minimally invasive plate osteosynthesis (MIPO) techniques (see Chapter 15). Minimally invasive techniques are utilized more often in the presence of comminution where reconstruction is not applicable (Operative Technique 23.6).

Regional anatomy dictates that the lateral aspect of the femur is most appropriate for plating; however, because of the normal procurvatum of the bone distally, a straight bone plate cannot readily be applied without inducing a recurvatum deformity. Thus the plate must be twisted and applied in a helical fashion to maintain anatomical alignment of the bone (Figure 23.7). Alternatively, more recent locking plate systems incorporating the potential for six degrees of freedom bending, such as string-of-pearls (SOP) or VetLOX™ systems are useful as they can easily be contoured to conform to the entire length of the lateral femur. In the cat, in which the femur has much less procurvatum distally, conventional 2.4 mm non-locking or locking plating systems or 1.5–2/2–2.7 mm veterinary cuttable plates, either singular or stacked, are appropriate.

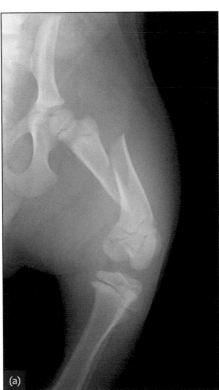
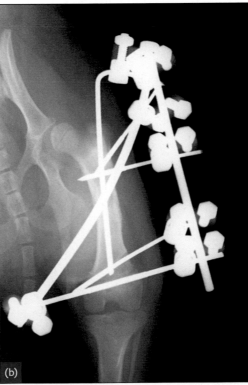
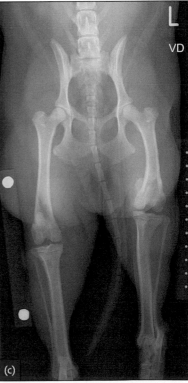

23.5 (a) Mid-diaphyseal oblique left femoral fracture in a 6-month-old Cairn Terrier. The fracture was stabilized with a modified type 1/2 linear external skeletal fixator with a tied-in IM pin. (b) Follow-up radiographs revealed the fracture to have healed after 6 weeks, at which time the fixator was removed. Note: the distal two femoral pins traverse the physis. The dog was presented 12 months later with medial patellar luxation, at which point (c) radiographs revealed multiple abnormalities including coxa vara, an elongated femoral neck, femoral shortening and distal femoral varus. The medial patellar luxation can also be appreciated.

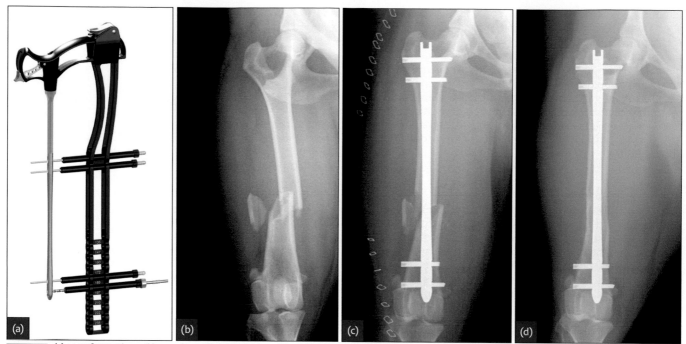

23.6 (a) I-LOC® ILN. The nail has an hourglass-shaped profile. A morse taper fit between the bolts and the nail gives angle stable fixation. (b) Craniocaudal radiograph of a 12-month-old female neutered Labradoodle with a closed comminuted fracture of the femoral diaphysis. Postoperative radiographic appearance (c) immediately and (d) 1 year following stabilization with a 7 x 160 mm I-LOC®.
(a, Courtesy of BioMedtrix; b–d, Courtesy of L Déjardin)

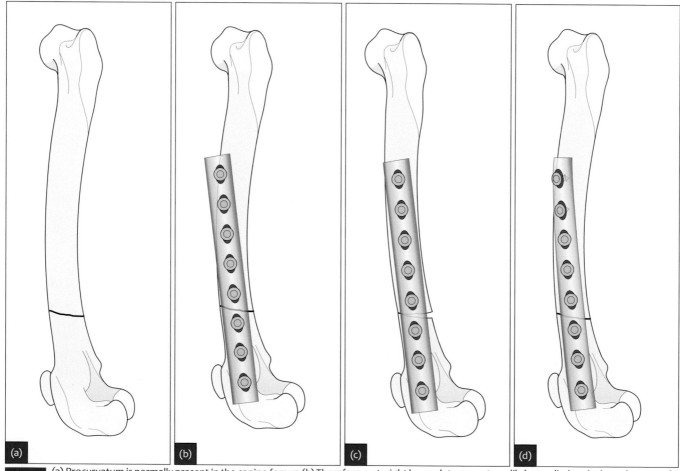

23.7 (a) Procurvatum is normally present in the canine femur. (b) Therefore, a straight bone plate cannot readily be applied to the lateral aspect of the femur as this will cause the plate to be malaligned proximally, compromising screw purchase. (c) Alignment of the femur along the straight bone plate can result in an iatrogenic recurvatum deformity and malreduction of the fracture. (d) To remedy this, the proximal extent of the plate can be twisted to lie on the craniolateral aspect of the femur; this is known as helical plating.

Combining a plate with an IM pin (pin–plate stabilization) has been shown to be a very effective system for biological osteosynthesis of comminuted femoral fractures in dogs and cats (Reems *et al.*, 2003) (Figure 23.8). Addition of the pin reduces plate strain two-fold with a corresponding ten-fold increase in plate fatigue life (Hulse *et al.*, 1997). Practically, a pin approximately 35–40% the diameter of the mid-diaphyseal isthmus is selected, but sizes as low as 30% still confer a mechanical advantage, albeit of lesser magnitude. Placement of the IM pin first facilitates distraction and axial alignment of the bone prior to subsequent plate placement. Original recommendations for this construct suggested one bicortical and three monocortical screws should be placed through the plate either side of the fracture; however, the optimum screw number and configuration is not entirely clear, especially when locking systems such as the locking compression plate are used. Locking compression plates have been shown to have similar stiffness to LC-DCPs in four-point bending and torsion for simulated femoral diaphyseal fractures (Aguila *et al.*, 2005).

Minimally invasive plate osteosynthesis

Regardless of the plating system employed, the surgeon must choose whether to place implants via a traditional open approach or via a minimally invasive approach (e.g. MIPO) (see Chapter 15). Pin–plate constructs can be created utilizing pre-contoured plates introduced through small incisions proximally and distally. Although guidelines for case selection are unclear, for comminuted fractures MIPO confers theoretical advantages and outcomes appear to be at least comparable to cases where implants are placed via an open approach.

External skeletal fixation

Type 1 and modified type 2 linear external skeletal fixation (ESF) systems (see Operative Technique 23.7) and hybrid fixation systems can be applied to the femur successfully; completely circular fixation systems are limited proximally by the trunk, and thus cannot be applied effectively. However, the femur is not ideally suited to stabilization with external fixation because of the muscle coverage around the limb, which can lead to significant pin tract morbidity. The surgeon must be mindful during the design and application of ESF to the femur to respect the appropriate corridors for pin placement (Marti and Miller, 1994), these being the trochanteric and condylar regions only. As the corridors for safe pin placement are limited to the proximal and distal extremities of the bone, an IM pin is a useful and almost universally necessary adjunct to counteract bending forces, the pin either being separate or 'tied-in' to the frame (see Figure 23.5).

Following fixation in immature animals with comminuted diaphyseal fractures, care should be taken to monitor for signs of quadriceps muscle contracture, manifesting with persistent extension and severely limited motion of the stifle (see Chapter 28). The condition is best avoided by appropriate rigid fracture stabilization and early postoperative weight-bearing. Once the condition becomes established, the prognosis is poor.

Fractures of the distal femur

Distal femoral fractures can be classified as metaphyseal, supracondylar and condylar in the mature patient, and epiphyseal in the juvenile (Figures 23.9 and 23.10). Collectively, distal femoral fractures are common in dogs and cats.

Distal femoral physeal fractures

The distal femur is the most common site of physeal fractures in immature dogs (37%), the majority of which are Salter–Harris types I and II. Topographically, the metaphyseal pitons of the distal femur interdigitate with the physis and these are useful anatomical landmarks by which to assess the accuracy of fracture reduction at surgery as well as providing a degree of translatory and rotational stability to the repair (Figure 23.11). Numerous stabilization techniques for these fractures have been described including a single IM pin, paired convergent pins, Rush pins and crossed metal or polyglycolic acid pins. *Ex vivo* analyses of these techniques reveal crossed metal pin constructs to sustain greatest load to failure (Sukhiani and

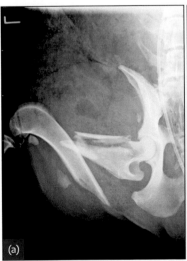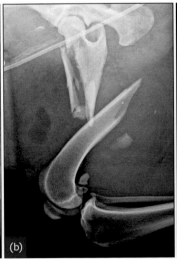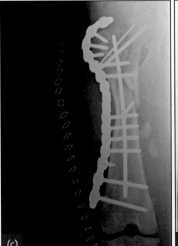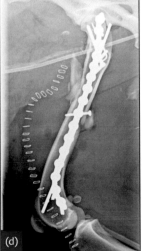

23.8 Preoperative (a) ventrodorsal and (b) mediolateral radiographs of an 18-month-old Jack Russell Terrier with a closed comminuted fracture of the femur with concurrent femoral neck fracture. Postoperative (c) cradiocaudal and (d) mediolateral radiographs. The diaphysis was stabilized with an IM pin and 3.5 mm SOP plate, and the femoral neck fracture with a lag screw and anti-rotational K-wire. Note how six-point bending of the SOP plate facilitates contouring of the plate distally to follow the normal procurvatum of the femur. Ideally, a larger IM pin should have been used.

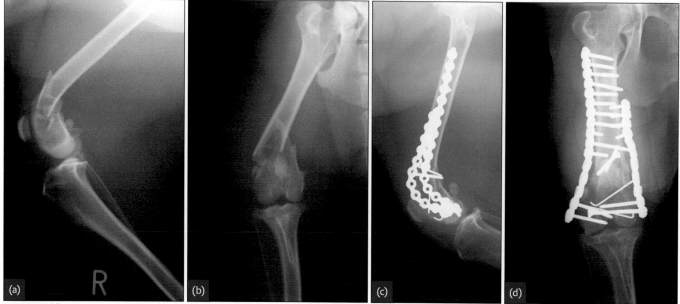

23.9 (a) Mediolateral and (b) craniocaudal radiographs of a closed, comminuted bicondylar fracture of the distal femur in a 6-year-old Dobermann. Postoperative (c) mediolateral and (d) craniocaudal radiographs. The fracture was stabilized with a transcondylar lag screw and bilateral 3.5 mm SOP locking plates.

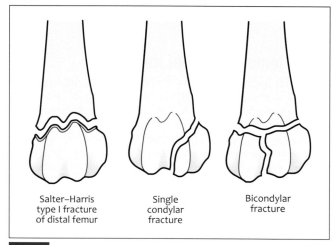

Salter–Harris type I fracture of distal femur

Single condylar fracture

Bicondylar fracture

23.10 Fractures of the distal femur.

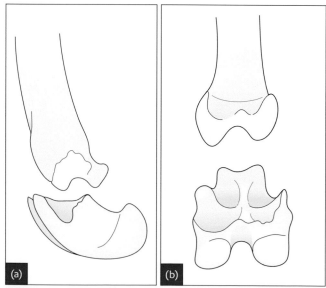

23.11 Views of the (a) medial and (b) caudocranial aspects of the canine distal femoral physis. Note the morphology of the metaphyseal pitons that interdigitate with the physis.

Holmberg, 1997). Studies have shown that Rush pins placed across the distal femoral physis of juvenile dogs without fracture do not appear to impede growth (Stone *et al.*, 1981), but naturally occurring physeal fractures usually disrupt the proliferative zone of the physis and thus the injury itself will often compromise future growth potential. This is supported by clinical case series where the potential for growth disturbance appears independent of the means of fixation employed (Berg *et al.*, 1984). Should premature physeal closure occur, compensatory growth of the tibia is reported with femoral length deficits of up to 23% being tolerated without an overt change in gait (Wagner *et al.*, 1987). Whether to use cross pinning or Rush pinning techniques is decided according to surgeon preference (see Operative Technique 23.8).

Supracondylar and condylar fractures

Supracondylar and condylar fractures in skeletally mature dogs and cats occur infrequently. In contrast to physeal injuries, supracondylar fractures can be challenging to manage due to frequent comminution, thin metaphyseal bone, significant disruptive forces and a short distal fragment that is eccentrically positioned caudally relative to the diaphysis. This morphology limits the use of IM pins and conventional bone plate purchase at this site. Reconstruction plates can be readily contoured and applied at this site; however, they may not be of sufficient strength for the treatment of a comminuted fracture requiring a bridging implant and are not advocated. Current strategies for fixation include application of an inverted human lateral tibial head fracture plate (Lidbetter and Glyde, 2000), a specific supracondylar femoral plate and bilateral plating (see Operative Technique 23.9). Locking plates permitting six degrees of freedom of screw placement can also readily be used (see Figure 23.9). Specific case series evaluating the efficacy of these implant systems *in vivo* for the treatment of supracondylar fractures are currently lacking. Use of the supracondylar plate has been reported in the context of stabilizing the distal femur following osteotomy for the correction of distal femoral varus with encouraging results. Similarly, hybrid

ESF, comprising a distal stretch ring coupled to a lateral linear connecting bar with or without an IM pin has been reported with excellent results in the majority of cases (Kirkby et al., 2008).

Fractures to either the medial or lateral portion of the femoral condyle appear to occur rarely, with the former being more common (Carmichael et al., 1989). Non-weight-bearing lameness following twisting of the limb or a fall with proximocaudal displacement of the medial portion of the condyle is typical. As these fractures are articular, prompt anatomical reduction and rigid internal fixation with a transcondylar screw and anti-rotational supracondylar implant(s) are required (see Operative Technique 24.10). Prognosis is good with prompt surgical management. Bicondylar fractures with a 'T' shaped configuration also occur uncommonly; these can be managed by reconstruction of the articular surfaces using lag screws and subsequent stabilization of the supracondylar component of the fracture using plates, pins or ESF.

References and further reading

Aguila AZ, Manon JM, Orlansky AS et al. (2005) In vitro biomechanical comparison of limited contact dynamic compression plate and locking compression plate. Veterinary and Comparative Orthopaedics and Traumatology 18, 220–226

Beale B (2004) Orthopedic clinical techniques femur fracture repair. Clinical Techniques for the Small Animal Practitioner 19, 134–150

Berg RJ, Egger EL, Konde LJ and McCurnin DM (1984) Evaluation of prognostic factors for growth following distal femoral physeal injury in 17 dogs. Veterinary Surgery 13, 172–180

Bernarde A, Diop A, Maurel N and Viguier E (2001) An in vitro biomechanical study of bone plate and interlocking nail in a canine diaphyseal femoral fracture model. Veterinary Surgery 30, 397–408

Burns CG, Litsky AS, Allen MJ and Johnson KA (2011) Influence of locking bolt location on the mechanical properties of an interlocking nail in the canine femur. Veterinary Surgery 40, 522–530

Carmichael S, Wheeler SJ and Vaughan LC (1989) Single condylar fractures of the distal femur in the dog. Journal of Small Animal Practice 30, 500–504

Craig LE (2001) Physeal dysplasia with slipped capital femoral epiphysis in 13 cats. Veterinary Pathology 38, 92–97

Daly WR (1978) Femoral head and neck fractures in the dog and cat: A review of 115 cases. Veterinary Surgery 7, 29–38

Dueland RT, Berglund L, Vanderby R Jr and Chao EY (1996) Structural properties of interlocking nail, canine femora, and femur-interlocking nail constructs. Veterinary Surgery 25, 386–396

Dueland RT, Johnson KA, Roe SC, Engen MH and Lesser AS (1999) Interlocking nail treatment of diaphyseal long-bone fractures in dogs. Journal of the American Veterinary Medical Association 214, 59–66

Duhautois B (2003) Use of veterinary interlocking nails for diaphyseal fractures in dogs and cats: 121 cases. Veterinary Surgery 32, 8–20

Evans HE (1993) The skeleton; Arthrology; The muscular system. In: Miller's Anatomy of the Dog, 3rd edn, ed. HE Evans, pp. 122–384. WB Saunders, Philadelphia

Fanton JW, Blass CE and Withrow SJ (1983) Sciatic nerve injury as a complication of intramedullary pin fixation of femoral fractures. Journal of the American Animal Hospital Association 19, 687–694

Hulse D, Hyman W, Nori M and Slater M (1997) Reduction in plate strain by addition of an intramedullary pin. Veterinary Surgery 26, 451–459

Johnson KA and Huckstep RL (1986) Bone remodelling in canine femora after internal fixation with the Huckstep nail. Journal of Veterinary Radiology 27, 20–23

Kalis RH, Liska WD and Jankovits DA (2012) Total hip replacement as a treatment option for capital physeal fractures in dogs and cats. Veterinary Surgery 41, 148–155

Kirkby KA, Lewis DD and Lafuente MP (2008) Management of humeral and femoral fractures in dogs and cats with linear-circular hybrid external skeletal fixators. Journal of the Americal Animal Hospital Association 44, 180–197

Lambrechts NE, Verstraete FJM and Sumner Smith G (1993) Internal fixation of femoral neck fracture in the dog – an in vitro study. Veterinary and Comparative Orthopaedics and Traumatology 6, 188–193

Lidbetter DA and Glyde MR (2000) Supracondylar femoral fractures in adult animals. Journal of the American Animal Hospital Association 22, 1041–1045

Marti JM and Miller A (1994) Delimitation of safe corridors for the insertion of external fixator pins in the dog 1: Hindlimb. Journal of Small Animal Practice 35, 16–23

Palmer RH, Aron DN and Purinton PT (1988) Relationship of femoral intramedullary pins to the sciatic nerve and gluteal muscles after retrograde and normograde insertion. Veterinary Surgery 17, 65–70

Piermattei DL and Johnson KA (2004) The hindlimb. In: An Atlas of Surgical Approaches to the Bones and Joints of the Dog and Cat, 4th edn, pp. 329–391. Saunders, Philadelphia

Pozzi A and Lewis DD (2009) Surgical approaches for minimally invasive plate osteosynthesis in dogs. Veterinary and Comparative Orthopaedics and Traumatology 22, 316–320

Reems MR, Beale BS and Hulse DA (2003) Use of a plate–rod construct and principles of biological osteosynthesis for repair of diaphyseal fractures in dogs and cats: 47 cases (1994–2001). Journal of the American Veterinary Medical Association 223, 330–335

Stone EA, Betts CW and Rowland GN (1981) Effect of Rush pins on the distal femoral growth plate of young dogs. American Journal of Veterinary Research 42, 261–265

Sukhiani HR and Holmberg DL (1997) Ex vivo biomechanical comparison of pin fixation technique for canine distal femoral physeal fractures. Veterinary Surgery 26, 398–407

Unger M, Montavon PM and Heim UF (1990) Classification of fractures of the long bones in the dog and cat: introduction and clinical application. Veterinary and Comparative Orthopaedics and Traumatology 3, 41–50

Vernon FF and Olmstead ML (1983) Femoral head fractures resulting in epiphyseal fragmentation. Results of repair in five dogs. Veterinary Surgery 12, 123–126

Wagner SD, Desch JP, Ferguson HR and Nassar RF (1987) Effect of distal femoral growth plate fusion on femoro-tibial length. Veterinary Surgery 16, 435–439

→ **OPERATIVE TECHNIQUE 23.2 CONTINUED**

EQUIPMENT EXTRAS

Appropriately sized bone screw set (1.5–2 mm for cats and small dogs, 2.4–4.5 mm for medium to giant-breed dogs); Langenbeck retractors; large and small Hohmann retractors; pointed reduction forceps; drill; K-wires; pin/wire cutters; pin benders; periosteal elevator.

SURGICAL TECHNIQUES

Approach

Craniolateral as described in Operative Technique 23.1.

Reduction and fixation

Outward rotation of the femur and placement of Hohmann retractors allows visualization of the fracture and the intertrochanteric region of the femur. The glide hole is then drilled retrograde or normograde from the femoral neck to the lateral subtrochanteric area (Figure 23.14). The use of an aiming guide can make this easier.

> **WARNING**
>
> When retrograde drilling, take care to protect the sciatic nerve from injury from the drill bit as it exits the bone

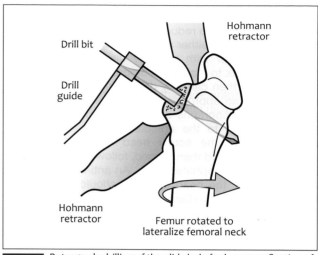

23.14 Retrograde drilling of the glide hole for lag screw fixation of femoral neck fractures.

A centring drill sleeve is inserted from laterally to medially and the femur internally rotated to reduce the fracture. The fracture is held in reduction either with pointed reduction forceps, or medial pressure on the femoral neck to manually compress the fracture. The thread hole is then carefully drilled through the centring drill sleeve to an appropriate depth, as measured from the preoperative radiographs, taking care not to penetrate the articular cartilage (Figure 23.15) When measuring the screw length, do not add 2 mm as would be the case for standard screw placement as this extra length could lead to penetration of the articular surface. When the lag screw has been placed, an anti-rotational K-wire is inserted parallel to the screw using a drill (Figure 23.16). The tip of the wire is then bent over and cut to prevent migration.

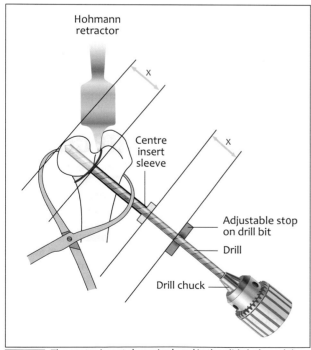

23.15 The centre insert sleeve is placed in the glide hole and the fracture reduced. An adjustable stop is attached to the drill bit a distance (x) corresponding to just less than the measured depth of the femoral head, such that articular penetration does not occur.

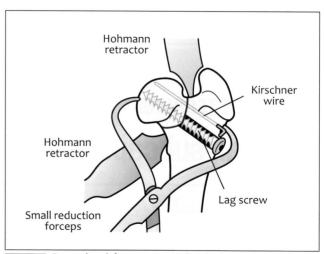

23.16 Femoral neck fracture repaired with a lag screw and anti-rotational K-wire. Pointed reduction forceps can be used to maintain reduction of a femoral neck fracture following the drilling of the screw glide hole (see text for details).

→ **OPERATIVE TECHNIQUE 23.2 CONTINUED**

Alternative technique

In immature patients or smaller mature animals, three K-wires can be placed instead of a screw and anti-rotational K-wire. The pins are similarly placed from the subtrochanteric region and carefully advanced the measured distance into the epiphysis before being cut (Figure 23.17). Either divergent or parallel pins can be used; parallel pins may be advantageous as these allow compression of the fracture during weight-bearing.

Wound closure

See Operative Technique 23.1.

POSTOPERATIVE MANAGEMENT

See Operative Technique 23.1.

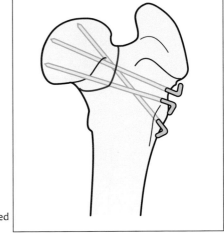

23.17 Femoral neck fracture repaired with three K-wires.

OPERATIVE TECHNIQUE 23.3

Fractures of the greater trochanter

PREOPERATIVE PREPARATION

Assessment of appropriate size of K-wires and orthopaedic wire for size of patient.

POSITIONING

Lateral recumbency with the affected limb quarter draped and uppermost.

ASSISTANT

Optional.

EQUIPMENT EXTRAS

Gelpi self-retaining retractors; K-wires; orthopaedic wire; pin/wire cutters; drill; reduction forceps; wire twisters.

SURGICAL TECHNIQUES

Approach

Incision over the greater trochanter directly on to the fracture.

Reduction and fixation

The fracture fragment is grasped with reduction forceps and tractioned distally, complete with its muscular insertions, back into position. Two parallel K-wires are then inserted diagonally through the trochanter in a distomedial direction, angled approximately 50 degrees distally, either engaging the medial cortex or being placed as IM pins. A hole is then drilled transversely in a craniocaudal orientation in the proximal femoral metaphyseal region. Orthopaedic wire is placed through this hole, looped around the K-wires proximally and twisted in a figure-of-eight orientation. The K-wires are bent dorsally to prevent migration and then cut (Figure 23.18). It is also possible to use a single lag screw for fixation in mature animals (Figure 23.19), the screw being inserted similarly at an angle of 50 degrees and engaging with the medial femoral cortex. The placement of an additional figure-of-eight tension-band wire, as used with pin fixation (Figure 23.18a), around the screw head may be beneficial.

→

➜ **OPERATIVE TECHNIQUE 23.3 CONTINUED**

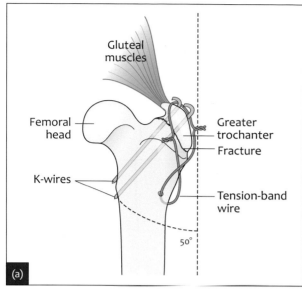

(a)

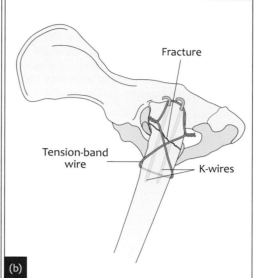

(b)

23.18 (a) Cranial and (b) lateral views of a fracture of the greater trochanter repaired with two K-wires and a figure-of-eight tension-band wire.

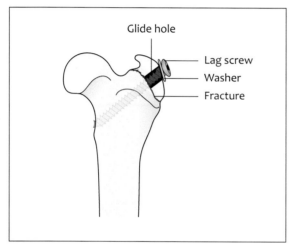

23.19 Cranial view of a fracture of the greater trochanter in a mature patient repaired with a single lag screw.

POSTOPERATIVE MANAGEMENT

See Operative Technique 23.1.

OPERATIVE TECHNIQUE 23.4

Intramedullary pinning of spiral/long oblique diaphyseal fractures

PREOPERATIVE PREPARATION

- The length of the bone is estimated based on radiographs of the intact contralateral femur.
- If a pin is being used in combination with cerclage wiring, its diameter should nearly impact the medullary canal at its narrowest point as determined by measurement of the orthogonal radiographs; this measurement should be confirmed in surgery prior to pin placement.
- If the pin is to be placed as an adjunct to a plate or external fixator, a pin width of 35–40% of the medullary canal width at its narrowest point is appropriate.
- The height of the greater trochanter relative to the trochanteric fossa should be measured on the craniocaudal radiograph.

POSITIONING

It is useful to traction the limb with the patient in dorsal recumbency as the patient is prepared for surgery, to overcome muscle contraction. For surgery, position in lateral recumbency, with the affected limb quarter draped and uppermost.

ASSISTANT

Optional. Useful for applying countertraction to the limb.

EQUIPMENT EXTRAS

Jacobs chuck; bone-holding forceps; appropriately sized IM pin; orthopaedic wire; wire twisters; pin/wire cutters; Gelpi self-retaining retractors.

SURGICAL TECHNIQUES

Approach

Wherever possible the pin should be placed by normograde insertion. A limited approach to the greater trochanter can be performed with direct incision of the skin over this site. A combination of limited blunt dissection and careful palpation with a pair of straight haemostats will allow identification of the intertrochanteric fossa, which is the site where the pin must enter the femur (Figure 23.20). A limited lateral approach to the diaphysis, of sufficient size to adequately visualize the fracture, should then be performed. Following a skin incision over the fracture site, incision of the fascia lata allows delineation of the vastus lateralis muscle cranially and biceps femoris muscle caudally; these are separated to reveal the fracture site (Figure 23.21). The adductor muscle attachments to the caudal femur are left undisturbed since these provide an important extraosseous blood supply to the bone.

Reduction and fixation

For normograde placement, the trochar tip is introduced into the intertrochanteric fossa, abutting the medial aspect of the greater trochanter. A Jacobs chuck or drill is then used to advance the pin into the bone, being mindful that the pin is oriented parallel with the long axis of the bone. On emergence of the pin at the fracture site, the trochar tip of the pin can be removed with bolt cutters prior to advancement into the distal fragment (Figure 23.22a) to reduce the risk of inadvertent penetration of the stifle joint, although this theoretically risks reducing the stability of the distal contact point. If the pin is being placed retrograde, bone-holding forceps are applied to the proximal femoral fragment and the femur manipulated such that the hip is both extended and mildly adducted. The pin should be introduced obliquely into the femur such

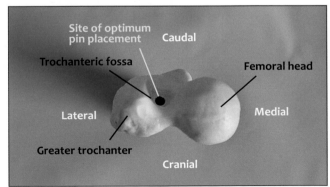

23.20 Proximal aspect of a disarticulated left femur showing the optimum entry/exit point for an IM pin in the trochanteric fossa.

→ **OPERATIVE TECHNIQUE 23.4 CONTINUED**

that it contacts the medial aspect of the femur at the fracture site (Figure 23.23a) and thus is guided towards the lateral aspect of the femur proximally, rather than the medial side (Figure 23.23b). This limb and pin position, prior to pin advancement proximally, will reduce the risk of iatrogenic sciatic nerve damage.

Following placement of the pin in the proximal bone fragment, the fracture is reduced and the pin driven into the distal femoral fragment until resistance is felt as the pin engages metaphyseal bone. Holding a pin of identical length next to the bone is a useful guide of how much further advancement is required to avoid penetration of the stifle joint.

The preoperative measurement of the depth of the trochanteric fossa is then used to ascertain the height that the IM pin should be cut (Figure 23.22b). With the pin fully seated in the bone the Jacobs chuck is attached to the pin at a height level with the greater trochanter. The pin is then reversed out of the bone 1–2 cm, the trochanteric fossa depth measured down the pin using the attachment of the Jacobs chuck as the reference point, and then the pin scored

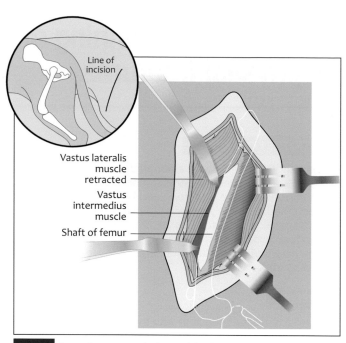

Vastus lateralis muscle retracted

Vastus intermedius muscle

Shaft of femur

Line of incision

23.21 Lateral exposure of a femoral diaphyseal fracture.

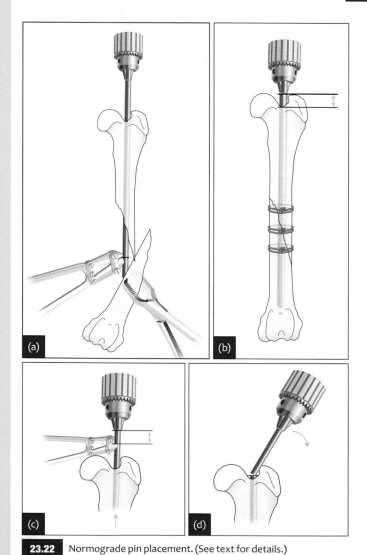

(a)

(b)

(c)

(d)

23.22 Normograde pin placement. (See text for details.)

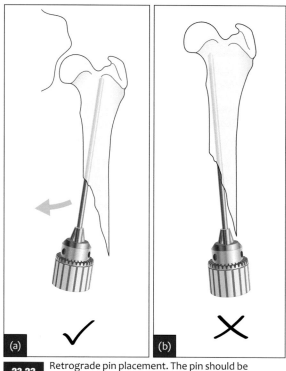

(a) ✓

(b) ✗

23.23 Retrograde pin placement. The pin should be purposely oblique within the bone during placement, touching the medial cortex distally so that the trochar tip tracks laterally away from the joint and the sciatic nerve.

→ **OPERATIVE TECHNIQUE 23.4 CONTINUED**

at the appropriate level 50–60% of its diameter, using implant cutters or a hacksaw (Figure 23.22c). The pin is then pushed back to its fully seated position and the remaining protruding pin bent cranially and caudally with the chuck until it breaks off at the level where it was scored (Figure 23.22d). The trochanteric fossa should be carefully palpated to ensure the pin is recessed; if this is incomplete, careful advancement with a punch and mallet can be performed to seat the pin correctly.

If the pin is to be left long and 'tied-in' to an ESF frame, a sufficient length of pin should be left protruding from the skin proximally to ensure the pin or any fixator clamps do not impinge on the skin.

Wound closure

The fascia lata is closed with an absorbable suture material in a simple continuous pattern; thereafter closure is routine.

POSTOPERATIVE MANAGEMENT

Cage/small room rest for 6 to 8 weeks followed by repeat radiographs. If healing is progressing satisfactorily, incrementally increasing exercise over the following 6- to 8-week period can ensue.

WARNING

An IM pin ± cerclage wire should never be used as the sole method of fixation of transverse or comminuted fractures of the femur as compressive, distractive and rotational forces are not adequately neutralized, predisposing to non-delayed union. Although cerclage wire can be used in conjunction with the IM pin for stabilization of long oblique or spiral fractures, in almost all cases more robust additional fixation using a plate or an external fixator is advisable

PRACTICAL TIPS

- Normograde pin placement is preferred in almost all cases. If the pin is placed in a retrograde fashion this should be performed with the hip in extension and mild adduction to reduce the risk of sciatic impalement
- Alignment of the edge of the adductor muscle on the caudal border of the femoral shaft is a useful check for correct rotational alignment of the limb distally following fracture reduction

OPERATIVE TECHNIQUE 23.5

Open bone plating of the diaphysis

PREOPERATIVE PREPARATION

Plates are applied to the lateral aspect of the femur, should span the length of the bone and should be contoured appropriately. Plates can be applied with difficulty to the cranial aspect of the femur proximal to the trochlear sulcus, if orthogonal plating is required.

POSITIONING

It is useful to traction the limb with the patient in dorsal recumbency as the patient is prepared for surgery, to counteract muscle contraction. For surgery, the patient is positioned in lateral recumbency, with the affected limb quarter draped and uppermost.

ASSISTANT

Useful for applying countertraction to the limb, and for fracture reduction and plate application.

EQUIPMENT EXTRAS

Appropriately sized screw and plate kit; plate-bending irons; bone-holding forceps; fragment forceps; self-retaining and hand-held retractors.

→ **OPERATIVE TECHNIQUE 23.5 CONTINUED**

SURGICAL TECHNIQUES

Approach

As for Operative Technique 23.4.

Reduction and fixation

Dependent on individual fracture configuration. Bone-holding forceps applied to the proximal and distal fragments by the assistant can allow accurate control of fracture fragment apposition. Placement of a temporary IM pin can also assist maintenance of reduction during plate application. The surgeon can assess torsional alignment accurately via the caudal surface of the femur, which is marked by a finely roughened line, the linea aspera. The appropriate length bone plate is selected, contoured and placed on the lateral aspect of the bone. The method of plate application (dynamic compression, neutralization or bridging; see Operative Techniques 11.9–11.11) is governed by the configuration of the fracture. The plate should be as long as possible to maximize resistance to disruptive forces.

If the fracture involves the proximal diaphysis the plate should be contoured over the greater trochanter; screws can then be directed distally into the trochanter as well as along the femoral neck for additional bone purchase.

Wound closure

As for Operative Technique 23.4.

POSTOPERATIVE CARE

As for Operative Technique 23.4.

PRACTICAL TIP

Take care to ensure that the torsional alignment of the limb is correct by assessing regional anatomy, fracture fragment orientation and movement of the hip, stifle and distal limb prior to and following implant placement

OPERATIVE TECHNIQUE 23.6
Pin–plate stabilization of comminuted diaphyseal fractures

BACKGROUND

Comminuted mid-diaphyseal fractures are best managed by spatial realignment of the bone fragments without an attempt to reconstruct the fracture. This can be achieved by an OBDNT limited approach to the fracture site, or less commonly, by a MIPO technique using small proximal and distal incisions without direct exposure of the fracture site (see Operative Technique 15.4). Due to the mechanical demands on the implants in a non-load sharing situation, the plate is best combined with an IM pin (Figure 23.24).

PREOPERATIVE PREPARATION

An appropriate size and length of plate should be chosen based on orthogonal radiographs of the contralateral femur. Conventional or locking plates can be used. The plate can be pre-contoured, with special attention being paid to contouring over the greater trochanter and if necessary to the procurvatum of the distal femur. An IM pin approximately 35–40% of the width of the diaphysis at its narrowest point should be selected.

POSITIONING

It is useful to traction the limb with the patient in dorsal recumbency as the patient is prepared for surgery, to counteract muscle contraction. For surgery, the patient is positioned in lateral recumbency, with the affected limb quarter draped and uppermost.

→ **OPERATIVE TECHNIQUE 23.6 CONTINUED**

ASSISTANT

Useful for applying countertraction to the limb and for fracture reduction and plate application.

EQUIPMENT EXTRAS

Appropriately sized screw and plate kit; plate-bending irons; bone-holding forceps; fragment forceps; self-retaining and hand-held retractors; IM pins; pin cutters; drill; Jacobs chuck.

SURGICAL TECHNIQUES

Approach

As for Operative Technique 23.4, with the addition of a 3–5 cm limited approach to the distal lateral femur. An additional approach may also need to be made to the lateral aspect of the greater trochanter in some cases. Alternatively, a single long incision can be made spanning the entire length of the femur.

Reduction and fixation

The IM pin is placed first; normograde pin placement is preferred. Attachment of bone-holding forceps to the proximal and distal fragments facilitates manipulation of the bone to allow engagement of the IM pin. No attempt is made to manipulate intermediate fragments. If multiple smaller incisions have been made, an epiperiosteal tunnel is created between them by blunt dissection, to allow introduction of the plate; clearly this is not necessary if a single long incision has been made. The plate is contoured and applied to the lateral aspect of the bone. Alignment of the limb is then assessed with particular care being taken to assess the torsional alignment. Two or three screws are then placed proximally and distally, with the aim of placing at least one bicortical screw in each major bone segment. If a locking plate and screws are used it can be useful to initially apply one non-locking cortical screw proximally and distally in an area of good bone contact with the plate, to pull the plate down on to the bone before the locking screws are placed.

Wound closure

As for Operative Technique 23.4.

POSTOPERATIVE MANAGEMENT

As for Operative Technique 23.4.

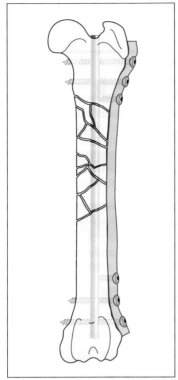

23.24 Pin–plate construct used to stabilize a comminuted mid-diaphyseal femoral fracture.

> **WARNING**
>
> Take care to ensure that torsional alignment of the limb is correct prior to placing screws in the plate, otherwise an internal or external rotational deformity of the distal limb will be induced

> **PRACTICAL TIP**
>
> Cutting the pin short before the screws are placed in the plate will limit the risk of multiple screw threads contacting the pin and making withdrawal of the pin for cutting impossible

→ **OPERATIVE TECHNIQUE 23.8 CONTINUED**

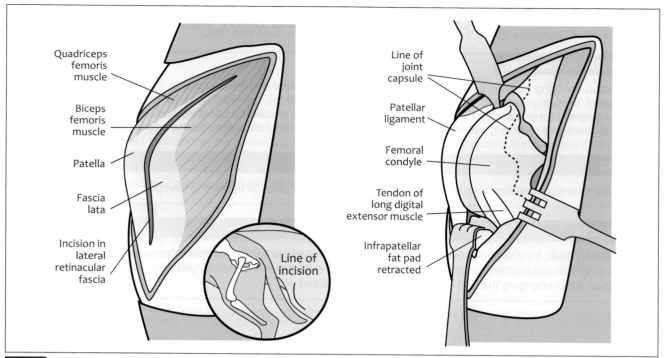

23.26 Exposure of a distal femoral fracture.

Reduction and fixation – crossed pins

The epiphysis is most often displaced caudally relative to the femoral metaphysis due to contraction of the hamstring muscles. The fragment can be reduced by indirect manipulation using the tibia as a 'handle', or by careful manipulation using a small Hohmann retractor or pointed reduction forceps placed transversely across the condyles. Reduction is easier with the stifle held in flexion. It is helpful to drill a small hole on the cranial aspect of the distal femoral diaphysis; this can be used as an anchor point for a small pair of fragment forceps placed between the hole and the intercondylar notch (Figure 23.27). K-wires are then placed. The lateral wire should enter the condyle just below the origin of the long digital extensor tendon and run obliquely to engage the medial cortex of the metaphysis. The medial K-wire should be placed in a corresponding symmetrical orientation from the medial portion of the condyle such that the wires cross within the bone proximal to the physis. The K-wires should then be bent to prevent migration. Care should be taken when bending these pins that they do not cut through the soft condylar bone (Figure 23.28). The patella is reduced, and patellar tracking and range of motion of the stifle assessed prior to closure.

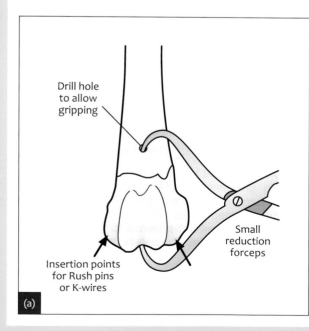

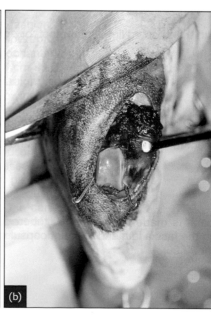

23.27 (a) Position of reduction forceps to hold distal epiphyseal separation of femur reduced with insertion points for Rush pins or K-wires. (b) Reduced epiphyseal separation in a cat showing position of Rush pins before they are seated completely.

→ **OPERATIVE TECHNIQUE 23.8 CONTINUED**

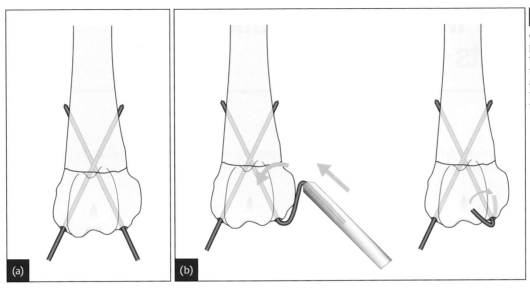

23.28 (a) Correct K-wire placement for distal femoral repair. (b) The pins are bent axially towards the femoral trochlea and then cut off. Wire twisters are used to straighten the tip of the pin away from the trochlea.

Reduction and fixation – Rush pins

Rush pins can be fashioned using K-wires or small Steinmann pins (see Chapter 10). Following exposure of the fracture site, a large pin is driven into the metaphysis of the femur through the fracture surface to create a tunnel for subsequent introduction of the Rush pins. Following reduction of the fracture, pilot holes are drilled in the epiphysis using K-wires the same size as the Rush pins. These pilot holes are started in the same location as described above for crossed pins, and aimed proximally and slightly obliquely. The Rush pins are then advanced through the pilot holes into the femoral metaphysis; final seating of the hook of the Rush pin against the bone can be done using a punch and mallet (Figure 23.29).

Wound closure

The joint capsule and fascia lata are closed. Subcutaneous and cutaneous tissues are closed routinely.

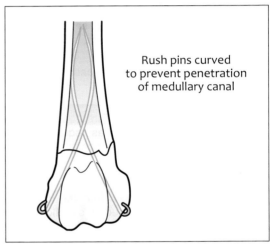

Rush pins curved to prevent penetration of medullary canal

23.29 Epiphyseal separation repaired with two Rush pins. Their hooks are above and clear of the bearing surface of the condyles.

POSTOPERATIVE MANAGEMENT

Strict rest for 4 weeks followed by repeat radiographs with an incremental increase in activity over the following 6-week period. Pins can be removed once the fracture has consolidated (normally 4 to 6 weeks postoperatively), although this is not necessary unless they are perceived to cause irritation.

WARNINGS

- Bone in this region is extremely soft and it is easy to cause significant damage with overzealous use of retractors and fragment forceps
- It is easy to under-reduce these fractures, especially when using crossed pins. Take care to ensure that reduction is anatomical prior to implant placement

PRACTICAL TIP

Once the K-wires are placed they should be bent in an axial direction towards the femoral trochlea and then twisted to lie parallel with the femoral shaft. Avoid bending the pins proximally or abaxially as they may cut through the bone as they bend

→ **OPERATIVE TECHNIQUE 23.10 CONTINUED**

Approach

See Operative Technique 23.8. Increased exposure may be gained by osteotomy of the tibial tuberosity and proximal reflection of the quadriceps muscle mass; this is rarely necessary.

Reduction and fixation

Fracture to the lateral or medial portion of the femoral condyle

The fractured portion of the condyle is cleared of fracture haematoma. A glide hole can then be drilled from 'inside-out' in the smaller portion of the condyle. The fractured portion of the condyle is then reduced and compressed in reduction with fragment forceps. A drill insert sleeve is placed in the glide hole and the glide hole drilled through the sleeve. The depth of the hole is measured and an appropriate length screw placed. An anti-rotational implant should be also be placed (either a second screw, a K-wire or a short plate and screws) (Figure 23.32).

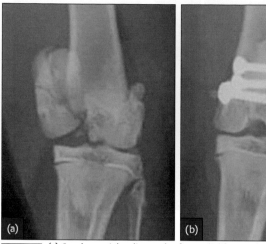

23.32 (a) Caudocranial radiograph of a medial femoral condylar fracture in an 11-month-old cat. (b) The fracture has been reduced and stabilized with three lag screws.
(Courtesy of T Gemmill)

Alternatively, for placement of the lag screw an 'outside-in' approach can be used as with the distal humerus (see Chapter 20); however, accurate screw placement may be more challenging.

T or Y fracture of the femoral condyle

So-called depending on the obliquity of the supracondylar fracture fragments. Reduction and fixation of the articular portion of the fracture is performed first, as described above. The condyle is subsequently reattached to the femoral metaphysis with crossed K-wires, a plate and K-wire or bilateral plates. If plates are applied, be mindful that distally it may be necessary to contour the plate to the natural procurvatum of the bone. Locking plates with six degrees of freedom bending are useful at this site.

Wound closure

As for Operative Technique 23.8.

Strict rest for 6 weeks followed by repeat radiographs, with an incremental increase in activity over the following 6-week period if radiographs show satisfactory healing.

Chapter 24

The tibia and fibula

Steven J. Butterworth

Fractures of the tibia and fibula are commonly seen in small animal practice. In one study, they represented 14.8% of 284 canine fractures and 5.4% of 298 feline fractures (Phillips, 1979). Such injuries are usually a result of road traffic accidents, but other causes include dog fights and trapping a paw whilst moving at speed.

Fractures of the proximal tibia and fibula

In the vast majority of cases these involve physes of skeletally immature patients.

Avulsion of the tibial tubercle

This injury is seen almost exclusively in animals less than 10 months of age (Figure 24.1). The Greyhound and terrier breeds are over-represented, with Staffordshire Bull Terriers being commonly affected in one study (Gower *et al.*, 2008). The tibial tubercle forms as a separate centre of ossification and serves as the point of insertion for the straight patellar tendon. Avulsion of the tubercle renders the dog unable to fix the stifle in extension during weight-bearing. Swelling will be present on the cranial aspect of the joint, the tubercle may be palpated proximal to its normal position and the patella will be positioned proximally in the trochlear groove. Radiography provides a definitive diagnosis.

In all cases where complete avulsion has occurred, open reduction and internal fixation using the tension-band principle are required to re-establish the integrity of the quadriceps complex (see Operative Technique 24.1).

If radiography shows only a partial avulsion, then the patient may be treated conservatively (von Pfeil *et al.*, 2012). Casting or splinting is unlikely to be effective, and management should comprise strict cage rest and monitoring in case the avulsion should become complete. The author's approach tends to be internal fixation to avoid the risk of the avulsion becoming complete. A Kirschner (K) wire is used alone or, more commonly, in combination with a tension-band. A figure-of-eight suture of absorbable material with a long half-life can be used in place of the wire tension-band, to try and reduce the likelihood of premature closure of the physis and subsequent abnormal development of the tibial crest.

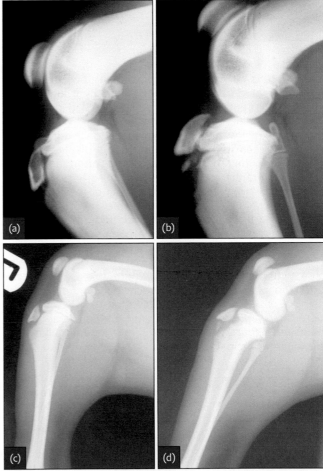

24.1 Avulsion of the tibial tubercle. (a) Mediolateral radiograph of the normal stifle of a 6-month-old Greyhound. (b) Contralateral joint of the same animal, showing complete avulsion of the tubercle. (c) Mediolateral radiograph of the normal left stifle in a 4-month-old Tibetan terrier. (d) Contralateral joint of the same animal, showing a partial avulsion of the tibial tubercle.

Separation of the proximal tibial physis

This is a relatively uncommon injury seen only in immature patients (Figure 24.2). It is associated with caudal rotation of the tibial plateau and craniomedial displacement of the proximal tibial metaphysis. The caudal rotation of the tibial plateau can be severely disabling since the stifle cannot be fully extended. Marked lameness will be seen, associated with pain and swelling around the stifle joint.

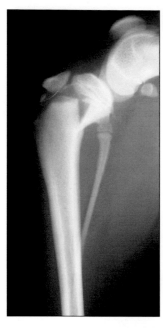

24.2 Mediolateral radiograph of the stifle of a 6-month-old Shetland Sheepdog showing a Salter–Harris type II fracture of the proximal tibial physis with caudal rotation of the epiphysis.

If there is only minimal displacement then the patient may be treated conservatively, particularly if the fibula is intact (Pratt, 2001; Clements *et al.*, 2003) (Figure 24.3). Casting or splinting may be considered but in most cases strict cage rest without external coaptation is appropriate.

In all cases where significant caudal displacement of the plateau has occurred, which is often associated with concurrent fracture of the fibula, early open reduction and internal fixation are required (see Operative Technique 24.2). In most cases, the tubercle remains attached to the plateau. In this situation one or two pins and a tension-band wire can be placed cranially as the only implants required to stabilize the fracture; this allows the implants to be seated away from the articular margins (see Figure 24.12a). In cases where this is inadequate then the plateau may additionally be secured in place using crossed K-wires, a combination of a K-wire and a bone screw where there is a large metaphyseal component (see Figure 24.12c), or a single intramedullary (IM) pin in larger patients.

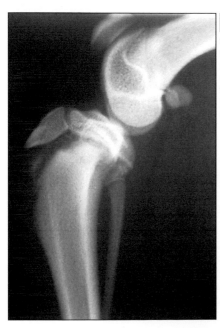

24.3 Mediolateral radiograph of the stifle of a 5-month-old Border Terrier showing a minimally displaced Salter–Harris type II fracture of the proximal tibial physis and an intact fibula.

Fracture of the proximal tibial metaphysis–diaphysis

An unusual fracture configuration of uncertain aetiology has been recognized that affects the proximal metaphyseal–diaphyseal region of the tibia. Usually caused by low impact injury, it may be seen bilaterally and tends to affect 3- to 7-month-old puppies. On a mediolateral radiograph the fracture line starts at the distal end of the tibial tuberosity and is usually curved in profile, with the proximal segment being concave (Figure 24.4a). Other configurations are occasionally encountered (Figure 24.4b). These fractures have been successfully managed using conservative measures, external skeletal fixation (ESF) and various methods of internal fixation. Interestingly, in a series of 26 dogs reported by Gritti *et al.* (2012), six developed valgus deformity that required corrective surgery. A similar, but slightly further distal, pattern of fracture has been noted in adult cats; these cats also commonly had non-union patellar fractures (Langley-Hobbs *et al.*, 2009).

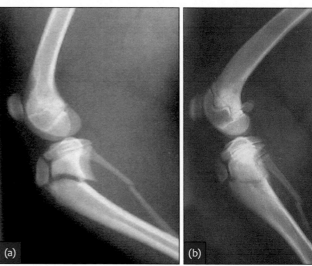

24.4 (a) Proximal metaphyseal–diaphyseal fracture in a 7-month-old Chinese Crested Dog that had fallen from its owner's arms, where the fracture surface of the proximal fragment is concave (most commonly reported). (b) A similar fracture in a 15-week-old German Shepherd Dog cross where the fracture surface of the proximal fragment is convex.

Fracture of the proximal fibula

These fractures occur rarely in isolation. If they result from a lateral blow to the limb then there may be pain or swelling on the lateral aspect of the stifle and pain on joint manipulation. The majority of these rare events are not associated with separation of the fibular head from the tibia and can be treated conservatively. Since the lateral collateral ligament of the stifle inserts on the fibular head, it is possible that lateral instability of the stifle can develop, although this is uncommon. If lateral instability is encountered, the fibular head can be reattached to the tibia using either a lagged bone screw or a pin and tension-band wire.

Fractures of the tibial and fibular diaphyses

These injuries usually occur in combination, but it is the tibial fracture that is the more important. The fibula bears little weight and shaft fractures of this bone alone may be treated conservatively. In cases where both bones are fractured, reduction and stabilization of the tibia will amply realign and protect the fibula during fracture healing. Where the fibula remains intact in the face of a tibial fracture, the support offered by the intact bone will support any fixation applied to the tibia.

The paucity of soft tissue coverage over the mid and distal tibial diaphysis results in an increased likelihood of such fractures being open, and may also lead to a reduced rate of fracture healing. However, surgical exposure of fractures is relatively straightforward. Owing to the natural twist in the tibia, fractures tend to spiral along the shaft and hairline fissures that extend beyond the radiographically visible fracture lines are not uncommon. The anatomy of the crus makes it feasible to employ a number of methods to stabilize tibial shaft fractures. These include casts (see Chapter 16), IM pins, ESF, interlocking nails and bone plates and screws (see Operative Techniques 24.3, 24.4 and 24.5). Combinations of these implants can also be employed, such as pin–plate or pin–ESF constructs. Deciding which fixation technique to use can be challenging; surgeons should carefully consider all principles of fracture treatment and choose the most appropriate technique for individual fractures (see Chapters 7, 8 and 11).

Fractures of the distal tibia and fibula

In skeletally immature patients the 'weak points' in this region are the distal physes, whereas in the older patient it is more likely that trauma will result in avulsion of the medial and/or lateral malleolus, which are the points of origin for the tarsocrural collateral ligaments. The importance of these fractures revolves around their influence on tarsocrural joint alignment and stability.

Distal physeal separation

This injury is seen in skeletally immature patients (Figure 24.5) and most often results from a medially directed blow to the lateral aspect of the distal crus which causes medial displacement of the distal tibial metaphysis and valgus deformity of the pes. Abrasions may be present; in some cases the distal tibial metaphysis might even break through the skin.

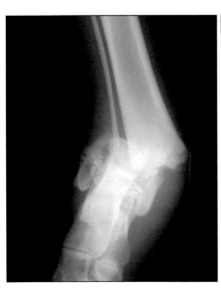

24.5 Dorsoplantar radiograph showing a displaced Salter–Harris type I fracture of the distal tibial physis and fibula in a 5-month-old Dobermann.

If closed reduction is possible with good anatomical reduction of the fracture, and the fracture then feels relatively stable, external coaptation may be employed with casting of the limb as far proximal as the stifle. However, great care must be taken to avoid the development of cast sores. If closed reduction cannot be achieved, or the site is considered unstable, then open reduction and internal fixation is indicated (see Operative Technique 24.6). Alternatively, the fracture can be stabilized using a transarticular ESF; this technique can be especially useful in cats where bone fragments can be very small and accurate implant placement is challenging.

Fractures of the lateral or medial malleolus

Such injuries are usually seen in skeletally mature patients resulting from road traffic accidents. They take the form of avulsion fractures caused by the distal limb being trapped under the wheel of a braking car. Shearing injuries are occasionally encountered; these can be seen in animals of any age. Apart from swelling and possible displacement of the pes, the main clinical finding following a malleolar fracture relates to tarsocrural instability due to loss of collateral support (Figure 24.6ab). Radiography may show gross displacement (Figure 24.6cd) but, in some cases, stressed views may be necessary to demonstrate the instability.

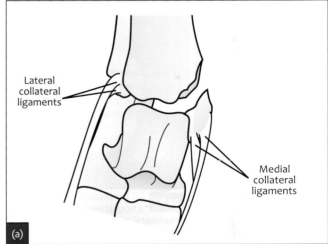

Lateral collateral ligaments

Medial collateral ligaments

(a)

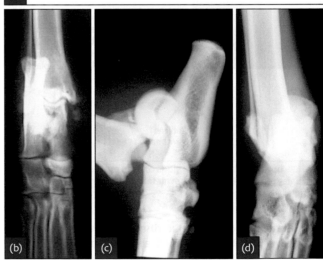

(b) (c) (d)

24.6 Malleolar fractures. (a) Fracture of the medial malleolus resulting in loss of collateral ligament support. (b) Dorsoplantar radiograph of a medial malleolar fracture in a 9-month-old Retriever cross. (c) Mediolateral and (d) dorsoplantar radiographs showing caudal luxation of the tarsocrural joint associated with fracture of the lateral malleolus in a dog.

→ **OPERATIVE TECHNIQUE 24.1 CONTINUED**

more proximally to utilize available bone stock. In these patients, either a single pin can be used with the tension-band wire positioned cranial to the tendon, or two pins side by side can be used with the tension-band wire positioned caudal to the tendon. Great care must be taken to avoid the tension-band wire damaging the tendon.

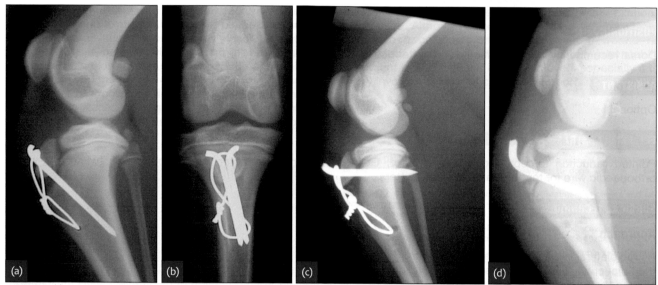

24.9 (a) Mediolateral and (b) caudocranial postoperative radiographs showing a repaired tibial tuberosity avulsion in a 5-month-old Airedale. The fracture was stabilized using two K-wires and a figure-of-eight tension-band wire. (c) Postoperative radiograph of a repaired tibial tuberosity avulsion in a 7-month-old Border Terrier. The fracture was stabilized using a single K-wire and a figure-of-eight tension-band wire. (d) Postoperative radiograph of a repaired partial tibial tuberosity avulsion in a 5-month-old Staffordshire Bull Terrier. The fracture was stabilized using a K-wire and figure-of-eight suture of polydioxanone.

In patients approaching skeletal maturity by the time the fracture has healed (i.e. 8 to 10 months of age), the implants may be left in place. However, in much younger patients implants should be removed after about 3 to 5 weeks to try to prevent early closure of the physis and subsequent drifting of the tubercle distally relative to the tibial shaft. Alternatively, in these young patients, or in patients with partial avulsion, absorbable implants may be used (e.g. biodegradable pins and/or figure-of-eight polydioxanone sutures in place of the wire tension band) (Figure 24.9d). However, premature closure of the physis probably results from the injury itself and deformity may be seen whatever treatment method is chosen, even if a tension-band is avoided or removed early (Figure 24.10).

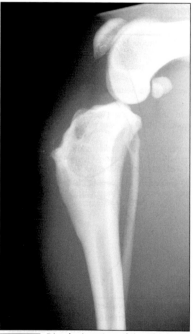

24.10 Distal migration of the tibial tuberosity due to premature growth plate closure following repair of a tibial tuberosity avulsion. The implants had been removed after 4 weeks.

PRACTICAL TIP

In cases where only a small part of the tubercle has become avulsed, reattachment of the patellar tendon to the tibia is best achieved by placement of sutures through the tendon and through transverse bone tunnels in the tibial tuberosity. These sutures can be protected by guard wires placed between bone tunnels drilled in the patella and the tibial crest and/or a transarticular external skeletal fixator positioned to place the stifle in an extended position for 6 weeks

---

Alternative technique

Some surgeons prefer to secure the tubercle in position with a lagged bone screw, with or without an anti-rotational K-wire and/or tension-band wire. Since such a technique will create static compression of the physis it can only be recommended in patients already approaching skeletal maturity. Great care must be taken when placing a screw in this location as it is possible to cause significant damage to the insertion of the patellar tendon.

→ **OPERATIVE TECHNIQUE 24.1 CONTINUED**

Wound closure

Should include reattachment of the fascia of the cranial tibialis muscle to the cranial aspect of the tibia.

POSTOPERATIVE MANAGEMENT

The joint may be supported in a padded bandage for 5 to 10 days and the patient should be rested until fracture healing has taken place, usually by 4 to 6 weeks. Although clinical union is probably much more rapid than this (as evidenced by consideration of implant removal after 3 weeks), it may be difficult to monitor this radiographically as a physis is involved and so restriction for longer is advisable as a precaution. Implant removal may have to be considered, as discussed above.

OPERATIVE TECHNIQUE 24.2

Separation of the proximal tibial physis

POSITIONING

Dorsal recumbency with the affected limb extended caudally.

ASSISTANT

Optional.

EQUIPMENT EXTRAS

Pointed reduction forceps; Hohmann retractor; Gelpi self-retaining retractor; chuck; pliers; K-wires; orthopaedic wire; pin/wire cutters.

SURGICAL TECHNIQUES

Approach

A craniomedial incision is made, extending from just below the level of the patella to about two-thirds of the way down the tibial crest. Soft tissue dissection should allow identification of the tibial plateau and removal of any organizing haematoma will expose the fracture surfaces. If a tension-band wire is to be applied then reflection of the cranial tibialis muscle from the lateral aspect of the tibia is required to expose the site for drilling of the transverse tibial tunnel.

Reduction and fixation

Reduction of the fracture is most easily achieved by holding the stifle in extension. If necessary, a small Hohmann retractor can be carefully placed into the fracture gap from the craniomedial aspect and gently levered to move the plateau forward (Figure 24.11); however this is rarely necessary.

WARNING

Take care when manipulating the tibial plateau; it may fracture if too much leverage is applied

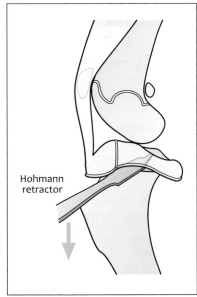

Hohmann retractor

24.11 The use of a Hohmann retractor to facilitate reduction of a proximal tibial physeal fracture.

→ **OPERATIVE TECHNIQUE 24.2 CONTINUED**

Digital pressure is usually the most practical way of holding the plateau in reduction whilst the implants are placed. In most cases the tibial tuberosity and proximal epiphysis remain as one and the simplest means of fixation is placement of a K-wire through the tuberosity along with a tension-band wire (Figure 24.12a) (see Operative Technique 24.1) (Pratt, 2001). Alternatively, additional fixation may be achieved by placement of crossed K-wires to secure the epiphysis. A K-wire in combination with a bone screw can be used if there is a large metaphyseal component (Figure 24.12bc). If at all possible, the pins should be bent over to avoid implant migration.

Wound closure

Should include reattachment of the fascia of the cranial tibialis muscle to the cranial aspect of the tibia.

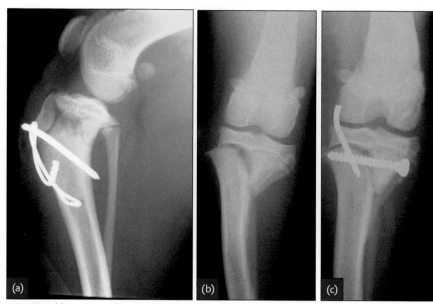

24.12 (a) Fracture of the proximal tibial physis in a 5-month-old West Highland White Terrier stabilized with a single K-wire and a figure-of-eight tension-band wire.
(b) Preoperative and (c) postoperative radiographs of a proximal tibial physeal fracture in a 7-month-old Boxer. The fracture has been stabilized with a combination of a K-wire medially and a bone screw laterally through the metaphyseal component.

POSTOPERATIVE MANAGEMENT

The joint may be supported in a padded bandage for 5 to 10 days and the patient should be rested until fracture healing has taken place, usually by 4 to 6 weeks. Implant removal may have to be considered, as discussed above. The implants, most notably K-wires placed through the epiphysis, are positioned close to the articular margins and may interfere with normal joint function, making it necessary for them to be removed.

OPERATIVE TECHNIQUE 24.3

Tibia – medial bone plating

POSITIONING

Lateral recumbency with the affected limb down, to allow access to the medial aspect. The contralateral limb is drawn out of the surgical field and a rope or bandage sling is secured to the table, passing medial to the affected limb proximally so that traction can be applied to the fracture site by pulling on the pes without this causing movement of the patient. Alternatively, the limb may be suspended from a ceiling hook, which allows 360 degree access to the crus, or the patient can be placed in dorsal recumbency with the affected limb extended caudally.

ASSISTANT

Useful, especially if traction is required to help maintain fragment alignment and to reduce the time taken for plate application.

EQUIPMENT EXTRAS

Pointed reduction forceps; other bone-holding forceps of the surgeon's choice such as Dingman or Lewin bone-holding forceps; Hohmann retractors; self-retaining retractors such as Gelpi or Weitlaner retractors; periosteal elevator; drill and bits; appropriate plate and screw instrumentation set.

→ **OPERATIVE TECHNIQUE 24.3 CONTINUED**

SURGICAL TECHNIQUES

Approach

A craniomedial skin incision is made along most (if not all) of the tibial length (Figure 24.13a). If the incision is made too medially then the closure will lie directly over the plate and increase the likelihood of problems with wound healing. Dissection through the subcutaneous fascia will expose the tibial shaft easily, with the cranial tibial muscle forming the cranial margin and the long digital flexor muscle the caudal margin. The only complicating structures are those of the cranial branch of the medial saphenous artery and vein which run alongside the saphenous nerve. All three structures cross the medial aspect of the tibia in a caudoproximal to craniodistal direction about half way along the diaphysis. Although it is preferable to preserve these structures, they can be ligated and sectioned if necessary without causing serious complications. Proximally, it may be necessary to elevate the pes anserinus, the aponeurosis comprising the insertion of the caudal sartorius, gracilis and semi-tendinosus muscles.

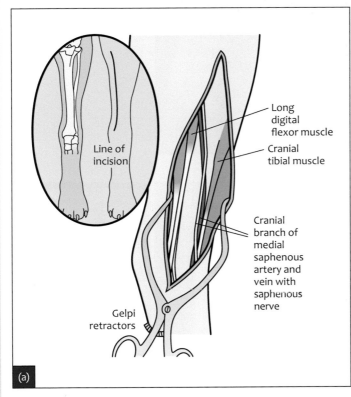

Long digital flexor muscle

Cranial tibial muscle

Line of incision

Cranial branch of medial saphenous artery and vein with saphenous nerve

Gelpi retractors

(a)

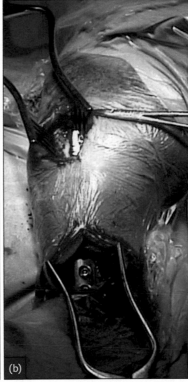

24.13 (a) Medial exposure of the tibial diaphysis. (b) Medial exposure of the proximal and distal segments of the tibia for application of a bridging plate to stabilize a comminuted fracture in a 6-year-old English Bull Terrier using a minimally invasive strategy.

(b)

If a plate is to be applied as a bridging plate (see Reduction and fixation) using a minimally invasive strategy, then it is possible to make two skin incisions to expose the proximal and distal bone segments, leaving the skin over the fracture site intact. This will allow a pre-contoured bone plate to be tunnelled through the fracture site and secured to the bone ends using plate screws with minimal invasion of the fracture envelope (Schmokel *et al.*, 2007) (Figure 24.13b; see Chapter 15).

Reduction and fixation

See Figures 24.14, 24.15, 24.16 and 24.17. Common mistakes in plate application include not exposing the tibia proximally enough where it is easy to believe the exposure must be close to the stifle when there is still one-third of the tibia further proximal (especially in obese patients), and not extending the plate distally enough for fear of compromising the tarsocrural joint. Proximal exposure is assisted by use of the groin sling and having an assistant to apply traction to the limb.

If the bone stock is poor proximally or distally then T-plates, L-plates or a tibial head buttress plate (McGuiness *et al.*, 2009) may enable adequate screw 'grouping' and thus implant purchase, although these tend to be available in only limited lengths and are often inadequate in comminuted fractures. Distally, as long as the plate does not extend beyond the origin of the medial collateral ligament and the distal-most screw is angled slightly proximally, there is little chance of interfering with talocrural joint function.

Inherently unstable fractures, such as comminuted fractures or fractures with a deficit in the lateral cortex (i.e. a defect on the compression side of the bone, which will predispose the plate to increased bending forces, which in turn can result in cyclic loading and eventual failure) require supplementation of the plate fixation. This can be →

→ **OPERATIVE TECHNIQUE 24.3 CONTINUED**

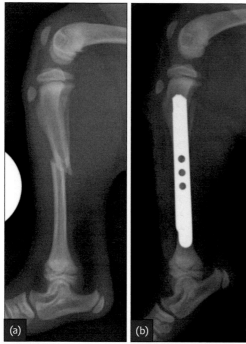

(a)

(b)

24.14 (a) Preoperative and (b) postoperative radiographs of a 4-month-old Pomeranian with a short oblique fracture of the tibia treated with stacked veterinary cuttable plates. Although the plate holes are round, it was possible to place screws slightly eccentrically in the plate holes leading to compression of the fracture during screw tightening.
(Courtesy of T Gemmill)

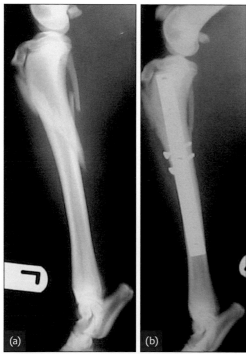

(a)

(b)

24.15 (a) Preoperative and (b) postoperative radiographs of an oblique tibial diaphyseal fracture in a 9-month-old Labrador Retriever, stabilized using lagged bone screws and a neutralization plate.

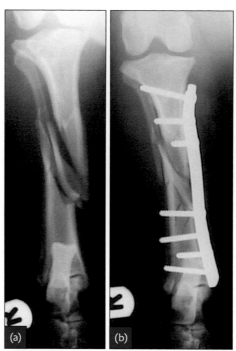

(a)

(b)

24.16 (a) Preoperative and (b) postoperative radiographs of a comminuted fracture in a 6-year-old English Bull Terrier managed with a bridging plate (same case as Figure 24.13b).

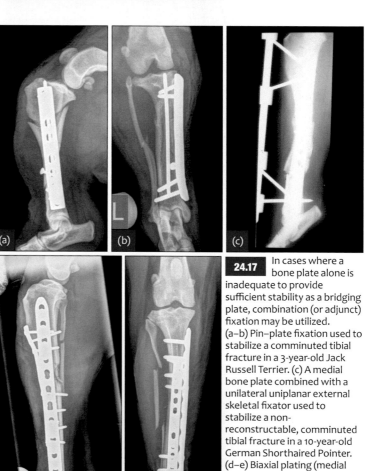

(a)

(b)

(c)

(d)

(e)

24.17 In cases where a bone plate alone is inadequate to provide sufficient stability as a bridging plate, combination (or adjunct) fixation may be utilized. (a–b) Pin–plate fixation used to stabilize a comminuted tibial fracture in a 3-year-old Jack Russell Terrier. (c) A medial bone plate combined with a unilateral uniplanar external skeletal fixator used to stabilize a non-reconstructable, comminuted tibial fracture in a 10-year-old German Shorthaired Pointer. (d–e) Biaxial plating (medial and cranial) of a non-reconstructable, comminuted tibial fracture in a 1-year-old crossbred dog.
(a,b,d,e, Courtesy of D Clements)

→

→ **OPERATIVE TECHNIQUE 24.3 CONTINUED**

achieved with an IM pin (Figure 24.17ab) (see Operative Technique 24.4), of 35–40% of the bone's diameter at the isthmus, placed before the medial plate is fixed to the bone, or with the addition of an external skeletal fixator (Figure 24.17c). Alternatively, second cranial plate can be applied (Figure 24.17de) after the medial plate is fixed to the bone. In all these situations, the ancillary fixation reduces the lateral bending forces on the medial plate during load bearing, significantly reducing the risk of implant failure.

Wound closure

Closure is achieved by apposition of the subcutaneous and/or subcuticular fascia and then the skin.

POSTOPERATIVE MANAGEMENT

In most cases it is preferable to apply a Robert Jones bandage for 3 to 7 days. Exercise restriction should be implemented until radiographic healing of the fracture is apparent – usually 4 to 8 weeks, depending on the nature of the fracture and age of the patient. The need to remove implants is a controversial issue. Generally, the author prefers to leave the implants *in situ* unless they cause problems. The most common reasons for removing the plate are caused by the lack of soft tissue cover in this region. The subcuticular implant may cause irritation, leading to lick granulomas (Figure 24.18), or lameness due to cooling in low environmental temperatures. Low environmental temperatures can cause differential shortening of the plate and bone; this causes stresses within the bone and hence pain (so-called cold or thermal lameness). If any such problems are noted then the implants are removed. Following removal of a plate the patient should be rested for about 6 weeks whilst bone remodelling accommodates any 'stress protection' afforded by the plate.

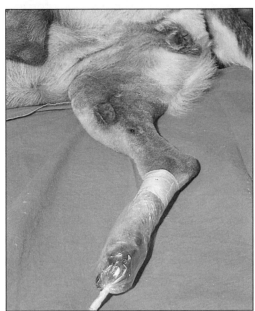

24.18 Local irritation over the tibial plate leading to lick granuloma formation. Implant removal and resection of the affected tissue led to an uneventful recovery.

OPERATIVE TECHNIQUE 24.4

Tibia – intramedullary pinning

POSITIONING

Dorsolateral recumbency with the affected limb down, to allow access to the medial aspect if IM pinning is to be combined with cerclage wiring or ESF (see Operative Technique 24.3). Access to the limb should be improved by supporting the limb on a sandbag so that it can be lifted, allowing manipulation of the stifle, for IM pinning. Alternatively, the dog can be positioned in dorsal recumbency with the limb extended caudally, as in Operative Technique 24.1.

PRACTICAL TIP

IM pinning alone has been described to manage cases of transverse fractures with some interdigitation of the fragments, to preclude rotation. However, IM pins should be used alone with great caution; it is safer to combine them with supplementary fixation such as cerclage wire or, far more reliably, combine them with an ESF construct or a bone plate to control rotational and axial forces

ASSISTANT

Optional. Most useful during reconstruction of comminuted fractures.

→ **OPERATIVE TECHNIQUE 24.4 CONTINUED**

EQUIPMENT EXTRAS

Pointed reduction forceps; other bone-holding forceps of the surgeon's choice (e.g. Dingman or Lewin bone-holding forceps); Hohmann retractors; self-retaining retractors (e.g. Gelpi or Weitlaner); periosteal elevator; appropriate Steinmann pins; large pin cutters; chuck; drill; orthopaedic wire for cerclage; pliers/wire twisters; ESF equipment (see Operative Technique 24.5) if a type 1 ESF frame is used as auxilliary fixation (see Figure 24.21a).

SURGICAL TECHNIQUES

Approach

The fracture site is exposed using a limited craniomedial approach (see Operative Technique 24.3).

Reduction and fixation

In the case of reconstructable comminuted fractures, the fragments are reduced and compressed into position using cerclage wires until a two-piece fracture is achieved. When applying these it must be ensured that the fibula is not included, since this will make it impossible to achieve adequate tension in the wire. The proximal part of the tibial diaphysis is wedge-shaped and to prevent slipping of the wire it may be necessary to create a notch in the surface of the bone or apply the wire in a hemicerclage fashion (see Chapter 11), but it is preferable to use an alternative fixation technique. If the wire is tightened by twisting the two ends around one another then it is usually necessary to bend the ends over, as there is inadequate soft tissue cover to consider the option of leaving them standing at right angles to the bone surface.

PRACTICAL TIP

Although, with care, retrograde pinning is possible, it is generally considered that normograde pinning is most appropriate for tibial fractures

The pin is introduced through a keyhole incision caudal to the straight patellar tendon alongside its medial border with the stifle held flexed. It enters the bone at the base of the tibial crest, cranial to the intermeniscal ligament (Figure 24.19ab). Although a Jacobs chuck can be used, a slow-speed power drill affords better control of placement and is less likely to be associated with the pin slipping off the proximal tibia. To prevent the pin slipping off the tibial plateau during insertion, a pilot hole can be made with a smaller diameter pin (a drill bit can be used but this tends to wrap up the soft tissues, and the limited access prevents satisfactory use of tissue guards). Alternatively, a power drill with an oscillating function will help to control pin slippage. Whenever possible the notch in a pre-cut pin is protected by being kept within the chuck in order to prevent premature breakage; alternatively, the pin can be advanced to near its full insertion in the tibia (using a second pin to compare the distance the distal end is in the bone) and then drawn back to facilitate cutting a notch half way through the pin with a hacksaw, before being fully seated in the tibia. The pin is driven into the distal metaphysis (Figure 24.19c). As the pin approaches the distal metaphysis it is preferable to use a Jacobs chuck as it provides better control, making it less likely that the tarsal joint will be entered. Once fully seated, the pin is bent over and broken off at the level of the pre-cut notch.

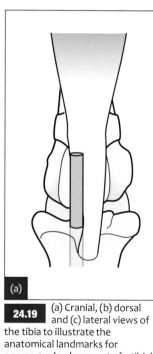

(a)

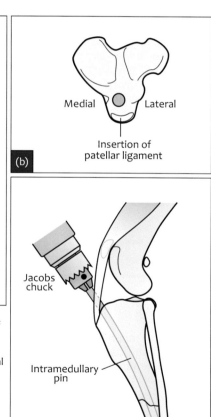

(b)

(c)

24.19 (a) Cranial, (b) dorsal and (c) lateral views of the tibia to illustrate the anatomical landmarks for normograde placement of a tibial IM pin.

Medial — Lateral

Insertion of patellar ligament

Jacobs chuck

Intramedullary pin

→ **OPERATIVE TECHNIQUE 24.4 CONTINUED**

Wound closure

Closure is routine with the addition of a single suture in the skin at the site of pin placement.

POSTOPERATIVE MANAGEMENT

A Robert Jones bandage may be applied for 3 to 7 days if appropriate. Exercise is restricted until radiographic healing of the fracture is apparent (usually 4 to 8 weeks, depending on the nature of the fracture and age of the patient).

Implant removal is a controversial issue. Whilst there is a justifiable fear that leaving implants *in situ* will result in them becoming totally encased within the growing bone in immature patients, making removal very difficult if problems become apparent, implants are generally left in place unless they cause problems. Therefore, in adult patients it may be better to pre-cut the pin so that it breaks close to the bone margin (Figure 24.20). In most cases cerclage wires are left in place.

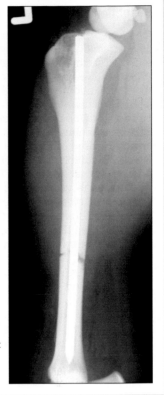

24.20 Postoperative radiograph showing repair of a transverse tibial fracture in an adult terrier using a single IM pin. Fracture configurations that lend themselves to use of an IM pin alone are uncommon. Adjunct fixation is normally required (see text).

OPERATIVE TECHNIQUE 24.5

Tibia – external skeletal fixation

POSITIONING

Lateral recumbency with the affected limb down, to allow access to the medial aspect (see Operative Technique 24.3) but with allowance to lift the leg off the table if full pins are being used. Alternatively, the limb may be suspended from a ceiling hook which allows 360 degree access to the crus, or the patient can be positioned in dorsal recumbancy with the affected limb extended caudally.

ASSISTANT

Useful, especially if traction is required to help maintain fracture alignment and also to assist in the assembly of the connecting bar and clamps.

EQUIPMENT EXTRAS

Appropriate ESF set; variable speed drill; large pin cutters (hacksaw as last resort); chuck; smaller diameter pins or drill bits and appropriate soft tissue guards if pre-drilling is performed.

SURGICAL TECHNIQUES

Approach

Closed or limited open approach (Operating Technique 24.3) to the fracture site.

→ **OPERATIVE TECHNIQUE 24.5 CONTINUED**

Reduction and fixation

Once the fracture has been reduced – either closed using traction, or by a limited open approach – the external skeletal fixator may be applied. The medial aspect of the tibia is most commonly used for placement of fixation pins. Two half pins will create a unilateral, uniplanar (type 1) fixator that is adequate to control rotational forces around an IM pin (Figure 24.21), whereas four (transverse fracture) or six (oblique with interfragmentary implants) half pins would be sufficient to stabilize relatively simple fractures either alone (Figure 24.22a) or in combination with cerclage wires or lagged bone screws (Figure 24.22b). Full pins, used to create a bilateral, uniplanar (type 2) ESF frame (Figure 24.22c), are generally only required when there is axial instability due to comminution where fragments have not been or cannot be reconstructed, and/or where limited load sharing by the tibia can be expected until the fracture heals. The use of full pins proximally is often associated with moderate morbidity relating to pin tract drainage caused by placement through the cranial tibialis muscle. In order to avoid this, and the potential risk of injury to the peroneal nerve, a unilateral, biplanar (type 1b) ESF configuration may be preferable and will achieve similar frame stiffness (Figure 24.23).

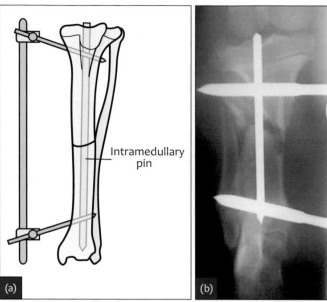

(a) (b)

24.21 (a) A two-pin unilateral, uniplanar (type 1) external skeletal fixator may be used as an adjunct to IM pinning in order to counteract rotational forces acting at transverse or short oblique fracture lines. (b) Postoperative radiograph of a tibial fracture in a 4-month-old Standard Dachshund, stabilized using an IM pin and a two-pin unilateral, uniplanar (type 1) external skeletal fixator.

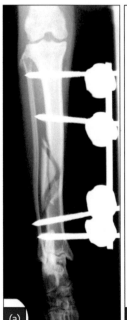
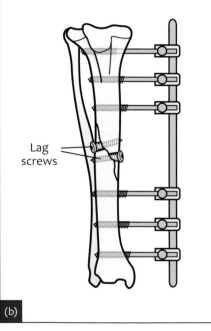
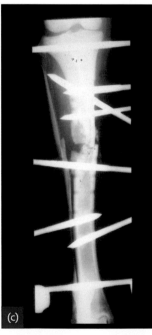

(a) (b) (c)

24.22 Use of ESF to stabilize relatively simple fractures either alone or in combination with lagged bone screws or cerclage wires. (a) Postoperative radiograph of a tibial fracture in a 2-year-old cat, stabilized using a four-pin, unilateral, uniplanar (type 1) ESF construct. Note the fibula is intact. (b) A six-pin unilateral, uniplanar (type 1) ESF frame used to stabilize a simple oblique fracture in combination with lagged bone screws. (c) Postoperative radiograph of a tibial fracture in a 5-year-old German Shepherd Dog, stabilized with an eight-pin, bilateral, uniplanar (type 2b) ESF construct. The fracture occurred 2 weeks earlier and had been stabilized with an 8-hole bone plate. Screw purchase had failed in the proximal segment and so management had been revised to use of an external fixator.

In cases with limited bone stock distally, it is usually possible to create a modification of type 1b and 2 ESF frame configurations whereby two distal pins are placed, one a half pin on the cranial aspect and one a full pin with the lateral end tied into the connecting bar (Figures 24.23 and 24.24). Bilateral, biplanar (type 3) frames are rarely required. They are most often used in situations where much bone stock has been lost and the fracture is open, i.e. where healing is expected to be slow, and this situation is most commonly associated with gunshot injuries. Circular (ring) ESF constructs can also be used to stabilize tibial fractures (Rovesti *et al.*, 2007) and may offer some advantages where there is limited bone stock proximally or distally.

→ **OPERATIVE TECHNIQUE 24.5 CONTINUED**

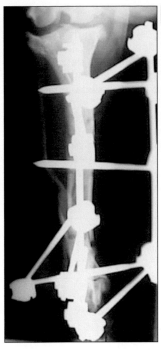

24.23 Postoperative radiograph of a revised (infected plate) fracture in an 8-year-old Labrador Retriever. The site has been stabilized with a modified bilateral, biplanar (modified type 1b) external skeletal fixator with only the distal fixation pin extending laterally and being 'tied back' into the cranial connecting bar.

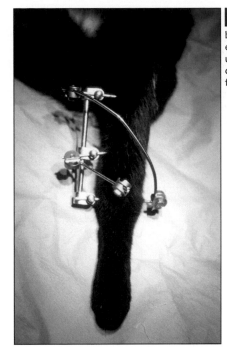

24.24 A modified bilateral, biplanar (modified type 1b) external skeletal fixator used to stabilize a very distal tibial diaphyseal fracture in a cat.

Wound closure

Routine.

POSTOPERATIVE MANAGEMENT

It is usually necessary to apply a padded bandage to the limb within the frame, including the foot, for 7 to 10 days, otherwise swelling of the limb and foot is often seen. Other care is routine (see Chapter 11). It is wise to restrict the patient's exercise until radiographic union is complete or until 3 to 4 weeks after frame removal.

OPERATIVE TECHNIQUE 24.6

Separation of the distal tibial physis

POSITIONING

Lateral recumbency with the affected limb down and the contralateral limb drawn cranially.

ASSISTANT

Optional.

EQUIPMENT EXTRAS

Gelpi self-retaining retractor; Hohmann retractor; small periosteal elevator; self-retaining pointed reduction forceps; K-wires or small Steinmann pins; chuck; pliers; pin/wire cutters.

SURGICAL TECHNIQUES

Approach

A medial approach is made to the distal tibia.

→ **OPERATIVE TECHNIQUE 24.6 CONTINUED**

Reduction and fixation

Reduction is achieved by toggling the fragments (Figure 24.25ab). This may be assisted by using a Hohmann retractor as a lever. Once reduced, the fracture will usually remain stable, provided the foot is not allowed to displace laterally. One or two K-wires or small Steinmann pins are then placed diagonally, at an angle of about 30 to 40 degrees to the longitudinal axis, in normograde fashion through the medial malleolus and distal tibia (Figure 24.25c and 24.26a). If required, a pin or K-wire can be placed in similar fashion through the lateral malleolus and into the distal tibia (Figure 24.26b). After placement of *each* pin, movement of the tarsocrural joint should be checked so that if an implant has compromised joint function it can be removed and relocated. The ends should then be bent over to prevent migration. Whether the pins are placed through the trans (far) cortex or whether the Rush pin principle is used is a matter of personal preference. Although theoretically the Rush pin principle is superior, in practical terms crossed pins are easier to apply and produce satisfactory results. Increased stability is then achieved by suturing torn soft tissues and may be further increased by placement of a K-wire through a keyhole incision over the lateral malleolus. In larger patients, tension-band wires can also be placed laterally and/or medially to neutralize bending forces (see Operative Technique 24.7).

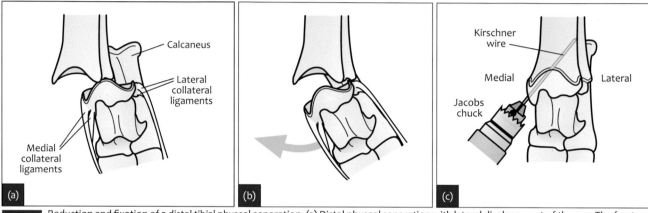

24.25 Reduction and fixation of a distal tibial physeal separation. (a) Distal physeal separation with lateral displacement of the pes. The fracture often feels 'locked' in this position. (b) The fracture is reduced by toggling the ends (see Chapter 11). A Hohmann retractor, placed in the fracture and used to lever the physis distally, is sometimes necessary. (c) Once reduced, fixation is achieved by normograde placement of one or two K-wires through the medial malleolus.

Alternative technique

Use of an IM pin has been described but this gains very little purchase in the distal epiphysis and it restricts articular function if it is passed across the tarsocrural joint to improve security. Alternatively, closed reduction can be performed and a transarticular external skeletal fixator applied. This technique is useful in cats when bone stock can be very limited.

Wound closure

Closure is by apposition of the subcutaneous and/or subcuticular fascia and then the skin.

POSTOPERATIVE MANAGEMENT

See Operative Technique 24.5.

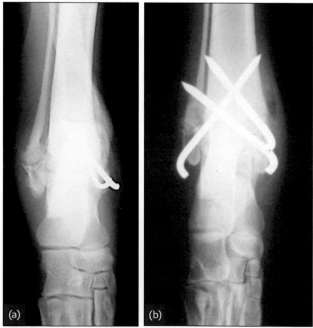

24.26 (a) Postoperative radiograph of a distal tibial physeal fracture in a 4-month-old Boxer, stabilized using two K-wires placed through the medial malleolus. (b) Postoperative radiograph of a distal tibial physeal fracture in a 5-month-old Dobermann, stabilized using K-wires placed through both the medial and lateral malleoli.

OPERATIVE TECHNIQUE 24.7

Fractures of the medial and lateral malleoli

POSITIONING

Lateral recumbency with the affected limb down and the contralateral limb drawn cranially, for exposure of a medial malleolar fracture; and with the affected limb uppermost, supported on a bolster, for exposure of a lateral malleolar fracture.

ASSISTANT

Optional.

EQUIPMENT EXTRAS

Gelpi self-retaining retractor; Hohmann retractor; small periosteal elevator; self-retaining pointed reduction forceps; K-wires; wire for tension band; chuck; pliers/wire twisters; pin/wire cutters; appropriate screw set and drill bits if a lag screw technique is used.

SURGICAL TECHNIQUES

Approach

A medial or lateral approach is made to the distal tibia/fibula.

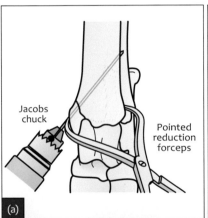

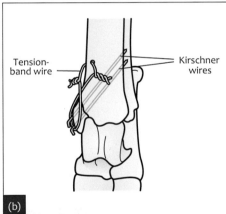

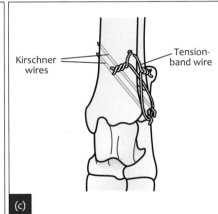

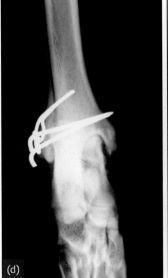

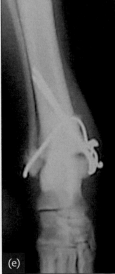

24.27 Reduction and fixation of malleolar fractures. (a) Reduced medial malleolar fracture; pointed reduction forceps can be used to maintain the malleolar fragment in position whilst a K-wire or pin is introduced. (b) A second K-wire or pin may then be placed and a figure-of-eight tension-band wire added. (c) Repaired lateral malleolar fracture. (d) Postoperative radiograph showing the use of two K-wires and a tension-band to repair a lateral malleolar fracture in a dog. (e) Postoperative radiograph showing the repair of medial and lateral malleolar fractures in a 9-month-old Jack Russell Terrier. The medial malleolus has been stabilized using two K-wires and a figure-of-eight tension-band wire. The lateral malleolus has been stabilized using a K-wire, which is more readily driven into the distal tibia than the fibular diaphysis. A tension-band is more difficult to place laterally and less necessary than medially because the lateral side of the joint tends to be under compression during weight-bearing.

→ **OPERATIVE TECHNIQUE 24.7 CONTINUED**

Reduction and fixation

Reduction is achieved by traction on the fragment and collateral ligament. Holding the fragment in reduction can be difficult; pointed reduction forceps may assist in holding the fragment (Figure 24.27a) or Allis tissue forceps may be used to grasp the ligament. One or two K-wires are then placed diagonally, at an angle of about 30 to 40 degrees to the longitudinal axis, through the medial or lateral malleolus and distal tibia (Figure 24.27bc). After placement of *each* pin, movement of the tarsocrural joint should be checked so that an implant can be removed and relocated if it has compromised joint function. The ends should then be bent over to prevent migration. The tension-band wire is then placed around the pin ends and through a tunnel drilled in the distal tibia. Increased stability may be achieved by suturing torn soft tissues.

Alternative techniques

A lagged bone screw may be used instead of the pin and tension-band wire. Where the fragment is too small to accommodate implants it may be more appropriate to use a bone screw and spiked washer to reattach the avulsed collateral ligament. Alternatively, a transarticular external skeletal fixator can be applied for around 6 weeks. This allows healing of traumatized tissues by fibrosis, which can restore tarsocrural stability. However, osseous healing of smaller malleolar fragments rarely occurs using this technique.

Wound closure

Closure is achieved by apposition of the subcutaneous and/or subcuticular fascia and then the skin.

POSTOPERATIVE MANAGEMENT

In general, the application of a Robert Jones bandage for 2 weeks, when the skin sutures may also be removed, is sufficient as long as the patient's exercise is restricted to cage/room rest and short lead walks for 6 weeks after surgery. Alternatively, the repair can be protected with a cast, but if adequate stability has been achieved then it should be possible to avoid casting and allow early return to controlled joint function.

Chapter 25

The carpus and tarsus

Alessandro Piras and Tomás Guerrero

Fractures of the carpus and tarsus are common in athletic dogs, but are encountered less frequently in pet dogs and cats. Most fractures of these joints have an articular component and they are often associated with concurrent ligamentous injury. Multiple carpal or tarsal bones and multiple joint levels may be injured concurrently.

A thorough knowledge of anatomy is imperative for the accurate diagnosis of fractures affecting the carpus or tarsus. Accurate diagnosis requires detailed clinical examination and high-definition diagnostic imaging. Common clinical findings during physical examination include soft tissue swelling, pain and decreased range of motion; there is often associated instability and crepitus. Radiographic examination should always include routine orthogonal views, although oblique and stressed views may be required to identify all the injuries present. Due to the intricate anatomy of these areas, more detailed imaging techniques such as computed tomography (CT) are recommended in complex cases, particularly if multiple bones are involved.

PRACTICAL TIPS

- A bony specimen can be a helpful reference for use during investigation, preoperative planning and surgery. Three-dimensional printing of CT images can also provide useful information about the nature and location of these fractures
- Hairline or incomplete fractures may be difficult to detect during radiographic examination immediately after injury. It can be useful to apply a Robert Jones bandage for 48 hours and repeat the radiographic study as fragment displacement may occur and make the fracture more visible; alternatively advanced imaging, such as CT scanning, can be considered

---

Careful preoperative planning should incorporate consideration of the fracture in relation to the age, breed and expected level of physical activity of the dog, the level of expertise of the surgeon and the availability of specific implants. In some cases, salvage by arthrodesis may be the most appropriate treatment option. Surgical approaches to the carpal and tarsal joints are usually made directly over the area of interest, with exposure of the underlying structures by sharp dissection. Combined approaches may be required for comminuted fractures or fractures involving more than one bone. Contrary to popular belief, the use of an Esmarch's bandage and tourniquet are not necessary to provide adequate haemostasis. Wrapping of the extremity with a sterile stockinette and cohesive bandage can be considered, however in most cases this is not required, providing haemostasis is performed quickly and carefully during the surgical procedure.

The carpus

Anatomy

Bony anatomy

The carpus is a complex joint composed of seven named bones arranged in two rows. The proximal row comprises the radial, ulnar and accessory carpal bones and the distal row comprises the first, second, third and fourth carpal bones, numbered from medial to lateral. A small sesamoid bone is located in the tendon of insertion of the abductor pollicis longus muscle on the medial side of the carpus; this should not be mistaken for a chip or avulsion fracture.

The carpus is a complex gynglimus joint which mainly allows flexion and extension. A small degree of internal and external rotation and valgus and varus movement is also present in the healthy joint. Limited craniocaudal translation can also be elicited. Three joints are responsible for the range of flexion and extension of the carpus. The antebrachiocarpal joint provides about 70% of the movement, the intercarpal joint about 25% and the distal carpometacarpal joint about 5%.

Ligaments of the carpus

A strong network of ligaments and fibrocartilage on the palmar side of the carpus prevents hyperextension. The palmar radiocarpal and ulnocarpal ligaments bridge the palmar aspect of the antebrachiocarpal joint and prevent hyperextension of this joint. Distally hyperextension is prevented by the accessoro–metacarpal ligament (running between the accessory carpal bone and the base of metacarpal bones 4 and 5), the radiocarpal–metacarpal ligaments (between the radial carpal bone and the base of the metacarpal 2 and 3) and a strong palmar fibrocartilage pad (attached to the palmar aspect of all the carpal bones, aside from the accessory carpal bone, and running to the bases of the metacarpal bones).

The collateral ligaments are strong, especially the radial ligament located on the medial surface of the radiocarpal joint, and are constantly under tension. The radial

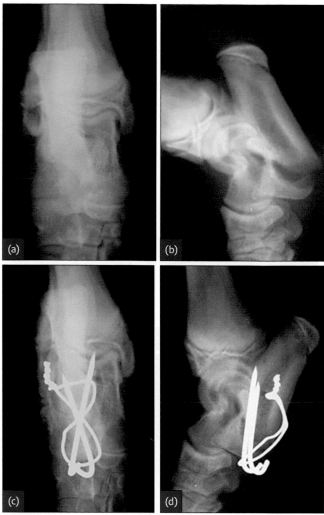

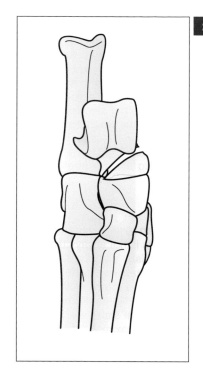

25.18 Fracture of the neck of the talus.

25.16 (a) Plantarodorsal and (b) mediolateral views of a fracture of the base of the calcaneus in a 6-month-old Greyhound. (c–d) The fracture was stabilized with a combination of K-wires and a figure-of-eight tension-band wire.

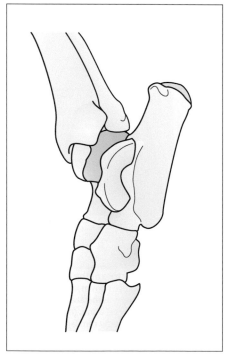

25.17 Fracture of the lateral ridge of the talus producing a large osteochondral fragment.

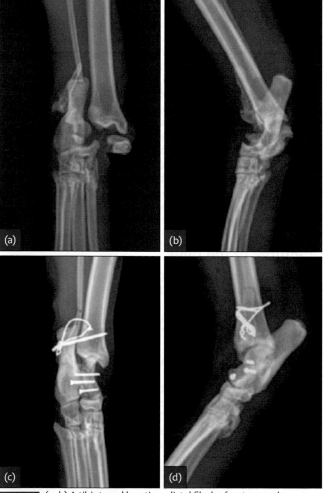

25.19 (a–b) A tibiotarsal luxation, distal fibular fracture and a fracture of the medial trochlea of the talus in a cat. (c–d) The distal fibular fracture was stabilized with a pin and tension-band wire, and the fracture of the talus was stabilized with a combination of mini lag screws and a threaded K-wire.

Fractures of the central tarsal bone

Although central tarsal bone fractures are most commonly seen in racing dogs, they have also been reported in other sporting or working breeds (Guilliard, 2007). These fractures are very rare in non-athletic dogs. In the racing Greyhound central tarsal bone fractures usually affect the right hindlimb because of the compressive stresses produced by racing in an anticlockwise direction. Fractures of the central tarsal bone have been classified into five types on the basis of their conformation (Boudrieau *et al.*, 1984) (Figure 25.20):

- **Type I** – dorsal slab fragment with no displacement
- **Type II** – dorsal slab fragment with displacement
- **Type III** – medial fragment with displacement
- **Type IV** – combination of dorsal slab fragment and medial slab fragment more or less displaced
- **Type V** – comminuted fracture with several fragments.

The most common central tarsal bone fractures are types I, II and IV. Clinical findings vary according to the severity of the fracture, but in most cases dogs are markedly lame or non-weight-bearing. In all cases pain is elicited on flexion of the hock. A mild swelling on the dorsum of the tarsus can be evident with type I and II fractures. Conversely, severe swelling with crepitus and varus deviation of the distal limb can be observed with type IV and V fractures.

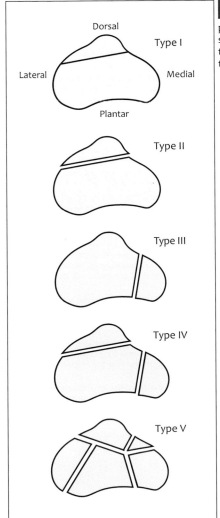

25.20 Schematic view of the proximal articular surface of the central tarsal bone to illustrate the fracture types.

Radiographic examination is mandatory to establish the severity and type of fracture. Plantarodorsal and mediolateral views are usually diagnostic; with type I fractures it can also be useful to obtain a mediolateral radiograph with the joint in full extension to enable better evaluation of the degree of displacement of the slab.

Oblique radiographic views allow more detailed evaluation of the degree of comminution and the shape of the fragments with type IV and V fractures. However, CT is the most sensitive imaging modality as it allows accurate evaluation of the degree of comminution and the involvement of other tarsal bones (Figure 25.21). With few exceptions, central tarsal bone fractures require open reduction and internal fixation to achieve anatomical reconstruction and realignment of the tarsus in order to improve post injury prognosis.

Single dorsal slabs (type I and II fractures) are stabilized with a dorsoplantar lag screw (usually 2 to 2.7 mm). Rarer type III fractures can be reduced and stabilized with a single mediolateral screw, although non-displaced type I fractures that are not detected on preoperative radiographs are often apparent at the time of surgery, and should be stabilized concurrently.

> **PRACTICAL TIP**
>
> When the fragment is too small, drilling a glide hole for a lag screw may cause iatrogenic splitting of the fragment. This can be avoided by inserting a positional screw. Interfragmentary compression can be achieved with pointed reduction forceps until screw insertion is complete. Failure to maintain appropriate reduction and compression will invariably leave a gap at the fracture site

Type IV fractures are stabilized with a mediolateral 4 mm partially threaded cancellous screw and dorsoplantar lag screws (see Operative Technique 25.6) (Figure 25.33). The mediolateral screw is inserted ensuring that the threaded portion is engaged in the fourth tarsal bone. Type V fractures can be stabilized with insertion of multiple lag screws and small washers to constrain very small, unstable fragments; alternatively, a small plate can be applied from the talus to the distal tarsal bones or proximal aspect of the second metatarsal bone to bridge across the comminuted area.

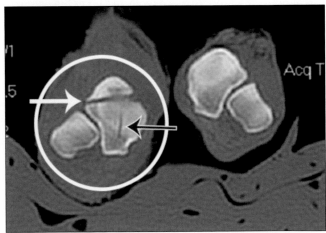

25.21 A CT image of a type IV central tarsal bone fracture. The mediolateral fracture (white arrow) was visible on radiographs; however, the dorsoplantar fissure (black arrow) was only identified on the CT scan. The contralateral intact bone is visible on the right.

After surgery the tarsus is supported with a cast or a splint for a period varying from 3 to 4 weeks, with strict rest required. The cast should be removed as soon as evidence of osseous healing is identified on radiographs, at which point physical therapy can be started.

Fractures of the plantar process of the central tarsal bone

This is a relatively common injury in active dogs; the Border Collie appears to be overrepresented. The fracture is seen in association with dorsomedial luxation of the body of the central tarsal bone. Diagnosis is straightforward based on assessment of orthogonal radiographs. The central tarsal bone is manually reduced and compressed against the fourth tarsal bone with pointed forceps. A positional screw (2.7 mm in a Border Collie-sized dog) is placed in a mediolateral direction from the central tarsal bone into the fourth tarsal bone to maintain reduction. The plantar process is not directly stabilized. Postoperative external coaption is provided for around 4 weeks.

Second, third and fourth tarsal bone fractures

Fracture of the third tarsal bone can be a solitary lesion, or can be associated with fracture of the second tarsal bone. This injury can be quite subtle and must be confirmed by radiographic evaluation using standard orthogonal views. Open reduction and internal fixation with a lag screw inserted in dorsoplantar direction is usually the best method of stabilization (Guilliard, 2010). Fractures of the second tarsal bone are quite rare and are usually associated with a fracture of the third tarsal bone. Dorsoplantar or plantarodorsal radiographic views are usually diagnostic, showing an increased joint space between the second and third tarsal bones. Again, open reduction and internal fixation with small lag screws is usually the treatment of choice. Postoperative coaptation for 3 to 4 weeks is recommended.

Fourth tarsal bone fractures are almost invariably associated with fractures of the central tarsal bone and are a consequence of collapse of the dorsomedial aspect of the joint due to compressive forces. Diagnosis is by clinical and radiographic examination. Reduction of the fourth tarsal bone is achieved indirectly by reconstructing the central tarsal bone; the prognosis is directly related to the nature of the central tarsal bone fracture. The fourth tarsal bone can be reconstructed with lag screw and/or plate fixation. Postoperative care is similar to that described for central tarsal bone fractures.

Shearing injuries of the tarsus

Shearing injuries of the tarsus and metatarsus are similar to those of the carpus and metacarpus in that they usually involve the medial aspect of the limb with loss of soft tissue coverage, collateral ligaments and, according to the severity of the lesion, varying amounts of bone.

Often shearing injuries of the tarsus result in subluxation or luxation of the tarsocrural joint, with exposure of the articular surface through a large dorsomedial wound. Primary care of shearing injuries consists of wound debridement, lavage and serial bandaging (see Chapter 12). Type 1 or 2 transarticular ESF constructs are particularly useful, as they offer excellent support to the injured joints and facilitate management of the open wound. The transarticular external skeletal fixator is usually left in place for 6 to 8 weeks followed by implant removal and gradual rehabilitation. Primary repair or replacement of collateral ligament injuries is rarely required, as the degree of fibrosis resulting from the period of immobilization with ESF is usually sufficient to provide good joint stability. Partial or pantarsal arthrodesis are occasionally required for these types of injuries, particularly if severe bone loss has occurred or marked joint instability persists after removal of the external skeletal fixator; however, this is uncommon.

Acknowledgements

The editors would like to thank John Houlton for allowing them to reproduce and modify Operative Techniques from the previous edition of this manual to accompany this chapter.

References and further reading

Boudrieau RJ, Dee JF and Dee LG (1984) Central tarsal bone fractures in the racing Greyhound. *Journal of the American Veterinary Medical Association* **184**, 1486–1491

Dee JF (1988) In: *Decision Making in Small Animal Orthopaedic Surgery*, ed. G Summer-Smith. BC Decker Inc., Philadelphia

Gnudi G, Mortellaro CM, Bertoni G *et al.* (2003) Radial carpal bone fracture in 13 dogs. *Veterinary and Comparative Orthopaedics and Traumatology* **16**, 178–183

Guilliard MJ (2007) Central tarsal bone fracture in the Border Collie. *Journal of Small Animal Practice* **48**, 414–417

Guilliard MJ (2010) Third tarsal bone fractures in the Greyhound. *Journal of Small Animal Practice* **51**, 635–641

Houlton JEF, Cook JL, Innes JF and Langley-Hobbs SJ (2006) *BSAVA Manual of Canine and Feline Musculoskeletal Disorders*. BSAVA Publications, Gloucester

Johnson KA (1987) Accessory carpal bone fractures in the racing Greyhound. Classification and pathology. *Veterinary Surgery* **16**, 60–64

Johnson KA and Piras A (2005) Fractures of the carpus. In: *AO Principles of Fracture Management in the Dog and Cat*, ed. AL Johnson *et al.*, pp 340–348. AO Publishing, Stuttgart

Li A, Bennett D, Gibbs C *et al.* (2000) Radial carpal bone fractures in 15 dogs. *Journal of Small Animal Practice* **41**, 74–79

Perry K, Fitzpatrick N, Johnson J and Yeadon R (2010) Headless self-compressing cannulated screw fixation for treatment of radial carpal bone fracture or fissure in dogs. *Veterinary and Comparative Orthopaedics and Traumatology* **23**, 94–101

Piermattei DL, Flo GL and DeCamp CE (2006) Fractures and other orthopedic conditions of the carpus, metacarpus, and phalanges. In: *Brinker, Piermattei, and Flo's Handbook of Small Animal Orthopedics and Fracture Repair*, pp. 382–428. WB Saunders Co., Philadelphia

Piermattei DL, Flo GL and DeCamp CE (2006) Fractures and other orthopedic injuries of the tarsus, metatarsus, and phalanges. In: *Brinker, Piermattei, and Flo's Handbook of Small Animal Orthopedics and Fracture Repair*, pp. 661–713. WB Saunders Co., Philadelphia

Voss K, Geyer H, Montavon PM (2003) Antebrachiocarpal luxation in a cat, a case report and anatomical study of the medial collateral ligament. *Veterinary and Comparative Orthopaedics and Traumatology* **16**, 266–270

OPERATIVE TECHNIQUE 25.1

Dorsal approach to the carpus

POSITIONING

The dog may either be placed in dorsal recumbency with the affected limb pulled caudally to lie alongside the thorax, or be placed in sternal recumbency with the limb drawn forwards. The limb can be covered in a sterile stockinette or cohesive bandage, if desired.

ASSISTANT

Required.

EQUIPMENT EXTRAS

Round tip periosteal elevator (dental type); Gelpi retractors; small Hohmann retractor.

SURGICAL TECHNIQUES

Approach

Following incision of the stockinette or cohesive bandage, the skin incision is made on the mid-dorsal surface of the joint, curving laterally at its distal end parallel with the accessory cephalic vein, allowing the latter to be retracted medially (Figure 25.22). The incision is continued between the tendons of the common digital extensor and the extensor carpi radialis muscles and through the periosteum of the distal radius. This is elevated on either side of the incision so that the tendons can be elevated without disturbing their sheaths. The tendons are retracted laterally and medially, respectively, with Gelpi retractors. The joint capsule is incised longitudinally, parallel to the tendons. The synovium attached to the dorsal surface of the carpal bones must be incised around the bones in question in order to expose them.

> **PRACTICAL TIP**
>
> Exposure is improved by suturing the margins of the skin incision to the stockinette and cohesive bandage, and by flexing the carpus

Wound closure

The subcutaneous tissues and skin are closed routinely.

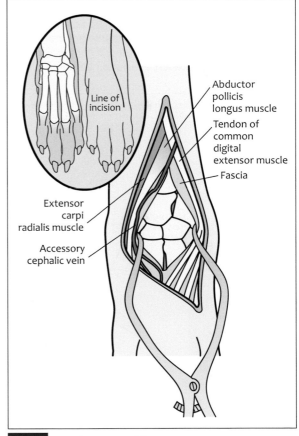

Line of incision

Abductor pollicis longus muscle

Tendon of common digital extensor muscle

Fascia

Extensor carpi radialis muscle

Accessory cephalic vein

25.22 Dorsal exposure of the carpus.

OPERATIVE TECHNIQUE 25.2

Palmaromedial approach to the radial carpal bone

POSITIONING

Dorsal recumbency with the affected limb drawn cranially so that the palmar surface of the foot is uppermost.

ASSISTANT

Required.

EQUIPMENT EXTRAS

Round tip periosteal elevator (dental type); Gelpi retractors; small Hohmann retractor; Rake-type retractors may be useful.

SURGICAL TECHNIQUES

Approach

A skin incision is made equidistant between the radial styloid process and the carpal pad. The underlying cephalic vein is ligated and transected (Figure 25.23). The flexor retinaculum is incised in a similar direction to expose the tendons of the flexor carpi radialis and the digital flexor muscles. The antebrachiocarpal joint space is identified with a 21 G needle and the deep fascia and joint capsule are incised at this level. There is a plethora of different vessels and nerves in this region, but most can be retracted if care is taken. The median artery and nerve, the ulnar nerve, and the deep palmar arch and palmar metacarpal arteries are the most important and must be preserved.

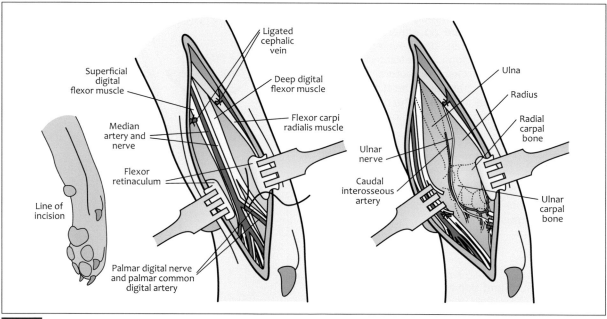

25.23 Palmaromedial exposure of the radial carpal bone.

PRACTICAL TIP

In order to increase visualization of the fracture line and verify the orientation of the implants, it is possible to combine the palmar approach with the standard dorsal approach described in Operative Technique 25.1

WARNING

This approach is not recommended for inexperienced surgeons

Wound closure

The flexor retinaculum is carefully apposed and the subcutaneous tissues and skin closed routinely.

OPERATIVE TECHNIQUE 25.3

Screw fixation of type I and II accessory carpal bone fractures

POSITIONING

Dorsal recumbency with the affected limb pulled cranially so that the palmar aspect of the foot is uppermost.

ASSISTANT

Required.

EQUIPMENT EXTRAS

Round tip periosteal elevator (dental type); mini Gelpi retractors (angled arms and short tips); small Hohmann retractor; 1.5 mm screw sets; mini power drill; small pointed reduction forceps.

SURGICAL TECHNIQUES

Approach

A palmarolateral approach is made. The skin incision is started at the caudomedial border of the distal ulna, taken around the accessory carpal bone, and ended distally over metacarpal 5 (Figure 25.24). The subcutaneous tissues are incised along the same line. The flexor retinaculum is carefully incised on its lateral aspect and retracted medially together with the superficial digital flexor tendon. Care should be taken to leave sufficient tissue at its insertion in order to facilitate repositioning and suturing.

The abductor digiti quinti muscle is lifted from the palmar aspect of the accessory carpal bone by sharp dissection. Care should be taken to not damage the accessoro–metacarpal ligaments. The muscle is reflected distally and a mini Gelpi retractor is inserted between the two accessoro–metacarpal ligaments. Care should be taken to avoid impingement of the neurovascular bundle that lies medially, just below the accessorometacarpal IV ligament. Visualization of the palmar aspect of the bone is increased by flexing the carpus and spreading the Gelpi retractors.

Reduction and fixation

Once the fragment is visualized it can be reduced either with a pair of small pointed reduction forceps, or by gentle pressure applied with the drill guide. The fragment is covered completely by the palmar ligament; the ligament origin must be respected and should not be elevated off the fragment. A 1.1 mm drill hole is started in the centre of the fragment. The hole should be drilled from the reduced fragment to the accessory carpal bone, perpendicular to the fracture line and parallel to the joint. A glide hole is then drilled using the 1.5 mm drill bit.

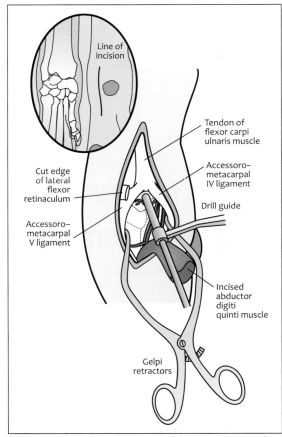

25.24 Palmarolateral exposure of the accessory carpal bone.

Labels in figure:
- Line of incision
- Cut edge of lateral flexor retinaculum
- Accessoro-metacarpal V ligament
- Tendon of flexor carpi ulnaris muscle
- Accessoro-metacarpal IV ligament
- Drill guide
- Incised abductor digiti quinti muscle
- Gelpi retractors

During over-drilling the fragment should be held in position using a pair of small forceps to prevent it rotating with the drill bit, which could potentially further damage the ligament. If it is difficult to hold the fragment securely, it is advisable to over-drill the fragment with a drill bit and hand chuck rather than using a power tool. The hole is measured using the depth gauge, and tapped with the 1.5 mm tap before placement of the screw. In order to facilitate compression without stressing the repair the carpal joint should be flexed to reduce the ligamentous tension on the fragment. During the drilling phases reduction is often lost. To facilitate accurate reduction and realignment, the screw can be reinserted into the glide hole with the tip protruding a few millimetres to enable its safe location into the pilot hole in the accessory carpal bone (Figure 25.25).

→

→ **OPERATIVE TECHNIQUE 25.3 CONTINUED**

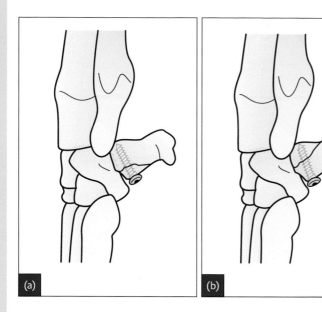

25.25 Screw fixation of (a) type I and (b) type II articular fractures of the accessory carpal bone.

Wound closure

The lateral flexor retinaculum is carefully apposed and the subcutaneous tissues and skin closed routinely.

POSTOPERATIVE MANAGEMENT

The carpus is cast in a flexion for around 6 to 8 weeks. Each second or third week the cast should be replaced and the joint re-cast in a less flexed position. At the end of this period, the carpus will have a restricted range of movement, which will improve with a gradual increase in exercise level.

OPERATIVE TECHNIQUE 25.4

Pin and tension-band fixation of calcaneal fractures

POSITIONING

Dorsal recumbency with the affected limb drawn forwards or lateral recumbency.

ASSISTANT

Optional.

EQUIPMENT EXTRAS

Round tip periosteal elevator (dental type); mini Gelpi retractors; K-wires; orthopaedic wire for tension-band; small chuck; pin/wire cutters; pliers/wire twisters; pointed reduction forceps; drill bits.

SURGICAL TECHNIQUES

Approach

A plantarolateral approach (Figure 25.26) is made to the calcaneus to avoid the point of the tuber calcanei. The skin incision begins on the lateral aspect of the Achilles tendon and curves distally. The deep fascia is incised lateral to and parallel with the superficial digital flexor tendon. Medial retraction of the superficial digital flexor tendon from the gastrocnemius tendon completes the exposure. ➡️

→ **OPERATIVE TECHNIQUE 25.4 CONTINUED**

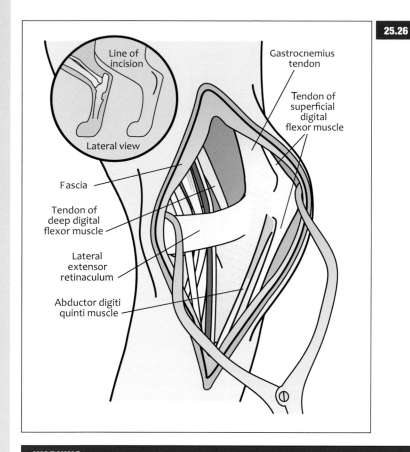

25.26 Plantarolateral exposure of the calcaneus.

Line of incision

Lateral view

Gastrocnemius tendon

Tendon of superficial digital flexor muscle

Fascia

Tendon of deep digital flexor muscle

Lateral extensor retinaculum

Abductor digiti quinti muscle

WARNING

It is unwise to use an Esmarch's bandage and tourniquet when repairing calcaneal fractures, as the tourniquet will apply tension to the Achilles tendon and hinder fracture reduction

---

Reduction and fixation

PRACTICAL TIP

Extension of the tarsus will assist fracture reduction

The transverse hole for the tension-band wire should be drilled first and the orthopaedic wire pre-inserted to avoid impingement on the pins. Retraction of the superficial digital flexor tendon medially with a small Hohmann retractor will enable the end of the wire to be grasped when it is placed through the bone tunnel.

When managing physeal separation in puppies, the K-wires should be driven side by side as far laterally and medially as possible. During this phase attention should be paid to the fluted shape of the calcaneus in order to prevent the K-wires exiting the medial or lateral cortices of the bone. The tension-band wire is then tightened, making sure that it is adjacent to the bone and under the tendon of the superficial digital flexor muscle. The ends of the K-wires must be bent over as close to the surface of the bone as possible, to minimize soft tissue irritation (Figure 25.27).

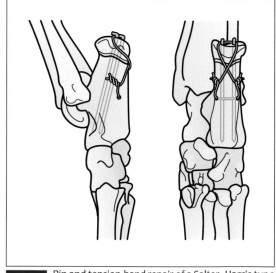

25.27 Pin and tension-band repair of a Salter–Harris type I fracture of the proximal calcaneal physis.

→ **OPERATIVE TECHNIQUE 25.4 CONTINUED**

In mature animals with mid-body fractures, counter-sunk pins can be used as these interfere less with superficial digital flexor tendon function and create fewer soft tissue problems. A single larger pin is adequate; the tension-band wire is passed through two transverse tunnels in the calcaneus, one proximal to and one distal to the fracture (Figure 25.28). Pre-drilling the calcaneus with a slightly smaller drill bit than the final pin is advised as the calcaneus is a very dense bone and can be challenging to penetrate with a trochar tip, which in turn can lead to excessive heat production during drilling.

> **PRACTICAL TIP**
>
> The tension-band wire should be made from two separate pieces of wire; one passed through the distal bone tunnel, the other taken around the ends of the K-wires. The ends can then be tightened. This ensures even tension across the entire tension-band wire and makes its placement easier

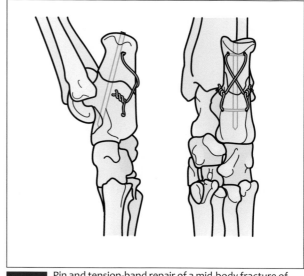

25.28 Pin and tension-band repair of a mid-body fracture of the calcaneus.

Alternative technique

Calcaneal fractures can also be stabilized using a bone plate applied to the lateral and/or caudal surface of the bone, with or without additional intramedullary pin and tension-band wire fixation (see Figures 25.12–25.14); the choice is governed by the configuration of the fracture. Plate fixation can be applied to the lateral surface of the bone through a lateral or plantarolateral approach. Although the caudal surface is the tension side of the bone, laterally applied plates are stronger by virtue of the fact that the plate is loaded 'on edge' (see Chapter 4). Plate size and type is selected on the basis of personal preference and availability. The cortices of the calcaneus are very dense, particularly at its proximal aspect, and this should be borne in mind when drilling holes for screws or other implants; sharp drill bits are required.

Wound closure

The deep fascia is repaired and the subcutaneous tissues and skin closed routinely.

POSTOPERATIVE MANAGEMENT

The tarsus is supported in slight extension for 6 to 8 weeks using a moulded splint or a fibreglass cast on a well padded bandage. In an athletic dog it is often necessary to remove implants such as plates, pins and wires, but screws can be left in place unless they are perceived to be causing irritation.

OPERATIVE TECHNIQUE 25.5

Internal fixation of articular fractures of the talus

POSITIONING

Medial or lateral recumbency, depending on which region of the talar surface is being exposed.

ASSISTANT

Required.

EQUIPMENT EXTRAS

Round tip periosteal elevator (dental type); mini Gelpi retractors; small Hohmann retractor; osteotome and mallet or preferably a mini oscillating saw; small chuck; K-wires; pointed reduction forceps; a 1/1.5/2 mm screw set; Rake-type retractors may be useful; a headlight can aid visualization of the surgical site.

SURGICAL TECHNIQUES

Approach

The skin is incised directly over the relevant malleolus, and an additional incision made into the joint capsule. Adequate exposure of larger fragments may not be possible without a malleolar osteotomy. To expose the medial talar ridge, the medial collateral ligament is isolated by incising either side of it and the malleolus removed with an osteotome (Figure 25.29). This is not straightforward as the osteotomy must be deep enough to include most of the origin of the malleolus, but not so deep as to involve the weight-bearing articular surface. Reference to an anatomical specimen or three-dimensional print of the distal tibia can be helpful. To expose the lateral talar ridge, the distal fibula is isolated by a transverse osteotomy (Figure 25.30a).

> **PRACTICAL TIP**
>
> Drill the fixation screw/K-wire holes before performing the osteotomy

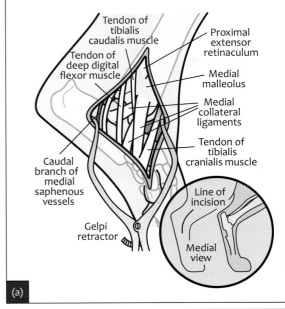

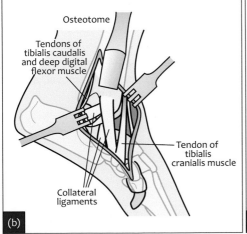
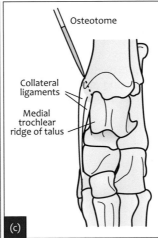
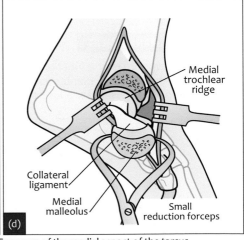

25.29 Medial exposure of the talocrural joint via osteotomy of the medial malleolus. (a) Exposure of the medial aspect of the tarsus. (b) Retraction of caudal tendons prior to osteotomy. (c) Position of osteotomy. (d) Distal reflection of medial malleolus to expose the medial trochlear ridge.

→ **OPERATIVE TECHNIQUE 25.5 CONTINUED**

Reduction and fixation

Large fragments should be reduced and stabilized with 1 mm to 2 mm lag screws countersunk into the articular surface. K-wires can be used for provisional fixation, but they do not represent a stable method of fixation, and should only be used when lag screw fixation is not possible (Figure 25.30). The use of biodegradable pins has also been suggested (see Chapter 9). Some parasagittal intertrochlear fractures may be amenable to lag screw fixation through subarticular bone.

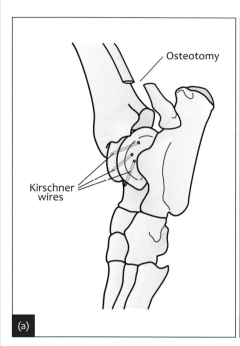

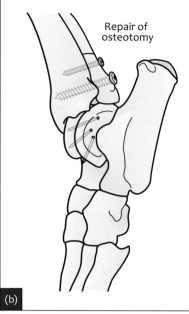

25.30 (a) Repair of a fracture of the lateral talar ridge using countersunk K-wires. The fracture is exposed via osteotomy of the distal fibula and lateral reflection of the malleolus. If possible small lag screws should be used rather than K-wires, since these provide better stability, although when used in small bone fragments there is a risk that the lag screws can cause further fragmentation. (b) The fibular osteotomy is repaired using two positional screws into the distal tibia.

> **PRACTICAL TIP**
>
> Small fragments can be manipulated by inserting a small gauge K-wire. The pin is used as a 'joystick' to reduce the fragment. Once reduced the pin is advanced to maintain fixation whilst a lag screw is placed. It is important to ensure that the position of the pin does not interfere with the ideal position of the lag screw

Wound closure

The malleolus is reattached with a lag screw or pin and tension-band wiring (see Chapter 19). If a lateral approach has been used with fibular osteotomy, the distal fibula can be stabilized using two positional screws directed into the tibia (Figure 25.30b).

POSTOPERATIVE MANAGEMENT

The tarsus is supported at a functional angle for approximately 5 weeks using a cast. The full cast can be bivalved and after 3 weeks the dorsal or plantar part used in isolation as a splint within the bandage. Following cast removal, activity is restricted to lead walking for a further 2 to 4 weeks, before gradually increasing the patient's exercise.

OPERATIVE TECHNIQUE 25.6

Internal fixation of central tarsal bone fractures

POSITIONING

Dorsal recumbency with the affected leg extended caudally. The base of the tail should be at the edge of the surgical table allowing the entire limb to overhang the table edge. A sterile stockinette or cohesive bandage can be applied to the limb, if desired.

PRACTICAL TIP

When positioning the dog, it is helpful to extend the limb so that the tarsus and pes are parallel to the ground. This aids accurate drilling in a dorsoplantar direction

ASSISTANT

Helpful.

EQUIPMENT EXTRAS

Round tip periosteal elevator (dental type); screw set ranging from 1.5 mm to 4 mm; drill; mini Gelpi retractors; small Hohmann retractor; small and large pointed reduction forceps.

SURGICAL TECHNIQUES

Approach

The surgical approach is dorsomedial (Figure 25.31). Following incision of the stockinette or cohesive bandage a skin incision is made from the medial malleolus to metatarsal 2 between the saphenous and medial saphenous vein, lateral to the tendon of insertion of the cranial tibial muscle. A small Hohmann retractor is used to retract the tendon medially and expose the dorsal surface of the central tarsal bone. Alternatively, a small Gelpi retractor can be placed between the tibialis cranialis tendon and the lateral side of the incision.

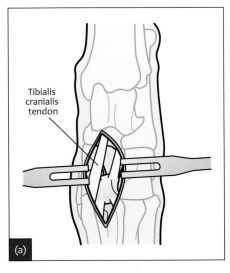

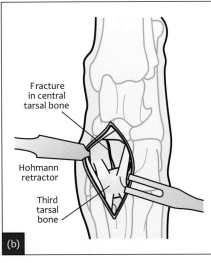

25.31 Dorsomedial exposure of the central tarsal bone. (a) Incision through skin and subdermal fascia. (b) Retraction of the tibialis cranialis tendon exposes the fracture.

PRACTICAL TIP

In order to increase soft tissue retraction the skin is incised and sutured to the stockinette and cohesive bandage

→ **OPERATIVE TECHNIQUE 25.6 CONTINUED**

Reduction and fixation

Type I and II fractures are repaired using a dorsoplantar 2.7 mm lag screw (Figure 25.32). The fracture is reduced by extending the tarsus and aligning the articular surfaces. The reduction is maintained with pointed reduction forceps; twin-point forceps can be particularly useful. Care should be taken to start the drill bit in the centre of the bone – too proximally and it will enter the talocentral joint. If the tarsus is parallel with the floor and the drill bit directed vertically, the screw will be in the correct dorsoplantar direction, aiming towards the plantar process of the bone.

Type IV fractures are repaired using a mediolateral 4 mm partially threaded cancellous bone screw placed from the central tarsal bone into the fourth tarsal bone, and a 2 mm to 2.7 mm lag screw through the dorsal slab. The use of a cancellous mediolateral screw helps to stabilize any concurrent compression fracture of the fourth tarsal bone, and the non-threaded portion within the central tarsal bone allows easier placement of the dorsoplantar screw as its shaft diameter is smaller than a standard 2.7 mm or 3.5 mm fully threaded screw (Figure 25.33). Screw placement is critical if both screws are to avoid the talocentral and centrodistal joint spaces. The mediolateral screw should be placed first, starting at the junction of the middle and distal third of the slab. The dorsoplantar screw is started at the junction of the proximal and middle third of the bone. If the mediolateral screw is inserted higher due to unusual fragment shape, dorsoplantar screw size can be reduced to 1.5 mm or 2 mm avoid conflict between the two implants.

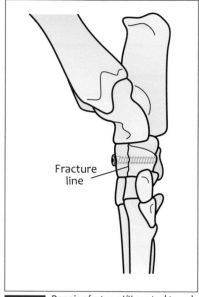

25.32 Repair of a type I/II central tarsal bone fracture using a dorsoplantar lag screw.

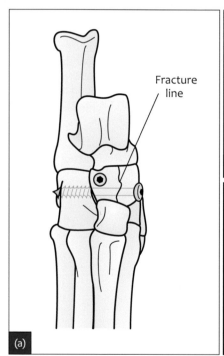

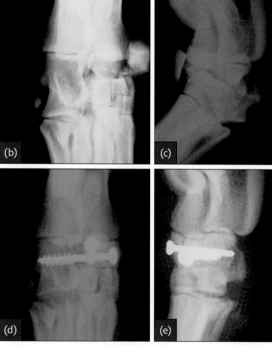

25.33 (a) Schematic to show screw position in the repair of a type IV central tarsal bone fracture. A mediolateral partially threaded cancellous screw is used to stabilize the medial slab; this allows more space for insertion of a dorsoplantar lag screw to stabilize the dorsal slab. (b) Plantarodorsal and (c) mediolateral views of a type IV central tarsal bone fracture in a Greyhound. (d) Plantarodorsal and (e) mediolateral postoperative views. The fracture has been stabilized with a mediolateral 4 mm partially threaded screw and dorsoplantar 2.7 mm lag screw.

PRACTICAL TIP

Reduction of the type IV fracture is facilitated by hyperflexion of the intertarsal joints and valgus leverage applied to the metatarsal bones. This manoeuvre will open the dorsal and medial joint space, allowing reduction of the fragments

→ **OPERATIVE TECHNIQUE 25.6 CONTINUED**

Pointed reduction forceps are carefully applied to gradually reduce the fragments. Avoid placing the pointed reduction forceps in the same position as the screws or on the periphery of the fragments, which could result in further fragmentation. Take care as, whilst the medial fragment is usually quite thick and robust, the dorsal fragment can be very thin and can fragment easily. The mediolateral screw should be oriented slightly in plantar direction (see Figure 25.33d) to avoid penetrating the dorsal aspect of the fourth tarsal bone. Sometimes an apparent type IV central tarsal bone fracture (as diagnosed by preoperative radiography) can be a type V, and have a number of small fragments in between the larger three main fragments. These prevent perfect reduction. In these cases the dorsal slab is carefully lifted, preserving the ligamentous attachments, and the fracture area is gently flushed to remove small chips, facilitating reduction; alternatively, a small plate can be applied from the distal aspect of the talus to the distal tarsal bones or the proximal aspect of the second metatarsal bone, bridging the fracture.

Wound closure

The subcutaneous tissues and skin are closed routinely.

POSTOPERATIVE MANAGEMENT

The tarsus is supported at a functional angle for 5 weeks using a fibreglass cast over a well padded bandage. The cast can be bivalved and reduced to a dorsal or plantar splint after 3 weeks.

Chapter 26

The distal limb

Mike Guilliard

Anatomy

The four main metacarpal (MC) and metatarsal (MT) bones, numbered 2 to 5 from medial to lateral, are arranged in a dorsally convex arcade. The central bones (MC/MT3 and 4) are the main weight-bearing bones. The first metacarpal bone (MC1) is the vestigial dewclaw on the medial aspect of the limb; the first metatarsal bone (MT1) is usually rudimentary with no external form. The base, or proximal part, of each metacarpal/metatarsal bone articulates proximally with the distal row of carpal/tarsal bones to form the carpometacarpal/tarsometatarsal joints, and provides the insertion points of the carpal/tarsal ligaments.

The body of each metacarpal/metatarsal bone has a greater dimension in the dorsopalmar/dorsoplantar plane than in the lateromedial plane. This allows easier placement of external skeletal fixation (ESF) pins in a lateromedial (or mediolateral) direction. Distally the metacarpal/metatarsal arcade becomes more convex and the bones diverge in the mediolateral plane, which can make placement of implants here more challenging. The head, or distal end, of each metacarpal/metatarsal bone articulates with the first phalanx. On the palmar/plantar aspect of the head lie pairs of proximal sesamoid bones within the tendons of the interosseous muscles. The sagittal condylar ridge separates the sesamoid bones from each other. The sesamoid bones are numbered 1 to 8 from medial to lateral.

Small single dorsal sesamoids lie within the extensor tendons at the metacarpophalangeal/metatarsophalangeal and the proximal interphalangeal joints, but are of no clinical significance.

Surgical considerations

Fractures of the distal limbs can affect the metacarpal and metatarsal bones, the sesamoid bones and the phalanges. In toy dog breeds and cats the bones are very small, making surgical fixation challenging. Postoperative soft tissue swelling is common and, with the limited skin extensibility of the distal limb, can result in severe oedema of the digits. This can be mitigated with the application of support dressings of orthopaedic padding, conforming bandage and an elastic bandage for several days after the surgery. Cats appear to be particularly prone to gross oedema of the digits but this generally resolves naturally over a few days.

The main vascular supply is within the palmar and plantar aspects of the distal limbs, with poor vascularity on the dorsal aspects, the main surgical approach. Over-tight external coaptation or postoperative dressings can rapidly lead to skin necrosis and infection.

Aseptic preparation of the paw is difficult due to the presence of the nails and pads. After aseptic preparation, isolation of these areas from the surgical site can be achieved by the application of a sterile elastic bandage that can also be extended to use as a tourniquet around either the distal antebrachium or distal tibia. This may be useful when using internal fixation techniques on the bones of the distal limb or for sesamoidectomy. Use of a tourniquet is not necessary when an external skeletal fixator is used alone.

Treatment by external coaptation

It is very important to apply well padded dressings that can incorporate a palmar/plantar splint. The digits should be separated using orthopaedic padding or cotton wool. Incorporating the paw into the spoon of a gutter splint gives good support and prevents excessive, uncontrolled weight-bearing (see Chapter 16).

> **WARNING**
>
> Dressing-induced ischaemic necrosis is a common complication. In the author's opinion, full distal limb casts should not be used. Dressings must be kept dry

Metacarpal and metatarsal bone fractures

Fractures of the metacarpus and metatarsus are common in both pet dogs and cats, accounting for 8.1% and 3.3% of fractures, respectively (Phillips, 1979), and are typically traumatic in origin. They are also common in the racing Greyhound, with metacarpal and metatarsal fractures accounting for 7% and 10% of distal limb fractures, respectively (Guilliard, 2012). In racing Greyhounds these are predominantly stress or fatigue fractures and there is often no history of any significant external trauma.

Fractures can involve single or multiple bones. In the metacarpus they tend to occur in the mid to distal diaphysis and in the metatarsus in the proximal diaphysis (Muir and Norris, 1997). Typically, these are simple transverse or oblique fractures with little or no comminution. The proximal fragment overrides the dorsal aspect of the distal fragment and with multiple bone fractures rotation of the digits is common. Comminuted single bone fractures are more common in the racing Greyhound.

Articular fractures are uncommon, but can occur proximally in association with carpal and tarsal hyperextension injury. The collateral ligaments of the carpometacarpal and tarsometatarsal joints attach medially and laterally to MC/MT2 and 5; proximal fractures can involve these ligament insertions, leading to joint instability in a valgus or varus direction.

Management of metacarpal and metatarsal fractures can be non-surgical or surgical. Surgical intervention should be considered when there is a likelihood of significant malalignment of the digits. Indications for surgical treatment include:

- More than two metacarpal or metatarsal bones fractured in the same limb
- Reconstructable fractures of MC/MT3 or 4 with substantial displacement of the fragments
- Open fractures and shear injuries.

Non-surgical treatment can be used for:

- Fracture of a single metacarpal or metatarsal bone
- Fractures of multiple bones with little displacement
- Comminuted single bone fractures in the racing Greyhound.

Non-surgical management has been shown to give similar results to surgery (Kapatkin *et al.*, 2000), although this may reflect the surgical techniques chosen in the case series. Non-surgical management for multiple bone fractures, whilst often resulting in acceptable clinical outcomes (Kapatkin *et al.*, 2000), almost invariably causes malunion with digital rotation, synostosis and sometimes non-union (Figure 26.1). Digital rotation can lead to soft tissue problems of the pads and interdigital skin including hyperkeratosis, corns, interdigital hyperplasia and dermatitis. These problems may not become clinically apparent for a number of years (Figure 26.2).

Many different surgical techniques for fracture repair have been described, with no single method becoming the gold standard.

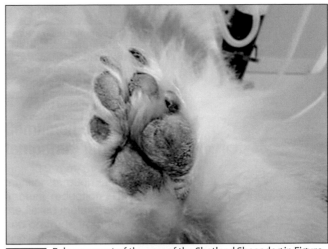

26.2 Palmar aspect of the paw of the Shetland Sheepdog in Figure 26.1. Note the hyperplasia of digital pad 5. This dog presented with acute onset lameness due to septic arthritis of the distal interphalangeal joint of digit 5.

Plates and screws

For both simple and comminuted fractures the veterinary cuttable plate or a mini-plate can be applied to the dorsal aspect of MC/MT3 and 4 (Figure 26.3), and to the abaxial aspects of MC/MT2 and 5. In addition, it may be possible to lag screw oblique fractures (Figure 26.4). The advantages of plates and screws are that good reduction is usually possible, and there is minimal risk of iatrogenic damage to articular surfaces proximally and distally. Disadvantages include financial cost, the potentially invasive nature of the surgical procedure, the necessity to use relatively small, weak implants because of the size of the bones, and the possibility that implant removal may be required if complications arise.

The use of a mini hook plate fashioned from the veterinary cuttable plate has been described for use in juxta-articular fractures in the racing Greyhound, giving more points of fixation. However, this is rarely required as almost all metacarpal and metatarsal fractures can usually be successfully managed by other less invasive approaches such as conservative management or ESF.

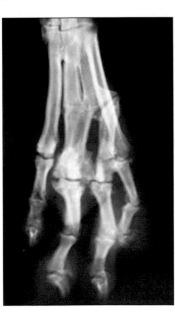

26.1 A dorsopalmar radiograph of the metacarpus of an 8-year-old Shetland Sheepdog that had sustained multiple fractures several years previously. A synostosis, a non-union fracture and severe osteoarthritis of the third metacarpophalongeal joint are present. Note the rotation of digits 3, 4 and 5.

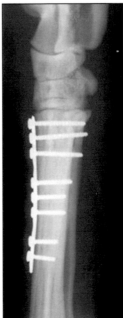

26.3 A fracture of the third metatarsal bone in a racing Greyhound treated with a veterinary cuttable plate applied to the dorsal aspect.

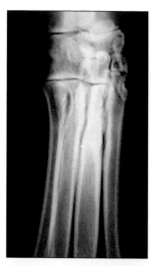

26.8 A dorsoplantar radiograph of the metatarsus of a racing Greyhound showing sclerotic changes of the proximal diaphysis of the third metatarsal bone, which represents a healing response to non-displaced cortical stress fractures. Continued rest resolved the lameness.

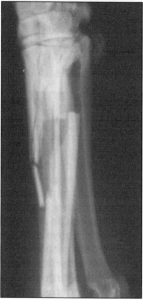

26.9 A comminuted, displaced fracture of the third metatarsal bone in a racing Greyhound. The treatment was kennel rest with no external support. The dog successfully returned to the track after 13 weeks.

fractures without external support has been shown to be highly successful with no loss of racing form (Guilliard, 2013). Recommended surgical treatment of simple displaced metacarpal and metatarsal fractures (Figure 26.10) is ESF with temporary IM pinning, which carries an excellent prognosis. Alternatively, reconstruction with a bone plate is relatively simple but in the racing dog may require implant removal due to stress concentration at the plate extremities.

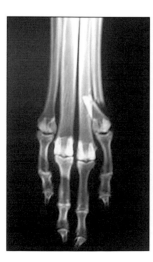

26.10 A displaced distal fracture of the fifth metatarsal bone in a racing Greyhound. This was aligned using a temporary IM pin followed by fixation with a type 1 external skeletal fixator for 6 weeks.

Highly comminuted fractures of single metacarpal or metatarsal bones will heal with conservative management, and surgical intervention may only be necessary if the digit is displaced. ESF or the application of a bridging plate are suitable treatment methods.

Fractures of the sesamoid bones

Fractures of the palmar and plantar sesamoid bones are rare and are seen primarily in the racing Greyhound. Bipartite and multipartite (fragmented) sesamoid bones have an unknown aetiology and can be confused with fractures. These are a common non-clinical finding in certain breeds including the Greyhound and the Rottweiler. Typically sesamoid bones 2 and 7 are affected (Figure 26.11).

Clinical signs of sesamoid bone fracture are acute onset lameness, joint swelling and pain on joint manipulation with focal pain present over the fractured sesamoid. There is a sharp demarcation of the fracture site with distraction of the fragment (Figure 26.12). Surgical removal of the displaced fragment or the complete sesamoid bone results in a return to successful racing. However, in the author's experience, conservative management gives a similar outcome to surgical removal.

It is uncertain whether fragmented sesamoids themselves are a cause of lameness, since they are often an incidental finding. However, it is possible they may predispose the dog to a strain injury of the associated interosseous tendon. They may be a coincidental finding associated with

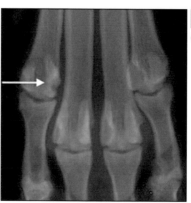

26.11 Bipartite second sesamoid bone (arrowed) in a Greyhound.

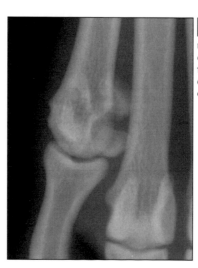

26.12 A fractured second sesamoid bone in a racing Greyhound. Note the distraction of the proximal fragment and the sharp demarcation of the fracture edges.

joint sprain. Surgical removal should only be considered when non-surgical management has failed and pain has been repeatedly localized over the sesamoid.

Sesamoidectomy

A surgical approach is made over the affected sesamoid bone with a longitudinal skin incision running abaxially to the metacarpal/metatarsal pad. The annular ligament is transected, and the underlying digital flexor tendons are displaced to expose the palmar/plantar aspect of the sesamoid. The fragment or entire bone can then be dissected from the interosseous tendon proximally and the sesamoidan ligaments. Closure of the subcutaneous tissues is with a synthetic absorbable suture material. Skin closure is routine. The foot should be bandaged for 10 days to protect the wound.

Fractures of the digits

Phalangeal fractures can affect any of the three phalangeal bones. The presenting signs are severe lameness and localized swelling of the digit. Diagnosis is by radiography.

Fractures of the first (P1) and the second (P2) phalanges can be simple, but are often oblique, spiral or comminuted. Articular involvement is common. Surgical reconstruction with lag screws can be demanding and is rarely necessary.

Non-surgical management is usually successful and external support may only be necessary for 2 weeks, or in some cases not at all as the soft tissue swelling is compartmentalized, the digit forming a natural splint.

Surgical intervention should be considered if there is misalignment of the digital pad. The application of an external skeletal fixator for 3 weeks gives good axial alignment. Pins sized 1.4 mm are suitable for the larger breeds of dog and are placed on the dorsal aspect, slightly abaxially (Figure 26.13). A transarticular configuration is often necessary including the seating of two pins in the third phalanx (P3) (Figure 26.14).

After pin insertion the pins are bent through 90 degrees, overlapping each other to allow application of acrylic putty. There should be a space of approximately 1 cm between the putty and the skin.

Common problems associated with the application of a fixator to the digits include:

- Premature loosening of the pins; this can be due to pin tract infection
- Osteomyelitis; this will resolve following pin removal and treatment with antibiotics
- Pin impingement on an adjacent digit from excessive protrusion from the trans (far) cortex
- Frame impingement on the soft tissues.

Articular fractures are *not* an indication for digital amputation as a pain-free ankylosis often develops.

Fracture of P3 is difficult to diagnose but should be suspected if the nail is loose. It is difficult to visualize

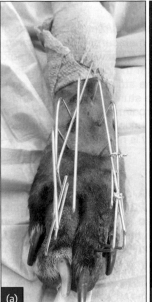
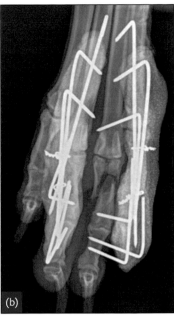

26.13 (a) An intraoperative photograph of a surgical repair of comminuted, articular fractures of the first phalanx of digits 3 and 4 of the right forelimb treated with transarticular external skeletal fixators before the application of the acrylic putty. (b) A postoperative radiograph showing the external skeletal fixators spanning both the metacarpophalangeal and proximal interphalangeal joints. The comminuted fractures involve the proximal articulations of both bones. Applying the fixators under tension has resulted in good reduction.

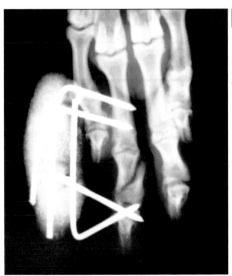

26.14 A spiral fracture of the second phalanx treated with a transarticular external skeletal fixator with two pins in the third phalanx.

radiographically. The differential diagnoses for swelling of the distal digit are:

- P2 or P3 fracture
- P2/P3 joint instability
- P3 osteomyelitis
- Neoplasia.

Treatment of P3 fractures, as well as P2/P3 joint instability and osteomyelitis, is permanent nail removal (ungual crest ostectomy; see Operative Technique 26.3).

Amputation of the digits

Amputation should be considered as a last resort when other treatments have failed.

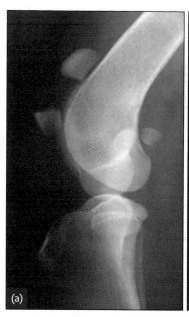

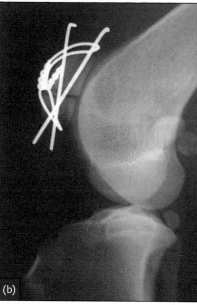

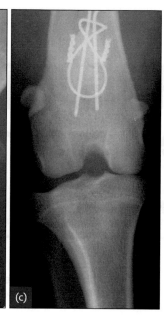

27.2 A patellar fracture in a Boxer. The dog had run into a wall and sustained a small wound over the stifle. When attempting to bear weight the dog was unable to maintain stifle extension. (a) Mediolateral view of a transverse fracture of the patella. (b) Postoperative mediolateral and (c) craniocaudal views of the fracture repaired with two K-wires and a figure-of-eight tension-band wire.

(Figure 27.1a). Patellar fractures are usually bilateral, but they generally occur several months apart rather than simultaneously. There may be radiographic evidence of sclerosis of both patellae prior to fracture. Other low-energy atraumatic avulsion-type fractures occur subsequently (or have occurred previously) in over half of the cats affected with patellar fractures, including pelvic fractures (bilateral or unilateral acetabular and ischial avulsion fractures), humeral condylar fractures and proximal transverse tibial fractures (Langley-Hobbs, 2009; Langley-Hobbs *et al.*, 2009) (see Figure 27.1b). Retained deciduous teeth or delayed dental eruption has also been reported in a high number of cats with patellar fractures. The bilateral nature of the fractures and the subsequent development of fractures of other bones in over half of affected cats gives credence to the likelihood that these fractures are insufficiency stress fractures occurring in pathologically weakened bone. The presence of retained deciduous teeth in many cats suggests that this syndrome may have a developmental or hereditary basis and further investigations are ongoing to determine if this is the case.

The optimal treatment method for stress fractures of the patella in cats is not known. Pin and tension-band fixation of feline patellar fractures results in a very high complication rate with 86% of cases resulting in additional fractures and fragment displacement (Langley-Hobbs, 2009), so this method of fixation cannot be recommended. Conservative treatment or a less invasive method of repair for widely displaced fractures such as an encircling wire or a figure-of-eight wire, without a pin, may be preferable. Even with surgical repair, the majority of patellar fractures will not heal but will form functional non-unions. Prognosis is guarded for a full return to function with more than 50% of cats having residual lameness.

The fabellae

The gastrocnemius muscle arises by distinct medial and lateral heads from the medial and lateral supracondylar tuberosities, respectively, of the femur. The fabella (Latin for 'little bean') is a small sesamoid bone; one is found embedded in each of the tendons of origin of the two heads of the gastrocnemius muscle. The fabellae sit adjacent to the caudoproximal aspects of the lateral and medial condyle of the femur. The two heads of the gastrocnemius muscle fuse distally and give rise to the large tendon that inserts on the calcaneus. The superficial digital flexor muscle is firmly attached to the deep surface of the lateral head of the gastrocnemius muscle and shares attachments to the lateral fabella, so avulsion of the origin of the lateral head of the gastrocnemius might also include injury to the superficial digital flexor muscle (Reinke *et al.*, 1993). The peroneal nerve may also be injured concurrently. Radiographs of the stifle joints of cats revealed a lack of mineralization in the medial fabella in a high percentage of domestic cats, although on post-mortem examination a small fibrocartilaginous structure was identified in most cats in the region of the medial fabella (Arnbjerg and Heje, 1993).

Various regions of the gastrocnemius muscle may be injured in the dog, including the origins of the lateral and medial heads or both (Chaffee and Knecht, 1975; Walker, 1977; Reinke *et al.*, 1982; Vaughan, 1985; Robinson, 1999; Ting *et al.*, 2006), the muscle belly, usually at the musculo-tendinous junction (Mitchell, 1980; Vaughan, 1985), and the tendon of insertion on the calcaneus (Reinke *et al.*, 1993). Injury to the gastrocnemius may also occur as part of a more complex injury to the Achilles mechanism (Vaughan, 1985; Meutstege, 1993). Injury proximally is less common than injury to the distal muscle and tendon. Reported problems of the fabellae in the literature include avulsion, fracture, or a combination of the two. Avulsion of both the medial and lateral fabellae has been reported (Chaffee and Knecht, 1975; Vaughan, 1979; Reinke *et al.*, 1982; Muir and Dueland, 1994; Walker, 1997; Ridge and Owen, 2005). Isolated fracture with minimal displacement of the gastrocnemius muscle bellies has also been reported (Houlton and Ness, 1993).

Isolated fracture of the fabella was associated with acute onset lameness during or after exercise in seven dogs, including four Border Collies or Collie crosses; the dogs varied in age from 6 months to 10 years (Houlton and Ness, 1993). In all dogs the lateral fabella was affected, in six dogs the condition was unilateral and in one dog bilateral. In all dogs the lameness worsened with exercise, and pain could be elicited on direct palpation over the caudolateral stifle joint. The dogs did not have a plantigrade stance, suggesting that the gastrocnemius muscle was still functional. Four of the cases were treated conservatively with restricted exercise and four with excision of the fabella and fragments. Chronic fabellar fractures take on an amorphous appearance (Houlton and Ness, 1993) (Figure 27.3). The dogs treated surgically became sound within approximately 1 month; the lameness in the dogs treated conservatively also resolved, but this took an average of 10 to 12 weeks (Houlton and Ness, 1993).

Avulsion of the gastrocnemius with displacement of the fabella usually results in the dog presenting with a plantigrade stance (Reinke *et al.*, 1982). This is seemingly dependent on the degree of damage and whether both muscle bellies are affected; avulsion of the lateral belly is more likely to result in a plantigrade stance than isolated avulsion of the medial belly. The condition has been

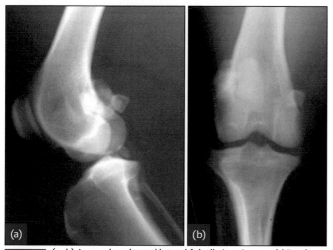

27.3 (a–b) A grossly enlarged lateral fabella in a 6-year-old Border Collie. The changes are suspected to be secondary to previous trauma or fracture that has healed with prolific callus formation.

reported in Beagles, a Schipperke, a Fox Terrier and the Golden Retriever (Chaffee and Knecht, 1975; Walker, 1977; Reinke *et al.*, 1982; Muir and Dueland, 1994; Robinson, 1999; Ridge and Owen, 2005). Avulsion of the lateral head of the gastrocnemius has also been reported in cats (Bali, 2011; Pratesi, 2012). Historical signs may include an acute onset of lameness after vigorous exercise, or a more chronic insidious onset of lameness (Vaughan, 1985). Clinical signs include pain on focal palpation over the region of the fabella, reduction in stifle range of motion, and pain particularly on stifle extension. Radiographs usually show distal displacement of the fabella; if a fracture is present the smaller fragment or fragments are usually more proximal. In one case a radiograph taken with the hock and stifle flexed was necessary to demonstrate the displacement of the fabella, which was in a normal position when radiographed with the hock and stifle in a more neutral extended position. West Highland White Terriers and some other terriers appear predisposed to, and have a high prevalence of, an abnormal mediodistal location of the medial fabella. The authors of this study suggested this is an incidental finding and should not be confused with true pathological fabellar displacement (Störk *et al.*, 2009).

There is limited information on the optimal treatment for proximal gastrocnemius muscle avulsions. Reported treatment options include reattachment of the avulsed fabella or muscle fascia by direct wire reattachment, figure-of-eight wire or suture via bone tunnels, or spiked washer and screws. This was combined with fixation of the hock joint in extension to neutralize forces on the repaired gastrocnemius muscle (Figure 27.4). Vaughan (1985) always applied a tibiocalcaneal screw prior to repair of the gastrocnemius, which aided reduction of the avulsed muscle, and then the screw was maintained for 6 weeks during muscle healing. A transarticular external skeletal fixator across the tarsus can also be used to maintain the hock at a standing angle and prevent hock flexion during the healing phase (Ridge and Owen, 2005).

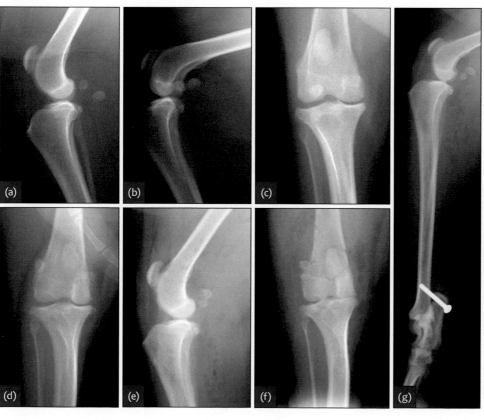

27.4 An overweight 7-year-old Shetland Sheepdog was presented with chronic right hindlimb lameness of 5 months' duration. The dog was mainly non-weight-bearing on the right hindlimb, but when it did bear weight, there was a plantigrade stance. On orthopaedic examination the right hock could be hyperflexed even with the stifle extended. Orthogonal mediolateral and craniocaudal radiographs of (a, c) the right and (b, d) the left stifle show that the right fabellae have displaced distally, suggesting a tear or rupture of the origin of the gastrocnemius muscle.
(e) Mediolateral and (f) craniocaudal postoperative radiographic views. Surgery was performed by placing sutures from the gastrocnemius muscle, anchored distal to the fabellae, to two bone tunnels in the areas of the gastrocnemius origin. At surgery there was an obvious tear in the lateral gastrocnemius belly, but the tear in the medial belly was less obvious. There was extensive fibrous tissue present, which was not unexpected given the duration of clinical signs. (g) A 2.7 mm calcaneotibial screw was placed, combined with external coaptation, to temporarily hold the hock in extension and therefore relieve tension across the gastrocnemius repair during the early phases of healing; the screw was removed after 6 weeks.

Conservative treatment has been used for partial proximal gastrocnemius muscle avulsions in dogs, with non-steroidal anti-inflammatory drugs, physical therapy and restriction of activity to a short leash or pulsed therapeutic ultrasonography (Muir and Dueland, 1994; Mueller *et al.*, 2009). The outcome is generally good for avulsion of the origin of the gastrocnemius muscle, although recovery can take several months.

The popliteal sesamoid

The popliteal sesamoid is found in the tendon of origin of the popliteal muscle. The popliteal tendon originates from a small depression on the lateral femoral condyle just medial and slightly cranial to the lateral collateral ligament, then courses in a caudomedial direction to the caudomedial border of the proximal tibia where the muscle belly inserts. The musculotendinous junction is located caudodistal to the tibial plateau. The popliteal sesamoid is found in the caudal portion of the long tendon of origin (Tanno *et al.*, 1996). The popliteal muscle functions to flex and internally rotate the stifle. On radiographs, the popliteal sesamoid is usually seen as a small, mineralized structure in the region of the caudolateral stifle. In a retrospective radiology study, the incidence of ossification of the popliteal sesamoid was 84% in dogs and 100% in cats (McCarthy and Wood, 1989). Distal displacement of the popliteal sesamoid is a useful parameter in the interpretation of tibial compression radiographs in cases of cranial cruciate ligament rupture in the dog. An accuracy of 99% and a specificity of 100% were achieved by assessing the localization of the sesamoid bone in the diagnosis of cruciate disease (Rooster and Bree, 1999).

Avulsion of the popliteal sesamoid is not a common injury in the dog. It usually affects young dogs around 4 months of age although it can be seen in older dogs. It has been reported in a Malinois, an Afghan Hound and a Labrador Retriever (Eaton-Wells and Plummer 1978; Tanno *et al.*, 1996). The lameness is usually marked and develops during a period of vigorous exercise. Avulsion of the popliteal tendon has also been reported in association with avulsion of the origin of the long digital extensor tendon and lateral patellar luxation (Bardet and Piermattei, 1983).

As contraction of the popliteal muscle causes internal rotation of the tibia and flexion of the stifle, Tanno *et al.* (1996) theorized that acute external rotation of the tibia relative to the femur whilst the stifle is positioned in partial flexion must occur in order for a dog to sustain an isolated rupture of the popliteus muscle. Radiographic changes include displacement of the popliteal sesamoid in a distal direction and an avulsion fracture from the tendon origin. Differential diagnoses include avulsion of the long digital extensor tendon, avulsion of the cruciate ligaments or stifle osteochondrosis; the diagnosis is made by careful consideration of the orthogonal radiographs and the precise location of the bone fragments. Other imaging modalities such as computed tomography or ultrasonography can be used to assist in making a diagnosis.

In most of the single case reports in the literature, surgery was performed to debride small avulsed bone fragments and reattach the larger fragments or tendon as near to the site of origin as feasible to allow a tension-free repair. In one case the tendon was reattached to the long digital extensor tendon (Eaton-Wells and Plummer, 1978). If the avulsion fracture fragment is large enough and displacement is minimal then the fragment can be reattached at its site of origin (Figure 27.5). The prognosis is generally good for a return to function.

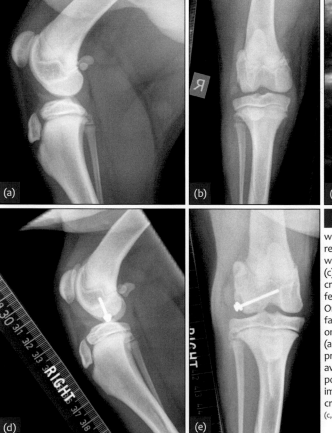

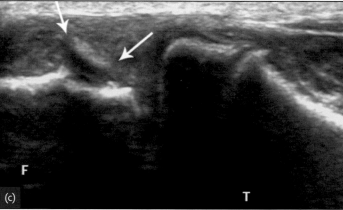

27.5 Popliteal avulsion in a 4-month-old Labrador Retriever puppy that was presented with sudden onset right hindlimb lameness after playing with another dog. Pain was localized to the right stifle joint. The cranial draw test revealed a normal degree of laxity in the cranial cruciate ligament compatible with the age of the dog. (a) Mediolateral and (b) craniocaudal radiographs and (c) an ultrasonogram of the lateral aspect of the stifle were performed. On the craniocaudal radiographic view there is a defect on the contour of the lateral femoral condyle, and lateral and adjacent to this defect is a mineralized opacity. On the mediolateral radiograph there is some decrease in size of the infrapatellar fat pad, compatible with a mild joint effusion. No bony abnormalities are present on the mediolateral radiograph. The ultrasonogram shows a bony opacity (arrowed) and an underlying concave defect on the femoral condyle just proximal to the tibial plateau. In this puppy it was possible to reattach the bony avulsion fragment with a 2 mm bone screw and washer. The 4-week postoperative (d) mediolateral and (e) craniocaudal radiographic views show the implants in position and evidence of bony callus around the screw head on the craniocaudal radiograph.
(c, Courtesy of N Rousset)

References and further reading

Alvarenga J (1973) Patellar fracture in the dog. *Modern Veterinary Practice* **54**, 43–44

Arnbjerg J and Heje NI (1993) Fabellae and popliteal sesamoid bones in cats. *Journal of Small Animal Practice* **34**, 95–98

Bali MS (2011) Avulsion of the lateral head of the gastrocnemius muscle in a cat. *Journal of Feline Medicine and Surgery* **13**, 784–786

Bardet JF and Piermattei DL (1983) Long digital extensor and popliteal tendon avulsion associated with lateral patella luxation in a dog. *Journal of the American Veterinary Medical Association* **183**, 465–466

Betts CW and Walker M (1975) Lag screw fixation of a patellar fracture. *Journal of Small Animal Practice* **16**, 21–25

Bleedorn JA, Towle HA, Breur GJ et al. (2006) What is your diagnosis? Avulsion of the popliteal tendon. *Journal of the American Veterinary Medical Association* **229**, 1885–1886

Bright SR and May C (2011) Arthroscopic partial patellectomy in a dog. *Journal of Small Animal Practice* **52**, 168–171

Chaffee VW and Knecht CD (1975) Avulsion of the medial head of the gastrocnemius in the dog. *Veterinary Medicine and Small Animal Clinician* **70**, 929–931

Eaton-Wells RD and Plummer GV (1978) Avulsion of the popliteal muscle in an Afghan Hound. *Journal of Small Animal Practice* **19**, 743–747

Harari JS, Person M and Berardi C (1990) Fractures of the patella in dogs and cats. *Compendium on Continuing Education for the Practicing Veterinarian* **12**, 1557–1562

Houlton JEF and Ness M (1993) Lateral fabellar fractures in the dog: a review of eight cases. *Journal of Small Animal Practice* **34**, 373–376

Langley-Hobbs SJ (2009) Stress fractures of the feline patella: 52 fractures in 34 cats. *Veterinary Record* **164**, 80–86

Langley-Hobbs SJ, Ball S and McKee WM (2009) Transverse stress fractures of the proximal tibia in 10 cats with non-union patellar fractures. *Veterinary Record* **164**, 425–430

Langley-Hobbs SJ, Brown G and Matis U (2008) Traumatic fracture of the patella in eleven cats. *Veterinary and Comparative Orthopaedics and Traumatology* **21**, 427–433

McCarthy PH and Wood AKW (1989) Anatomical and radiological observations of the sesamoid bone of the popliteus muscle in the adult dog and cat. *Anatomia, Histologia, Embryologia* **18**, 58–65

McCurnin DM and Slusher R (1975) Tension-band wiring of a fractured patella (a photographic essay). *Veterinary Medicine and Small Animal Clinician* **70**, 1321–1323

McKee WM and Cook JL (2006) The stifle. In: *BSAVA Manual of Canine and Feline Musculoskeletal Disorders*, ed. JEF Houlton, JL Cook, JF Innes and SJ Langley-Hobbs, pp. 350–395. BSAVA Publications, Gloucester

Meutstege FJ (1993) The classification of canine Achilles' tendon lesions. *Veterinary and Comparative Orthopaedics and Traumatology* **6**, 57–59

Mitchell M (1980) Spontaneous repair of a ruptured gastrocnemius muscle in a dog. *Journal of the American Animal Hospital Association* **16**, 513–516

Mueller MC, Gradner G, Hittmair KM et al. (2009) Conservative treatment of partial gastrocnemius muscle avulsions in dogs using therapeutic ultrasound – a force plate study. *Veterinary and Comparative Orthopaedics and Traumatology* **22**, 243–248

Muir P and Dueland T (1994) Avulsion of the origin of the medial head of the gastrocnemius muscle in a dog. *Veterinary Record* **135** , 359–360

Piermattei DL and Johnson KA (2004a) Approach to the lateral collateral ligament and caudolateral part of the stifle joint. In: *An Atlas of Surgical Approaches to the Bones and Joints of the Dog and Cat, 4th edn*, pp. 356–357. Elsevier, USA

Piermattei DL and Johnson KA (2004b) Approach to the medial collateral ligament and caudomedial part of the stifle joint. In: *An Atlas of Surgical Approaches to the Bones and Joints of the Dog and Cat, 4th edn*, pp. 360–363. Elsevier, USA

Pond MS and Losonsky JM (1976) Avulsion of the popliteus muscle in the dog: a case report. *Journal of the American Animal Hospital Association* **12**, 60–63

Pratesi A, Grierson J and Moores AP (2012) The use of a stifle flexion device to manage avulsion of the lateral head of the gastrocnemius muscle in a cat. *Veterinary and Comparative Orthopaedics and Traumatology* **25**, 246–249

Reinke JD, Kus SP and Owens JM (1982) Traumatic avulsion of the lateral head of the gastrocnemius and superficial digital flexor muscles in a dog. *Journal of the American Animal Hospital Association* **18**, 252–262

Reinke JD, Mughannam AJ and Owens JM (1993) Avulsion of the gastrocnemius tendon in 11 dogs. *Journal of the American Animal Hospital Association* **29**, 410–418

Ridge PA and Owen MR (2005) Unusual presentation of avulsion of the lateral head of the gastrocnemius muscle in a dog. *Journal of Small Animal Practice* **46**, 196–198

Robinson A (1999) A traumatic bilateral avulsion of the origins of the gastrocnemius muscle. *Journal of Small Animal Practice* **40**, 498–500

Robinson GW (1966) What is your diagnosis? *Journal of the American Veterinary Medicine Association* **148**, 1419–1420

Rooster HD and Bree HV (1999) Popliteal sesamoid displacement associated with cruciate rupture in the dog. *Journal of Small Animal Practice* **40**, 316–318

Rutherford S, Bell JC and Ness MG (2012) Fracture of the patella after TPLO in 6 dogs. *Veterinary Surgery* **41**, 316–318

Stahl C, Wacker C, Weber U et al. (2010) MRI features of gastrocnemius musculotendinopathy in herding dogs. *Veterinary Radiology and Ultrasound* **51**, 380–385

Störk CK, Petite AF, Norrie RA et al. (2009) Variation in position of the medial fabella in West Highland White Terriers and other dogs. *Journal of Small Animal Practice* **50**, 236–240

Tanno F, Weber U, Lang J et al. (1996) Avulsion of the popliteus muscle in a malinois dog. *Journal of Small Animal Practice* **37**, 448–451

Ting D, Petersen SW, Mazzaferro EM and Worth LT (2006) Avulsion of the origin of the gastrocnemius muscle. *Journal of the American Veterinary Medical Association* **228**, 1497–1498

Vaughan LC (1979) Muscle and tendon injuries in dogs. *Journal of Small Animal Practice* **20**, 711–736

Vaughan LC (1985) The management of tendon injuries in dogs. *Journal of Small Animal Practice* **26**, 133–142

Walker (1977) What is your diagnosis? *Journal of the American Veterinary Medical Association* **170**, 843–844

White RA (1977) Bilateral patellar fracture in a dog. *Journal of Small Animal Practice* **18**, 261–265

OPERATIVE TECHNIQUE 27.1

Fracture of the patella

POSITIONING

Dorsal recumbency.

ASSISTANT

Optimal to have an assistant.

EQUIPMENT EXTRAS

Jacobs chuck and K-wires; air or battery-powered drill; orthopaedic wire and wire twisters; pointed reduction forceps.

SURGICAL TECHNIQUES

Approach

An approach to the stifle is performed as described by Piermattei and Johnson (2004ab). A skin incision is made on the craniolateral or craniomedial aspect of the stifle extending from the distal femur to the proximal tibia. Subcutaneous tissues are dissected through and retracted. An incision in the fascia parallel to the patellar ligament can be used to assess reduction of the articular surface intraoperatively.

Reduction and fixation

A **traumatic** fracture of the patella in a dog (if the bone has fractured into two similarly sized fragments) can be managed with pin and tension-band wire fixation. A sharp (new) drill bit is required to drill through the dense bone of the patella; it may be helpful to 'map out' the patella using hypodermic needles as the regional soft tissues may obscure the bone. If the bone is of sufficient size then it is optimal to place two parallel pins. It is preferable to use fairly small K-wires rather than risk causing further fracturing of the sesamoid by placement of an oversized pin. Orthopaedic wire (0.8–1.25 mm) is then twisted around the K-wire(s) in the patella in a figure-of-eight pattern. Positioning the stifle in extension will facilitate reduction of the patella. Pre-drilling the hole for the K-wires with a sharp drill bit is advisable as the patellar bone is very hard (Figure 27.6).

If the fracture is suspected to be a **stress** fracture in a cat then it is not advisable to place K-wires but to use only a figure-of-eight tension-band wire or an encircling wire (Figure 27.7). The bone is very brittle and liable to fracture if holes or wires are drilled through it. Wire is placed either through the patellar tendon proximal and distal to the patella and tightened in a figure-of-eight configuration, or in a purse-string fashion and tightened as a loop. Use of a hypodermic needle pre-placed through the quadriceps tendon can facilitate placement of the wire (Figure 27.6c).

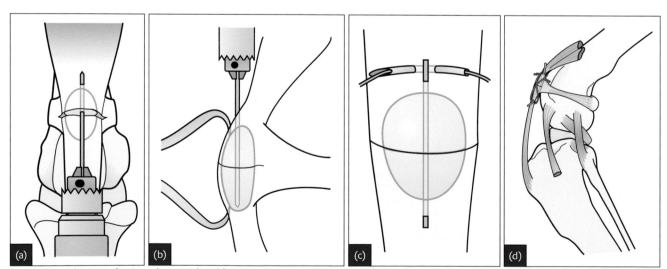

27.6 Application of a pin and tension-band for a transverse patellar fracture. (a) Retrograde placement of a pin in the proximal fragment. A pilot hole can be made first with a drill bit. (b) Fracture held in reduction using small pointed reduction forceps. The pin is advanced into the distal fragment. (c) A wire is passed through the patellar ligament and behind the K-wire at each pole through the lumen of a pre-placed suitably sized hypodermic needle. The needle can be bent slightly to facilitate placement. (d) The tension-band is tightened in a figure-of-eight or loop pattern.

→

→ **OPERATIVE TECHNIQUE 27.1 CONTINUED**

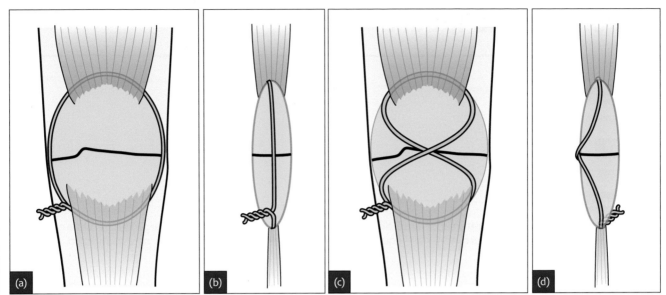

27.7 Wiring techniques for repair of transverse patellar fractures in the cat. (a) Cranial and (b) lateral views of circumferential wire. (c) Cranial and (d) lateral views of figure-of-eight wire. In both cases the orthopaedic wire is passed through the patellar ligament and distal quadriceps muscle. The wire can be placed in a similar fashion as shown in Figure 27.6c, facilitated by placing a hypodermic needle first.

Whether using orthopaedic wire in isolation or in combination with K-wires, it is important not to overtighten the orthopaedic wire as this will open up the fracture gap on the articular surface – this will result in micromotion at the fracture gap during weight-bearing and predispose to premature implant fatigue and breakage. Check the articular cartilage congruity prior to soft tissue closure.

If the fragments are small polar or apical pieces of bone and if the quadriceps mechanism is still functional then these fragments can be removed by sharp dissection.

If there is disruption of the quadriceps mechanism in association with small unreconstructable fracture fragments then this injury will need treating primarily as a tendon rupture (McKee and Cook, 2006). The tendon will need reattachment using tendon sutures such as a Bunnell suture or locking loop. The repair may need augmentation with autogenous tissue such as a fascia lata graft. The repair then needs protection using internal methods, such as a musculotendinous–tibial tuberosity wire (Figure 27.8) or suture, or external methods such as a transarticular external skeletal fixator. External coaptation can be attempted with the leg splinted in extension, but this may be inadequate.

After any patellar fracture repair, consideration should be given to whether the repair would benefit from internal or external protection as described in the paragraph above. The nature of the fracture and the patient, and the advantages and disadvantages of the additional fixation devices, should all be taken into consideration.

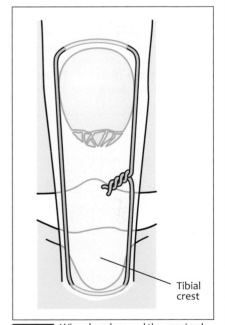

Tibial crest

27.8 Wire placed around the proximal patella and through the tibial tuberosity to protect a patellar fracture repair or patella tendon repair associated with an unreconstructable patellar fracture.

Wound closure

If there is disruption of the parapatellar fibrocartilages then these should be sutured with mattress sutures of non-absorbable or slowly absorbable suture material. The muscles and fascia are closed using polydioxanone, the subcutaneous tissue with rapidly absorbable suture material, such as poliglecaprone, and the skin by interrupted sutures of monofilament nylon.

POSTOPERATIVE MANAGEMENT

The repair should be protected by exercise restriction or internal or external coaption for 4 to 12 weeks. The prognosis for fracture healing is guarded, but a functional non-union may result. Radiographs should be taken at 4- to 6-weekly intervals. Healing, when it occurs, can take over 3 months, so further radiographic evaluation at a later date is recommended.

OPERATIVE TECHNIQUE 27.2

Avulsion of the fabella

POSITIONING

Sternal/lateral recumbency.

ASSISTANT

Optimal but not essential.

EQUIPMENT EXTRAS

Jacobs chuck and pins; air or battery-powered drill; orthopaedic wire and wire twisters; large gauge suture material (nylon leader line or braided suture material); equipment for placement of a calcaneotibial screw; pointed reduction forceps.

SURGICAL TECHNIQUES

Approach

Lateral fabella

An approach to the stifle is performed as described by Piermattei and Johnson (2004a). A skin incision is made on the craniolateral aspect of the stifle extending from the distal femur to the proximal tibia (Figure 27.9a). Subcutaneous tissues are dissected through and retracted. An incision is made in the aponeurosis of the biceps femoris muscle directly cranial to the muscle fibres (Figure 27.9b) and the muscle is retracted caudally. It is not necessary to enter the joint unless it is deemed necessary to inspect the cruciate ligaments for concurrent injury. The lateral fabella can be palpated in the lateral belly of the gastrocnemius muscle (Figure 27.9c).

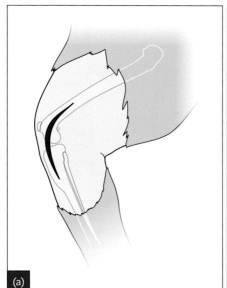 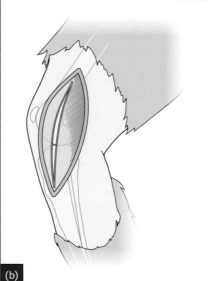 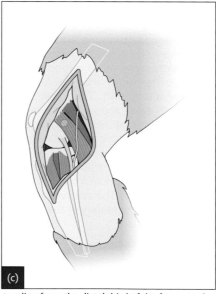

27.9 Surgical approach to the lateral fabella. (a) A skin incision is made over the lateral stifle extending from the distal third of the femur to the level of the tibial tuberosity. (b) An incision is made through the fascia along the cranial aspect of the biceps femoris muscle. (c) After retraction of the biceps femoris muscle the lateral fabella is palpable in the gastrocnemius muscle. The peroneal nerve may be encountered caudally.

Medial fabella

An approach to the stifle is performed as described by Piermattei and Johnson (2004b). A skin incision is made on the craniomedial aspect of the stifle extending from the distal femur to the proximal tibia (Figure 27.10a). Subcutaneous tissues are dissected through and retracted. An incision is made in the aponeurosis of the caudal sartorius muscle and the muscle is retracted caudally (Figure 27.10b). It is not necessary to enter the joint unless it is deemed necessary to inspect the cruciate ligaments for concurrent injury. The medial fabella can be palpated in the medial belly of the gastrocnemius muscle (Figure 27.10c). ➡️

→ **OPERATIVE TECHNIQUE 27.2 CONTINUED**

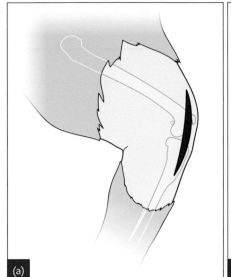 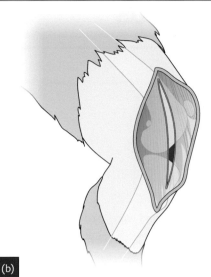 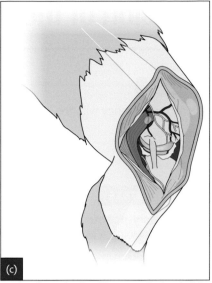

27.10 Surgical approach to the medial fabella. (a) A skin incision is made over the medial stifle extending from the distal femur to the level of the tibial tuberosity. (b) The dissection is continued by division between the cranial and caudal bellies of the sartorius muscles. (c) After retraction of the caudal sartorius muscle the medial fabella is palpable in the medial belly of the gastrocnemius muscle, below the branches of the saphenous nerve and femoral artery.

Reduction and fixation

Sutures are placed from the gastrocnemius muscle, anchored distal to the fabellae, to bone tunnels in the region of the supracondylar tuberosities at the gastrocnemius origins (Figure 27.11). Stainless steel wire, monofilament nylon leader line or braided suture material such as braided polyester or polyethylene can be used. Mattress sutures or other tendon repair sutures can be used to repair muscle tears.

To optimize the healing environment, tension should be removed from the repair by temporarily stabilizing the hock in extension. This can be achieved by use of a calcaneotibial screw (see Figure 27.4g) or transarticular ESF frame (see Chapter 25). A cast used alone is unlikely to provide sufficient immobilization and movement of the hock in the cast may lead to cast sores. To place a calcaneotibial screw, firstly a small incision is made over the caudal aspect of the calcaneus. The medial retinaculum securing the superficial digital flexor tendon to the calcaneus is cut and the tendon retracted medially. Then a large pair of pointed reduction forceps is placed across the calcaneus to the tibia, which holds the hock in extension and maintains the position between the calcaneus and tibia. This also makes it easier to find the holes in the two bones after drilling. A hole is drilled from the calcaneus into the tibia using an appropriately sized drill bit (the same size as the screw shaft). The depth of the hole is measured and a suitably sized tap is then used to pre-cut the thread for the screw, and the calcaneotibial screw is placed. A positional screw is usually used.

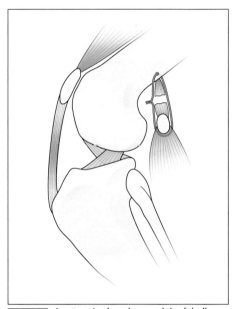

27.11 A suture is placed around the fabella distally and anchored to a bone tunnel in the region of the supracondylar tuberosities at the origin of the gastrocnemius muscle.

Alternative technique

Conservative treatment can also be considered (see text).

Wound closure

The muscles and fascia are closed using polydioxanone, the subcutaneous tissue with poliglecaprone and the skin by interrupted sutures of monofilament nylon.

POSTOPERATIVE MANAGEMENT

After placement of a calcaneotibial screw, a cast is placed from the toes to the level of the mid-tibia to maintain the hock in extension and protect the screw from breakage. The screw and cast are removed after 6 weeks and then the leg bandaged in extension for a further 2 weeks. If a transarticular ESF frame has been used then the frame should be removed after around 6 weeks.

OPERATIVE TECHNIQUE 27.3

Avulsion of the popliteus

Lateral recumbency with the affected leg uppermost.

ASSISTANT

Not essential.

EQUIPMENT EXTRAS

Air or battery-powered drill; orthopaedic wire and wire twisters; pointed reduction forceps; equipment for screw insertion if placing a lag screw and washer.

SURGICAL TECHNIQUES

Approach

An approach to the lateral collateral ligament and caudolateral part of the stifle is performed as described by Piermattei and Johnson (2004a), and described in Operative Technique 27.1 (see Figure 27.9ab). It is not necessary to enter the joint unless it is deemed necessary to inspect the cruciate ligaments for concurrent injury. The retraction of the biceps femoris muscle exposes the lateral collateral ligament and the tendon of the popliteus muscle (see Figure 27.9c), although the latter is still covered by fascia that needs to be dissected through (Figure 27.12).

Reduction and fixation

If the fragment is of a large enough size for reattachment then the corresponding defect on the femur is exposed and debrided of fibrous tissue. The fragment is carefully reduced using a pair of pointed reduction forceps and then secured in place with a small lag screw and washer (see Figure 27.5de). Care should be taken not to break the soft fragment with either overzealous tightening of the reduction forceps, too large a screw or excessive tightening of the screw. Additional sutures can be placed between the tendon and the periosteum and lateral collateral ligament.

Alternative techniques

The avulsed fracture fragment can be reattached to the femur in a more caudo-ventral location if it is not possible to reduce it accurately. If the avulsion fracture fragment is small it can be resected and the tendon reattached to the lateral collateral ligament or joint capsule using mattress sutures or locking loop sutures.

Wound closure

The muscles and fascia are closed using 2 or 3 metric polydioxanone and the skin by interrupted 3 metric multifilament nylon.

POSTOPERATIVE MANAGEMENT

Orthogonal radiographic views of the repair should be taken to ensure correct screw placement. Bandaging the limb in flexion for 10 days until suture removal has been recommended (Tanno et al., 1996); alternatively the dog can be discharged on cage rest with restricted lead-only walks for 3 to 4 weeks. Radiographs should be repeated after 3 to 4 weeks before gradually allowing a return to normal exercise.

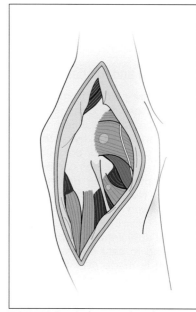

27.12 Surgical approach to the popliteus muscle. Following a lateral approach to the caudolateral aspect of the stifle (see Figure 27.9), the deep fascia is dissected to reveal the popliteus muscle immediately caudal to the lateral collateral ligament.

Chapter 28

Fracture disease

Carlos Macias

The term 'fracture disease' was first used by Müller (1963) to describe suboptimal limb function following fracture treatment. Fracture disease is commonly characterized by muscle atrophy and/or contracture, joint stiffness and osteoporosis. These changes persist well past documented bone healing times and, in some cases, are irreversible. Fracture disease is frequently associated with prolonged limb immobilization.

The Arbeitsgemeinschaft für Osteosynthesefragen (AO) group was founded in 1958 to study and develop surgical techniques and instrumentation that facilitated improvements in fracture reduction and stabilization (see Chapter 1). In turn, these techniques resulted in improved limb use during the early postoperative healing period, thus minimizing the risk of fracture disease. The AOVET group was founded in 1969 to apply similar concepts in the veterinary field. Since then, the benefits of internal or external surgical stabilization, avoiding limb immobilization and allowing early weight-bearing, have become well accepted in small animal orthopaedic medicine.

Despite significant advances, irreversible fracture disease still occasionally occurs in dogs and cats. This is most commonly a consequence of inappropriate decisions regarding initial fracture management or as a result of complications following surgical stabilization. Young animals are more susceptible to fracture disease than adults. Quadriceps contracture associated with femoral fracture is one of the most severe forms of fracture disease; another severe example is carpal contracture and concurrent reduction in the range of movement of the elbow, which is occasionally seen secondary to fractures involving the elbow joint. However, it should be borne in mind that the term fracture disease covers a spectrum of problems, which range from mild and temporary to severe and permanent, and thus any outcome which is less than ideal should be considered to be a manifestation of fracture disease.

Aetiology

Prolonged immobilization is known to cause muscle and tendon atrophy and osteoporosis in addition to joint stiffness. Temporary limb and joint immobilization in the absence of trauma leads to structural changes affecting tendons, muscles, bone and cartilage within as little as 3 weeks. This may be reversible if mobilization is restored (Shires *et al.*, 1982), but irreversible changes will occur if immobilization is maintained any longer.

Poor limb use and suboptimal joint and muscle function following fracture treatment may be the result of inadequate surgical stabilization of fractures (Figure 28.1), excessive postoperative pain, or the use of inadequate or prolonged external coaptation.

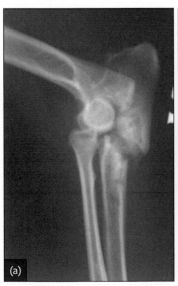
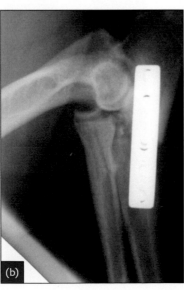
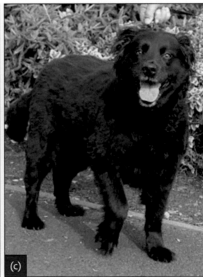

28.1 Fracture disease affecting the forelimb of a skeletally mature dog as a result of inadequate fracture management. (a) A proximal ulnar fracture with concomitant radial head luxation (Monteggia fracture). (b) The fracture was treated with a plate applied to the ulna, without appropriate reduction and stabilization of the radial head. (c) This led to the loss of elbow function with concurrent carpal flexor contracture.

Non-union, delayed union and osteomyelitis are not uncommon complications that can lead to fracture disease due to inadequate limb use. Poor reduction and inadequate stability of articular fractures predisposes to joint stiffness as the healing response triggers excessive development of fibrous tissue and adhesion formation. The effect of soft tissue and muscle trauma, either at the time of initial fracture or at surgery, on the development of fracture disease is unclear. However, excessive soft tissue trauma will undoubtedly increase the risk of development of delayed unions or surgical infections because of compromised vascularity; it will also increase postoperative pain, which will discourage early limb use.

If the limb is immobilized, severe joint stiffness is frequently observed affecting the stifle and elbow; this may be due to the greater number of muscles crossing over the joint compared to more distal joints.

Clinical signs of fracture disease

Severe or non-weight-bearing lameness following fracture stabilization should alert the clinician to the possibility of the animal developing fracture disease. Following appropriate surgical stabilization, animals will usually start weight-bearing within a few days of surgery and should not have significant pain on palpation or manipulation, especially if adequate analgesia has been provided. Once the postoperative inflammation has subsided, limb use should steadily improve and movement should gradually mimic that of a normal limb.

The severity of the changes observed in dogs and cats with fracture disease will depend on the duration of clinical signs. In addition to lameness, features such as marked muscle atrophy, loss of joint range of motion and pain on forced manipulation of joints are key aspects. Abnormal limb angulation, especially in dogs and cats with quadriceps contracture, can also be seen.

External coaptation is sometimes used to treat distal limb injuries and non-displaced fractures, but should only be considered if removal is expected in a relatively short period of time. Casts and bandages usually immobilize adjacent joints, and thus their use can lead to varying degrees of disuse muscle atrophy and temporary loss of joint range of motion in adult animals. Conversely, in growing animals excessive laxity of the carpal and tarsal joints can be seen following cast removal, although this resolves rapidly in most cases without any specific treatment. Loss of bone density can be observed on radiographs of bones immobilized with casts, even when fracture healing is uneventful, more so in the younger animal. This change, although undesirable, is considered normal following cast application and will usually be reversible without further attention. These temporary effects will be minimized if casts or dressings are applied in a manner which allows weight-bearing on the limb (see Chapter 16).

Pathophysiology

The effects of limb immobilization have been studied experimentally in dogs and cats, showing changes in bone, muscles, articular cartilage and ligaments (Shires *et al.*, 1982; Akeson *et al.*, 1987; Keller *et al.*, 1994).

Loss of healthy bone

Decreased bone mass leading to osteopenia occurs secondary to limb disuse, according to Wolff's law (see Chapter 3). Thinning of the cortices with increased medullary cavity diameter has been described. The distal bones appeared more susceptible to loss of bone mass, and younger animals are more likely to show early changes (Figure 28.2). Lack of muscle activity and increased blood supply are considered important initiating factors, combined with a lack of mechanical stimuli associated with not bearing weight on the limb (Leighton, 1981). Following remobilization, the production of new bone occurs at one-tenth the rate of bone removal and the loss of bone mass may not be fully reversible (Bardet and Hohn, 1983).

Muscle atrophy and contracture

A decrease in muscle size and strength occurs within 3 to 5 days of immobilization. Muscles with slow fibres (type I) atrophy to a greater extent than muscles with fast fibres (type II); postural (anti-gravity) muscles are more severely affected. Muscle atrophy without contracture is completely reversible, although recovery can take between two and four times the duration of immobilization.

In humans, an imbalance between agonist and antagonist muscles can occur due to neurological disorders and lifestyle or postural habits. A decrease in muscle tone leads to muscular atrophy. The constant contraction of the agonist muscle with minimal resistance can subsequently result in a contracture (Farmer and James, 2001). This mechanism may also occur in small animals.

Histologically, irreversibly contracted muscles show an increase in fibre size variability, prominence of subsarcolemmal nuclei, increased perimysial and endomysial

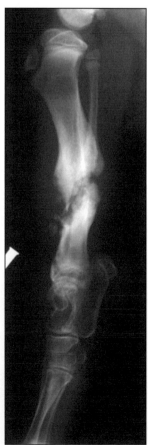

28.2 Mediolateral radiograph of the tibia in a 10-week-old Labrador Retriever 3 weeks after cast immobilization to treat a distal diaphyseal fracture. The poor contrast between the bone and soft tissues distally is suggestive of loss of bone density and cortical thinning, consistent with a diagnosis of disuse osteopenia.

connective tissue, focal fibre necrosis and fatty infiltration (Braund et al., 1980). The viscoelastic elements of muscle are replaced with fibrous tissue, resulting in a non-extensible, constricting, cord-like structure (Leighton, 1981).

Articular and peri-articular changes

Prolonged immobilization can lead to fibrous tissue proliferation, which can impinge on a joint. Fibrous adhesion formation and a loss of tissue extensibility can contribute to loss of joint range of motion (Farmer and James, 2001).

The effects of immobilization on joints have received more detailed attention than those on other structures. Lack of movement alters the morphological, biochemical and biomechanical characteristics of various components of synovial joints. Prominent among the changes that result are proliferation of fibrous connective tissue within the joint space, adhesions between synovial folds, adherence of fibrous connective tissue to cartilage surfaces, atrophy of cartilage, ulceration at points of cartilage–cartilage contact, disorganization of cellular and fibrillar ligament alignment, and weakening of ligament insertion sites owing to osteoclastic resorption of bone and Sharpey's fibers. Collagen mass in bone declines by about 10%. In the cartilage, collagen turnover increases with accelerated degradation and synthesis. Formation of reducible collagen crosslinks increases. Content of proteoglycan, notably hyaluronic acid, falls and water content is correspondingly reduced (Akeson et al., 1987).

These changes can be reversible if remobilization occurs within 4 to 6 weeks. However, some changes may be permanent despite progressive remobilization, and can lead to progressive osteoarthritis. The angle of joint fixation appears to have a significant effect on the development of degenerative changes (Ouzounian et al., 1986). If immobilization is performed in flexion the changes are less severe than if the joint is immobilized in extension.

Growth disturbances

Lack of mechanical stimulation decreases osteoblastic activity and reduces epiphyseal bone growth. Hip subluxation, increased femoral torsion and bone hypoplasia have been described after 8 weeks of cast immobilization of the pelvic limb with the stifle in extension, as well as medial patellar luxation and poor development of the femoral trochlear groove (Bardet, 1987).

Quadriceps contracture

Quadriceps contracture, seen in association with femoral fractures, is one of the most dramatic manifestations of fracture disease. This complication usually has severe and irreversible consequences and therefore all precautions should be taken to avoid its occurrence.

Fortunately, increased awareness and improved surgical techniques have reduced the incidence of quadriceps contracture. External splints with the limb held in extension were used extensively in the past to immobilize femoral fractures, frequently leading to this complication. It is now clear that use of Schroeder–Thomas devices to splint femoral fractures has no place in modern veterinary orthopaedic medicine.

Younger dogs with distal femoral fractures appear to have a greater risk of developing quadriceps contracture,

but the condition has also been described following mid-diaphyseal fractures in the cat as well as in the mature dog. Risk factors include severely comminuted fractures and persistent instability, especially when intramedullary (IM) pins alone are employed. Inappropriately applied cerclage wire contributes little to stability and can cause further soft tissue damage (Figure 28.3). Instability can lead to excessive callus formation, especially in younger animals; fibrous adhesions of the vastus muscle groups to the fracture callus are observed. Following adhesion formation, all heads of the quadriceps undergo further contraction and atrophy. If not resolved, myofibre necrosis will occur after as little as 3 weeks.

The majority of cases are associated with inadequate weight-bearing or implant-related complications (Fries et al., 1988; Wilkens et al., 1993; Liptak and Simpson, 2000; Moores and Sutton, 2009). Sciatic neuropraxia is common in the reported cases, often secondary to inappropriate use of IM pins; as in humans, it is has been suggested that loss of biceps femoris muscle activity (quadriceps antagonist) leads to a relative increase in quadriceps muscle tone resulting in stifle hyperextension and subsequent contracture. Hyperextension leads to stifle joint fibrosis and cartilage atrophy. In time, genu recurvatum, hip dislocation, tarsal hyperextension and flexion of the digits occur (Bardet, 1987; Moores and Sutton, 2009).

Clinical signs

The clinical appearance of dogs with quadriceps contracture is dramatic and pathognomonic (Figure 28.4). Severe, often non-weight-bearing, lameness is noted. Genu recurvatum and medial patellar luxation can be present. The stifle cannot be flexed, the tarsus is held in extension, and the digits are flexed. If the animal does attempt to bear weight, dorsal excoriation of the paw may be observed. Pain can be elicited if flexion of the stifle is attempted and may also be a feature on palpation of the

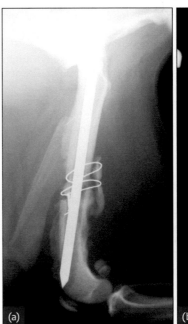
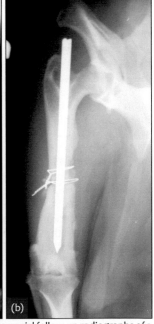

28.3 (a) Mediolateral and (b) caudocranial follow-up radiographs of a femoral fracture inappropriately stabilized with an IM pin and cerclage wires. The distal aspect of the pin has penetrated the craniodistal femoral cortex. An area of radiolucency surrounding the distal aspect of the pin indicates pin loosening. Inadequate fracture stability will increase the risk of quadriceps contracture.

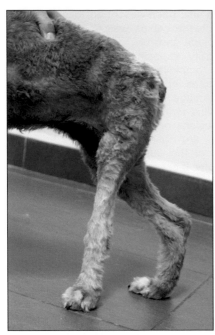

28.4 Quadriceps contracture following inappropriate femoral fracture treatment. Stifle and tarsal hyperextension and genu recurvatum are present.

allow some degree of active physiotherapy (Wilkens et al., 1993; Liptak and Simpson, 2000). Moores and Sutton (2009) described a simple static apparatus in a 4-month-old Golden Retriever. Two loops of monofilament nylon were anchored at the ischial tuberosity and at the calcaneus and were joined by inelastic bandage material, holding the stifle in flexion for 5 days. The stifle was released twice daily to allow physiotherapy sessions under sedation until stifle flexion and limb use were restored. Restoration of good limb function were reported.

The prognosis for dogs with established quadriceps contracture is very poor, with amputation being the only salvage option available. Arthrodesis of the stifle joint has been proposed but will often result in a poor functional outcome due to concurrent and continuing hip sublaxation and the hock hyperextension. A return to acceptable limb function is therefore unlikely.

femur at the level of the original fracture. Discomfort can also be present proximally, especially if sciatic nerve impingement is present.

Radiographically, generalized osteopenia, hip sublaxation, increased femoral torsion and medial patellar luxation can often be appreciated, especially in younger dogs.

Treatment and prognosis

Treatment of quadriceps contracture is generally unrewarding and poor functional results are common. In the cat, acceptable limb function can be observed despite quadriceps contracture in some cases. Therefore, if limb function is adequate, conservative treatment may be appropriate (Fries et al., 1988). Surgical treatment will not be successful if genu recurvatum, femoral torsion and hip joint subluxation have occurred, leaving amputation as the only viable option in many patients.

In less severely affected cases, several surgical techniques have been described (Leighton, 1981; Bardet, 1987). These techniques have included partial quadriceps myotomy, myoplasty, releasing adhesions and implantation of plastic sheeting to avoid reformation, sliding myoplasty and vastus excision. However, the prognosis is poor in most animals. Femoral head and neck excision does little to improve clinical function even if subluxation of the hip is noted, and is usually not recommended.

Successful treatment will only be achieved if surgery is performed early before significant bone, joint and muscle changes occur. Addressing femoral fracture instability in cases of non-union or implant failure and freeing adhesions between the quadriceps and the callus are mandatory. Removal of IM pins is advocated regardless of whether or not they are thought to be causing sciatic nerve impingement; rigid stabilization of the fracture using plates and screws is ususally performed. Flexion of the stifle should be achieved at least partially at the time of surgery, by gentle manipulation and by freeing fibrous adhesions. Aggressive analgesia and physiotherapy will be required in the postoperative period to avoid recurrence.

Successful surgical management has been described in dogs and cats using dynamic or static external skeletal fixators that allow the stifle joint the be held in flexion and

Avoiding fracture disease

The concept of 'prevention is better than cure' is especially applicable to fracture disease. Fracture disease can be avoided by strict adherence to the principles of fracture treatment. Careful surgical technique to avoid unnecessary muscle and joint trauma, provision of adequate fracture site stability, meticulous implant placement and rapid return to mobility are mandatory. In the immature animal, these principles are even more critical so the surgeon should ensure all necessary steps are followed. Dogs should be monitored carefully in the postoperative period and any complications addressed promptly and effectively.

On occasions fractures are encountered that require external coaptation, either as the sole method of stabilization or to protect internal fixation. When used, casts or splints should be maintained for the minimum required time to achieve bone healing, and the limb should be bandaged in flexion or in a physiological position to allow weight-bearing (see Chapter 16). The clinician should avoid splinting the limb in extension. Splints and casts should be re-examined and changed on a regular basis; whenever possible splint and cast changes should be done with the patient under sedation to avoid disrupting the healing fracture callus.

The importance of adequate stability at the fracture site cannot be overemphasized. Fracture stability is vital to allow early weight-bearing, and therefore stabilization techniques should address and neutralize all forces acting at the fracture site. Plating techniques will usually address these forces better than any other internal or external stabilization techniques, and are advocated for most diaphyseal femoral fractures whenever possible. Whilst possible, the use of external skeletal fixation for femoral fractures frequently causes higher morbidity due to the limited pin corridors available, especially in dogs. The use of IM pins to stabilize femoral fractures without supplementary fixation is rarely, if ever, indicated, as pins fail to resist fracture collapse and rotational instability. In addition, inappropriate use of IM pins can lead to sciatic neuropraxia. If an IM pin is used in combination with a plate, the surgeon should introduce the pin in a normograde fashion and ensure that the pin is appropriately positioned, well seated in the intertrochanteric fossa, to avoid sciatic impingement (see Chapter 23). If sciatic impingement is noted, the pin should be removed immediately. Any implants interfering with joint movement must be removed and replaced.

If transarticular fixation is required the use of an external skeletal fixator with dynamic hinged systems will facilitate intermittent range of movement or passive manipulations, which may help reduce joint stiffness (Figure 28.5).

The role of medical therapy to ameliorate the effects of joint immobilization has been studied experimentally (Keller *et al.*, 1994). The use of non-steroidal anti-inflammatory drugs does not have a direct effect on joint stiffness but helps to reduce post-traumatic swelling. Adequate analgesia following trauma is essential to ensure early weight bearing, and therefore adequate and prolonged analgesia should be provided in all trauma cases to reduce the detrimental effect of postoperative pain on limb function.

Following surgery, early mobilization and weight-bearing are key aspects in the prevention of fracture disease. Controlled activity should be encouraged as early as possible, progressing to more active exercise as bone healing and fracture stability allows. The role of physiotherapy to encourage limb use, reduce postoperative pain and increase joint mobility has received more attention in recent years, although its role in small animals is somewhat controversial. Swimming is an excellent form of exercise in the postoperative period, and can encourage early use of the limb. Goniometry can be used to measure the range of motion of joints and monitor progress (Millis, 2006).

The clinician should be aware of the increased risk of developing fracture disease when managing femoral fractures and periarticular elbow fractures, especially in the young patient. Close monitoring and follow-up should be performed and aggressive action should be taken if the onset of fracture disease is suspected.

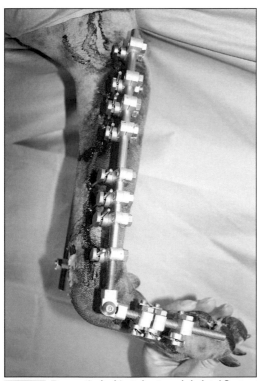

28.5 Transarticular hinged external skeletal fixator. Hinged fixators can be used to allow passive or active joint movement. In this case, the fixator was used to protect a collateral ligament repair allowing flexion and extension of the carpus whilst preventing medial, lateral or rotational displacement.

References and further reading

Akeson WH, Ameil D, Avel M, Garfin SR and Woo SL (1987) Effects of immobilization on joints. *Clinical Orthopaedics and Related Research* **219**, 28–37

Bardet JF (1987) Quadriceps contracture and fracture disease. *Veterinary Clinics of North America: Small Animal Practice* **17**, 957–973

Bardet JF and Hohn RB (1983) Quadriceps contracture in dogs. *Journal of the American Veterinary Medical Association* **183**, 680–685

Braund KG, Shires PK and Mikeal RL (1980) Type I fiber atrophy in the vastus lateralis muscle in dogs with femoral fractures treated by hyperextension. *Veterinary Pathology* **17**, 164–176

Farmer SE and James M (2001) Contracture in orthopaedic and neurological conditions: a review of causes and treatment. *Disability and Rehabilitation* **23**, 549–558

Fries LF, Binnington AG and Cockshutt JR (1988) Quadriceps contracture in four cats: a complication of internal fixation of femoral fractures. *Veterinary and Comparative Orthopaedics and Traumatology* **1**, 91–96

Keller WG, Aron DA, Rowland GN, Odend'hal S and Brown J (1994) The effect of trans-stifle external skeletal fixation and hyaluronic acid therapy on articular cartilage in the dog. *Veterinary Surgery* **23**, 119–128

Leighton RL (1981) Muscle contracture in the limbs of dogs and cats. *Veterinary Surgery* **10**, 132–135

Liptak JM and Simpson DJ (2000) Successful management of quadriceps contracture in a cat using a dynamic flexion apparatus. *Veterinary and Comparative Orthopaedics and Traumatology* **13**, 44–48

Millis DL (2006) Postoperative management and rehabilitation. In: *BSAVA Manual of Canine and Feline Musculoskeletal Disorders*, eds. JEF Houlton, JL Cook, JF Innes and SJ Langley-Hobbs, pp. 193–211. BSAVA Publications, Gloucester

Moores AP and Sutton A (2009) Management of quadriceps contracture in a dog using a static flexion apparatus and physiotherapy. *Journal of Small Animal Practice* **50**, 251–254

Müller ME (1963) Internal fixation for fresh fractures and for non-union. *Proceedings of the Royal Society of Medicine* **56**, 455–460

Ouzounian TJ, Kabo JM, Grogan TJ, Dorey F and Meals RA (1986) The effects of pressurization on fracture swelling and joint stiffness in the rabbit hind limb. *Clinical Orthopedics and Related Research* **210**, 252–256

Shires PK, Braund KG, Milton JL and Liu W (1982) Effect of localized trauma and temporary splinting on immature skeletal muscle and mobility of the femorotibial joint in the dog. *American Journal of Veterinary Research* **43**, 454–460

Wilkens BE, McDonald DE and Hulse DA (1993) Utilization of a dynamic stifle flexion apparatus in preventing recurrence of quadriceps contracture: a clinical report. *Veterinary and Comparative Orthopaedics and Traumatology* **6**, 219–223

Chapter 29

Implant failure

Gordon Brown

The aim of fracture stabilization is to restore a bone's structure and function temporarily whilst fracture healing restores it permanently. The implants used in fracture repair must initially bear all or part of the load usually carried by the bone. In optimal conditions, the relative load borne by the implants reduces whilst that taken by the bone increases over the healing period. If the bone fails to heal within a reasonable time then the implants undergo cyclic fatigue and may ultimately fail. It is essential that the orthopaedic surgeon takes account of all of the biological and mechanical factors (see Chapters 4 and 8) that can influence the rate of bone healing when selecting either individual or combinations of implants for fracture stabilization. It should be remembered that the major cause of implant failure in orthopaedic surgery is technical error as a result of improper selection or application of implants, rather than the implants' inherent material weakness.

Implant material failure

The majority of implants used in small animal fracture repair are manufactured from 316L stainless steel. The material structure and mechanical properties of 316L stainless steel are discussed in detail in Chapter 10 but in summary it is a non-toxic biocompatible material that provides a good balance between high strength and stiffness with good ductility and adequate fatigue and corrosion resistance. Titanium alloy implants are less stiff and more corrosion resistant, but significantly more expensive, than 316L stainless steel. This has largely precluded their use for the majority of veterinary osteosynthesis applications to date.

In the clinical situation it must be remembered, firstly, that orthopaedic implants are fixed to bone. They are part of a bone–metal composite, and from a mechanical viewpoint the size and distribution of stresses through the implant will be enormously influenced by their relationship with the bone. Secondly, implants function within an adverse bioenvironment continually bathed in extracellular fluid that is potentially corrosive.

Four mechanisms may cause the failure of a metallic implant in the clinical situation:

- Mechanical failure due to metallurgic imperfections or manufacturing faults
- Acute overload failure
- Fatigue failure
- Corrosive degradation.

These processes do not occur in isolation and it is not unusual for several processes to be acting concurrently and often synergistically. The situation can then be further exacerbated by technical errors, such as inadequate fracture reduction, inappropriate implant choice, errors in application and unsympathetic tissue handling leading to delay in fracture healing.

Mechanical failure due to metallurgic imperfections or manufacturing faults

Stainless steel (316L) is a relatively simple material to manufacture. The metal is extensively forged, worked and polished under strict quality control before being delivered as a high quality finished product. The potential for an implant made from an imperfect material getting as far as the surgeon is small, although this relies on the quality control procedures implemented by the manufacturer. Implant failure due to metallurgic imperfection is correspondingly rare.

Acute overload failure

Early acute material failure of a metal implant is analogous to the fracture of cortical bone as a result of acute overloading and is extremely uncommon. Such sudden and catastrophic failure of a metal implies the development and immediate propagation of a crack in the material in response to the rapid application of a load that exceeds the ultimate strength of the implant. When compared with fracturing bone, large forces and massive amounts of energy are required to propagate a crack in metal as strong as 316L stainless steel and consequently this type of failure is rarely seen in small animal orthopaedics. This is in contrast to the failures sometimes seen in equine long bone fracture repair, when plates can fracture as the patient attempts to rise following surgery. The considerable stresses generated in the plate by the uncoordinated efforts of the horse to stand are sufficient to initiate a crack in the implant.

An example of acute implant failure that may be encountered in small animal orthopaedics is that of a screw head shearing off as the screw is over-tightened (Figure 29.1). A screw is a simple machine that converts a small torque into a much larger axial force. During insertion, the screw head becomes restrained against the cortex or bone plate. Further torque merely increases tensile force in the shaft of the screw resulting in a stress

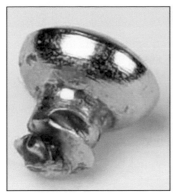

29.1 Fractured cancellous screw head from a clinical case. The surgeon had mistakenly used this screw in conjunction with a plate where a cortical screw would have been more appropriate. Note the plastic deformation in the thread prior to core failure. The radius (r) of the core is significantly smaller than in a cortical screw and core resistance to torque stress is proportional to r^4 (see Chapter 4). Relative over-tightening led to acute material failure.
(Courtesy of D Strong)

riser where the thread cuts into the screw shaft proximally. Over-tightening causes the screw head to snap off. This is an example of acute material failure as a result of technical error. However, in most cases it is not that the screw is too weak, but that the surgeon is too strong.

Fatigue failure

Fatigue failure is by far the most important mode of failure encountered in small animal orthopaedics.

Implant failure as a result of fatigue usually occurs some weeks after an apparently successful fracture repair. Typically, the patient will have shown an uneventful early return to function and will have appeared to be recovering well until the implant 'suddenly' fails. Fatigue failure occurs after an implant has been exposed to repetitive cyclic loads that in isolation would not result in material deformation (i.e. loads below the material's yield strength; see Chapter 4), but which can cause progressive, microscopic damage to the metal's material structure. Initially there is dislocation or slippage along planes within the crystalline microstructure of the metal, leading to micro-cracking, which is progressively advanced, perhaps by only a fraction of a micron, each time the stress is reapplied. The micro-cracks will continue to propagate in the face of continued repetitive loading until the crack reaches a length beyond which the remaining material cannot withstand applied stress. At this point the implant will fail by propagation of the crack through the cross-section of the implant.

The fatigue characteristics for a metal can be determined experimentally and described graphically (Figure 29.2). Under fatigue conditions the number of stress cycles that a metal implant can withstand is inversely proportional to the magnitude of the stress. If the magnitude of the stress is reduced the fatigue life of the implant will be extended. Conversely, if relatively high stresses are applied repetitively then the fatigue life will be shortened. If these stresses exceed the material's yield strength but are insufficient alone to cause acute overload failure then deformation of the relatively ductile implant material becomes plastic (permanent) and it will bend before ultimately failing.

In orthopaedic practice, repetitive cyclic stress is applied to a load-bearing (or sharing) metal implant during weight-bearing over the fracture healing period prior to full bony union being achieved. In response the surgeon may select stronger implants that will be less prone to fail before bony union is achieved, or consider restricting the patient's activity in an attempt to maximize implant longevity. In practice, however, the extent to which we can vary implant size or levels of patient activity in clinical cases is limited and as such may have only a relatively small effect

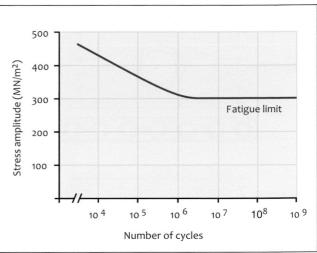

29.2 Curve for stress *versus* number of cycles, determined for 1045 carbon steel. The fatigue limit is a level of stress that will never cause material failure regardless of how often the stress is applied. The curve shows that even quite modest increases in stress amplitude can greatly reduce the number of cycles to failure: a 50% increase in stress might reduce the life of the material by a factor of 10 or more. Much larger stresses (higher than those recorded on this curve) will lead to plastic deformation or even acute fracture of the material.
(Redrawn from Radin et al., 1992)

on implant stress levels and longevity. Of greater significance in this respect is an understanding of the effect of stress concentration, which has the potential to increase local stresses by several orders of magnitude, significantly reducing the time (number of cycles) to failure. If a tensile force is applied to a metal bar, the stresses will be spread equally across the bar (Figure 29.3). If a hole or notch is cut into the bar, the same stresses will be distributed less evenly and areas of stress concentration will arise (Figure 29.4). Areas where stress concentration occurs are known as stress risers. Recently plate designers have adopted strategies to minimize stress concentration around and between screw holes whilst also making contouring easier (see Chapter 10).

The importance of stress concentration on implants should not be underestimated: sharp, deep defects in a metal plate can result in local stresses being increased 1000 times or more. Most plates and wires in small animal orthopaedics are placed on the tension aspect of long bones and are therefore subjected mainly to tensile stresses; stainless steel is relatively resistant to pure tensile forces. Repeated bending stresses, which are a frequent precursor to implant failure, can be considered as cyclic tensile stresses applied to the convex surface of the implant, with the largest tensile stresses being recorded at the abaxial surface of the implant. Applying this information to the example of a bone plate on the lateral (tension) surface of a dog's femur, we can appreciate that the tensile stresses on the outer aspect of the plate will be exaggerated (Figure 29.5), especially if

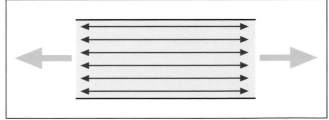

29.3 When a metal bar is placed under tension, the stress (shown here by lines of force) is spread evenly across the bar.

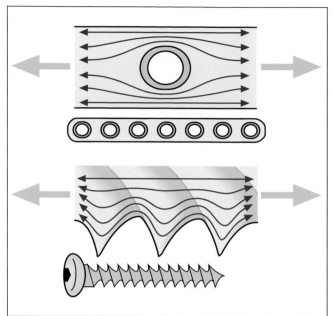

29.4 With the bar under tension, the number of lines of force at any cross-section must remain constant. Cutting a hole or notch into the bar will lead to stress concentration around the hole or at the extremity of the notch. The similarities between these hypothetical models and bone plates and screws are obvious.

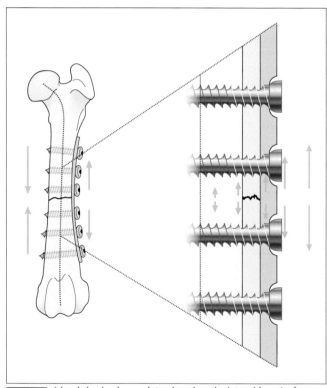

29.5 A load-sharing bone plate placed on the lateral (tension) surface of a dog's femur experiences cyclic tensile (bending) stresses of greater magnitude at the abaxial surface of the implant compared to those applied to the underside surface.

the bending forces are concentrated on a small portion of the plate at the fracture site. The screw holes will further enhance the stress concentration. Consequently, some of the metal making up the plate will be subjected to stresses many times greater than could be expected if only the patient's weight and the cross-sectional area of the plate were taken into consideration. The concept of stress concentration is essential to the understanding of why implants of seemingly reasonable size can fail.

Recommendations to use complex (rather than simple) unilateral single bar external skeletal fixator frames in inherently unstable fractures, or to use larger implants when applying a bridging plate, represent a recognition that in some circumstances there is an increased risk of implant fatigue failure. Intuitively, we know that a plate over a poorly reduced fracture will be exposed to greater stresses than a plate over an anatomically reconstructed bone, but the full consequence in terms of the amount of increased stress may not be immediately obvious. Area moment of inertia (AMI), discussed in Chapter 4 in relation to the biomechanics of fracture repair, is an expression of a structure's ability to resist bending. AMI depends on the distance of the material making up the construct from the neutral axis of the structure. The neutral axis is that part of a structure under bending (or eccentric axial loading) which is exposed to neither tensile nor compressive force. Figure 29.6a shows an anatomically reduced fracture fixed with a plate applied to the lateral (tension) aspect of the femur. The neutral axis is displaced laterally but remains within the bone. In Figure 29.6b the neutral axis lies within the plate itself; consequently, the AMI in this example is low, not only because the bone does not contribute, but also because the material of the plate is close to the neutral axis.

The low resistance to bending (low AMI) that accelerates fatigue failure (Figure 29.6b) will at the same time permit movement at the fracture. This may delay fracture healing and therefore further increase the risk of implant failure. The possibility of implant failure in this situation must be recognized by the orthopaedic surgeon who will avoid leaving a gap in the opposite cortex. When unavoidable, the use of cancellous bone autografts or osteoinductive bone graft substitutes will prompt new bone formation, thus restoring mechanical competence to the opposite cortex and easing the stress acting through the implant. In addition, supplementary implants can be placed which increase the AMI of the construct and protect the plate from bending forces.

An example of fatigue failure resulting from stress concentration in an implant caused by the lack of a mechanically competent opposite cortex is shown in Figure 29.7. The plate size appears appropriate and although a larger implant might have delayed failure, it probably would not have prevented it as the implant remains mechanically challenged. Had the lateral cortex been reducible and load bearing, the AMI would have been increased and the stress levels in the plate consequently decreased. As well as application of a bone graft to decrease anticipated healing time, one option for 'protecting' the medial plate in this example would have been the addition of an intramedullary pin (pin–plate fixation) to increase the AMI. In Figure 29.8 the surgeon has failed to account for the considerable stresses

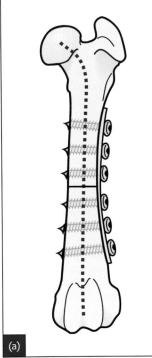
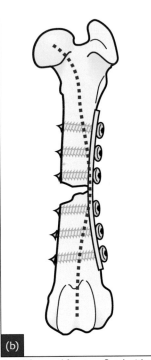

29.6 (a) An anatomically reduced mid-femoral fracture fixed with a plate and screws. The dashed line represents the estimated location of the neutral axis. This bone and plate composite is inherently stable and has a high AMI as a result of the location of the mass of material (bone plate laterally and cortex medially) at some distance from the neutral axis. (b) A mid-femoral fracture, without the benefit of a mechanically competent medial cortex. Here the neutral axis lies within the plate itself and as such the AMI of the bone and plate composite is very much lower. Load-bearing will cause cyclic stress to be concentrated in the small area of plate overlying the fracture, leading to fatigue failure.

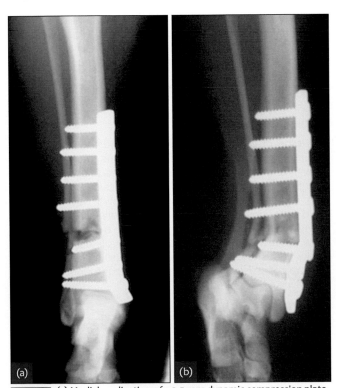

29.7 (a) Medial application of a 3.5 mm dynamic compression plate to manage this mildly comminuted, distal tibial fracture in an active Labrador Retriever. Here the surgeon has underestimated the effect of the gap in the opposite cortex, resulting in (b) fatigue failure of the implant and collapse of the lateral fracture gap 4 weeks postoperatively.

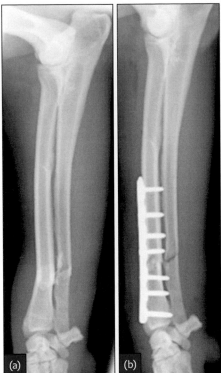
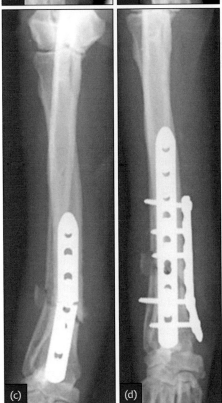

29.8 (a) This mildly comminuted fracture of the distal radius and ulna in a Golden Retriever (b) was managed initially using only a 3.5 mm locking compression plate and screws applied to the cranial aspect of the distal radius. (c) Fatigue failure occurred 3 weeks postoperatively. (d) The application of an orthogonal radial plate, as undertaken at the review, or separate fixation of the fractured ulna would almost certainly have prevented this complication.

applied to the cranially applied bone plate during early load bearing in the presence of a fractured ulna. The application of an orthogonal radial plate (as undertaken at the review; Figure 29.8d) or separate fixation of the fractured ulna would almost certainly have prevented this complication.

Corrosion degradation

All metallic implants have the potential to undergo a degree of chemical or electrochemical corrosion due in part to their natural reactivity and compounded by the complex and corrosive nature of their clinical bioenvironment. In addition to more complex compounds and proteins, extracellular fluid contains water, dissolved oxygen and large amounts of sodium (Na^+) and chloride (Cl^-) ions in a 0.9% solution together with electrolytes such as bicarbonate and small amounts of potassium, calcium, magnesium, phosphate and sulphate. Ionic compounds perform numerous functions that include the maintenance of the extracellular fluid pH and participation in electron transfer, reduction and oxidation (redox) reactions. At the time of implantation and for some time thereafter, the bioenvironment is disturbed, initially by the local trauma of the fracture process and subsequently by surgical intervention. The inflammatory process that results and continues into the healing period produces a wide range of potentially protective or destructive biochemical mediators that can locally alter the composition and reactivity of the bioenvironment.

Corrosion alone is unlikely to result in extensive damage to implants. The primary importance of the various localized forms of corrosion is their role in potentiating other forms of implant failure. Corrosion creates two problems: firstly, it results in damage to regions of the implant surface that weaken the structure and subsequently act as stress risers and, secondly, it releases corrosion products that can adversely affect biocompatibility causing pain, inflammation and focal bone necrosis.

PRACTICAL TIP

If plate contouring is required then this should be undertaken sympathetically avoiding sharp bends and twists that concentrate forces, and avoiding surface scratches and marks which might risk corrosive attack

---

Galvanic corrosion

Galvanic corrosion occurs as a result of the electrochemical potential created between two metals when immersed in a conductive medium. The key chemical reaction is that of a more active metal displacing a less active metal from solution. The net result of this chemistry is loss of substance, and therefore strength, from the implant. Implants of differing composition should never be mixed; however, as almost all small animal orthopaedic implants are made from 316L stainless steel, significant electrochemical corrosion is an uncommon occurrence. Whilst there may be differences in manufacturing and finishing methods when plates and screws are obtained from different implant manufacturers, the differences are unlikely to be sufficient to elicit a galvanic response provided the implants are made of medical grade (standard) implant material. Inadvertent use of titanium plates with 316L stainless steel screws (and *vice versa*) carries a theoretical risk of inducing galvanic corrosion, although the evidence for this occurring clinically is lacking. The use of non-standard implants or non-implant quality drill bits, which may snap and be left *in situ,* should be discouraged.

Intergranular corrosion is a form of galvanic corrosion within the substance of the implant due to impurities or inclusions within the metallic alloy. Production standards for medical grade metallic implants are very high and therefore intergranular corrosion is rare.

Pitting corrosion

The metallic surface of implants is self-protected by the spontaneous formation of a thin oxide film. Whilst it is only a few nanometers thick, it is a highly protective passive barrier between the metal surface and its aggressive bioenvironment. Its protectiveness against corrosion is dependent on its integrity, resistance to mechanical damage and to the rate and extent of repassivation following damage.

In 316L stainless steel it is primarily the formation of chromium oxide that imparts surface passivity. The nickel component of the alloy is credited with improved adhesion of the oxide layer. The spontaneous reaction of chromium with the oxygen in air to produce the oxide film can be summarized as:

$$4Cr + 3O_2 \rightarrow 2Cr_2O_3$$

Under certain conditions, localized breakdown of passivity leads to focal corrosion at sites of localized inhomogeneity of the material (such as scratches, defects or wear) or where there are local variations in, for example, oxygen tension, electrolyte concentrations or changes in pH that alter the reactivity potential of their environment. Metals in environments with differing oxidation–reduction (redox) potentials will display different levels of reactivity and consequently can become involved in electrochemical reactions.

The redox reaction can be summarized (M = metal) as:

$$M - e^- \rightarrow M^+$$

and:

$$O_2 + 2H_2O + 4e^- \rightarrow 4OH^-$$

The key chemical reaction is:

$$2Fe + 2H_2O + O_2 \rightleftharpoons 2Fe(OH)_2$$

The reaction is driven by the higher oxidation potential on the left side of the equation. The net result is loss of elemental iron (metal) into solution under conditions of low oxygen tension, with the formation of hydrated metal oxides and hydroxides. This is manifested as corrosion of the metallic implant.

Pitting corrosion is a localized form of open surface corrosion caused by focal loss of the passive film as a result of minor scratches and abrasions, areas of reduced polish or surface impurities. It results in the formation of focal cavities surrounded by an intact passive film.

Crevice corrosion

This type of corrosion is closely related to pitting corrosion, but occurs preferentially in regions where the local bioenvironment is more adverse as a result of interference with the 'free flow' of tissue fluids. Reduced oxygen tension, lower pH and increased electrolyte levels lead to rapid activation of the metal surface following dissolution of the passive layer. Crevice corrosion occurs in shielded sites such as the underside of bone plates or between screw heads and plates (Figure 29.9) or in crevices within the implant created by unsympathetic contouring.

Fretting corrosion

This occurs at contact sites between implant materials where there is relative micromotion under loading, resulting in mechanical wear damage. Fretting results in focal dissolution of the passive layer and prevention of its reformation, exposing the fretted surface to electrochemical corrosion. In fracture repair, fretting most commonly occurs at the screw head/plate interface. It is the form of localized corrosion that is most likely to be associated with the production of wear debris. This debris results in a host inflammatory and immune response that may further

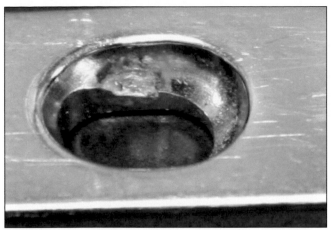

29.9 Crevice corrosion occurring at a typical location within the screw hole of a 316L stainless steel bone plate. Note the resulting focal, irregular loss of material substance and the production of superficial orange–brown deposits of hydrated metal oxides and hydroxides.

adversely alter the local bioenvironment. Debris that cannot be degraded and excreted will be encased in a cellular fibrous lining with the potential for a reduction in the security of the bond between the bone and the implant.

Corrosion fatigue

Corrosion fatigue is an accelerated form of fatigue failure that occurs because of the combined interaction of electrochemical reactions and cyclic loading. This can result from exposure of unprotected slippage planes by corrosion, resulting in stress risers that are mechanically disadvantageous. Conversely, cyclic mechanical damage can result in surface damage that is then a focus for corrosion. The combination of corrosive damage and subsequent formation of stress risers within the implant compounds the effect of cyclic mechanical fatigue, resulting in a marked reduction in the number of cycles to failure. As a result the implant may fail far earlier than could be predicted from simple *in vitro* mechanical testing.

Bearing in mind that fatigue failure as a result of incorrect choice or application is by far the most common cause of implant failure; it is clear that most implant failures can be avoided by appropriate decision making. An awareness of the mechanisms of material failure and synergistic electrochemical corrosion, together with a sound knowledge of fracture repair techniques and fracture healing, will help the aspiring fracture surgeon to avoid the technical errors that culminate in implant failure.

References and further reading

Einhorn TA, O'Keefe RJ and Buckwalter JA (2007) *Orthopaedic Basic Science, 3rd edn.* American Academy of Orthopaedic Surgeons, Rosemont

Jacobs J, Gilbert JL and Urban RM (1998) Current concepts review – Corrosion of metal orthopaedic implants. *Journal of Bone and Joint Surgery (American Volume)* **80**, 268–282

Nordin M and Frankel VH (1989) *Basic Biomechanics of the Musculoskeletal System, 2nd edn.* Lea and Febiger, Philadelphia

Perren SM and Rahn BA (1978) Biomechanics of fracture healing. *Orthopaedic Survey* **2**, 108–143

Radin EL, Rose RM, Blaha JD and Litsky AS (1992) *Practical Biomechanics for the Orthopaedic Surgeon, 2nd edn.* Churchill Livingstone, New York

Sumner-Smith G (1982) *Bone in Clinical Orthopaedics.* WB Saunders, Philadelphia

Virtanen S, Milosev I, Gomez-Barrena E *et al.* (2008) Special modes of corrosion under physiological and simulated physiological conditions. *Acta Biomater* **4**, 468–476

Chapter 30

Osteomyelitis

Angus Anderson

Osteomyelitis is defined as inflammation of the bone cortex and marrow. Osteitis, myelitis and periostitis refer to inflammation involving the bone cortex, marrow and periosteum, respectively. Although most commonly caused by bacteria, fungi may also cause the disease and corrosion of metallic implants may initiate inflammatory responses in bone.

Osteomyelitis is often classified as being haematogenous or post-traumatic in origin. Post-traumatic osteomyelitis develops following the direct inoculation of bacteria into a fracture site. This may occur in the following ways:

- Iatrogenic (surgery)
- Trauma (typically road traffic accidents and less commonly falls, bites, gunshot injuries)
- Extension of infection from adjacent soft tissues (bite wounds, migrating foreign bodies).

Post-traumatic osteomyelitis is usually focal and monostotic (confined to a single bone). Unfortunately, the most common reason for the development of osteomyelitis in small animals is the open reduction of fractures. Haematogenous osteomyelitis is an uncommon disease that results from blood-borne bacteria localizing to bones, but the source of these bacteria is frequently unknown. The disease may be monostotic or polyostotic (affecting multiple bones).

Although there is no satisfactory definition that distinguishes acute from chronic forms of the disease, acute osteomyelitis usually develops within 2 to 3 weeks of the trauma or surgery and is characterized by the classical signs of inflammation (namely heat, pain and swelling, leading to disuse) and sometimes systemic illness. Chronic osteomyelitis usually develops within several months of trauma or surgery. The classical signs of inflammation are less apparent and systemic signs of illness are unusual. Chronic osteomyelitis is usually characterized by the presence of avascular cortical bone and requires surgical intervention for the disease to resolve. Some bacteria (e.g. *Mycobacterium* spp.) and some fungi give rise to a disease that is chronic in nature.

Pathogenesis of post-traumatic osteomyelitis

Osteomyelitis caused by introduction of bacteria during orthopaedic surgery is the commonest form of the disease. In order to understand how the disease should be treated, the clinician must have a thorough understanding of its pathophysiology and the factors that may contribute to its development. Normal bone is relatively resistant to infection and studies of animal models of osteomyelitis have shown that chronic disease can only be generated if a number of factors are present. These include:

- Sufficient numbers of pathogenic bacteria (this will vary depending on the local environment and the ability of the host to resist colonization)
- Avascular cortical bone
- A favourable environment for bacterial colonization and multiplication (e.g. metallic implants, haematomas, necrotic soft tissue).

Chronic osteomyelitis is unlikely to develop if these three factors are not present (Braden *et al.*, 1987).

During surgery, bacteria from the animal's skin, the atmosphere or the surgeon frequently contaminate the exposed tissues and the surface of metallic implants (Smith *et al.*, 1989). From the time of implant placement there is a 'race for the surface', with bacteria competing with integrating host tissue for dominance of this surface environment. Bacteria have been found to grow predominantly in biofilms and their formation is a crucial step in the pathogenesis of many subacute and chronic infections (Zoubos *et al.*, 2012). A biofilm can be defined as a microbially derived sessile environment where bacteria are embedded in a matrix, attached to each other or a substrate and have an altered phenotype (gene expression, growth, protein production) (Budsberg, 2012). The first stage in the development of biofilm is adsorption of host-derived macromolecules to the implant (conditioning film). These proteins may also be present as residues on an implant surface following its production. Some bacteria (e.g. staphylococci) express surface adhesion molecules that promote attachment to host extracellular matrix proteins such as fibronectin and laminin that are present in the conditioning film on the implant (Vercelotti *et al.*, 1985). Initially, binding is reversible, but rapidly becomes irreversible and bacteria then multiply and produce exopolysaccharides (glycocalyx) (Gristina *et al.*, 1985) that trap nutrients and planktonic (free-living) bacteria. This glycocalyx may impede the diffusion of antibiotics to their target and prevent entry of components of the host immune response such as antibodies and complement. The physical environment (pH, altered partial pressures of CO_2 and O_2) created within the biofilm may also render antibiotics less effective.

Neutrophils can penetrate some biofilms, but are usually unable to clear the bacteria and the release of cytotoxic and proteolytic substances contribute to tissue injury and periprosthetic osteolysis. Over time, the biofilm matures; there is a depletion of nutrients and accumulation of waste products and bacteria enter a slow-growing or stationary state, rendering them up to 1000 times more resistant to antibiotics compared to their planktonic counterparts. Bacteria in this state may differentiate into phenotypically resistant forms, but some may revert to planktonic forms and leave the biofilm (Figure 30.1). Some *Staphylococcus* species may become intracellular within host cells, rendering them less susceptible to antibiotics. Another strategy to evade eradication that is common amongst some species (e.g. *Escherichia coli* and *Pseudomonas aeruginosa)* is plasmid-mediated transmission of multidrug-resistant traits.

In the acute inflammatory phase of infection, exudate may be forced along the Haversian and Volkmann canals of the cortex, under the periosteum (particularly in young animals where the periosteum is more loosely attached to underlying cortical bone) and into the medullary canal (Figure 30.1). Obliteration of the blood supply results in ischaemia and bone necrosis. Fragments of cortical bone that have lost their blood supply (sequestra) may become surrounded by exudate and act as persistent foci of infection. The periosteum and endosteum of cortical bone adjacent to a sequestrum may attempt to wall off this infected material by depositing new bone (involucrum)

around it. Infected areas of bone that are devoid of a blood supply become refractory to treatment because they are isolated from the host immune responses and the effects of antibiotics.

Despite the high incidence of contamination during surgery, osteomyelitis only develops in a small proportion of cases (Smith *et al.*, 1989). Factors that increase the likelihood of the development of infection include:

- Excessive trauma to soft tissues
- Periosteal stripping resulting in devascularization of cortical bone
- Fracture instability
- The presence of individual host factors that may alter local defences (e.g. malignancy, diabetes mellitus).

Fracture instability is an important mechanism potentiating infection. Lysis of cortical bone adjacent to implants, as a result of the infection, may lead to implant loosening and increased interfragmentary movement. This effect may be compounded by excessive movement at the fracture site caused by inadequate fracture fixation or technical errors in implant application. Motion at the fracture site impedes neovascularization. The resulting triad of infection, cortical bone resorption and fracture instability usually leads to delayed fracture healing or non-union (Johnson, 1994).

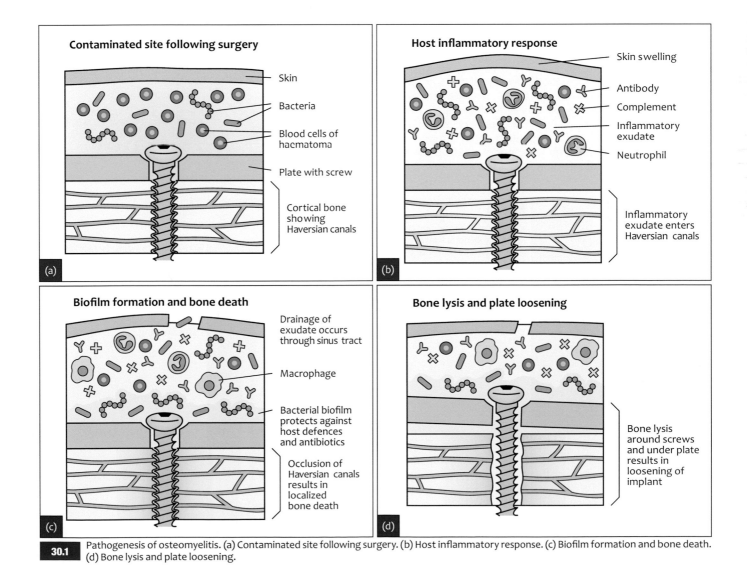

30.1 Pathogenesis of osteomyelitis. (a) Contaminated site following surgery. (b) Host inflammatory response. (c) Biofilm formation and bone death. (d) Bone lysis and plate loosening.

Diagnosis

A diagnosis of osteomyelitis is suggested from the history, clinical signs and radiographic findings. Confirmation requires bacteriological culture of the causative organism(s).

History

As the majority of cases of osteomyelitis develop as a result of open reduction of fractures, there is usually a history of fracture surgery. Where osteomyelitis develops as a result of extension of infection from an adjacent site, the most common sources of infection include bite wounds, teeth, nail beds and the middle ear (Caywood *et al.*, 1978; Muir and Johnson, 1992). Spinal osteomyelitis has also been associated with migrating foreign bodies (Pratt *et al.*, 1999; Sutton *et al.*, 2010). In haematogenous osteomyelitis, clinical evidence of a septic focus elsewhere in the body may be present (e.g. prostate, uterus, lungs), although frequently the source of the infection remains unknown.

Clinical and laboratory findings

Clinical signs depend on the stage of the disease process and the bone(s) affected. During the acute stage of the disease the affected animal may show:

- Pain on palpation of the bone and associated soft tissues
- Swollen, inflamed soft tissues (Figure 30.2)
- Pyrexia, anorexia, lethargy
- Discharge from sinus tracts.

Haematological examination may reveal a neutrophilia with a left shift. Differentiating acute osteomyelitis from deep wound infection may be very difficult because radiographic changes in bone will not appear immediately following infection. Needle aspiration from around the fracture site may reveal large numbers of neutrophils with bacteria, suggestive of infection involving the bone.

During the more chronic stages of the disease process, systemic signs are usually absent and haematology is usually normal. The main clinical findings are:

- Lameness
- Discharging sinus tracts
- Pain on palpation of the bone
- Disuse muscle atrophy
- Instability at the fracture site
- Intermittent soft tissue swelling.

Radiography and other imaging modalities

The radiographic appearance of osteomyelitis is variable and depends on the stage of the disease process. During the acute stages, the only visible changes may be soft tissue swelling. More rarely, gas shadows may be present if the causative organism is a gas-producer (e.g. some *Clostridium* spp.) (Figure 30.3). It may take up to 2 weeks for radiographic changes to appear in the bone. As the disease becomes more chronic additional features may be evident (Figures 30.4, 30.5 and 30.6).

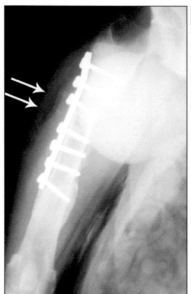

30.3 Craniocaudal radiograph of a femur showing gas in the soft tissues (arrowed) overlying a fracture stabilized with a bone plate. Gas production was due to infection with *Clostridium novyi*.
(Courtesy of AC Stead)

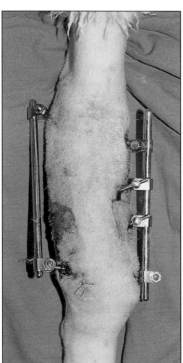

30.2 Acute osteomyelitis following application of a modified type 2 external skeletal fixator to stabilize an osteotomy of the distal radius and ulna. The limb is swollen and purulent material is discharging through the skin incision on the lateral aspect of the limb.

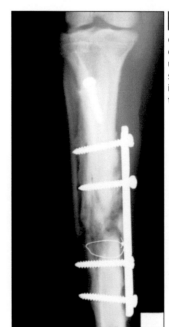

30.4 Craniocaudal radiograph of a tibia showing chronic osteomyelitis following application of a bone plate. There is lysis of bone under the plate and around the screws, fracture non-union, an irregular periosteal reaction and soft tissue swelling.

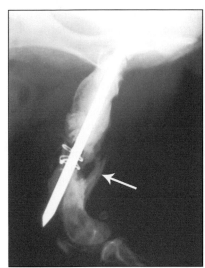

30.5 Mediolateral radiograph of a femur showing chronic osteomyelitis following fracture fixation with an intramedullary pin. There is extensive periosteal new bone on the proximal fragment, fracture non-union and large periosteal spurs on the distal fragment (arrowed).

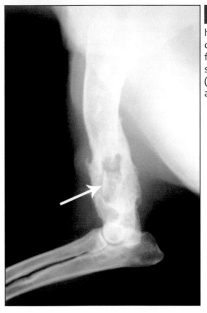

30.6 Mediolateral radiograph of a humerus showing chronic osteomyelitis. Although the fracture has healed, a large sequestrum is present (arrowed) surrounded by an involucrum.

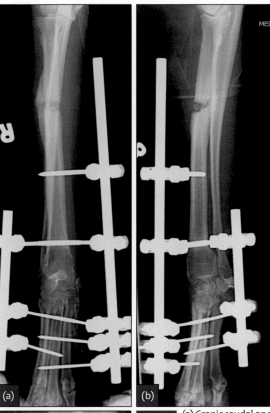

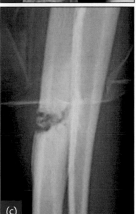

30.7 (a) Craniocaudal and (b) mediolateral radiographs of a ring sequestrum at the site of an external skeletal fixator transfixation pin placement. (c) The circular necrotic bone sequestrum can be identified on closer inspection.
(Courtesy of T Gemmill)

These additional features may include:

- Bone lysis (usually focal or adjacent to metallic implants)
- Periosteal new bone (smooth or irregular)
- Sclerosis
- Cortical thinning
- Involucrum (identified as an area of sclerotic bone surrounding a sequestrum)
- Delayed fracture healing or non-union
- Sequestrum (identified as a radiodense fragment of cortical bone surrounded by a zone of radiolucency).

Sequestra are sometimes difficult to visualize and repeated radiographic examination may be necessary for their identification, together with oblique views in addition to the standard views in two planes. They may vary in size from very small fragments to large segments of the diaphyseal cortex. Sequestra adjacent to external skeletal fixator pin tracts have been referred to as ring sequestra because of their characteristic radiographic appearance (Kantrowitz *et al.*, 1988). They may be caused by excessive thermal necrosis at the time of pin insertion, movement of the pin and localized infection (Figure 30.7).

Injection of water-soluble contrast media into discharging sinus tracts (sinography) may help to confirm the location of foreign bodies (e.g. surgical swabs), if these are the cause of the disease (Caywood, 1983), or to delineate sequestra.

Where osteomyelitis has developed as a result of infection spreading from adjacent tissues, the initial radiological manifestation is usually a periosteal reaction (Figure 30.8). It must be emphasized that the radiographic features of osteomyelitis are not peculiar to this disease, and have to be differentiated from normal bone healing and disease processes such as neoplasia, vascular infarction and trauma.

Radionuclide scintigraphy using technetium 99m-methylene diphosphonate (^{99m}Tc-MDP) may facilitate the early diagnosis of osteomyelitis (Aliabadi and Nikpoor, 1994) and reveal foci of active inflammation in chronic disease (Lamb, 1987). Use of this technique may reveal areas of increased activity in affected bones within 3 days of infection, considerably in advance of radiographic changes. Although the sensitivity of ^{99m}Tc-MDP bone scanning is high (90%), its specificity is relatively low (60–70%). This specificity can be increased by using gallium 67 or white blood cells labelled *in vitro* with indium (III) oxide. However, because of

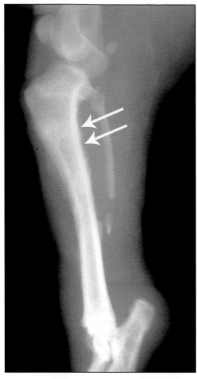

30.8 Mediolateral radiograph of a tibia showing chronic osteomyelitis following extensive soft tissue trauma to the limb. Arrows show an irregular periosteal response.

a widespread lack of availability, these tests are rarely performed in veterinary practice. Computed tomography (CT) and magnetic resonance imaging (MRI) have been found to be of value in the diagnosis and early detection of osteomyelitis and in the detection and localization of sequestra (Aliabadi and Nikpoor, 1994) and may be of value where the presence of foreign bodies is suspected. The use of CT and MRI can be confounded by the presence of stainless steel implants.

Bacteriology

Bacterial infections of bone may be mono- or polymicrobial. The majority of infections are reported to be mono-microbial (Caywood et al., 1978; Hirsh and Smith, 1978) and the most commonly isolated organisms are shown in Figure 30.9, the majority of which are beta-lactamase producers. The most common organism to be isolated is Staphylococcus pseudintermedius (originally classified, and in many earlier reports referred to, as S. intermedius (Bond and Loeffler, 2012)). Polymicrobial infections may involve Gram-negative and Gram-positive organisms, aerobes and anaerobes. Occasionally infections are caused by multidrug-resistant bacteria such as Pseudomonas aeruginosa, Escherichia coli, Proteus and methicillin-resistant Staphylococcus pseudintermedius (MRSP).

Tissue samples for culture should ideally be obtained from the affected bone, adjacent soft tissues or implants

Aerobes	Anaerobes
• Staphylococcus spp.	• Bacteroides spp.
• Streptococcus spp.	• Fusobacterium spp.
• Escherichia coli	• Actinomyces spp.
• Pseudomonas aeruginosa	• Clostridium spp.
• Proteus spp.	• Peptostreptococcus spp.
• Klebsiella spp.	
• Pasteurella spp.	
• Nocardia spp.	

30.9 Bacteria isolated from dogs with osteomyelitis.
(Hirsh and Smith, 1978; Muir and Johnson, 1992; Stead, 1984)

that are removed during debridement. In situations where debridement is not performed, a sample of bone may be obtained by a closed needle biopsy technique using a Jamshidi or similar bone marrow biopsy needle. However, studies in humans have shown that this is a less reliable method of obtaining the causative organism(s) than culture of tissues removed at open debridement (Perry et al., 1991). Similarly, swabs taken from discharging sinuses may not isolate the causative organism(s), particularly where an infection is polymicrobial or where anaerobes are present (Perry et al., 1991). Gram staining of smears made from swabs taken from the bone or discharging sinuses may give some indication of the causative bacteria, prior to obtaining the results of culture.

Anaerobic bacteria may be present alone or in combination with aerobic bacteria. The most common sites of isolation have been reported to be the radius/ulna, mandible and tympanic bulla (Muir and Johnson, 1992). The presence of anaerobes may be suggested by the presence of fight wounds, malodorous discharge, gas shadows on the radiographs (indicating the presence of gas-forming organisms such as Clostridium spp.) and the failure to isolate bacteria by aerobic culture when they have been identified on Gram-stained smears. Tissue samples for anaerobic culture should be exposed to an anaerobic environment promptly because failure to do so will reduce the rate at which these organisms are isolated. Advice on the appropriate media should be sought from the laboratory where the sample is to be sent. Fungal culture should be considered where there is evidence of polyostotic disease, particularly in breeds known to be predisposed to these infections (e.g. German Shepherd Dogs) and if there is a history of importation from countries where these diseases have been reported (e.g. USA and Australia).

Histopathology

Histopathological examination of affected bone is rarely necessary to obtain a diagnosis of osteomyelitis following trauma. Where there is no history of trauma it is sometimes performed to help differentiate infection from other disease processes such as neoplasia and metaphyseal osteopathy. The morphological identification of bacteria or neutrophils with engulfed bacteria is considered diagnostic (Braden et al., 1989). Fungal hyphae may be identified if these agents are the cause of the disease.

Treatment of post-traumatic osteomyelitis

Successful management of post-traumatic osteomyelitis usually requires a combination of surgery and a prolonged course of antibiotics. There are several basic principles that apply to the treatment of the disease:

• Surgical debridement to remove all dead and necrotic soft tissue and bone
• Allow drainage and obliterate dead space
• Provide absolute stability at the fracture site if necessary
• Prolonged course of antibiotics based on the results of culture and sensitivity.

These basic guidelines should be tailored to each individual case. Essentially, the same principles are applied to the management of acute and chronic osteomyelitis. However, chronic osteomyelitis is often characterized by the presence of avascular cortical bone that requires removal for resolution of the infection, and is usually associated with fracture site instability, delayed fracture healing or non-union.

Surgical debridement and drainage

Acute infections will normally appear within a few days of trauma or surgery and infection of the bone may be impossible to differentiate from soft tissue infection. Early aggressive treatment is essential to limit the spread of infection within the bone, prevent widespread cortical necrosis and prevent the disease from becoming chronic. Treatment may require copious lavage, drainage, debridement of necrotic tissue and rigid stabilization of the fracture site. Samples should be submitted for culture and systemic antibiotic therapy initiated. Establishing drainage from the infected site may be achieved by sterile open wound management or insertion of drains. Antibiotic treatment is normally continued for a minimum of 4–6 weeks.

In chronic disease, if sequestra are present they are normally identifiable on radiographs, but problems may sometimes be encountered locating them during surgery. Although rarely performed, this may be facilitated by instilling 2% methylene blue into the sinus tracts where these are present, 24 hours prior to surgery. Avascular tissue will not clear the dye within this period and hence will appear blue, allowing differentiation of viable from nonviable bone. Sequestra are usually 'free-floating' and can be identified *in situ* by their characteristic appearance (initially ivory-like, later becoming discoloured and pitted) (Figure 30.10). Where a sequestrum is surrounded by an

involucrum, some of this new bone may require removal (using rongeurs or a mechanical burr) to enable the sequestrum to be removed (Figure 30.11). This may significantly weaken the bone, predisposing it to fracture (Figure 30.12). Although it has been recommended that ring sequestra are surgically removed (Kantrowitz *et al.*, 1988), they may resolve spontaneously following external skeletal fixator pin removal.

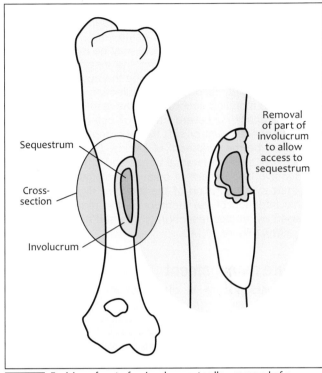

30.11 Excision of part of an involucrum to allow removal of a sequestrum. The bone may require subsequent support with a fixation device if sequestrum removal has significantly weakened the bone (see Figures 30.12 and 30.17).

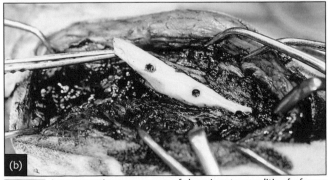

30.10 Intraoperative appearance of chronic osteomyelitis of a femur following application of a bone plate for fracture stabilization. (a) Sequestered cortical bone is visible beneath the bone plate (black arrow); viable cortical bone is denoted by the white arrow. (b) The sequestrum is more clearly visible following removal of the bone plate.

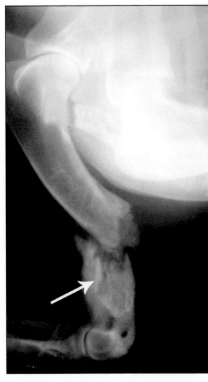

30.12 Mediolateral radiograph of a humerus following an attempt to remove a sequestrum. The sequestrum (arrowed) was not found and the weakening of the bone resulted in its fracture.

Where new bone deposition has obliterated the medullary canal, channels should be made through this bone with a reaming device or a large drill bit (Figure 30.13). This will facilitate the ingrowth of new blood vessels and hasten resolution of infection and fracture healing. Although some authors recommend debridement of sinus tracts, provided all the avascular, infected cortical bone is removed and other principles of treatment applied, discharge from these sinuses should quickly disappear. How the resulting wound is managed will depend on the degree of discharge and the location of the affected bone. Where there is significant discharge, aseptic open wound management (see the *BSAVA Manual of Canine and Feline Wound Management and Reconstruction*) may be indicated or the wound may be closed following the insertion of closed suction or Penrose drains. Antibiotic therapy should be initiated immediately following the collection of samples for culture, and modified according to the results.

Occasionally, in severe cases of osteomyelitis where there are serious joint or soft tissue complications, amputation may be the treatment of choice. Chronic infections of the metacarpal/metatarsal bones and digits where there is extensive involvement of adjacent soft tissues are best managed by amputation of the affected digit(s). Similarly, chronic infection of the sternebrae and mandible can be managed by *en bloc* resection of affected tissues (Fossum *et al.*, 1989) (Figure 30.14).

Fracture management

Chronic osteomyelitis is often associated with delayed union or non-union and prolonged rigid fracture stabilization is essential if the infection is to resolve and the fracture is to heal. It is important to remember that fractures will generally heal in the presence of infection provided they are stable. Where the fracture has not healed, removal of any existing implants may not be required if the implants are providing adequate stability. If the fracture site is unstable

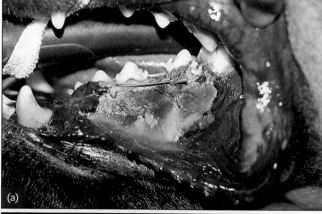

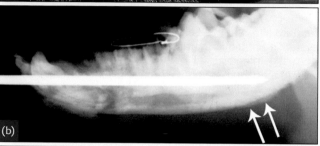

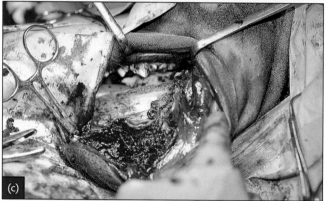

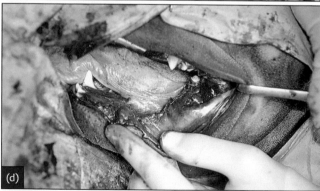

30.14 (a) Chronic osteomyelitis with sequestration of a large segment of the mandible following the insertion of a pin into the mandibular canal to stabilize a fracture. (b) Lateral radiograph of the mandible showing an irregular periosteal response adjacent to the distal end of the pin (arrowed). (c–d) Treatment for the dog involved rostral hemimandibulectomy to remove all dead, infected cortical bone.

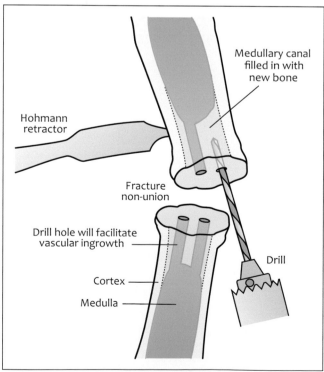

30.13 Reaming of the medullary canal (obliterated by new bone formation following infection) to facilitate vascular ingrowth and fracture healing.

the existing implants should be either supplemented or more commonly removed and replaced. Historically, external skeletal fixation (ESF) has often been used because the pins can often be placed some distance from the fracture site, limiting the amount of foreign material in the infected area, and their removal is quick and easy (Figure 30.15). However, they often need to be in place for an extended period because of prolonged healing times (Ness, 2006)

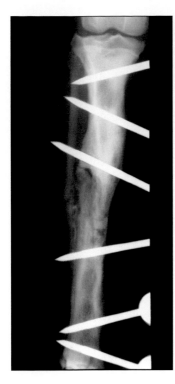

30.15 Craniocaudal radiograph of a tibia following application of a type 1 external skeletal fixator to stabilize an infected fracture.
(Courtesy of J Ferguson)

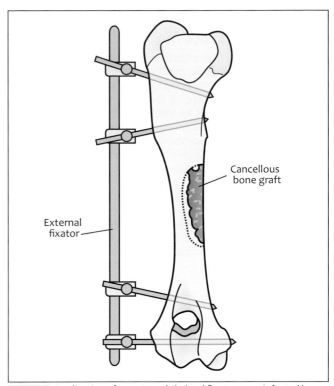

30.17 Application of an external skeletal fixator to an infected bone to provide additional support following removal of a sequestrum. The defect has been packed with a cancellous bone graft.

and premature pin loosening is relatively common, often necessitating further surgery. Alternatively, bone plating provides excellent stability, but requires more extensive surgery for application. In most cases bone plate fixation is preferred; however, owners should be warned that implant removal may be required following fracture healing because of persistence of infection associated with the implant (Figure 30.16). Intramedullary devices such as pins and nails are probably best avoided because they may provide a conduit for bacterial spread along the medullary canal and if used alone may not provide sufficient stability for bone healing in the presence of infection.

If the fracture has healed but following sequestrectomy and debridement the strength of the bone appears to be compromised, the use of an appropriate bone graft or bone graft substitute and a period of supplemental support with an ESF frame (or bone plate) may be advisable (Figure 30.17). In chronic low-grade infections where the fracture has healed, implant removal and a prolonged course of antibiotics may be all that is necessary for the infection to resolve (Figure 30.18).

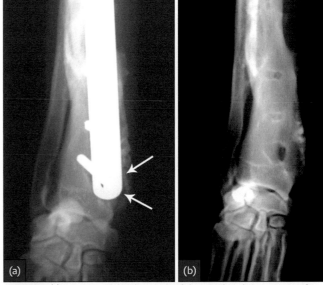

30.18 (a) Craniocaudal radiograph of the antebrachium 2 years after the application of a bone plate to stabilize a fractured radius. The fracture has healed but there is evidence of low-grade osteomyelitis. An irregular periosteal response is present on the distal radius (arrowed). (b) Following removal of the plate and a prolonged course of antibiotics, the infection resolved.

Bone grafting

The value of cancellous bone grafting in the management of delayed and non-union fractures is well established (see Chapter 14). Cancellous bone grafting can be performed either immediately following debridement or as a delayed procedure if there is significant discharge present (Bardet *et al.*, 1983). These grafts can survive in the presence of infection, though their value is likely to be compromised in the presence of inflammatory exudate or where the local blood supply has been compromised. Where large cortical

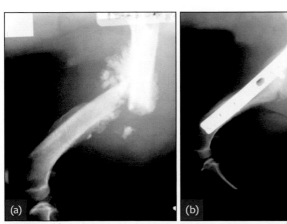

30.16 (a) Mediolateral radiograph of a femur showing an infected non-union fracture. (b) The fracture healed with a malunion following stabilization with a bone plate.

defects exist and large quantities of bone graft are needed to fill these areas, cancellous bone graft may need to be harvested from more than one donor site. Great care must be taken to ensure that infection is not transferred from the infected bone to the bone graft donor site.

The use of devascularized cortical allografts is contra-indicated in the treatment of large segmental cortical defects in the presence of an infection. Synthetic bone graft substitutes are available, but their efficacy in the presence of infection may be compromised. Demineralized bone matrix impregnated with antibiotics has been investigated for the treatment of infected non-union fractures. This has the potential advantage of stimulating osteoinduction and osteoconduction as well as treating infection (Beardmore et al. 2005).

Bone transport osteogenesis using a linear or circular ESF frame can be used to fill large cortical defects following debridement in chronic osteomyelitis (Lesser, 1994; Ting et al., 2010).

Antibiotic therapy in osteomyelitis

The effectiveness of antibiotics in the treatment of osteomyelitis is not just dependent on the virulence and antibiotic sensitivity of the causative organism, but also the viability and stability of the bone and the condition of the associated soft tissues. Antibiotics alone cannot be expected to resolve an infection in the presence of necrotic bone, and indeed such situations will increase the likelihood of the development of resistant microbial populations. The appropriate choice of antibiotic is based on the results of culture and sensitivity. High doses are usually used to treat osteomyelitis to facilitate drug penetration to areas with poor perfusion.

In acute osteomyelitis, samples for bacteriology should be obtained and treatment started immediately. Knowledge of the organisms most likely to be present dictates the initial choice of antibiotic which should be broad-spectrum and bactericidal (Figure 30.19). As beta-lactamase-producing Staphylococcus spp. are the most common cause of osteomyelitis, suitable first choices include cefalexin or amoxicillin/clavulanate (co-amoxiclav). If the presence of anaerobes is suspected the addition of metronidazole will broaden the spectrum to include the majority of these organisms. This choice of antibiotic can be modified when the results of culture and sensitivity have been obtained. Bacteriostatic antibiotics such as lincosamides are probably best avoided unless specifically indicated from culture and sensitivity because they may not eliminate infection.

In chronic osteomyelitis, antibiotic therapy should be started after samples have been obtained for culture during debridement. Initiating therapy intraoperatively will limit the effects of any 'bacteriological shower' during surgery and will ensure high levels of antibiotics in any haematomas that form. Where antibiotics have been administered prior to surgery, they should be discontinued 2–3 days beforehand to increase the likelihood of isolating the causative organism(s). Therapy should continue for a minimum of 4–6 weeks; some refractory cases may require even longer (3–4 months). Fungal osteomyelitis often requires several months of therapy.

Infections caused by multidrug-resistant organisms such as MRSP are becoming more common in veterinary practice and they have been reported following orthopaedic surgery (McLean and Ness, 2008; Schwartz et al., 2009). Other bacteria that often show multidrug resistance include the Gram-negative organisms Pseudomonas aeruginosa, Enterobacter spp., Escherichia coli and Proteus spp. and their treatment can present significant problems (Papich, 2013). Animals infected with these bacteria should be isolated to reduce the risk of nosocomial and zoonotic transmission and they should be handled using dedicated protective outerwear (e.g. gowns, gloves). Infected wounds should be kept covered with clean, dry bandages. For more detailed information on the management of MRSP, readers are directed to the BSAVA website (www.bsava.com/Resources/MRSA).

Although some drugs used in humans, such as carbenicillin, ticarcillin and second and third generation cephalosporins (e.g. ceftazidime), may be effective against these organisms, these are not currently licensed for use in small animals, may be very expensive and usually require injection. Systemic use of gentamicin over an extended period (2 weeks) can result in kidney damage. This serious side effect can be overcome by local implantation of gentamicin-impregnated beads (Figure 30.20) or collagen sponge (Renwick et al., 2010; Hayes et al., 2013), although the precise elution characteristics of these products in

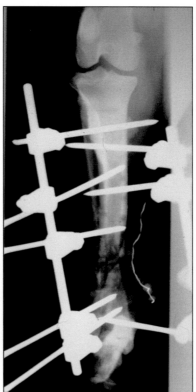

30.20 Craniocaudal radiograph of an infected tibial fracture stabilized with an external skeletal fixator. Gentamicin-impregnated beads have been implanted at the fracture site.
(Courtesy of S Langley-Hobbs)

Drug	Dose (mg/kg)	Route	Frequency
Amoxicillin/clavulanate	12–25	oral	q12h
Cefalexin	10–20	s.c., i.m., oral	q12h
Cefazolin[a]	20–25	i.v.	q8h
Clindamycin	5–11	oral	q12h
Enrofloxacin	2.5	oral	q12h
Gentamicin[b]	2	i.v., i.m., s.c.	q8h
Metronidazole	10–15	oral	q12h

30.19 Antibiotics commonly used in the treatment of osteomyelitis. [a] = Cefazolin is not licensed for use in small animals. However, because it can be used intravenously it is commonly used prophylactically during orthopaedic surgery. [b] = Gentamicin is nephrotoxic and should not be used for more than 1 week. Renal function should be monitored whilst it is being administered. Gentamicin is also available impregnated in polymethylmethacrylate beads or collagen sponges though these products are not licensed for use in animals.

infected canine tissue are not well defined. It has been recommended that beads are removed once the infection has resolved to reduce the risk of bacterial resistance developing (Hayes *et al.*, 2013). Some strains of *Pseudomonas aeruginosa* show susceptibility to fluoroquinolones (marbofloxacin or enrofloxacin) and their generally low toxicity and oral dosing may provide significant advantages over drugs such as gentamicin. Enrofloxacin should be used with caution in cats because of the risk of retinal blindness.

Factors affecting the development of osteomyelitis

Surgical site infections associated with orthopaedic surgical procedures can be devastating. They can increase morbidity and costs and result in outcomes that are frequently worse than those of uninfected cases. To minimize the risk of infections the clinician must consider preoperative, intraoperative and postoperative factors and interventions.

Animals that may be at a greater risk of infection include those suffering from comorbidities such as diabetes mellitus, renal failure, hyperadrenocorticism or malnutrition, or those on immunosuppressive therapy. If bacterial skin disease is present in the surgical field elective surgery should be delayed until this has been treated effectively. Open wounds associated with a fracture may increase the risk of infection and wherever possible surgical approaches or techniques (e.g. minimally invasive surgery) should be used that minimize the risk of contamination of the fracture site. Where fractures are open, the risk of infection developing increases with the grade of soft tissue/bone trauma and contamination (see Chapter 12).

Following induction of general anaesthesia, meticulous attention should be paid to aseptic technique to minimize the risk of bacterial contamination of the surgical site. In the operating theatre the greatest source of airborne bacteria is from theatre personnel. Numbers of airborne bacteria can be minimized by use of appropriate ventilation systems. Positive pressure ventilation creates a pressure gradient forcing air from clean to contaminated areas of a theatre suite. In human orthopaedic operating theatres vertical laminar air flow through high-efficiency particulate air filters has been shown to reduce the rate of surgical site infections, but their cost is likely to be prohibitive in veterinary practices (Fletcher *et al.*, 2007; Bosco *et al.*, 2010). Simpler ways to reduce theatre bacterial contamination include minimizing numbers of staff and traffic through the theatre, appropriate gowning and the use of hats and masks.

Following surgery, all wounds should be covered with an adhesive dressing for at least 24 hours to provide protection until a fibrin seal has formed. If any dressings become wet or soiled they should be changed promptly to avoid strike-through contamination. If drains have been inserted as part of treatment for osteomyelitis they should be maintained using strict aseptic technique to avoid the risk of nosocomial infection.

Perioperative antibiotics

The use of antibiotic prophylaxis in clean orthopaedic surgery in humans and veterinary patients has been shown to be beneficial in reducing the risk of infection (Whittem *et al.*, 1999; Eugster *et al.*, 2004; Fletcher *et al.*, 2007). For broad-spectrum bactericidal activity against likely Gram-positive (including *Staphylococcus* spp.) and Gram-negative pathogens, including some activity against anaerobes, amoxicillin/clavulanate and first and second generation cephalosporins are common choices (see Figure 30.19). These drugs should be administered 30–60 minutes prior to surgery and are generally continued for up to 24 hours following surgery. For lengthy surgical procedures additional doses of antibiotic can be administered (every 2 hours for amoxicillin/clavulanate and every 3–4 hours for cefazolin at the same dose as given prior to surgery). There is some evidence that extending the duration of antibiotics beyond 24 hours is of benefit in some clean veterinary orthopaedic procedures such as tibial plateau levelling osteotomy (Fitzpatrick and Solano, 2010). For joint replacement surgery where cemented implants are used, the use of antibiotic-loaded cement will reduce the risk of infection.

Effect of implant design

Veterinary metallic orthopaedic implants are normally made from 316L stainless steel. Some studies have shown that implants made from titanium alloys may be less prone to infection, but the subject remains controversial (Hayes *et al.*, 2013). The size, shape and topography of the implanted devices are also significant variables that may influence risk of infection. Bone plates whose design minimizes disruption to cortical vascularity (e.g. limited contact dynamic compression plates) may reduce the risk of bacterial infection. An essential early stage in the establishment of bacterial infection is adhesion of bacteria to the metallic implant and this has been shown to be influenced by its physical surface characteristics (Wu *et al.*, 2011). Smooth polished implants are generally more resistant to bacterial adhesion and growth compared to those with rougher surfaces, but their use may be disadvantageous if osseous integration of the implant is desirable.

As a consequence of the morbidity and costs of dealing with infections and the increasing incidence of multidrug-resistant infections in humans, there is considerable research into applying coatings to metallic implants that may minimize the risks of infection. These include antibiotic coatings such as gentamicin and vancomycin (Antoci *et al.*, 2007) and applications of silver compounds and nitrogen ions that have been shown to minimize bacterial adhesion (Ketonis *et al.*, 2012). These coatings may be combined with factors that stimulate osteogenesis (Goodman *et al.*, 2013). Use of implants with these coatings is likely to become more common in human orthopaedics, but their cost may prove to be prohibitive in veterinary orthopaedics in the near future.

Haematogenous and fungal osteomyelitis

Osteomyelitis that arises other than following extension of infection from adjacent tissues, trauma or the migration of foreign bodies is presumed to be haematogenous in origin although the primary focus of infection is often not apparent. This is a rare condition in small animals and whilst it has been identified in adult dogs (Caywood *et al.*, 1978; Rabillard *et al.*, 2011), it is more common in skeletally immature dogs (Dunn *et al.*, 1992) and animals with abnormal immune systems. It has also been reported in the cat (Dunn *et al.*, 1983).

Affected animals are usually presented with a history of lethargy, anorexia and lameness or stiffness. Pyrexia, pain and swelling localized to the affected areas of bone (usually the metaphyses of multiple long bones in skeletally immature dogs) are usually present, and infection may spread into adjacent soft tissues or joints, resulting in a septic arthritis. Occasionally, the infection may result in a pathological fracture of the affected bone (Emmerson and Pead, 1999).

The susceptibility of the metaphyseal regions may be due to the capillary buds lacking a basement membrane and having a discontinuous endothelium. During an episode of bacteraemia, bacteria may embolize through these gaps and be less accessible to inflammatory cells.

Radiographic findings include diffuse areas of bone lysis and periosteal reactions (Figure 30.21). Advanced imaging techniques such as technetium scintigraphy usually show an increase in uptake at infected sites and may be helpful in detection of multiple sites of infection. MRI offers superior sensitivity compared to scintigraphy and may allow earlier detection of infection and detect extraosseous complications. Bacteriological culture of blood and aspirates from bone may fail to identify the causative organisms, but they should be attempted. Urinary tract infection may also be associated with this disease and urine culture should be performed. Treatment consists of broad-spectrum antibiotics (see Figure 30.19) and exercise restriction for 6 weeks. If the infection extends into adjacent soft tissues the area should be drained and flushed. The prognosis is reported to be good.

Discospondylitis is an infection of the intervertebral disc space that extends into the adjacent vertebral bodies, although some dogs may show evidence of infection of the vertebral endplates in the apparent absence of infection in the intervertebral disc (Jimenez and O'Callaghan, 1995) (Figure 30.22). Extension of infection into the neural canal can result in neurological signs. This disease is more common than the forms of haematogenous osteomyelitis described above. Vertebral osteomyelitis has been associated with migrating foreign

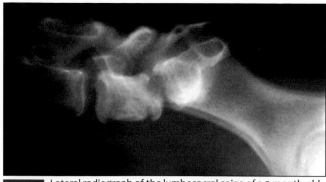

30.22 Lateral radiograph of the lumbosacral spine of a 5-month-old dog with discospondylitis at the L7/S1 intervertebral disc space. There is widening of the affected disc space with lysis of the adjacent vertebral endplates.

bodies. Treatment of discospondylitis with a prolonged course of antibiotics (6–8 weeks) is usually successful but some animals may require curettage of the affected disc space or vertebral stabilization (Gage, 1975; Kornegay and Barber, 1980; Renwick *et al.*, 2010).

Although not uncommon in some southern and western areas of the USA (Nunamaker, 1975), fungal osteomyelitis is very rare in the UK. In the USA the most commonly isolated causative agents are *Coccidioides immitis, Blastomyces dermatitidis, Histoplasma capsulatum* and *Cryptococcus neoformans* (Nunamaker, 1975). The main portal of entry is the respiratory tract, and in addition to respiratory signs affected animals may develop neural, ocular and skeletal lesions. Osteomyelitis caused by *C. neoformans* has been reported in the UK (Brearley and Jeffrey, 1992). Radiographic lesions resemble those previously described for chronic bacterial osteomyelitis (Figure 30.23). Diagnosis is based on the characteristic histological appearance of affected bone and isolation of the organism. Treatment with ketoconazole (10 mg/kg per day for 2 months, reducing to 5 mg/kg per day for a further 2 months) has been reported to be effective (Brearley and Jeffrey, 1992).

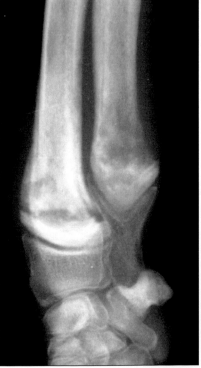

30.21 Mediolateral radiograph of the distal radius and ulna from a dog with haematogenous osteomyelitis. Focal areas of lysis are present in the metaphyses of both bones.
(Courtesy of J Houlton)

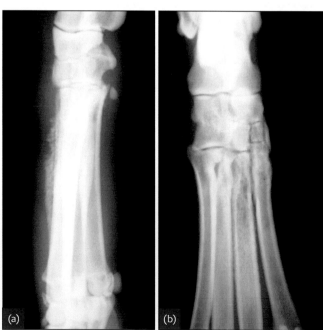

30.23 (a) Mediolateral and (b) dorsoplantar radiographs of the metatarsus of a dog with osteomyelitis caused by *Cryptococcus neoformans*. There is an irregular periosteal response and areas of lysis of the third metatarsal bone.
(Courtesy of M Brearley)

Osteomyelitis caused by *Aspergillus* spp. has also been reported in the USA and the UK (Butterworth *et al.*, 1995; Hotston Moore and Hanna, 1995). Although usually confined to the nasal cavity and paranasal sinuses, *Aspergillus* spp. can disseminate to other body systems, including the skeletal system. Female German Shepherd Dogs are predisposed to this disease, with infection usually causing discospondylitis at multiple sites. The organism may be cultured from affected intervertebral discs and from urine sediment. Frequently, affected animals will not have serum antibodies to the organism (Watt *et al.*, 1995). Treatment with ketoconazole (10–15 mg/kg q12h (at time of publication not available in the UK)) or itraconazole (17 mg/kg q24h) may control the infection in some dogs, but affected animals will need to be kept on medication permanently (Watt *et al.*, 1995). The prognosis is poor.

References and further reading

Aliabadi P and Nikpoor N (1994) Imaging osteomyelitis. *Arthritis and Rheumatism* **37**, 617–622

Antoci V, Adams CS, Hickok NJ *et al.* (2007) Vancomycin bound to Ti rods reduces periprosthetic infection: Preliminary study. *Clinical Orthopaedics and Related Research* **461**, 88–95

Bardet JF, Hohn RB and Basinger R (1983) Open drainage and delayed autogenous bone grafting for treatment of chronic osteomyelitis in dogs and cats. *Journal of the American Veterinary Medical Association* **183**, 312–317

Beardmore AA, Brooks DE and Wenke JC (2005) Effectiveness of local antibiotic delivery with an osteoinductive and osteoconductive bone graft substitute. *Journal of Bone and Joint Surgery (American Volume)* **87A**, 107–112

Bond R and Loeffler A (2012) What's happened to *Staphylococcus intermedius*? Taxonomic revision and emergence of multi-drug resistance. *Journal of Small Animal Practice* **53**, 147–154

Bosco JA, Slover JD and Haas JP (2010) Perioperative strategies for decreasing infection. *Journal of Bone and Joint Surgery (American Volume)* **92**, 232–239

Braden TD, Johnson CA, Gabel CL *et al.* (1987) Posologic evaluation of clindamycin, using a canine model of posttraumatic osteomyelitis. *American Journal of Veterinary Research* **48**, 1101–1105

Braden TD, Tvedten HW, Mostosky UV *et al.* (1989) The sensitivity and specificity of radiology and histopathology in the diagnosis of posttraumatic osteomyelitis. *Veterinary and Comparative Orthopaedics and Traumatology* **3**, 98–103

Brearley MJ and Jeffrey N (1992) Cryptococcal osteomyelitis in a dog. *Journal of Small Animal Practice* **33**, 601–604

Budsberg SC (2012) Osteomyelitis. In: *Veterinary Surgery: Small Animal,* ed. KM Tobias and SA Johnston, pp. 669–675. Elsevier, Canada

Butterworth SJ, Barr FJ, Pearson GR and Day MD (1995) Multiple discospondylitis associated with *Aspergillus* species infection in a dog. *Veterinary Record* **136**, 38–40

Caywood DD (1983) Osteomyelitis. *Veterinary Clinics of North America: Small Animal Practice* **13**, 43–53

Caywood DD, Wallace LJ and Braden TD (1978) Osteomyelitis in the dog. *Journal of the American Veterinary Medical Association* **172**, 943–946

Dunn JK, Dennis R and Houlton JEF (1992) Successful treatment of metaphyseal osteomyelitis in the dog. *Journal of Small Animal Practice* **33**, 85–89

Dunn JK, Farrow CS and Doige CE (1983) Disseminated osteomyelitis caused by *Clostridrium novyi* in a cat. *Canadian Veterinary Journal* **24**, 312–316

Emmerson TD and Pead MJ (1999) Pathological fracture of the femur secondary to haematogenous osteomyelitis in a weimaraner. *Journal of Small Animal Practice* **40**, 233–235

Eugster S, Schawalder P, Gaschen F *et al.* (2004) A study of postoperative surgical site infections in dogs and cats. *Veterinary Surgery* **33**, 542–550

Fitzpatrick N and Solano MA (2010) Predictive variables for complications after TPLO with stifle inspection by arthrotomy in 1000 consecutive cases. *Veterinary Surgery* **39**, 460–474

Fletcher N, Sofianos D, Berkes MB and Obremskey WT (2007) Prevention of perioperative infection. *Journal of Bone and Joint Surgery (American Volume)* **89**, 1605–1618

Fossum TW, Hodges CC, Miller MW and Dupre GP (1989) Partial sternectomy for sternal osteomyelitis in the dog. *Journal of the American Animal Hospital Association* **25**, 435–441

Gage ED (1975) Treatment of discospondylitis in the dog. *Journal of the American Veterinary Medical Association* **166**, 1164–1170

Goodman SB, Yao Z, Keeney M *et al.* (2013) The future of biologic coatings for orthopaedic implants. *Biomaterials* **34**, 3174–3183

Gristina AG, Oga M, Webb LX and Hobgood CD (1985) Adherent bacterial

colonisation in the pathogenesis of osteomyelitis. *Science* **228**, 990–993

Hayes G, Moens N and Gibson T (2013) A review of local antibiotic implants and applications to veterinary orthopaedic surgery. *Veterinary and Comparative Orthopaedics and Traumatology* **26**, 251–259

Hirsh DC and Smith TM (1978) Osteomyelitis in the dog: microorganisms and susceptibility to antimicrobial agents. *Journal of Small Animal Practice* **19**, 679–686

Hotston Moore A and Hanna FY (1995) Mycotic osteomyelitis in a dog following nasal aspergillosis. *Veterinary Record* **137**, 349–350

Jimenez MM and O'Callaghan MW (1995) Vertebral physitis: a radiographic diagnosis to be separated from discospondylitis. *Veterinary Radiology and Ultrasound* **36**, 188–195

Johnson KA (1994) Osteomyelitis in dogs and cats. *Journal of the American Veterinary Medical Association* **204**, 1882–1887

Kantrowitz B, Smeak D and Vannini R (1988) Radiographic appearance of ring sequestrum with pin tract osteomyelitis in the dog. *Journal of the American Animal Hospital Association* **24**, 461–465

Ketonis C, Parvizi J and Jones LC (2012) Evolving strategies to prevent implant-associated infections. *Journal of the American Academy of Orthopaedic Surgeons* **20**, 478–480

Kornegay JN and Barber DL (1980) Discospondylitis in dogs. *Journal of the American Veterinary Medical Association* **177**, 337–341

Lamb CR (1987) Bone scintigraphy in small animals. *Journal of the American Veterinary Medical Association* **191**, 1616–1622

Lesser AS (1994) Segmental bone transport for the treatment of bone deficits. *Journal of the American Animal Hospital Association* **30**, 322–330

McLean CL and Ness MG (2008) Meticillin-resistant *Staphylococcus aureus* in a veterinary orthopaedic referral hospital: staff nasal colonisation and incidence of clinical cases. *Journal of Small Animal Practice* **49**, 170–177

Muir P and Johnson KA (1992) Anaerobic bacteria isolated from osteomyelitis in dogs and cats. *Veterinary Surgery* **21**, 463–466

Ness MG (2006) Treatment of inherently unstable open or infected fractures by open wound management and external skeletal fixation. *Journal of Small Animal Practice* **47**, 83–88

Nunamaker DM (1975) Management of infected fractures: Osteomyelitis. *Veterinary Clinics of North America* **5**, 259–271

Papich MG (2013) Antibiotic treatment of resistant infections in small animals. *Veterinary Clinics of North America: Small Animals* **43**, 1091–1107

Perry CR, Pearson RL and Miller GA (1991) Accuracy of cultures of material from swabbing of the superficial aspect of the wound and needle biopsy in the preoperative assessment of osteomyelitis. *Journal of Bone and Joint Surgery (American Volume)* **73**, 745–751

Pratt JNJ, Munro EAC Kirby BM (1999) Osteomyelitis of the atlanto-occipital region as a sequel to a pharyngeal stick injury (1999) *Journal of Small Animal Practice* **40**, 446–448

Rabillard M, Souchu L, Niebauer GW and Gauthier O (2011) Haematogenous osteomyelitis: clinical presentation and outcome in three dogs. *Veterinary and Comparative Orthopaedics and Traumatology* **24**, 146–150

Renwick AIC, Dennis R and Gemmill T (2010) Treatment of lumbosacral discospondylitis by surgical stabilization and application of a gentamicin-impregnated collagen sponge. *Veterinary and Comparative Orthopaedics and Traumatology* **23**, 266–272

Schwartz M, Boettcher IC, Kramer S and Tipold D (2009) Two dogs with iatrogenic discospondylitis caused by methicillin-resistant *Staphylococcus aureus*. *Journal of Small Animal Practice* **50**, 201–205

Smith MM, Vasseur PB and Saunders HM (1989) Bacterial growth associated with metallic implants in dogs. *Journal of the American Animal Hospital Association* **195**, 765–767

Stead AC (1984) Osteomyelitis in the dog and cat. *Journal of Small Animal Practice* **25**, 1–13

Sutton A, May C and Couglan A (2010) Spinal osteomyelitis and epidural empyema in a dog due to migrating conifer material. *Veterinary Record* **166**, 693–694

Ting D, Petersen W and Déjardin LM (2010) Bone transport osteogenesis for treatment of canine osteomyelitis. *Veterinary and Comparative Orthopaedics and Traumatology* **23**, 134–140

Vercelotti GM, McCarthy JB, Lindholm P *et al.* (1985) Extracellular matrix proteins bind and aggregate bacteria. *American Journal of Pathology* **120**, 13–20

Watt PR, Robins GM, Galloway AM and O'Boyle DA (1995) Disseminated opportunistic fungal disease in dogs: 10 cases (1982–1990). *Journal of the American Veterinary Medical Association* **207**, 67–70

Whittem TL, Johnson AL, Smith CHW *et al.* (1999) Effect of perioperative prophylactic antimicrobial treatment in dogs undergoing elective orthopaedic surgery. *Journal of the American Veterinary Medical Association* **215**, 212–216

Williams J and Moores A (2009) *BSAVA Manual of Canine and Feline Wound Management and Reconstruction, 2nd edn.* BSAVA Publications, Gloucester

Wu Y, Zitelli JPP TenHuisen KS, Yu X and Libera MR TenHuisen KS (2011) Differential response of *Staphylococci* and osteoblasts to varying titanium surface roughness. *Biomaterials* **32**, 951–60

Zoubos AB, Galanakos SP and Soucacos PN (2012) Orthopaedics and biofilm-what do we know? A review. *Medical Science Monitor* **18**, 89–96

Chapter 31

Complications of fracture healing

Bill Oxley

Normal bone healing is the result of an elegant and ordered sequence of biological events, initiated by the inflammatory response inherent to fracture and culminating in the restoration of normal bone architecture. Specific disruptions to this process, often as a result of inappropriate fracture mechanics or biology, are implicated in the development of delayed unions, non-unions and malunions. Although some factors contributing to defective bone healing are beyond the surgeon's control, poor surgical planning, execution or follow-up are frequently responsible. Therefore, an appreciation of the optimum conditions for bone healing enables the surgeon not only to identify and correct underlying problems when faced with defective bone healing, but also to plan primary interventions to minimize the risk of such problems occurring.

Definitions

Bone union is the term used to indicate that a fracture has healed. However, due to the relatively slow nature of bone healing, complete fracture healing is rarely documented, and thus intermediate stages in the process are identified to aid clinical decision making. The precise definition of **radiographic union** varies but, typically for diaphyseal fractures, implies bridging of all four cortices on orthogonal views. The fracture gap may still be apparent on radiographs, but it should exhibit blurring and infilling with mineralized material (Figure 31.1). In these instances, although bone healing is incomplete, the development of subsequent complications is unusual. **Clinical union** implies sufficient progression of fracture healing to permit essentially normal function, with no evidence of pain or instability at the fracture site and, in the case of appendicular fractures, minimal lameness. Clinical union can occur before radiographic union. However, since well stabilized but biologically inactive fractures can satisfy some of the criteria for clinical union, radiographic assessment of healing is mandatory.

Delayed union is the term used to describe the situation when radiographic progression of fracture healing is slower than expected, but the fracture is expected to go on to heal. Clearly, the rate of anticipated healing will vary widely dependent on factors unique to the patient, fracture and management approach, and definitive differentiation between slow but normal healing and early non-union can be difficult.

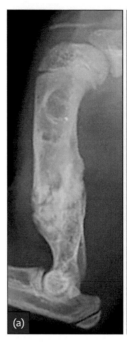
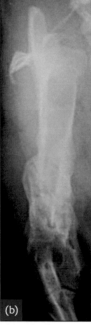

31.1

(a) Mediolateral and (b) craniocaudal views of radiographic union of a comminuted distal diaphyseal humeral fracture in a 4-month-old kitten, 5 weeks following external skeletal fixation. Although fracture lines are still visible these are blurred and exhibit infilling with mineralized material. Callus is crossing the fracture at all four cortices.

Non-union describes a fracture that is not expected to heal without additional intervention. Non-unions are classified as **viable** when biological activity is maintained at the fracture site and there is attempted bone healing, and **non-viable** when these features are absent.

Malunion refers to a fracture that has healed but with abnormal conformation of the affected bone; in the case of articular fractures there is imperfect restoration of the articular surface. Mild malunions are relatively common and are rarely of concern when function is normal; in this case the term **functional malunion** is appropriate. Conversely, the term **non-functional malunion** is used when deformity prevents normal function or results in a secondary debilitating problem such as patellar luxation.

Causes of defective bone healing

Although numerous, seemingly disparate, factors can affect the rate and quality of bone healing, their effects are ultimately modulated through positive or negative influences on fracture site mechanics and/or biology.

When inadequate, the relative quality of the mechanical and biological environments determines the type of non-union that develops.

Fracture site mechanics

From a biomechanical perspective, the primary influence on bone healing is the interfragmentary strain (IFS) within the fracture gap (see Chapters 4 and 5). Following surgical stabilization of a fracture the IFS is primarily influenced by the size of the fracture gap and the rigidity of the fixation applied. A low level of IFS will result in micromotion at the fracture gap, which is an important stimulus to bone healing via direct effects on mesenchymal stem cell (MSC) proliferation and differentiation (Kraus and Kirker-Head, 2006). It follows that when IFS is excessively low there may be insufficient stimulation of cells within the fracture gap to drive an appropriate healing response (as well as in local normal bone, where remodelling is not maintained and osteopenia results). This situation is termed **stress protection** and is unusual, but is occasionally encountered in cats and dogs, usually of toy breeds, following application of excessively stiff fixation to diaphyseal fractures (Figure 31.2).

Excessively high IFS occurs more frequently, and is an important cause of delayed unions and viable nonunions. The classic process of bone healing via endochondral ossification entails the sequential formation of

31.2 A distal radial fracture in a 4-year-old Greyhound stabilized with a lag screw and stacked T-plates. (a) The fracture appeared to be healing 4 months postoperatively, although a radiolucent line could still be identified at the fracture site. A decision was made to remove the plates because of recurrent implant-associated sepsis. (b) The fracture recurred 3 days following plate removal. Note the extensive bony remodelling proximal to the site of plate application, and the relative osteopenia of the distal radius under the plates. It is likely that excessive stiffness of the implants resulted in stress protection of the fracture site, which may have impeded healing. The recurrence of the fracture was a technical error on the part of the surgeon; the plates should not have been removed, or ancillary fixation should have been placed at the time of plate removal.
(Courtesy of D Clements)

haematoma, granulation tissue, cartilage and, finally, bone. Stability increases at each stage, paving the way for the next more rigid, but strain sensitive, tissue type. The strain tolerances of granulation tissue, cartilage and bone have been estimated at 100%, 10% and 2%, respectively (Perren, 1979) (see Chapters 4 and 5) and although such values are useful as guides only, it is clear that bone will not form in a fracture gap subject to persistently high IFS. This may occur when strain is concentrated at a very small fracture gap, or when fixation is too flexible. The potentially adverse effect of a high strain environment in a very small fracture gap can lead to inhibition of callus formation and longer term cyclic loading of implants, in turn leading to implant failure through fatigue even when strong and relatively rigid fixation has been applied (Sommer et al., 2004) (see Chapter 29). This appears to be an emerging complication of bridging fixation using locking plates to simple fractures; interfragmentary compression is optimal in this situation (Wilber and Baumgaertal, 2007). Insufficiently rigid fixation is the more common cause of excessively high IFS as a direct result of poorly controlled motion at the fracture gap. This may be due to poor surgical planning or technique, for example not applying compression to a simple transverse fracture, or due to complications leading to loss of integrity of an osteosynthesis. The type of fixation selected must provide not only appropriate immediate stability but must maintain this for a sufficient period to allow for bone healing; when this period is expected to be extended due to adverse biological factors, stronger implants capable of withstanding a longer period of cyclic loading should be used. Poorly placed implants will not provide the anticipated mechanical support and postoperative radiographs should be critically assessed. Loss of integrity of osteosynthesis may result from loosening at the implant–bone interface (e.g. due to poor surgical technique, infection or chronic overuse) or implant failure (acute or fatigue failure).

Unfortunately, the optimum level of IFS for a given fracture is almost impossible to estimate in clinical cases. For this reason the surgeon must rely on a sound grasp of the principles of fracture stabilization (see Chapter 8), combined with a critical assessment of each fracture, to judge the most appropriate form of fixation. Fortunately, experimental studies indicate that within a favourable biological environment bone healing will progress within a relatively wide range of IFS. In one experimental study, satisfactory callus formation occurred in a 1 mm ovine metatarsal osteotomy gap stabilized with a custom-built external skeletal fixator with IFS between 7 and 31%. The higher strains resulted in a higher volume of callus and a stronger union (Claes et al., 1997). Larger osteotomy gaps exhibited less vigorous callus formation, which was adversely affected by higher IFS. These considerations are particularly relevant with respect to the recent trend towards closed reduction as part of a minimally invasive approach to fracture management; whilst the inherent biological benefits are undoubted, appropriate IFS and fracture reduction remain of key importance and must not be neglected.

Fracture site biology

The importance of a biologically optimal fracture environment has received considerable recent attention. The basic biological unit responsible for fracture healing is the cell; initially MSCs, and later the more differentiated cells responsible for matrix elaboration (see Chapter 5). The first prerequisite for bone healing is a sufficient cell population. The second is that these cells are supplied with their requirements for optimal function; these include a good blood supply, appropriate cell signalling via growth factors and cytokines, and a suitable extracellular matrix. When biological activity at a fracture is insufficient for bone healing, non-viable non-union results; identification of inadequacies in these key biological elements facilitates appropriate intervention and improves the likelihood of a successful clinical outcome. Equally importantly, assessment of these features in a fresh fracture allows the surgeon to identify cases where compromised biological activity may adversely affect bone healing and modify treatment accordingly. It is useful to consider factors influencing key biological elements as either intrinsic (those inherent to the patient and fracture) or extrinsic (those determined by the treatment selected).

Cell population

Following fracture, MSCs are recruited from the periosteum, bone marrow, local soft tissues and blood as a result of cytokines released during the early inflammatory process. Intrinsic factors affecting the supply of MSCs include age (older animals have fewer periosteal MSCs with lower activity) and fracture location (the relative volume of local bone marrow and the quality of the local blood supply). Extrinsic factors include iatrogenic periosteal injury during surgery and any surgical disruption of the fracture haematoma. MSC chemotaxis wanes as a fracture moves from the inflammatory to proliferative stages of healing, and MSC numbers are not therefore indefinitely maintained if healing progresses poorly.

Blood supply

The importance of a good blood supply to fracture healing cannot be overemphasized, as a well vascularized oxygen-rich environment stimulates MSC proliferation and differentiation. The normal medullary and periosteal circulation is disrupted after fracture, with blood supply to the fracture site predominantly dependent on angiogenesis; new vessels develop rapidly following fracture from intact vessels within the adjacent periosteum and other local soft tissues.

Intrinsic factors affecting blood supply following fracture include the extent of injury to these tissues and their relative abundance, and the normal vascularity of the affected bone. Local soft tissue injury may be obvious, for example in shearing injuries or open fractures, but it can also be extensive but unapparent following high-energy fractures (typically associated with a high degree of comminution). Revascularization will be slower where local soft tissue cover is sparse, for example the antebrachium. Studies have demonstrated decreased vascular density at the distal diaphyseal–metaphyseal junction in toy breeds compared to large-breed dogs (Welch et al., 1997), and reduced arborization of the tibial medullary vasculature in cats versus dogs (Dugat et al., 2011), features which may impair fracture site blood supply.

Extrinsic factors include the extent of periosteal elevation during surgery, vascular compromise due to excessive exposure or rough tissue handling, and the type of fixation used (e.g. locking plates disrupt the periosteal circulation less than conventional plating). Postoperative complications may have significant effects on blood supply. Implant loosening frequently indicates mechanical instability, but may also disrupt vasculature; loose cerclage wires, for example, will circumferentially disrupt periosteal vessels and can promote oligotrophic or dystrophic non-union.

Cell signalling

Numerous cytokines and growth factors modulate the activity of cells within the fracture site. These mechanisms are complex, are intrinsic to the normal progression of bone healing, and remain incompletely elucidated, although certain key factors such as bone morphogenetic protein 2 (BMP2) are recognized. Following fracture, the immediate inflammatory response initiates the sequential expression of numerous factors, the pattern of which evolves and changes as healing progresses. This dynamic signalling environment will not persist if bone healing fails, and must be reinitiated if an established non-viable non-union is to be successfully treated. It should be noted that although the administration of exogenous cytokines such as BMP2 and BMP7 have demonstrated clinical efficacy (Pinel and Pluhar, 2012) (see Chapter 14), they cannot mimic the full range and temporal evolution of endogenous cytokine expression found in normal fracture healing.

Extracellular matrix

This is necessary for cell adhesion and proliferation. The normal process of fracture healing allows for the generation of novel extracellular matrix within the fracture gap. However, this ability is limited and large defects will not heal; inadequate cell signalling, MSC invasion and blood supply also contribute to this problem. The minimum gap that will not heal naturally is termed a critical defect. Due to the range of factors affecting bone healing this is impossible to quantify accurately in different patients; in general, gaps approaching the diameter of the bone are unlikely to heal. However, even small fracture gaps will adversely affect bone healing, and reduction should not be neglected even when fracture site biology is preserved during minimally invasive osteosynthesis or other approaches employing closed reduction.

Non-union

Diagnosis

Clinical and radiographic features must be considered in the diagnosis of fracture non-union. In the majority of cases non-unions are associated with pain, which in the case of appendicular fractures can cause lameness. The primary cause of pain is instability at the fracture site, which usually results from either inappropriate initial fixation or its progressive failure secondary to poor progression of bone healing. Clinical examination often reveals disuse muscle atrophy and pain at the fracture site on palpation or manipulation. Gross instability and limb malalignment may be apparent; however, the absence of these features does not preclude the presence of defective bone healing.

The key radiographic feature of non-union is a fracture gap or line persisting at an interval greater than that expected for normal or even delayed bone healing, with minimal or no mineralization of the defect. Failure to demonstrate progression of bone healing on serial radiography can help confirm the diagnosis. Additional radiographic features of non-union may include evidence of implant failure, excessive or absent callus formation, cortical atrophy, and osteopenia; these features can permit classification of the non-union as either viable or non-viable.

Radiographic features of viable non-unions

Viable non-unions retain reasonable fracture site biology but are prevented from healing by a poor mechanical environment, usually instability. This is reflected in their classic radiographic appearance where excessive mineralized periosteal and endosteal callus forms on either side of a fracture gap filled with radiolucent fibrous or cartilaginous callus. The relative volume of the periosteal, non-bridging callus is subjectively used to subdivide viable non-unions (Figure 31.3).

- Hypertrophic (or elephant's foot) non-unions exhibit marked mineralized callus formation (Figures 31.3a and 31.4).
- Moderately hypertrophic (or horse's hoof) non-unions exhibit less mineralized callus (Figures 31.3b and 31.5).
- Oligotrophic non-unions exhibit minimal or no mineralized callus formation, and fracture edges may appear sclerotic and rounded (Figures 31.3c and 31.6).

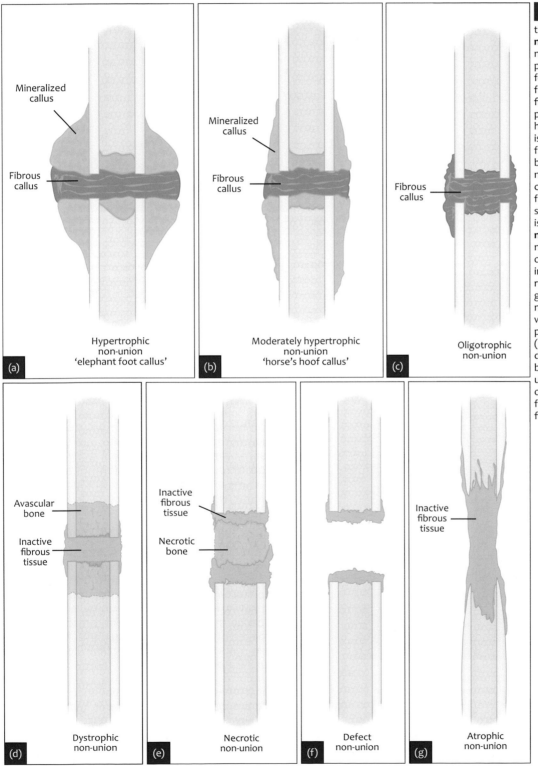

31.3 Schematic representation of the forms of non-union. **Viable non-unions:** (a) Hypertrophic non-union: significant periosteal and endosteal callus forms but cannot bridge the fracture gap when fibrous or fibrocartilaginous callus persists. (b) Moderately hypertrophic non-union: there is less callus formation but the fracture surfaces retain a good blood supply. (c) Oligotrophic non-union: a reduced fibrous callus forms; although the fracture surfaces retain a blood supply, the biological response is inadequate. **Non-viable non-unions:** (d) Dystrophic non-union: the blood supply to one or both fracture surfaces is interrupted and the biological response within the fracture gap is poor. (e) Necrotic non-union: a necrotic fragment within the fracture gap prevents healing. (f) Defect (gap) non-union: a critical defect exists which cannot be bridged. (g) Atrophic non-union: osteolysis and osteopenia predominate; the fracture gap contains mature fibrous tissue.

(a) Mineralized callus / Fibrous callus — Hypertrophic non-union 'elephant foot callus'

(b) Mineralized callus / Fibrous callus — Moderately hypertrophic non-union 'horse's hoof callus'

(c) Fibrous callus — Oligotrophic non-union

(d) Avascular bone / Inactive fibrous tissue — Dystrophic non-union

(e) Inactive fibrous tissue / Necrotic bone — Necrotic non-union

(f) Defect non-union

(g) Inactive fibrous tissue — Atrophic non-union

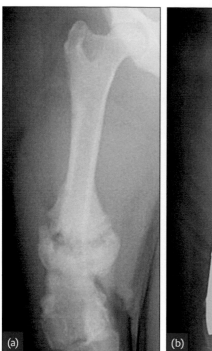
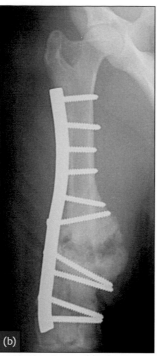

31.4 A hypertrophic fracture non-union in a 4-year-old Labrador Retriever. Initial stabilization of a distal diaphyseal femoral fracture had been with a four-pin external skeletal fixator which had loosened and had been removed. (a) A significant volume of callus has formed proximal and distal to the fracture gap, which remains apparent. (b) Malalignment was corrected and a bridging dynamic compression plate applied laterally; the fracture gap was not debrided.
(Courtesy of T Gemmill)

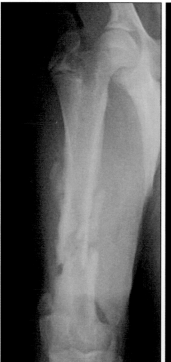
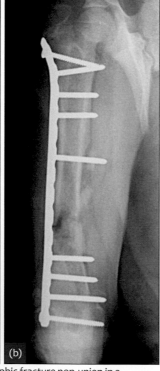

31.5 (a) A moderately hypertrophic fracture non-union in a 6-month-old Border Collie. The non-union developed following stabilization of a distal diaphyseal femoral fracture with an intramedullary pin. Loosening of the pin and rotational instability at the fracture site prevented fracture healing, although there was moderate mineralized callus formation. (b) Malalignment was corrected and a bridging locking compression plate applied laterally; the fracture gap was not debrided. The long distal screw in the proximal fragment extends into medial fibrocartilaginous callus.

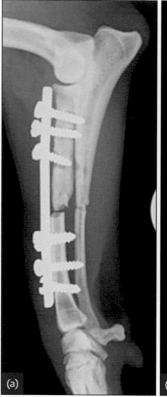
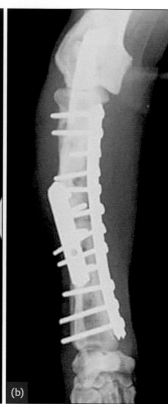

31.6 (a) An oligotrophic or dystrophic fracture non-union in a 5-year-old Cairn Terrier. An inappropriate plate has been applied and there is evidence of screw loosening proximally. There is minimal callus formation at both the radial and ulnar fracture gaps. (b) Revision surgery comprised removal of the original implants, limited ostectomy of the fracture surfaces with debridement of the fracture gap, placement of a bone graft, and orthogonal compression plating.

Oligotrophic non-unions are classified as viable non-unions since they retain a blood supply; however, in contrast to the hypertrophic forms their biology is compromised to a point where mineralized callus formation is minimal. Thus in practice the aetiology, radiographic appearance and treatment requirements of oligotrophic non-unions are more akin to non-viable non-unions than hypertrophic non-unions. Therefore differentiation from the non-viable form via quantification of fracture site vascularity using modalities such as nuclear scintigraphy is rarely indicated.

A pseudoarthrosis is an unusual form of hypertrophic non-union where a cavity lined with synovium producing synovial fluid forms within the fracture gap.

Radiographic features of non-viable non-unions

Non-viable non-unions have a poor fracture site biological environment. Fracture healing is therefore minimal and radiographs reveal a persistent fracture gap, often with sclerotic cortical margins, which exhibits no associated mineralized callus formation. Additional radiographic features may define the type of non-union present and may include evidence of necrotic bone fragments, bone loss, a large fracture gap and signs of infection. Four types of non-viable non-union are described.

- Dystrophic non-union. Severe disruption to the blood supply to one or both fracture surfaces has occurred. When only one fracture surface is avascular the other may exhibit callus formation and appear variably hypertrophic. Healing of one end only of a segmental fracture is a common form of dystrophic non-union.

Radiographic features include sclerotic rounded fracture edges with no evidence of callus formation; it is in many cases difficult to differentiate oligotrophic and dystrophic non-unions (see Figures 31.3d and 31.6).

- Necrotic non-union. A necrotic segment of bone (a sequestrum) is present within the fracture gap preventing healing. Sequestra may arise from comminuted fracture fragments which have lost their soft tissue attachments and thus vascular supply; radiographically they appear as sclerotic, isolated fragments of bone. The formation of sequestra is very rare (see Figures 31.3e and 31.7).
- Defect (gap) non-union. A critical defect exists which is too large for callus to bridge. This may occur due to poor reduction or bone loss (either at the time of injury, due to surgical fragment removal, or as a result of necrosis or resorption) (Figures 31.3f and 31.8).
- Atrophic non-union. This is an end-stage condition which occurs after a transition from a failed reparative response to a resorptive response. Radiography reveals loss of bone from the fracture surfaces and osteopenia of the remaining bone (Figures 31.3g and 31.9). This type of non-union can be encountered commonly following inadequate stabilization of distal diaphyseal radial fractures in toy breeds.

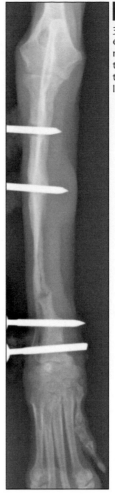

31.9 Atrophic non-union. A transverse fracture of the radius and ulna in a 3-year-old Yorkshire Terrier was treated with an external fixator. After 6 weeks the fracture had not healed and there was evidence of atrophy at the fracture site. Note the radiolucency around the transfixation pins suggestive of implant loosening.

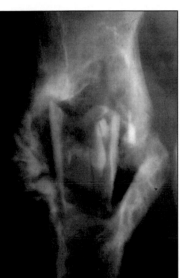

31.7 Necrotic non-union. An open comminuted humeral fracture in a 5-year-old terrier was treated using an external fixator. The fixator was removed after 6 weeks, but lameness persisted and a draining sinus tract was present over the fracture site. A radiodense sequestrum is present at the fracture site.

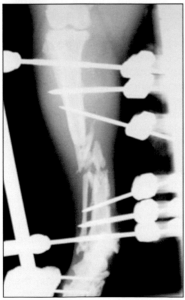

31.8 Defect non-union. A comminuted tibial fracture in an 8-year-old cat was treated by closed reduction and application of an external fixator. After 8 weeks the fracture had not healed; a gap is present at the fracture site. Note the radiolucency around multiple transfixation pins suggestive of implant loosening.

Additional radiographic features

Additional radiographic features may also influence treatment and should be assessed; these include the direction and extent of any malreduction, any evidence of infection, the location of the non-union (diaphyseal, metaphyseal or epiphyseal), and whether indications of implant failure are present.

Infection may be present in any form of non-union but is more common in non-viable non-unions due to their poor blood supply and the frequent presence of necrotic material. Radiographic changes suggestive of infection are reviewed in Chapter 30; however, key features include periosteal new bone formation (often extending some distance from the fracture site), osteolysis at the fracture surfaces and bone–implant interfaces, and local soft tissue thickening (Figure 31.10). The surgeon should bear in mind that infection can be present in the absence of specific radiographic changes.

Treatment

Management of a non-union fracture should have two key goals; the surgeon should aim to create an optimal environment at the fracture site for restoration of the normal process of bone healing, whilst maintaining normal bone conformation so that a return to appropriate mechanical function is possible. A key principle in the management of non-union fractures is the early identification and targeted treatment of the underlying cause or causes of failure of the normal bone healing process.

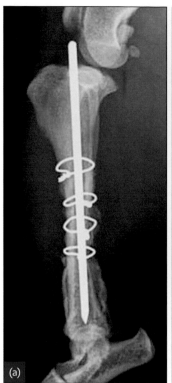
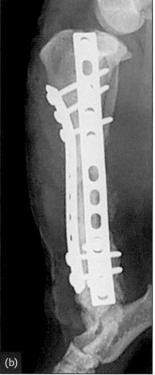

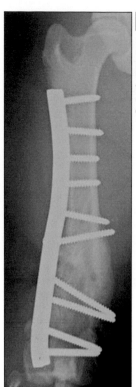

31.11 Healing of a hypertrophic non-union. Follow-up radiograph obtained 12 weeks following surgical management (pre- and postoperative radiographs are shown in Figure 31.4). There is bridging of the fracture gap by remodelled mineralized callus.
(Courtesy of T Gemmill)

31.10 (a) An infected oligotrophic non-union. Note the extensive periosteal new bone formation and the region of cortical osteolysis at the level of the distal cerclage wire. Note the inappropriate position of the intramedullary pin in the stifle joint, which occurred because it was placed in a retrograde manner. (b) Revision surgery comprised removal of the original implants, limited ostectomy of the fracture surfaces with debridement of the fracture gap, placement of a bone graft and a gentamicin-impregnated collagen sponge, and orthogonal compression plating. Healing was uncomplicated and the infection resolved; implant removal was not necessary.

Viable non-unions

Hypertrophic non-unions are typically associated with an inappropriate mechanical environment; most frequently instability at the fracture site results in a level of IFS that prevents the formation of mineralized callus within the fracture gap. Fracture site instability may occur due to poorly planned or applied primary fixation or subsequent implant failure. The cause of mechanical failure should be identified and considered when planning revision fixation, which must be capable of stabilizing the fracture for a sufficient time to permit bone healing. Since this may be an extended period, revision using internal fixation, typically a bone plate and screws, is often advisable. Following restoration of optimal IFS the fibrocartilage within the fracture gap will progress through the later stages of endochondral ossification leading to fracture union (Marsh *et al.*, 1994) (Figure 31.11). Debridement of this tissue is therefore not necessary, and may in fact impair healing due to further disruption of the biological environment (Rodriguez-Merchan and Forriol, 2004). As the fracture is biologically active, the placement of a bone graft at the fracture site (or other form of biological augmentation) and compression across the fracture site may be beneficial but are not absolute requirements for treatment success (Rodriguez-Merchan and Forriol, 2004). Plate application in such cases can be challenging due to adhesions, altered soft tissue and bone anatomy, and an irregular surface for plate application; the use of locking plates may facilitate application.

Treatment of hypertrophic non-unions may be complicated by the presence of clinically significant malalignment, pseudoarthrosis or infection. Where malalignment exists this should be corrected concurrently with placement of revision fixation. In the case of angular or torsional malalignments the fracture gap may be sufficiently pliable to permit realignment without debridement. Otherwise, the fracture must be mobilized with an additional limited ostectomy of one or both fracture surfaces, facilitating alignment. This also permits direct apposition of the bone ends and application of a compression plate. Cases with significant overriding of the fracture fragments are much harder to manage; restoration of normal bone length may be impossible due to adhesions and muscle contracture, and shortening of the affected bone may be necessary. This can have a clinical effect on gait in some cases. Pseudoarthroses may in some cases be functional, and the surgeon should balance the potential benefit of surgical intervention against the morbidity and risks inherent to this approach. When surgery is considered necessary, all fibrous and synovial tissue should be excised, possibly with limited ostectomies, and compression plating employed. Significantly greater surgical disruption of the fracture site is inevitable with these approaches and placement of an autogenous cancellous bone graft or other form of biological augmentation (see Chapter 14) should be considered.

Infected viable non-unions are unusual due to their relatively well preserved biological environment. Mechanical instability may be due to inadequate primary fixation, or can result from implant loosening secondary to the infection. Removal of the loose implants and provision of mechanical stability with robust revision fixation is usually sufficient in such cases. Bacterial culture of tissue samples and implants should be performed and topical antibiotics placed (e.g. gentamicin-impregnated polymethylmethacrylate (Ethell *et al.*, 2000), plaster of Paris (Santschi and McGarvey, 2003) or collagen (Chaudhary *et al.*, 2011)). Although recolonization of new implants may occur, these can be removed if necessary after fracture healing.

Oligotrophic non-unions maintain a vascular supply but have an impaired biological environment and an inadequate healing response; these are best managed similarly to non-viable non-unions.

Non-viable non-unions

Non-viable non-unions have an inadequate biological environment; a sufficiently vigorous healing response is not established, and bone union cannot be achieved. In most cases interventions aim to stimulate all aspects of the biological response. Not every non-viable non-union has a poor mechanical environment; however, this is a common feature and most cases require stabilization in addition to restoration of favourable fracture biology.

Restoration of an active biological environment is dependent on a number of key interventions. Implants which are loose or associated with persistent infection, or those not positively contributing to fracture stability, must be removed. Loose implants, especially loose cerclage wires (see Figure 31.10a), may adversely affect blood supply to the fracture and provide a focus for infection. Debridement of necrotic material is essential, whether infected or not, since this will prevent the establishment of an active healing response. This should always include fibrous tissue and sequestra within the fracture gap, as well as any avascular bone at the fracture surfaces. The extent of bone debridement may be quite minimal, for example in oligotrophic non-unions, but may be more extensive in dystrophic or atrophic cases. A degree of bone shortening is usually inevitable, and this should be considered prior to surgery; if limb function is likely to be compromised, a strategy for osteogenesis or amputation should be planned from the outset. This is particularly important when treating atrophic non-unions. Blood supply to the fracture site may be improved by drilling channels from the sclerotic fracture ends into the medullary canal (osteostixis), and by careful tissue handling and preservation of the periosteum during surgery. A bone graft, or other form of biological augmentation, should be placed (see Chapter 14). Finally, provision of appropriate and durable fracture stability usually necessitates application of plates and screws, which are placed following correction of any malalignment. The management of non-viable non-unions is technically challenging, but can be associated with a good prognosis provided the underlying causes are addressed. Atrophic non-unions are the exception; these can be very challenging to manage and are associated with a poor prognosis.

The management of infected non-viable non-unions follows similar principles, with removal of loose implants, debridement, bone grafting and provision of stability the key elements (see Figure 31.10). Tissue samples and implants should be cultured, and topical antibiotics placed. Provision of drainage is rarely indicated. Rigid fixation is essential and must be sufficiently durable to support the fracture through a potentially extended healing period; for this reason plate and screw fixation is usually optimal. The risk of recolonization of these implants is generally outweighed by their mechanical advantages; since fracture healing will progress when sufficient stability is maintained and infection controlled, implant removal can be performed later if necessary. In all such cases extended postoperative antibiotic treatment based on culture results is recommended, usually for at least 8 weeks.

Articular non-unions

Principles of treatment of articular non-unions are identical to those discussed for diaphyseal non-unions; however, restoration of normal joint congruity and function is an additional essential, and frequently challenging, objective. Fracture fragment remodelling is typical in non-union cases, potentially associated with both bone loss and callus formation, and can render perfect reduction difficult or impossible. Additional difficulties include the frequent presence of cartilage pathology associated with abnormal loading, periarticular fibrosis, and disuse muscle atrophy, which will hamper recovery of normal function. As with other non-unions, debridement and rigid internal fixation are key requirements; the provision of bone grafts or graft substitutes is not recommended unless this can be applied at a site distant to the articular surface (e.g. the epicondylar component of a fracture of the lateral portion of the humeral condyle). In severe cases, salvage procedures such as total joint replacement, excision arthroplasty or arthrodesis should be considered from the outset.

Non-surgical treatment modalities

Low intensity pulsed ultrasonography, extracorporeal shock wave therapy and pulsed electromagnetic fields have all been used in the treatment of fracture non-unions. The mode of action of pulsed ultrasonography is unclear, but may be similar to shock wave treatment where transfer of acoustic energy to bone is thought to stimulate healing, possibly due to inflammation resulting from microtrauma. Although some studies have shown positive results in human viable non-unions (Xu *et al.*, 2009), a recent systematic review found no evidence to support the routine use of either modality in this setting (Griffin *et al.*, 2012a).

Piezoelectric fields generated within bone during loading play an important role in normal remodelling (see Chapter 5), with bone deposition stimulated by negative potentials at sites of compression. Indirect electrical stimulation uses a magnetic field to create a secondary electric field at the fracture site, and has shown efficacy in some human studies of viable, but not non-viable, non-unions (Ito and Shirai, 2001). There is, however, no current evidence to support the use of pulsed electromagnetic fields in the treatment of canine or feline non-unions.

Delayed union

The feature differentiating delayed union from non-union is that the former will eventually progress to union without specific intervention, whilst the latter will not. It is self-evident that, due to the huge potential variation in intrinsic and extrinsic factors between cases, the anticipated period for fracture healing will vary between a few weeks and many months. The surgeon must therefore judge clinical and radiographic progress in the light of a balanced assessment of the anticipated rate of progression of bone healing. When doubt exists it is essential that identifiable factors predisposing to poor bone healing are excluded as early as possible, and that regular reassessments are scheduled. Whilst often tempting, undue delay in the face of mounting evidence of poor progression of bone healing may make subsequent management more challenging; it must be remembered that every non-union at some stage would have satisfied the criteria for delayed union.

The causes of delayed union are the same as non-union, albeit that in the former case the adverse effects are less severe and retard, rather than prevent, bone healing. Therefore when delayed union is suspected a critical assessment of fracture mechanics and biology should be made. The most common mechanical cause of delayed union is excessive motion at the fracture site. Clinically such patients commonly exhibit persistent lameness and muscle atrophy, pain at the fracture site and, occasionally, gross instability. Following appropriate surgical fixation, canine and feline fracture patients are expected to consistently bear weight on the affected limb within a few days, with lameness typically relatively mild after a few weeks; persistent or recurrent severe lameness should prompt investigations. Radiographs should be assessed for alteration in the relative orientation of the fracture fragments, implant failure and any evidence of loosening of the implants. Any such features should be critically assessed even if radiographic evidence of active callus formation is present; implant revision in a biologically active, non-displaced, early delayed union is technically easier and carries a much better prognosis than treatment of a chronic, displaced, non-viable non-union.

Early clinical and radiographic indications of poor fracture biology may be less obvious. From a clinical perspective lameness and fracture pain are features of instability rather than poor biological activity, and when mechanical stability is maintained progress may appear good. For this reason, in cases where at initial surgery intrinsic and extrinsic influences on fracture biology were considered adverse, follow-up radiographic assessments should be commenced before the anticipated time of bone healing and continued until satisfactory evidence of healing is documented. In such cases a large volume of mineralized callus may not be expected, but an absence of callus at a reasonable interval should prompt concern. Failure of progressive load sharing between implants and a healing fracture will inevitably lead to implant failure, compounding the difficulty of subsequent treatment. When made early, interventions can often be straightforward, for example application of bone graft or graft substitute at the fracture site in combination with limited local debridement. If radiography reveals evidence of a specific impediment to fracture healing, such as a sequestrum or a large, non-healing fracture gap, this must be addressed.

Infection will have adverse effects on both fracture stability (via implant loosening) and fracture biology (e.g. via reduced local oxygen tension and persistence of an inflammatory milieu at the fracture site). Although there is something of a dogma that fractures will heal in the presence of infection, this requires that appropriate stability be maintained and that infection is at least suppressed. Whilst in some cases extended antibiotic treatment based on culture of aspirated material is sufficient, more aggressive interventions are not infrequently indicated including surgical debridement and lavage, placement of topical antibiotics, revision of loose implants and implant exchange (Rightmire *et al.*, 2008).

Malunion

A malunion is a fracture that has healed but with abnormal resultant conformation of the affected bone. Malunion can occur in any plane and multiplanar deformities are common. Angular and torsional deformities occur when the fracture ends are in contact but malaligned during healing, whereas translational and shortening deformities occur when they are offset perpendicular or parallel to the long axis of the bone. Malunions may result from natural fracture healing, conservative management, poor surgical fracture reduction and postoperative implant failure or premature removal. The natural fracture healing process has evolved into a robust mechanism capable of achieving bone union even under significantly adverse conditions; however, appropriate alignment is rarely maintained due to disruptive muscle forces (Figure 31.12). When fracture healing is managed, malunions may still result if optimal alignment cannot be achieved or maintained. Optimal fracture realignment during surgery can be difficult to achieve especially when there is comminution, if small juxta-articular fragments are present, when closed reduction is used, or when bone anatomy is altered (e.g. non-union or angular limb deformity corrections). Intraoperative image intensification can be very helpful but is not widely available; critical assessment of postoperative radiographs and limb alignment are otherwise mandatory.

The recent trend towards biological osteosynthesis in canine and feline fracture management has de-emphasized perfect fracture reconstruction, with the result that a higher proportion of fractures heal with mild malalignment. Similar

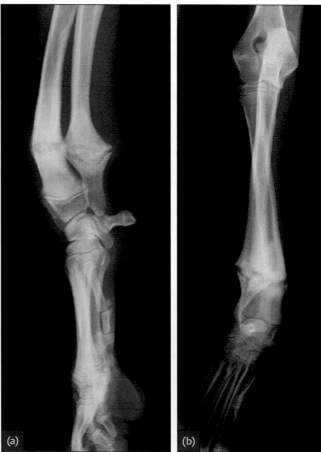

31.12 (a) Mediolateral and (b) craniocaudal views of radial malunion in a 4-month-old puppy. A vigorous healing response had occurred in this young dog and the fracture is progressing towards union; however, there is moderate caudal and valgus malalignment.

mild malunions are also expected following more traditional closed reduction and external coaptation or external skeletal fixation. Such malunions rarely impede function, and it is important to bear in mind that the significance of any malunion should be judged on the basis of clinical assessment rather than an isolated analysis of bone conformation. In general, malunions may cause clinically significant dysfunction in two ways.

Firstly, mechanical dysfunction will occur if the paw strikes the ground in a significantly abnormal position or orientation, or if marked compensatory gait changes are necessary to achieve reasonable paw placement. Mild limb shortening and craniocaudal angular deformities are usually well tolerated, since compensation via altered joint angles has a minimal effect on function. Small translations can also be well tolerated, since sagittal paw placement can still occur and relatively normal joint loading and function is maintained. Torsional and mediolateral (valgus and varus) angular deformities are relatively poorly tolerated as the scope for functional gait compensation is much more limited.

Secondly, joint pain due to abnormal loading or altered joint function may result in lameness. For example, joints distal to an angular deformity may experience abnormal tensile and compressive loading, potentially leading to chronic ligament sprains and cartilage pathology, which in turn can result in the development of osteoarthritis. An important example of potentially debilitating altered joint function following malunion is patellar instability due to a mediolateral or torsional femoral deformity (Figure 31.13). It follows that a careful assessment of the relative contributions of both mechanical and pain-related lameness should be made in such cases, as this may impact on decision making. For example, a mild mechanical lameness without evidence of joint pain may be considered acceptable by some owners, whereas a similar lameness associated with joint pain or patellar instability may warrant surgical intervention.

Surgical planning

Precise quantification of the location, plane and severity of a non-functional malunion is a prerequisite for surgical planning. This process can be considered in three stages: the acquisition of imaging data, its analysis to yield descriptive values for the deformities present and the use of this information in the creation of a surgical plan. Well positioned orthogonal radiographs are often sufficient, although in complex cases computed tomography (CT) examination can be very helpful.

Precise quantification of long bone conformation from imaging data can be complex, although a standardized system for its assessment in humans has been described (Paley, 2002); a similar system has been adopted for dogs (Fox and Tomlinson, 2012). This approach relies on the determination of standardized axes which define the orientation of the proximal and distal segments of a bone in a given plane (Figure 31.14). Some angular difference between axes is typical although normal values are hard to define, being dependent on individual variation, breed and

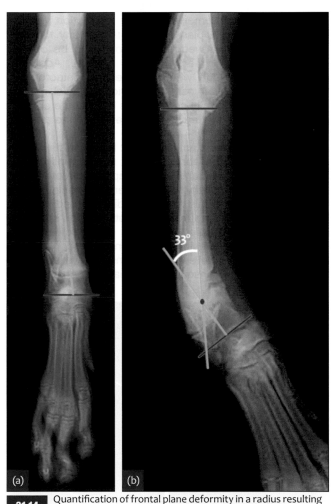

31.14 Quantification of frontal plane deformity in a radius resulting from fracture malunion in a 6-month-old Border Collie. (a) The contralateral limb is used as a normal reference. The green line represents the anatomical axis of the radius; since the radius is relatively straight when viewed cranially this axis is straight throughout the length of the bone. The red lines represent the proximal and distal joint orientation lines (the angles at their intersection with the anatomical axis define the anatomical joint orientation angles; note that these are not 90 degrees). (b) The affected radius has a varus deformity. The proximal and distal anatomical axes (green lines) are drawn through the proximal and distal parts of the bone. The centre of rotation of angulation (CORA; red dot) is the point of intersection of the proximal and distal anatomical axes; the angle between the axes is the correction angle required to restore normal frontal plane alignment – 33 degrees in this case.

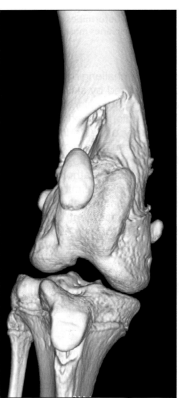

31.13 A volume rendered CT image of a femoral fracture malunion in a 1-year-old crossbreed dog. Lateral patellar luxation resulted from a combination of internal torsion and valgus angulation of the distal femur with subsequent malalignment of the quadriceps mechanism relative to the trochlear groove. The patella in this image is subluxated, but complete luxation was apparent on clinical examination.

Index

Page numbers in *italic* indicate figures
Page numbers in **bold** indicate Operative Techniques